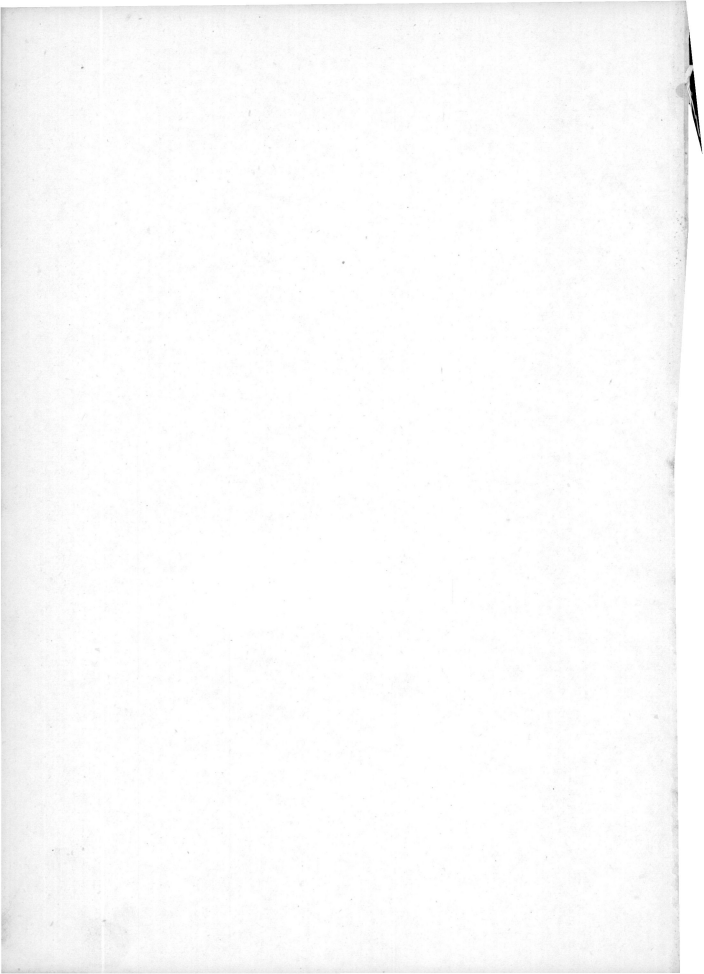

…CED TE…TBOOK ON …ONAL CHINESE MEDICINE AND PHARMACOLOGY

Vol. II

- PHARMACY
- PRESCRIPTION

NEW WORLD PRESS BEIJING, CHINA

First Edition 1995

ISBN 7-80005-262-1
Published by
New World Press
24 Baiwanzhuang Road, Beijing 100037, China

Distributed by
China International Book Trading Corporation
35 Chegongzhuang Xilu, Beijing 100044, China
P.O. Box 399, Beijing, China

Printed in the People's Republic of China

FOREWORD

In order to promote international exchange in the field of traditional Chinese medicine and to meet the needs of increasingly large numbers of foreign students studying traditional Chinese medicine, the Foreign Affairs Bureau of the State Education Commission and the Department of Traditional Chinese Medicine under the Ministry of Public Health (now the State Administration of Traditional Chinese Medicine and Pharmacy) held a meeting in Guangzhou in April 1986 to examine and approve textbooks of traditional Chinese medicine for foreign students. Eight textbooks for use by foreign students were examined during the meeting, including *Basic Theory of Traditional Chinese Medicine* and *The History of Traditional Chinese Medicine* compiled by the Beijing College of Traditional Chinese Medicine, *Traditional Chinese Internal Medicine* and *The Chinese Language* compiled by the Shanghai College of Traditional Chinese Medicine, *Chinese Pharmacy* and *The Science of Traditional Chinese Prescriptions* compiled by the Nanjing College of Traditional Chinese Medicine, and *Traditional Chinese Diagnostics* and *The Science of Acupuncture and Moxibustion* compiled by the Guangzhou College of Traditional Chinese Medicine.

The four colleges of traditional Chinese medicine involved in the compilation of the textbooks have been teaching foreign students for from five to ten years, during which time they have accumulated a great deal of experience. Most of the editors have experience in compiling textbooks in their fields of study used nationwide by full-time colleges of traditional Chinese medicine. Many of these textbooks have long been used in teaching foreign students. As a result, they are both comprehensive and applicable.

This series of textbooks draws on the contents of the fourth and fifth editions of national textbooks used by full-time colleges of traditional Chinese medicine and takes into consideration the fact that foreign students have a relatively short time for classroom studies and that there are differences in cultures and traditions. Such aspects as the depth and range of the contents, and the scientific, ideological and advanced level of the textbooks have been carefully considered. Efforts have been made to shorten and simplify while preserving the essence of traditional Chinese medicine and its systematic theories.

The publication of these textbooks marks a great achievement in the dissemination of traditional Chinese medicine. Training foreign students is an important way of spreading traditional Chinese medicine throughout the world. We hope that teachers and students will comment on any shortcomings they discover in this series of textbooks so that we may alter and improve subsequent editions.

State Administration of Traditional
Chinese Medicine and Pharmacy
1991

GENERAL CONTENTS

BOOK ONE
TRADITIONAL CHINESE PHARMACY

BOOK TWO
SCIENCE OF TRADITIONAL CHINESE PRESCRIPTION

BOOK ONE

TRADITIONAL CHINESE PHARMACY

Written by: Huang Yarong
Translated by: Li Liangyu
English text finalized by: Hou Can

CONTENTS

INTRODUCTION

Traditional Chinese pharmacology is a science that studies the basic theories, sources, methods of collection and processing, property, action and application of various Chinese medicinal materials.

Chinese pharmaceuticals are an important means employed by traditional Chinese medicine to prevent and treat diseases. They constitute an important component of traditional Chinese medicine and have made great contributions to maintaining the health of the Chinese people and the prosperity of the Chinese nation.

The drugs originate from plants, animals and minerals; most are raw, and only a few are processed. As most of them are from plants, medical books on Chinese materia medica through the ages have conventionally termed them "*ben cao*" (herbalism). China has extremely rich pharmaceutical resources, and the drugs have been applied under the guidance of the basic theories of traditional Chinese medicine. Therefore, Chinese pharmacology has its own unique theoretical system and methods of application.

CHAPTER ONE

THE SOURCES, COLLECTION, AND PREPARATION OF CHINESE DRUGS

Section 1

The Sources

The distribution and production of natural drugs are closely related to natural conditions. China is a country with a vast territory and the natural and geographical conditions vary greatly from place to place; so do the ecological factors, such as the water, soil, climate, amount of light and biological distribution. Therefore, the production of various kinds of crude drugs, whether in quantity or quality, has to some extent a regional feature, that is, the same drug produced in different places may be different in both output and quality. That is why past physicians all attached great importance to using *"didao"* (genuine) drugs. By genuine drugs, they meant drugs produced in areas which have been known for high yield, fine quality and excellent therapeutic effects of these drugs. Some examples are Rhizoma Coptidis, Bulbus Fritillariae Cirrhosae and Radix Aconiti Lateralis Preparata produced in Sichuan Province; Radix Angelicae Sinensis produced in Gansu Province; Fructus Lycii produced in the Ningxia Hui Autonomous Region; Radix Glycyrrhizae produced in the Inner Mongolia Autonomous Region; Radix Ginseng produced in Jilin Province; Radix Astragali and Radix Codonopsis Pilosulae produced in Shanxi Province; Rhizoma Dioscoreae, Radix Achyranthis Bidentatae and Radix Rehmanniae produced in Henan Province; Herba Menthae and Rhizoma Atractylodis produced in Jiangsu Province; Rhizoma Atractylodis Macrocephalae and Radix Paeoniae Alba produced in Zhejiang Province; Radix Notoginseng produced in Yunnan Province; Cortex Cinnamomi produced in Guangxi Zhuang Autonomous Region; and Fructus Amomi and Pericarpium Citri Reticulatae produced in Guangdong Province.

With the continuous development of science and technology as well as increasing demand for Chinese herbal drugs, great efforts have been made to introduce new fine species and domesticate some medicinal herbs while working hard to increase the output of "genuine" herbal drugs in a planned way. Nevertheless, the introduction and domestication of new fine species of medicinal herbs is a very complicated project which is, first of all, required to guarantee the quality of the drugs. Their production can only be expanded after repeated trials in planting, testing and verification. So far, however, some encouraging achievements have been obtained.

Section 2
The Collection

All the parts of plants for medical use, such as their root, stem, leaf, flower, fruit and seed have different periods of maturation; and the content of effective effects and properties of the mature and immature parts of the plants differs. Therefore, collecting them at the right time has a very important bearing on the therapeutic results. Only when the drugs are collected at the right season when they contain the most effective ingredients can they produce the desired therapeutic results. The following is a general account of the right periods of collection of medicinal herbs:

(1) **Roots**

It is advisable to collect the roots in early spring before the plants put forth buds or sprout, or in late autumn when the aerial part of the plants begins to wither. This is because during these periods the plants are dormant and their nutrients are mostly stored in the roots which contain more effective ingredients and are of good quality. Take Radix Puerariae for example. The root collected in late autumn is solid, starchy and of good quality; while that collected in late spring and early summer contains less starch and is more fibrous and of poor quality. But there are exceptions. Take Radix Pseudostellaria, Rhizoma Pinellia and Rhizoma Corydalis for example. Their aerial parts wither in summer and it is better to collect them then.

(2) **Barks of Trees and Roots**

It is advisable to collect tree barks in late spring or early summer when the plants are growing luxuriantly with ample sap, for their barks collected at this time contain more nutrients and can be easily peeled off from the woody parts. As for the barks of the roots, the collection should be conducted in autumn. For instance, Cortex Moutan Radicis collected in autumn is starchy and of good quality.

(3) **Whole Plants, Stems, Branches and Leaves**

Most are collected when the plants are growing luxuriantly with branches and leaves, or in full bloom. For perennial plants, the aerial parts are cut and collected; for plants with weak and tender stems and branches, or those short and small ones and plants that must be used together with the roots, the whole plant including the root is dug up; and the leaves of some plants are collected in autumn and winter, such as Folium Mori and Folium Eriobotryae.

(4) **Flowers**

It is advisable to collect flowers when they are in buds or just beginning to bloom, so as to avoid the dispersion of their fragrance and the loss of the petals. For instance, Flos Lonicerae, Flos Sophorae and Flos Chrysanthemi are collected during this period. Flos Carthami is collected at several separate occasions because it blooms at different times. It would be best to collect the flowers in fine weather so that they can be dried in the sun or by airing.

(5) **Fruits**

Generally speaking, fruits should be collected when they are ripe. Some, however, are collected before they are ripe, such as Pericarpium Citri Reticulatae Viride and Fructus Aurantii Immaturus; and some are collected when they are old, such as Fructus Trichosanthis and Retinerus Luffae Fructus. Juicy fruits like berries, which get rotten easily, should be collected in due time and dried afterwards. One example is Fructus Lycii.

(6) **Seeds and Kernels**

Seeds and kernels, such as Semen Raphani, Semen Armeniacae Amarum and Semen Trichosanthis, are collected when they are completely mature and aged. Fruits that would crack and lose their seeds are collected on sunny days as soon as they ripe but have not yet cracked.

Section 3
The Preparation

Preparation means to process crude drugs and make them into certain forms or preparations for clinical use. It includes the general processing of most natural drugs and the special preparation of some. Special preparation refers to a kind of high-temperature stir-baking, both the general processing and special preparation are called "*pao zhi*" in Chinese. As most Chinese drugs are raw, many of them need to be prepared beforehand to meet the requirements for medication and bring their therapeutic effects into full play.

1. The Purposes of Preparation

(1) To remove or reduce the toxicins or side effects of the drugs. For example, Fructus Crotonis has a strong purgative action. If processed into powder and defatted, the toxicins are reduced. Olibanum and Myrrha, if applied raw, causes nausea, but, stir-baked preparation reduces this undesired reaction.

(2) To change the properties of the drugs to meet the needs of treatment. Processing changes the effects of some drugs. For example, raw Radix Rehmanniae is mainly used to purge heat, cool the blood and promote the generation of body fluids. When processed into Radix Rehmanniae Preparata, it acquires a slightly warm property and become especially effective for enriching blood. Radix Polygoni Multiflori, when used raw, lubricates the large intestine and relieves constipation; it no longer relieves constipation and becomes especially effective for nourishing the liver and kidney.

(3) To enhance the therapeutic effects of the drugs. For example, Rhizoma Corydalis processed with vinegar has greater analgesic effect; Cortex Eucommiae, if stir-baked with slices of Radix Dipsaci, has its effect of nourishing the liver and kidney strengthened.

Moreover, processing can remove the non-medicinal parts from the crude drugs and make them convenient for preparation and storage.

2. Methods of Processing

During processing, a general treatment is given to crude drugs to remove foreign matters, soak and soften them, or cut them into small pieces ready for decoction. Then, different methods are required; the common ones are as follows:

(1) Stir-baking (*chao*): This means to bake the crude drugs in a pan with constant stirring. The method of stir-baking for different drugs may vary in terms of time and temperature, and the drugs can be baked until yellow, until brown, or until carbonized. For example, Rhizoma Atractylodis Macrocephalae, when baked until yellow, has its ability to strengthen the spleen; Radix Sanguisorbae, when carbonized by baking, enjoys improved hemostatic effect.

(2) Stir-baking with adjuvants (*zhi*): This means to bake the drugs with liquid adjuvants such as honey, vinegar, wine, ginger juice and salt water, and make the liquids soak into or attach to the drugs. The adjuvant liquids produce some kinds of therapeutic effects themselves and drugs processed with them have their own therapeutic effects enhanced. For example, Flos Farfarae stir-baked with honey produces an enhanced effect in moistening the lung and relieving cough; Radix Astragali seu Hedysari stir-baked with honey produces a improved effect in strengthening the middle *jiao* and replenishing *qi*; and Folium Eriobotryae mixed with ginger juice and stir-baked becomes more effective in relieving vomiting. In addition, there are other methods of stir-baking, such as stir-baking with sand. Here, the sand is stir-baked in a pan until it is hot and then the drugs are mixed with the heated sand to make them light and crispy. This method is mainly used for crustaceous drugs with hard shells, such as Squama Manitis, Plastrum Testudinis and Carapax Trionycis.

(3) High-temperature stir-baking (*pao*): This method means basically the same as that mentioned above, but it is done quickly over high heat to make the drugs loose and cracked. For instance, Rhizoma Zingiberis is processed in this way into Rhizoma Zingiberis Preparata to reduce its pungent and dispersive property so it can be used to warm the middle *jiao*. Some drugs, such as Radix Aconiti Lateralis Preparata and Semen Strychni, are heated in hot charcoal ashes until brown and cracking but not yet carbonized.

(4) Calcining (*duan*): This means to burn a drug directly or indirectly over fire to make it light, crispy and easily crushable so as to bring out all its therapeutic effects. The mineral or shellfish drugs are usually calcined directly until they turn red. The examples are Magnetitum and Concha Ostreae. Indirect calcining means to burn the drugs in an airtight refractory container. For example, Vagina Trachycarpi Carbonisatus and Crinis Carbonisatus are processed this way.

(5) Wet-coated baking or roasting (*wei*): This means to bake or roast the drugs coated with wet paper or wet dough in an oven until these coatings turn black. This reduces the fat and moderate the actions of some drugs. Two examples are Rhizoma Zingiberis Recens Preparata and Semen Myristicae Preparata.

(6) Steaming (*zheng*): This means to steam the drugs together with other adjuvants over a slow fire until they are cooked. For example. raw Radix Rehmanniae has a cold nature and acts to purge heat, cool the blood, replenish *yin* and promote the generation of fluids. Steaming it with wine changes its cool nature into a warm one and makes it effective in replenishing *yin* and blood. Radix et Rhizoma Rhei, processed by steaming and mixed with rice wine, has a reduced purgative effect and is more effective in activating blood circulation and removing *qi* and blood stagnation.

(7) Boiling (*zhu*): This means to boil the drugs in water or boil them together with adjuvants. Two examples are Radix Aconiti, boiled together with beancurd, and Flos Genkwa, boiled in vinegar. In both cases, the toxicins of the raw drugs are reduced.

(8) Grinding in water (*shui fei*): This means to crush the insoluble mineral and shellfish drugs into pieces and grind them under water into very fine powder which remain suspended. Then, the water is removed and the deposit is collected for use. Some examples are Cinnabaris, Talcum and Calamina.

There are other methods to process drugs, such as fermenting, germinating and powdering. Examples are Massa Fementata Medicinalis, Fructus Hordei Germinatus and Semen Crotonis Pulveratum.

CHAPTER TWO
THEORY OF THE PROPERTIES OF CHINESE DRUGS

By properties of drugs, they refer to the therapeutic effects and actions of medicinal materials. Generally speaking, they include three aspects: the four *qi* and five tastes; the ascending, descending, floating and sinking properties; attributive meridians; and the toxicins. The theory concerning the properties of Chinese drugs has been developed over the long history of medical practice in China in line with basic theory of traditional Chinese medicine.

The onset and development of a disease mean a loss of balance between *yin* and *yang*, the growth or decline of the pathogenic and antipathogenic *qi*, and the hyperactive or hypoactive state of physiological activities resulting from the dysfunctions of the *zang-fu* organs. Every drug has its own specific therapeutic effects, and it is through them that Chinese drugs regulate *yin* and *yang*, strengthen antipathogenic *qi* and eliminate pathogenic *qi*, restore the normal functions of the *zang-fu* organs and alleviate the symptoms and signs of excess or deficiency.

Section 1
The Four *Qi* and Five Tastes

The four *qi* (*si qi*) and five tastes (*wu wei*) constitute the main components of the theory of drug properties.

The four *qi* refer to the four properties of drugs, namely, cold, hot, warm and cool. The cold and cool properties differ in nature from the hot and warm properties. While cold and cool pertain to *yin*, warm and hot pertain to *yang*. But, cold and cool only vary in degree, so do warm and hot; cool refers to slightly cold and warm refers to slightly hot. Most cold and cool drugs purge heat and fire and lessen the virulence of any pathogenic organism; they are suitable for diseases whose nature is hot. Most warm and hot drugs dispel cold and invigorate *yang*; they are mainly indicated for cold diseases. Some drugs are not marked as cold or hot, and are considered as mild drugs. Actually, they must be slightly cool or slightly warm. Therefore, the properties of all drugs fall into the four categories.

The four *qi* of drugs were recognized and mastered by physicians by observing the reactions of the human body after these drugs were administered. The cold or hot nature of a disease reflects an impairment of the relative balance between *yin* and *yang* in the human body, which can be corrected by prescribing drugs hot or cold in property. For instance, in a hot case accompanied by such symptoms as high fever, irritability and thirst, if the symptoms can be relieved by administering Gypsum Fibrosum and Rhizoma Coptidis, we know that these drugs have cold properties; and in cases of diarrhea due to an attack of cold along with watery stools and abdominal pain alleviated by the application of warmth, and absence of thirst, and if these cold symptoms can be relieved after the administration of Rhizoma Zingiberis Recens and Rhizoma Zingiberis, we know these drugs are of a warm or hot nature. The principles of prescribing drugs, i. e. , "treating cold diseases with hot drugs" and "treating hot diseases with cold drugs," as stated in the "Prologue" of *Shen Nong's Classic of Herbalism*, were established on the basis of these observations. In providing treatment, only when the cold or hot nature of a disease and drugs are clearly understood can proper drugs be prescribed and desired therapeutic results achieved. For instance, Rhizoma Zingiberis and Rhizoma Coptidis both can be used in treating diarrhea, but Rhizoma Zingiberis is hot and it is indicated for diarrhea of a cold nature, while Rhizoma Coptidis is cold and is indicated for diarrhea of a hot nature. Without a clear understanding of the differences in drug properties, indiscriminate administration of drugs cannot obtain the desired therapeutic results. Worse still, negative results might be produced.

The five tastes refer to the drugs' five different flavors: acrid, sweet, sour, bitter and salty. Since the flavors of drugs have an intrinsic relationship with their efficacies, understanding the characteristics of the five tastes is of great importance in guiding the administration of drugs. They are as follows: The acrid flavor has a dispersive effect and also the effect to activate *qi* circulation. Drugs such as Folium Perillae and Herba Menthae for inducing perspiration and relieving exterior syndrome, and Pericarpium Citri Reticulatae and Radix Aucklandiae for activating *qi* circulation, are all acrid. The sweet flavor remedies deficiency, relieves spasms and convulsions and moistens dryness. Drugs such as Radix Astragali and Radix Rehmanniae Preparata for remedying deficiency, Radix Glycyrrhizae for relieving spasms and convulsions and moderating drug actions, and Mel for moistening the lung to stop cough and lubricating the large intestine to relax the bowels, are all sweet. The bitter flavor removes pathogenic dampness and purges and suppresses fire. Drugs such as Cortex Magnoliae Officinalis for removing dampness and suppressing *qi*, Rhizoma Coptidis and Radix Scutellariae for purging heat, removing dampness and purging fire, are all bitter. The sour flavor astringes the flow of fluid and *qi*. Drugs such as Fructus Mume and Fructus Schisandrae for stopping cough and diarrhea are sour. The salty flavor softens hard masses. Drugs such as Thallus Laminariae seu Eckloniae and Sargassum for resolving phlegm and softening hard masses are salty. In addition to these five tastes, there are the bland (almost tasteless) and the astringent flavors. Usually, however, the term of "five tastes" is used to cover all the tastes of drugs. The bland taste seems insipid but is actually slightly sweet, and so it is usually grouped together with the sweet taste as sweet-bland (*gan dan*). The bland flavor promotes diuresis, such drug as Poria and Rhizoma Alismatis is exemplified by a bland taste. The astringent flavor, similar to the sour flavor, astringes the flow of fluid and *qi*. Drugs of astringent flavor include Os Draconis and Concha Ostreae.

For a particular group of drugs, they may have the same taste, but the taste may vary in degree. Usually, such terms as "very" and "slightly" are used to distinguish them. Those with a strong taste usually are more effective.

Qi (property) and *wei* (taste) are found in every drug. For instance, Herba Ephedrae is acrid in taste and warm in property and Rhizoma Coptidis is bitter in taste and cold in property. Some drugs have the same property but different tastes, while others have the same taste but different properties. Therefore, these drugs may have similar yet varied actions. For example, Rhizoma Coptidis and Radix Rehmanniae are both cold drugs with similar action, namely, both purge heat. But Rhizoma Coptidis is bitter and removes dampness; it is indicated for syndromes of dampness-heat. Radix Rehmanniae, on the other hand, is sweet and replenishes *yin* and promotes fluid secretion; it is indicated for syndromes of *yin* deficiency that leads to heat. Another example is Folium Perillae and Herba Menthae. Both are pungent with the same actions, promoting diaphoresis and relieving exterior syndrome. But Folium Perillae is warm and it is indicated for exterior syndrome due to wind-cold, while Herba Menthae is cool and used for exterior syndrome caused by wind-heat. Therefore, when studying and identifying drug properties, *qi* and *wei* must not be separated.

Section 2
Ascending, Descending, Floating and Sinking Properties

Ascending (*sheng*), descending (*jiang*), floating (*fu*) and sinking (*chen*) are terms used to describe the direction of a drug's action. On the basis of differences in the trends of pathogenesis and affected parts of the body, physicians make the best use of the directional actions of drugs to expel and eliminate the pathogenic factors, or regulate the affected *qi* flow of the *zang-fu* organs and restore the physiological activities to normal. As far as pathological changes in the human body are concerned, there are differences in the body parts affected, that is, the upper and lower, exterior and interior, as well as differences of pathogenesis, that is, abnormal ascent and descent. Ascending and descending as well as floating and sinking form two pairs of opposite actions. Drugs with ascending actions are used to treat diseases which develop downwards. Two examples of such drugs are Radix Astragali and Rhizoma Cimicifugae, both of which can be used to cure cases due to *qi* collapse in the middle *jiao* characterized by the prolapse of the anus and uterus. Drugs with descending actions are able to treat vomiting and hiccup due to abnormal ascent of stomach *qi*, cough and asthma due to abnormal ascent of lung *qi*, and vertigo and headache due to the upward disturbance of hyperactive liver *yang*. For example, Haematitum has a descending property and can be applied to stop vomiting and asthma, and pacify liver *yang*. Drugs with the floating action are able to disperse and drive out pathogenic factors and so are used to treat diseases at the surface of the body. For example, in an exterior syndrome due to exogenous pathogenic factors, drugs of light weight with floating and dispersive actions are required to dispel the pathogenic factors from the surface. Sinking means to drive downwards. Drugs which treat diseases in the interior possess the action of sinking. For example, purgatives, diuretics, and drugs for purging fire all fall into this category.

In short, all ascending and floating drugs are characterized by upward and outward actions and have lifting and dispersive effects, while all sinking and descending drugs are characterized by downward and inward actions and have the effects of suppressing abnormal ascent, causing purgation, facilitating urination and purging fire.

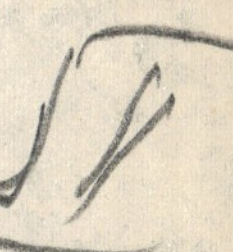

The ascending, descending, floating and sinking actions of the drugs are to some extent related to the four *qi* and five tastes as well as the texture of drugs. Drugs that are acrid and sweet, and warm and hot are mostly ascending and floating in action. Drugs that are bitter, sour and salty, and cool and cold are mostly sinking and descending in action. Flower and leaf drugs and drugs light in weight are mostly ascending and floating, while heavy drugs, such as seeds and minerals, are mostly sinking and descending.

In addition, the ascending, descending, floating and sinking actions may also be influenced by processing. In compound prescriptions, the potential action of one drug may be affected or restrained by other ingredients, and this warrants attention in clinical practice.

Section 3
Attributive Meridians

The theory of attributive meridians (*gui jing*) of drugs generalizes the domains of drug actions in accordance with the theories of the *zang-fu* organs and meridians, so as to show that a certain drug performs the major therapeutic effect on a certain *zang-fu* organ by entering the related meridian. The therapeutic actions of drugs have certain domains of their own in the human body. For example, although cold drugs all purge heat, their domains of action, however, are different: some mainly purge heat from the lung, others from the liver, still others from the stomach, so on and so forth. On the basis of generalizing the drug efficacies and inferring the domains in accordance with the theories of the *zang-fu* organs and the meridians, the theory of attributive meridians of drugs developed.

The meridians connect the interior and exterior parts of the human body. Pathological disorders of the body surface may affect the *zang-fu* organs in the interior, while disorders of the latter may in turn manifest themselves on the surface. Therefore, through the theory of meridians, a comprehensive understanding of the pathological changes in various parts of the body is acquired; and through observing reactions to drugs, the domain of a given drug, i. e., the attributive meridians can be inferred. For instance, cough, chest pain and sore throat manifest pathological changes in the Lung Meridian, and Radix Platycodi and Semen Armeniacae Amarum are indicated for such cases; thus the Lung Meridian is considered the attributive meridian of these drugs. Distensive pain in the hypochondrium and breasts and hernia pain show pathological changes in the Liver Meridian; Radix Bupleuri and Pericarpium Citri Reticulatae Viride are used for such cases, and so this meridian is thought to be the attributive meridian of them.

The summary of drug actions according to the theories of *zang-fu* organs and meridians is conducive to understanding the drug properties and selecting the right drugs in clinical practice. But this does not mean that diseases of a given meridian must be treated by drugs only from those that enter the given meridian. Since the *zang-fu* organs and the meridians are interrelated, both must be considered when administering drugs clinically. Take lung disease for example. If it is accompanied by spleen deficiency, drugs nourishing the spleen are often added to help the lung get adequate nourishment and make the patient recover sooner. Again for example. In a case caused by the upward displacement of hyperactive liver *yang* due to kidney *yin* insufficiency, drugs nourishing kidney *yin* are usually added to nourish the liver and pacify the hyperactive liver *yang* caused by *yin* deficiency.

The theories of attributive meridian, the four *qi* and five tastes, as well as ascending, descending, floating and sinking, expound drug properties from different angles; they complement one another. Since pathological changes of the same *zang-fu* organ or meridian may be different in nature and drugs assigned to the same meridian may have different effects, the theory of attributive meridian should be studied in combination with other theories. For example, Herba Ephedrae, Radix Scutellariae and Radix Glehniae all perform their actions through the Lung Meridian to treat cough. But Herba Ephedrae is acrid and floating, and acts to disperse cold, so it is especially effective for cough caused by the attack of wind-cold; Radix Scutellariae is bitter, cold and has a descending action, it is suitable for purging heat and indicated for cough due to heat in the lung; Radix Glehniae is sweet, cold and causes descent; it is especially effective in replenishing *yin* and treating cough due to *yin* deficiency.

Section 4
Toxicity of Drugs

Toxicity (*du xing*) refers to the harmful effects produced by drugs on the human body, including excessive therapeutic effects and unfavorable non-therapeutic reactions. It is of great significance to know whether a drug is toxic or not and whether its toxicins are mild or strong. Physicians of traditional Chinese medicine have always attached great importance to this point.

The toxicity of drugs differs in degree. In all books on Chinese materia medica, toxic drugs are usually marked with "very poisonous" or "slightly poisonous" to indicate the different degrees of toxicity. Very poisonous drugs must be administered with great care, because any improper use might cause serious damage to the human body or even death. Moreover, the drugs with mild toxicity, if taken in too large a dosage or over a long time, might also result in toxicosis. Therefore, the problem of how to handle toxic drugs properly, especially those with strong toxicity, merits special attention. In general, attention should be paid to the following aspects:

(1) Control the dosage: Drug toxicosis easily happens. When prescribing drugs with strong toxicity, the dosage should not be increased at will. In the beginning, the dosage should be small, and can be increased later in line with the patient's response. Continuous use of a drug for a long time should be avoided to prevent toxicosis from the accumulation of toxicins. As for drugs that are applied externally, it is not advisable to apply them over

too large an area so as to prevent toxicosis from absorption.

(2) Use only processed toxic drugs: The toxicity of most drugs can be reduced through processing. Generally speaking, processed drugs are milder in toxicity and safer than raw ones. With regard to drugs that can be applied in both raw forms and processed forms, attention should be paid to differences in indication, dosage and methods of use.

(3) Pay attention to different ways in using toxic drugs: The methods of applying poisonous drugs vary. Some can only be applied externally, others can only be taken in form of pills, powders or capsules but not decoctions, and still others can only be applied in compound prescriptions but not alone.

Besides, a full understanding should be gained of the compatibility, indications and contraindications of drugs.

The toxicity of drugs is harmful to the body. However, some drugs treat diseases just because of their toxicins. "Using poison to counteract poison" means exactly to combat pathogenic factors with the toxic substances. Poisonous drugs, if used according to established norms and with great care, can produce excellent therapeutic results.

One more remark should be made. Ancient physicians sometimes considered the extreme property of drugs as their "toxicity." For example, Zhang Jingyue, a famous physician in the Ming Dynasty, said, "It is the toxicity of drugs that makes them effective in treating diseases. Toxic drugs are so-called because of their excellent quality in the four *qi* and five tastes. . . . Those that combat pathogenic factors and reinforce antipathogenic *qi* can all be called toxic drugs." It is obvious that the "toxic drugs" he talked about are different from the toxic drugs this book discusses and they should not be confused with each other.

CHAPTER THREE
THE APPLICATION OF CHINESE DRUGS

The application of drugs covers compatibility, contraindication, dosage and use of drugs.

Section 1
Compatibility of Drugs

The compatibility of drugs (*yao wu pei wu*) means to match and combine more than two drugs compatibly and purposely in line with the specific conditions of a disease, the requirements of treatment and the drug properties and actions. A major form in the application of Chinese drugs, it constitutes the foundation to form prescriptions.

The conditions of diseases are very complicated and changeable. Sometimes one disease may be accompanied by several others, or both the exterior and interior of the body can be diseased, or else deficiency and excess, or cold and heat can be involved in the same case. In such cases, the use of only one drug usually fails to produce the desired therapeutic results, requiring the application of a number of drugs in a compatible combination. Such combined administration can enhance the therapeutic effects, cure more disorders and reduce the toxic and side effects.

In their medical practice, ancient physicians discovered that the combined use of drugs could produce a variety of complicated changes, such as increase or reduction of drug efficacies, inhibition or elimination of toxic and side effects, increase of toxicity, and unfavorable reactions. *Shen Nong's Classic of Herbalism* summarized these changes into seven categories, which are euphemistically termed as the following "seven emotions":

Single application (*dan xing*): Meaning administering a drug individually.

Synergism (*xiang xu*): This means to use drugs with similar properties to reinforce their effects. For example, both Radix et Rhizoma Rhei and Natrii Sulfas are purgatives; if used together, the purgative effect can be enhanced; Flos Lonicerae and Fructus Forsythiae both purge heat, and if used in combination, their effects can be increased.

Mutual enhancement (*xiang shi*): This means to use a drug as the principal ingredient and some others as the supplementary to assist and enhance the effects of the principal ingredient. These drugs may have different properties. For example, Radix Astragali, which replenishes *qi* and strengthens the spleen, is used together with Radix Stephaniae Tetrandrae, which has the diuretic effect, to treat weakness of the spleen accompanied by edema; Gypsum Fibrosum, which purges heat and purges fire, is used in combination with Radix Achyranthis Bidentatae, which conducts fire downward, to treat toothache due to stomach fire.

Mutual inhibition (*xiang wei*): The side effects or toxicity of a drug can be reduced or counteracted by another drug. For instance, Rhizoma Pinelliae and Rhizoma Arisaematis can inhibit Rhizoma Zingiberis Recens.

Mutual detoxication (*xiang sha*): One drug can reduce or eliminate the toxicity or side effects of another drug when used in combination. For instance, Rhizoma Zingiberis Recens can reduce or eliminate the side effects of Rhizoma Pinelliae if applied in combination.

Mutual antagonism (*xiang wu*): When two drugs are applied in combination, the original efficacies of one are reduced or even eliminated by that of the other. For example, if Radix Ginseng is used together with Semen Raphani, its effect of replenishing *qi* will be lost.

Incompatibility (*xiang fan*): The use of two drugs together results in toxic or side effects.

Clinically, "synergism" and "mutual enhancement" can be utilized to improve therapeutic effects. When applying drugs with toxic or side effects, "mutual detoxication" and "mutual inhibition" can be applied to relieve the toxic and side effects. Drugs with "mutual antagonism" and "incompatibility" should not be used together to prevent reduction of efficacies or the possible occurrence of an unfavorable reaction.

Section 2
Contraindications

Apart from their effects in preventing and treating diseases, Chinese herbal drugs can also produce harmful side effects. Therefore, it is necessary not only to acquire a clear understanding of the positive effects in preventing and treating diseases but also the possible harmful side effects. For example, drugs with cold and cool properties can purge heat, yet they may also produce damage to *yang qi*; hot drugs can eliminate cold, but may also consume *yin*; drugs with powerful purgative actions can eliminate pathogenic factors, and impair the antipathogenic *qi* as well; tonic drugs strengthen the antipathogenic *qi* yet may also agitate pathogenic *qi* and make them linger; drugs with ascending and lifting actions, if used in cases of *yang* hyperactivity, may make the situation even worse; and drugs for suppressing the abnormal ascent of *qi*, if applied in cases of prolapse of *qi*, may cause the cases deteriorate further. In order to be sure in administering drugs, it is necessary, on the other hand, to reduce or moderate the excessive qualities of drugs through processing, seeking proper combinations in making prescriptions, reducing dosage and improving methods of drug administration, and on the other, to have a clear understanding of the contraindications of drugs.

(1) Contraindications in forming prescriptions: It was recorded in ancient Chinese literature on herbal medicine that some drugs are incompatible with each other and can never

be used in the same prescriptions or else toxic reactions or weakened therapeutic effects will result. Records concerning the contraindications of drugs in forming prescriptions through the ages often do not agree one another. The most influential ones are the "eighteen incompatible drugs" and "nineteen antagonistic drugs." The "eighteen incompatible drugs" (*shi ba fan*) are as follows: Radix Aconiti is incompatible with Radix Pinelliae, Fructus Trichosanthis, Bulbus Fritillariae Cirrhosae, Radix Ampelopsis and Rhizoma Bletillae; Radix Glycyrrhizae is incompatible with Sargassum, Radix Euphorbiae Pekinensis, Radix Kansui and Flos Genkwa; and Rhizoma et Radix Veratri is incompatible with Radix Ginseng, Radix Adenophorae, Radix Salviae Miltiorrhizae, Radix Scrophulariae, Herba Asari and Radix Paeoniae Lactiflorae. The "nineteen antagonistic drugs" (*shi jiu wei*) are: Sulfur antagonizes Natrii Sulfas; Hydrargyrum antagonizes Arsenicum; Radix Euphorbiae Fischerianae antagonizes Lithargyrum; Fructus Crotonis is antagonistic to Semen Pharbitidis; Flos Caryophylli antagonizes Radix Curcumae; Radix Aconiti and Radix Aconiti Kusnezoffii are antagonistic to Cornu Rhinocerotis; Nitrum Depuratum is antagonistic to Rhizoma Sparganii; Cortex Cinnamomi antagonizes Halloysitum Rubrum; and Radix Ginseng is antagonistic to Faeces Trogopterori.

With regard to "eighteen incompatible drugs" and "nineteen antagonistic drugs," there is a discrepancy between the records and the clinical practice for some of them. This has been discussed by physicians of various ages. Although preliminary modern research has been done on some of these drugs, further experiments and research remain to be done. Before a definite conclusion is drawn, we'd better follow the traditional methods of prescription.

(2) Contraindications in drug application for the pregnant: During pregnancy, improper use of some drugs may cause damage to primordial *qi* that is vital for the development of the fetus, or else cause abortion, and so our predecessors attached great importance to drug contraindications for the pregnant. Drugs with strong toxicity or purgative effects, and aromatic drugs with motive and dispersive actions should generally be forbidden or applied with great care. These include Radix Euphorbiae Pekinensis, Flos Genkwa, Radix Kansui, Fructus Crotonis, Semen Pharbitidis, Radix et Rhizoma Rhei, Rhizoma Sparganii, Rhizoma Zedoariae, Hirudo, Tabanus, Mylabris, Radix Achyranthis Bidentatae, Semen Persicae, Flos Carthami, Radix Aconiti Lateralis Preparata, Cortex Cinnamomi and Moschus. However, for a pregnant woman who is seriously ill and whose disease cannot be treated without one or more of these drugs, they can be prescribed with great care according to the personal conditions of the patient.

Section 3
Dosage

In treating diseases with herbal drugs, attention should be paid to the dosage as it has a direct bearing on the therapeutic effects. Too small a dosage for a serious case would fail to obtain the desired result, while too large a dosage for a mild case would usually cause damage to the antipathogenic *qi* and result in wasting the medical substances. Therefore, proper dosage is of great importance for satisfactory therapeutic result. Usually, drug dosage is calculated by weight, though a few are calculated by quantity or volume. Over the long history of China, a traditional weight system was developed, in which one *jin* equaled 16 *liang* and one *liang* equaled 10 qian. The metric system was adopted recently, and it is now the standard system of weights in China. For convenience, an appropriate value can generally be adopted in concerting the traditional Chinese system of weights to the present metric system, namely: 1 *liang*= 30 g; 1 *qian*= 3 g; 1 *fen*= 0.3 g; and 1 *li* = 0.03 g.

The dosage for each drug quoted in this book usually means the dosage of a decoction for an adult patient. However, the dosage of herbal drugs is often influenced by other factors and therefore shows a certain flexibility in application. It is consequently necessary to have a clear understanding of the relationship between the dosage and these factors:

(1) Relationship between the properties of drugs and dosage: For drugs with mild properties, the dosage can be large; for toxic and potent drugs, it should be small; for drugs light in weight, it should be small; and for non-toxic drugs heavy in weight, such as minerals and shells, it should be large. In addition, for effective yet very expensive drugs, such as Cornu Rhinocerotis, Moschus and Calculus Bovis, the dosage should be small so as not to cause waste or unnecessary financial burden to the patient. For fresh medicinal herbs that usually contain some water, the dosage should approximately double that of the dried ones.

(2) Relationship between the dosage and forms of prescriptions: For a single-drug prescription, the dosage is usually large. In compound prescriptions, it is decided according to the number of ingredients in the prescriptions: in compounds with more drugs, the dosage of each is relatively smaller, while those with fewer ingredients have a larger dosage. The dosage of the chief drug is generally larger than that of the adjuvant ingredients. The dosage of the same drug may vary in different preparations, that for a decoction should be larger than that of pills and powders. Take Cortex Cinnamomi for example. If it is prescribed for a decoction, the usual dosage is 3 g.; if it is prescribed for a powder, the dosage should be just 0.5 to 1.5 g.

(3) Relationship between the dosage and the patient's condition, constitution and age: In severe and acute cases the dosage should be large, while in mild and chronic cases it should be small; the dosage for patients with weak constitution should be small, while that for those with strong constitutions it can be larger. The dosage for children and old patients should in general be small. In addition, attention should be paid to the dosage of toxic drugs.

In summary, three aspects should be taken into consideration in deciding the dosage of drugs. The three aspects are drugs, prescriptions and patients. In other words, the dosage should be in line with these three aspects. At the same time, the dosage should be adjusted according to variations in individual constitutions, geographical location as well as climatic and seasonal conditions.

Table 1. Drug Dosage Conversion Rate for the Young and the Old

AGE	DOSAGE
From newborn to 1 month	1/18—1/14 of the adult
Over 1 month to 6 months	1/14—1/7 of the adult
Over 6 months to 1 year	1/7—1/5 of the adult
1—2 years	1/5—1/4 of the adult
2—4 years	1/4—1/3 of the adult
4—6 years	1/3—2/5 of the adult
6—9 years	2/5—1/2 of the adult
9—14 years	1/2—2/3 of the adult
14—18 years	2/3 to total of the adult
18—60 years	total to 2/3 of the adult
Over 60 years	3/4 of the adult

Section 4
Preparation and Administration

Chinese herbal drugs can be used internally or externally. External use includes moxa application, bathing with medicinal decoction, insufflation to the throat, dropping into the eyes, powder pyrogenic dressing, suppository, etc. The forms of preparation depend on the conditions of the disease and the properties of the drugs. For example, Radix Kansui and Gemma Agrimoniae should be prepared into pills and powders since their effective ingredients do not dissolve easily in water. Aromatic drugs, such as Moschus and Borneolum Syntheticum, normally are not boiled in water in order to prevent the loss of the fragrance and effective ingredients. For cases of rheumatic pain and traumatic injuries, medicinal liquors is recommended so that their ability to activate blood circulation and remove stagnation from the meridians can be brought into full play. For chronic cases, pills or extracts should be prescribed to achieve a gradual cure. In addition to these traditional forms of preparations, there are many other forms, such as tablets, medicinal granules, aerosols, injections, etc.

In traditional Chinese medicine, decoction is the most frequently used form of preparation. In this respect, attention should be paid to the methods of decoction and administration.

(1) Methods of preparing a decoction: A ceramic pot is preferred to decoct drugs. The drugs should be soaked in cold water for half an hour before they are decocted. The amount of water should be proper, just submerge the drugs. Generally, one dose is decocted twice. For tonic drugs, it can be decocted thrice. The proper amount of the decoction should be about 250-300 ml.

The temperature should be controlled according to the properties of the drugs. For instance, aromatic drugs should be decocted over a strong fire and done quickly in 3-5 minutes because otherwise their effects will evaporate and reduce. Tonic drugs with dense texture should be decocted over a gentle fire for a longer period of time. Otherwise, it would be difficult to obtain their effective ingredients.

Different drugs in the same prescriptions may call for different decocting methods, and so clear instructions should also be given in the prescriptions so that both the pharmacologists and patients can follow them. These instructions can be summed up as follows:

Decoct first (*xian jian*): This suits mineral and shellfish drugs as they are hard in texture and their effective ingredients cannot be brought out easily. These should be crushed into small pieces and decocted first for over ten minutes before other drugs are added. Such drugs include Gypsum Fibrosum, Carapax Trionycis and Concha Haliotidis. Toxic drugs, such as Radix Aconiti Lateralis Preparata and Radix Aconiti, should be decocted first to have their toxicity reduced.

Decoct later (*hou xia*): This suits aromatic drugs or drugs whose effective ingredients would be easily destroyed if decocted together with other drugs for the same duration of time. They should be added when other drugs in the prescriptions are almost done. Such drugs include Herba Menthae Fructus Amomi, Ramulus Uncariae cum Uncis and crude Radix et Rhizoma Rhei.

Wrapped and decocted (*bao jian*): This method is used for those drugs that easily make the decoctions turbid and unpleasant to taste, or shells of some seed drugs which, when cracked, float on the surface of the decoction, or drugs with down or fine hairy growths which irritate the throat. These drugs should be wrapped in pieces of gauze and decocted. Examples are Halloysitum Rubrum, Talcum (ground in water), Flos Inulae and Semen Plantaginis.

Stew or decoct separately (*ling jian*): This is specially for precious drugs, such as Radix Ginseng and Cornu Saigae Tataricae, and is used in order to avoid having their effective ingredients absorbed by other drugs if decocted in the same container.

Melt in boiled solution (*yang hua*): This suits sticky and gluey drugs which melt easily, such as Colla Corii Asini and Saccharum Granorum. This method prevents these drugs from sticking to other drugs in the prescription or to the container. They should be put into the decoction of the other drugs free from residues and gently boiled until melted.

(2) Directions for use: Generally speaking, one dose (two decoctions) should be taken twice per day. For acute, severe or emergency cases, two doses (four decoctions) or more may be given per day at an interval of four hours. For chronic cases, one dose can be taken for two days (one decoction per day). Drugs for stopping vomiting can be taken repeatedly in small doses. For unconscious patients and those with lockjaw, the decoction can be applied via nasal feeding. Diaphoretics and purgatives should be suspended as soon as the patients begin to sweat or have bowel movements, so as not to cause excessive sweating or purgation which may damage the antipathogenic *qi*. Powder should be taken with boiled warm water; drugs prescribed in large dosage, with strong unpleasant smell or which would evoke choking can be taken with honey.

With regard to the time of administration, tonic drugs should be taken before meals, those irritant to the stomach and intestine after meals. Anthelmintics should be taken when the stomach is empty, and drugs for calming the mind should be taken before sleep.

Anti-malarial drugs should be taken two hours before the attack. For acute diseases, there is no restriction on the time of administration.

CHAPTER FOUR

DRUGS FOR RELIEVING EXTERIOR SYNDROME

Drugs that dispel exogenous pathogenic factors from the surface of the body and relieve exterior syndrome are known as "drugs for relieving exterior syndrome" (*jie biao yao*).

These drugs are divided into two kinds: Drugs for dispelling wind-cold (*fa san feng han yao*), and drugs for dispelling wind-heat (*fa san feng re yao*). The former, which are acrid and warm and act to dispel wind-cold, are indicated for exterior syndrome due to wind-cold marked by chills that are more obvious than fever, absence of thirst, and thin and white tongue coating. And the latter, which are acrid and cold and act to dispel wind-heat, are indicated for exterior syndromes marked by fever more predominant than chills, thirst, and white or yellow tongue coating. In addition, some of them also eliminate wind, promote the eruption of rashes and relieve edema.

Such drugs can be applied in combination with others in line with the specific conditions of the disease. For instance, in treating exterior syndrome complicated by cough with profuse sputum, they can be applied in combination with drugs that activate *qi* circulation and relieve chest symptoms; for exterior syndrome marked with dampness syndrome, they can be applied in combination with drugs for eliminating dampness; for exterior syndrome complicated by heat syndrome, they can be used in combination with drugs for purging heat; and exterior syndrome with accompanying weak constitution, they can be applied in combination with tonics so as to treat both the exterior syndrome and the underlying deficiency syndrome by strengthening the antipathogenic *qi* and eliminating pathogenic factors.

The proper dosage of drugs for relieving exterior syndrome causes slight perspiration; overdose can cause excessive perspiration, damage *yang qi* and consume body fluid. In summer or hot days when people perspire easily, the dosage should be decreased. For patients with spontaneous sweating, night sweating or blood loss, these drugs should be applied with great care even though the patients suffer from exterior syndromes due to attack by exogenous pathogenic factors.

Most drugs for relieving exterior syndrome are aromatics and contain volatile oils, and so should not be decocted for a long time, otherwise their therapeutic effects will be reduced.

Section 1
Drugs for Dispelling Wind-Cold

Herba Ephedrae (麻黄 *ma huang*)

Herba Ephedrae is the dried stem or branch of herb-like shrublets of Ephedra sinica Stapf, E. intermedia Schrenk et C. A. Mey, and E. equisetina Bge. of Ephedraceae. Mainly produced in Shanxi, Hebei, Liaoning and Gansu provinces as well as the Inner Mongolia Autonomous Region, it is collected from the Beginning of Autumn to Frost's Descent, dried in the shade and cut into segments.

Taste and Property: Acrid, slightly bitter and warm.
Attributive Meridian: Lung and urinary bladder meridians.
Actions and Indications:

(1) To induce perspiration and dispel cold. It is indicated for exterior excess syndrome due to wind-cold marked by anhidrosis, chills, aversion to cold, headache and general achiness. It is often used together with Ramulus Cinnamomi to form the Decoction of Ephedrae to strengthen the diaphoretic effect.

(2) To promote the dispersive function of the lung and relieve asthma. It is indicated for the accumulation of pathogenic *qi* in the lung that impairs its dispersive function. It is often used together with Semen Armeniacae Amarum and Radix Glycyrrhizae to form the Three Crude Drugs Decoction. If cold fluid is retained in the lung, drugs for warming the lung, such as Herba Asari and Rhizoma Zingiberis, are used together with it. If there is accumulated heat in the lung, it is used together with drugs for purging heat from the lung, such as Gypsum Fibrosum.

(3) To promote diuresis and relieve edema. It is particularly effective in treating edema which is more serious in the upper part (above the waist) of the body and accompanied by exterior syndrome due to wind. To treat such cases, it is often used together with Rhizoma Atractylodis Macrocephalae and Rhizoma Zingiberis Recens.

Dosage and Preparation: 1.5-10 g. As the crude drug has a stronger diaphoretic effect and the honey stir-baked has a weaker one, the former is often used for relieving exterior syndrome through diaphoresis, and the latter is usually used for stopping cough and relieving asthma.

Precaution: Contraindicated for patients with spontaneous sweating due to exterior deficiency or hypertension; and special care should be taken when prescribing it for patients with insomnia.

Remarks: The lung controls respiration and dominates the skin and hair over the entire body. Attack of the body surface by exogenous wind-cold impairs the opening and closing of the pores, leading to chills and fever; and impaired dispersive function of the lung leads to asthma and cough. Herba Ephedrae is effective in dispelling wind-cold and dispersing pathogenic factors in the lung. When wind and cold are dispelled, the exterior syndrome is relieved, and when the dispersive function of the lung becomes normal, asthma and cough stop. The lung is said to be the upper source of water metabolism; this drug restores the dispersive function, it also facilitates water metabolism and relieves edema. In short, all diseases Herba Ephedrae cures are related to the Lung Meridian. Hence, Li Shizhen, a great medical scientist in the Ming Dynasty, said, "Herba Ephedrae is the drug particularly effective for disorders of the Lung Meridian."

APPENDIX:

Radix Ephedrae (麻黄根 *ma huang gen*)

Radix Ephedrae is the root and rhizome of Ephedra sinica Stapf, E. intermedia Schrenk et C. A. Mey. or E. equisetina Bge. It is sweet in taste and mild in property, acts to stop perspiration, and has been proved effective in treating spontaneous sweating and night sweating; it is often used in combination with Radix Astragali, Fructus Tritici Levis (light) and Concha Ostreae. Its recommended dosage is 3-10 g. It can either be decocted for orally use or made into a powder for external application.

Ramulus Cinnamomi (桂枝 *gui zhi*)

Ramulus Cinnamomi is the dried tender twig of Cinnamomum cassia Prsel, an evergreen tree of Lauraceae. Produced in Guangdong, Yunnan and Sichuan provinces, as well as the Guangxi Zhuang Autonomom Region, it is collected in summer and autumn, dried in the sun or in the shade, and cut into thin pieces or small segments.

Taste and Property: Acrid, sweet and warm.
Attributive Meridian: Heart, lung and urinary bladder meridians.
Actions and Indications:

(1) To induce perspiration and dispel cold. It is indicated for exterior syndrome due to wind-cold either with or without sweating. For exterior deficiency syndrome with sweating, it is often combined with Radix Paeoniae Alba, as in Decoction of Ramulus Cinnamomi; and for exterior excess syndrome with anhidrosis, it is often used together with Herba Ephedrae.

(2) To warm the meridians. It is indicated for: (a) *Bi*-syndrome due to wind-dampness, especially with pain in the upper limbs, Rhizoma et Radix Notopterygii and Radix Ledebouriellae are often used together with it; (b) Irregular menstruation and amenorrhea due to cold retention and blood stagnation, and it is often used with Radix Angelicae Sinensis, Rhizoma Chuanxiong and Flos Carthami to activate blood circulation and remove obstruction in the meridians.

(3) To warm and invigorate *yang*. It is indicated for: (a) Internal cold and fluid retention, as in the lung (leading to asthmatic cough with dilute sputum) and in the stomach (leading to watery regurgitation). This drug is applied to warm and invigorate *yang* in order to relieve internal retention of cold and fluid; in the former case, it is often combined with Herba Ephedrae, and in the latter with Rhizoma Atractylodis Macrocephalae. (b) Dysfunction of the urinary bladder marked by dysuria and edema; it is often used in combination with diuretics, such as Poria, Polyporus Umbellatus and Rhizoma Alismatis, as in

Powder of Five Drugs Containing Poria. Besides, it can also be used for cases in which the decline of thoracic *yang* leads to chest pain.

Dosage: 3-10 g.

Precaution: This drug is quite warm, and can activate blood circulation and consume *yin* fluid as well. It is contraindicated for febrile diseases, cases of *yin* deficiency and bleeding. For pregnant women and women with menorrhagia, it is used with great care.

Remarks: The diaphoretic effect of Ramulus Cinnamomi is not as strong as that of Herba Ephedrae, while its ability to dispel cold is strong indeed. It can be applied for both exterior and interior cold syndrome. Moreover, it can go deep into the blood system, warm the meridians and remove obstruction in them; this is why it is often used in disorders caused by cold retention and blood stagnation. Besides, pathogenic cold tends to obstruct and block the flow of *yang qi*, Ramulus Cinnamomi can dispel cold and promote *yang-qi* circulation. Therefore, it is often used to treat cold and fluid retention as well as dysuria.

Folium Perillae(紫苏叶 *zi su ye*)

Folium Perillae refers to the dried tender twig and leaf of Perilla frutescens (L.) Britt., an annual herb of Labiatae. Produced mainly in Jiangsu, Anhui and Henan provinces, it is collected in autumn, with the root removed and dried in the sun.

Taste and Property: Acrid, and warm.

Attributive Meridian: Lung, spleen and stomach meridians.

Actions and Indications:

(1) To induce perspiration and dispel cold. It is indicated for exterior syndrome due to wind-cold marked by chills, fever and anhidrosis. As it can also activate *qi* circulation and harmonize the middle *jiao*, it is especially indicated for exterior syndrome accompanied by *qi* stagnation. It is often used together with Rhizoma Zingiberis Recens to strengthen the effect of dispelling wind-cold. For exterior syndrome due to wind-cold accompanied by cough, it is used with Semen Armeniacae Amarum and Radix Peucedani.

(2) To activate *qi* circulation and harmonize the middle *jiao*. In treating distention and fullness in the epigastrium and abdomen, poor appetite, nausea and vomiting due to spleen and stomach *qi* stagnation, it is often used in combination with Rhizoma Pinelliae and Pericarpium Citri Reticulatae. For cases marked by vomiting due to stomach heat, it can be used together with Rhizoma Coptidis to purge heat from the stomach and harmonize the middle *jiao*. It is also effective in activating *qi* circulation and appeasing the fetus, treating morning sickness and restlessness of the fetus; in such cases, it is often combined with Fructus Amomi.

This drug also relieves crab allergy marked by abdominal pain, vomiting and diarrhea. In such cases, it is decocted either singly or together with Rhizoma Zingiberis Recens for oral intake.

Dosage: 8-10 g.

APPENDIX:

Caulis Perillae(苏梗 *su geng*)

Caulis Perillae refers to the old stem of Perilla frutescens (L.) Britt. It is acrid and warm. With the action of activating *qi* circulation and harmonize the middle *jiao*, it is indicated for disharmony between the stomach and liver, and spleen and stomach *qi* stagnation.

Dosage: 5-10 g.

Remarks: Folium Perillae is diaphoretic and activates *qi* circulation and harmonizes the middle *jiao*. It is not only effective in relieving exterior syndrome due to wind-cold, but also frequently used in treating cases accompanied by spleen and stomach *qi* stagnation. Its effect in appeasing the fetus is also related to the pharmacologic action to activate *qi* circulation. Caulis Perillae is characterized by a weaker acrid flavor and dispersive action but stronger ability to activate *qi* circulation.

Rhizoma Zingiberis Recens(生姜 *sheng jiang*)

Rhizoma Zingiberis Recens is the fresh rhizome of Zingiber officinale (Willd.) Rosc., which is a perennial plant of Zingiberaceae. Produced mainly in Sichuan, Guangdong, Shandong and Jiangsu provinces, it is collected in autumn and winter, with the fibrous roots and soils removed.

Taste and Property: Acrid, and slightly warm.

Attributive Meridian: Lung, spleen and stomach meridians.

Actions and Indications:

(1) To induce perspiration and dispel cold. It is indicated for exterior syndrome due to wind-cold. It can be decocted singly or together with other acrid and warm drugs to relieve exterior syndrome.

(2) To warm the middle *jiao* and stop vomiting. It is indicated for various kinds of vomiting, especially those due to cold in the stomach. It can be decocted or crushed into a juice for drinking, or used together with Rhizoma Pinelliae to strengthen the antemetic effect. For vomiting due to stomach heat, it can be used in combination with Rhizoma Coptidis, which purges stomach heat. It can also be used as an adjuvant ingredient for such antemetic drugs as Rhizoma Pinelliae and Rhizoma Coptidis, so as to enhance their antemetic effect. Owing to its ability to warm the middle *jiao*, it is also indicated for epigastric and abdominal pain and diarrhea due to attack of the spleen and stomach by cold.

(3) To reduce or remove the toxicity of such drugs as Rhizoma Pinelliae, Rhizoma Arisaematis, Radix Aconiti Lateralis Preparata, Radix Aconiti, etc. It is either used together with these drugs or used as an adjuvant in their processing. Its decoction can treat poisoning by the above drugs. In addition, it can also relieve fish and crab allergy.

Dosage and Preparation: Cut into small pieces and take 2-3 pieces or 5-10 g for decoction; or pounded into juice and drink 3-10 drops with boiled water.

Remarks: Both Folium Perillae and Rhizoma Zingiberis Recens can dispel wind-cold and regulate spleen and stomach functions, but the former is more effective in promoting *qi* circulation, while the latter is more effective in warming the middle *jiao* and is an important antemetic.

Herba Elsholtziae(香薷 *xiang ru*)

Herba Elsholtziae refers to the dried aerial part with flower spikes of Elsholtzia splendens Nakai ex F. Maekawa or M. chinensis Maxim, which is an annual herbaceous plant of Labiatae. It is mainly produced in Jiangxi, Hebei and Henan Provinces. In summer when its fruits are ripe, the aerial part is cut and dried in the sun or in the shade.

Taste and Property: Acid, and warm.
Attributive Meridian: Lung and stomach meridians.
Actions and Indications:

(1) Promoting diaphoresis and eliminating summer-heat and dampness. It is often used in combination with Cortex Magnoliae Officinalis and Semen Dolichoris Album, as in the Decoction of Elsholtziae to treat summer-heat-dampness syndrome marked by fever, chills, anhidrosis, abdominal pain, vomiting and diarrhea.

(2) Diuretic and antedemic. For such cases, it is often used together with Rhizoma Atractylodis Macrocephalae.

Dosage: 3-10 g.
Remarks: This drug is acrid, warm and aromatic; it dispels pathogenic cold in the surface or dissolves turbidity and dampness and regulates spleen and stomach functions, and thus is commonly used for summer-heat-dampness syndrome due to attack of exogenous pathogenic cold or endogenous injury caused by too much intake of raw and cold food. It is not indicated for summer-heat stroke with high fever, severe thirst and profuse sweating.

Herba Schizonepetae(荆芥 *jing jie*)

Herba Schizonepetae refers to the aerial part of the annual herb Schizonepeta tenuifolia Briq. of Labiatae. Mainly produced in Jiangsu, Zhejiang, Jiangxi and Henan provinces, it is cut and collected when the spikes are green and dried in the sun.

Synonym: *Jia su*.
Taste and Property: Acrid, and warm.
Attributive Meridian: Lung and liver meridians.
Actions and Indications:

(1) To eliminate wind and relieve exterior syndrome. For exterior syndrome due to wind-cold, it is often used in combination with Folium Perillae, Rhizoma seu Radix Notopterygii and Radix Ledebouriellae. For exterior syndrome due to wind-heat, it is usually used together with Herba Menthae, Flos Lonicerae and Fructus Forsythiae. As this drug can eliminate wind, it is also indicated for headache due to attack of pathogenic wind and urticaria.

(2) To promote eruptions. It is indicated for the initial stage of infantile measles in

combination with Herba Menthae, Fructus Arctii and Periostracum Cicadae.

(3) To stop bleeding. The carbonized drug by stir-baking is indicated for hematemesis, epistaxis, hematochezia and uterine bleeding. In such cases, it can be used together with other hemostatics.

Dosage and Preparation: 3-10 g. To stop bleeding, the drug should be carbonized by stir-baking. For other purposes, it is used raw.

Remarks: This drug is warm but not dry, and its action is mild. Owing to its acrid property, it is mainly used for dispelling wind. It is indicated for exterior syndrome due to either wind-cold or wind-heat. The drug enters the blood system, and after carbonization by stir-baking, it becomes bitter and astringent; hence it can be used to check bleeding.

Radix Ledebouriellae(防风 *fang feng*)

Radix Ledebouriellae refers to the root of the perennial plant Ledebouriella divaricata (Turcz.) Hiroe of Umbelliferae. Mainly produced in Liaoning, Heilongjiang and Hebei provinces as well as the Inner Mongolia Autonomous Region, its root is collected in spring and autumn before the pedicels sprout, with the fibrous roots and soil removed and dried in the sun.

Taste and Property: Acrid and sweet, and warm.

Attributive Meridian: Urinary bladder, liver and spleen meridians.

Actions and Indications:

(1) To relieve exterior syndrome by dispelling wind. It is indicated for exterior syndrome due to wind-cold, and especially for cases caused by severe attack of pathogenic wind with serious headache and general achiness. It is often used together with Rhizoma et Radix Notopterygii, Radix Angelicae Dahuricae and Herba Schizonepetae.

(2) To relieve pain by eliminating wind. It is indicated for: (a) *Bi*-syndrome due to wind, cold and dampness, and painful joints, especially cases caused mainly by pathogenic wind; in such cases, it is often used with Rhizoma et Radix Notopterygii and Ramulus Cinnamomi. (b) Headache due to wind-cold or "head-wind" (persistent and recurrent headache), in which it is often combined with Rhizoma Chuanxiong, Radix Angelicae Dahuricae and Rhizoma et Radix Notopterygii.

(3) To relieve convulsion by eliminating wind. It is indicated for tetanus with lockjaw and opisthotonos. In such cases, Rhizoma Arisaematis, Rhizoma Typhonii and Bombyx Batryticatus are often used with it to increase the spasmolytic effect through eliminating wind.

(4) To relieve itching by eliminating wind, such as in cases of urticaria and pruritus.

The drug can also be used to treat abdominal pain and diarrhea due to disharmony between the liver and spleen.

Dosage and Preparation: 3-10 g; generally used raw, and stir-baked for abdominal pain and diarrhea.

Remarks: Radix Ledebouriellae is an important drug for eliminating wind, as reflected in relieving exterior syndrome, stopping pain and relieving convulsion and itching. Most drugs for eliminating wind are warm and dry, while this one is slightly warm but not dry. Hence, it is known as the "moistening drug among the drugs for eliminating wind."

In relieving exterior syndrome due to pathogenic wind, this drug is often used together with Herba Schizonepetae. Herba Schizonepetae has a stronger diaphoretic effect, however, while Radix Ledebouriellae is more effective in eliminating wind and stopping pain.

Rhizoma seu Radix Notopterygii(羌活 *qiang huo*)

Rhizoma seu Radix Notopterygii refers to the rhizome or root of the perennial plant Notopterygium incisum Ting. ex H. T. Chang or N. forbesii Boiss. of Umbelliferae. Mainly produced in Sichuan and Gansu provinces, it is dug out and cut into pieces in the spring and autumn.

Taste and Property: Acrid and bitter, and warm.
Attributive Meridian: Urinary bladder and liver meridians.
Actions and Indications:

(1) To relieve exterior syndrome by dispelling cold. It is indicated for exterior syndromes due to wind-cold, especially those with severe headache and general achiness. In treating such cases, it is often used together with Radix Ledebouriellae, Radix Angelicae Dahuricae and Folium Perillae.

(2) To eliminate wind-dampness and relieve pain. It is indicated for *bi*-syndrome due to wind, cold and dampness and painful joints, especially cases marked by pain in the upper part of the body. It can also be used together with Radix Ledebouriellae to cure headache due to wind and cold.

This drug is also effective in relieving itching by eliminating wind and additionally treating pruritus.

Dosage: 3-10 g.

Remarks: Both Ledebouriellae and Notopterygii can eliminate wind and they can be used together for syndromes due to exogenous wind. But Ledebouriellae is more effective in eliminating wind, and it is moist and mild in dispersive action; Notopterygii is warm and dry and has a stronger action in eliminating cold and dispelling dampness.

Radix Angelicae Dahuricae(白芷 *bai zhi*)

Radix Angelicae Dahuricae refers to the root of the perennial herb Angelicae dahurica (Fisch. ex Hoffm.) Benth. et Hook. f., or A. dahurica (Fisch. ex Hoffm.) Benth. et Hook. f. var. formosana (Boiss.) Shan et Yuan. The former is produced mainly in Heilongjiang, Jilin, Liaoning and Sichuan provinces; and the latter is produced mainly in Zhejiang, Jiangsu and Taiwan provinces. It is collected between summer and autumn when the leaves turn yellow, then dried in the sun or in a low temperature and cut into pieces.

Taste and Property: Acrid and warm.
Attributive Meridian: Lung, and stomach meridians.

Actions and Indications:

(1) To relieve exterior syndrome by eliminating wind. It is indicated for exterior syndrome due to wind-cold, especially that with severe headache. For such cases, it is often used together with Rhizoma seu Radix Notopterygii and Radix Ledebouriellae.

(2) To relieve pain by eliminating wind. It is indicated for headache due to pathogenic wind, pain around the superciliary ridge as well as toothache. It is especially effective for frontal headache, and can be made into pills for oral use or be ground into powder and insufflated into the nose. In compound prescription, it is often used with Notopterygii, Ledebouriellae and Rhizoma Chuanxiong. In treating toothache caused by cold, it is used with Herba Asari; for toothache caused by heat, it is used with Gypsum Fibrosum.

(3) To remove nasal obstruction. The drug is indicated for rhinorrhea, sinusitis and chronic rhinitis with nasal obstruction and discharge, distensive pain in the head or forehead. It can be used singly in powder form which is blown into the nose, or else used together with Asari and Fructus Xanthii in decoctions.

This drug also has a curative effect for carbuncles and swellings in the early stage; additionally, it dries dampness and is used to treat leukorrhagia.

Dosage: 3-10 g.

Remarks: Radix Angelicae Dahuricae is acrid, warm and aromatic, mainly enters the stomach meridian, which circulates via the head and face. This is why it stops pain by eliminating wind and removing nasal obstruction; it is indicated for diseases in the head and face, such as frontal headache, pain around the superciliary ridge, toothache and rhinorrhea. This is where the difference lies between this drug and Ledebouriellae as well as Notopterygii.

Fructus Xanthii(苍耳子 *cang er zi*)

Fructus Xanthii refers to the dried mature fruit with involucres of the annual herb Xanthium sibiricum Patr. of Compositae. Produced throughout the country, mainly in Jiangsu and Fujian provinces, it is collected in autumn when the fruit is ripe, and with the stems and leaves removed.

Taste and Property: Acrid and bitter, and warm; toxic.

Attributive Meridian: Lung meridian.

Actions and Indications:

(1) To remove nasal obstruction by dispelling wind-cold. It is indicated for rhinorrhea with constant turbid nasal discharge and impaired sense of smell, and often used together with Flos Magnoliae and Radix Angelicae Dahuricae, as in Powder of Fructus Xanthii. If a case is accompanied by heat, it is used with Radix Scutellariae and Herba Menthae. Since it dispels wind and cold, it can also be used to treat headache due to wind-cold, in which it is often used in combination with Radix Ledebouriellae and Dahuricae.

(2) To eliminate wind and dampness. It is indicated for treating rheumatic pain. Here, it is often used together with other anti-rheumatic drugs. It is also indicated for urticaria and pruritus.

Dosage and Preparation: 3-10 g for oral use, and a moderate amount for external use. In treating rhinorrhea, it can be applied in the forms of oily drops, emulsion or powder.
Precaution: Overdose may cause intoxication.

Flos Magnoliae(辛夷 *xin yi*)

Flos Magnoliae is the flower bud of the deciduous shrub Magnolia biondii Pamp. and M. denudata Desr., or M. sprengeri Pamp. of Magnoliaceae. Mainly produced in Henan, Anhui and Sichuan provinces, it is collected in late winter and early spring when the buds are not open or not fully open, then dried in the shade.

Synonym: *Mu bi hua*.
Taste and Property: Acrid, and warm.
Attributive Meridian: Lung and stomach meridians.
Actions and Indications:

It dispels wind and cold and removes nasal obstruction. It is a commonly used drug in treating rhinorrhea. In cases of rhinorrhea complicated by nasal obstruction, impaired sense of smell, persistent turbid nasal discharge, dizziness and headache, it can be used singly or in combination with Fructus Xanthii. If cold is more predominant, it is often used with Herba Asari and Radix Angelicae Dahuricae; if heat predominates, it is used together with Radix Scutellariae and Herba Menthae.
Dosage and Preparation: 3-10 g for oral use and a moderate amount for external application. The drug should be decocted with wrappings to avoid irritating the throat. For external use, it can be prepared into oil, emulsion or powder.

Section 2
Drugs for Dispelling Wind-Heat

Herba Menthae(薄荷 *bo he*)

Herba Menthae refers to the dried stem and leaf of the perennial herb Menthae haplocalyx Briq. of Labiatae. Mainly produced in Jiangsu, Zhejiang and Jiangxi provinces, its aerial part is cut and collected in summer and the new growth is collected once again in autumn. They are partially dried in the sun, then tied into bundles and dried again.

Taste and Property: Acrid, and cool.
Attributive Meridian: Lung and liver meridians.
Actions and Indications:

(1) To dispel wind-heat. It is indicated for exterior syndrome due to wind-heat with such manifestations as fever, slight aversion to cold, headache and anhidrosis, in which it is often used together with Herba Schizonepetae, Flos Lonicerae and Fructus Forsythiae.

(2) To purge heat from the head and eye and to soothe the throat. It is often used together with Folium Mori, Flos Chrysanthemi and Schizonepetae to treat headache, con-

gested eyes and sore throat.

(3) To promote rash eruption. It is often used together with Schizonepetae and Periostracum Cicadae to promote the eruption of infantile measles.

This drug also regulates liver *qi*. It is indicated for syndromes due to liver *qi* stagnation, for which a small amount of Menthae is added, as in *Xiaoyao* Powder.

Dosage and Preparation: 2-6 g. When used in a decoction, it should be decocted afterwards.

Fructus Arctii(牛蒡子 *niu bang zi*)

Fructus Arctii is the ripe fruit of the biennial herb Arctium lappa L. of Compositae. To be found throughout the country, mainly in northeastern China as well as Zhejiang and Jiangsu provinces, it is collected in autumn when the fruit is ripe and then dried in the sun.

Synonym: *Wu shi*, *shu zhan zi*, *da li zi*.

Taste and Property: Acrid and bitter, and cold.

Attributive Meridian: Lung, stomach and large intestine meridians.

Actions and Indications:

(1) To dispel wind-cold and soothe the throat. It is indicated for exterior syndromes due to wind-heat, especially cases marked with cough and sore throat. In treating such cases, it is often used in combination with other drugs for dispelling wind-heat.

(2) To promote eruption of measles. For such cases, it is often used together with other drugs for promoting eruptions, such as Herba Schizonepetae and Herba Menthae. In addition, it is also effective in purging heat and toxicins and indicated for boils and ulcers due to toxic heat.

Dosage: 5-10 g.

Remarks: The dispersive effect of Fructus Arctii is not as strong as its ability to purge heat from the lung and relieve cough, and purge heat and eliminate toxicins. It can also slightly facilitate bowel movement, and so is particularly indicated for wind-heat syndromes marked by cough or constipation due to toxic heat.

Periostracum Cicadae(蝉蜕 *chan tui*)

Periostracum Cicadae refers to the exuviae of nymph during Cryptotympana pustulata Fabr., an insect of cicadidae. Mainly produced in Shandong, Henan, Hebei and Jiangsu provinces, it is collected in summer and autumn, and dried in the sun with soil and other foreign matters removed.

Synonym: *Chan yi*, *chan ke*.

Taste and Property: Salty and slightly sweet, and cold.

Attributive Meridian: Lung and liver meridians.

Actions and Indications:

(1) To chiefly dispel wind-heat. It is indicated for exterior syndromes due to wind-heat or attack of the lung by wind-heat, marked by sore throat and hoarseness of voice. To treat such cases, it is often used in combination with Herba Menthae and Fructus Arctii.

(2) To relieve spasms and convulsions. It is indicated for: (a) Tetanus, for which it is used singly, or taken after being decocted with rice wine, or being ground into powder and taken with rice wine; or it is used together with Rhizoma Arisaematis and Scorpio; (b) Infantile convulsion, for which it is often used with Ramulus Uncariae cum Uncis and Scorpio.

It relieves itching by eliminating wind, and is indicated for urticaria and pruritus. Moreover, it relieves optic nebulaes and congestion of the eye.

Dosage: 3-30 g; and 15-30 g for tetanus.

Remarks: This drug can dispel wind-heat and is commonly used to treat loss of voice due to attack of the lung by wind-heat. Its ability to relieve spasms, convulsions and eye nebula distinguishes it from Herba Menthae and Fructus Arctii.

Semen Sojae Preparatum(淡豆豉 *dan dou chi*)

It refers to the processed product after fermentation of the ripe seeds of Glycine max (L.) Merr. of Leguminosae. The steps of processing are as follows: Take 70-100 g of Folium Mori and Herba Artemisiae Annuae each and boil them in water; and the filtrate is mixed with 1,000 g of soybeans; until the liquid is fully absorbed, the beans are steamed, aired for sometime, covered by the previously decocted Folium Mori and Artemisiae Annuae and fermented in a container until yellow hairs grow all over it; wash them clean (with residue removed); put in the container again for 15-20 days until fully fermented and the sweet smell comes out; then take them out, steam for a while and dry them.

Taste and Property: Acrid, sweet and slightly bitter, and slightly cold.

Attributive Meridian: Lung and stomach meridians.

Actions and Indications:

(1) Diaphoretic. It is indicated for exterior syndrome due to exogenous pathogenic factors. Since its diaphoretic action is relatively weak, it is often used together with other diaphoretics. For exterior syndrome due to wind-cold, it is used with Bulbus Allii Fistulosi, as in Decoction of Allii Fistulosi and Sojae Preparatum; for exterior syndrome due to wind-heat, it is used with Herba Menthae, Flos Lonicerae and Fructus Forsythiae.

(2) To relieve irritability. It is indicated for febrile diseases with affection of *qifen* by pathogenic heat, marked by fever, stuffiness in the chest, irritability and insomnia. For such cases, it is often prescribed together with Fructus Gardeniae, as in Decoction of Gardeniae and Sojae Preparatum, to dispel the pathogenic factors, purge heat and relieve irritability.

Dosage: 10-15 g.

Remarks: There are two kinds of fermented soybeans: one is salty and cannot be used as a drug; the other medical kind is not salty.

Folium Mori(桑叶 *sang ye*)

Folium Mori is the leaf of the deciduous tree Morus alba L. of Moraceae. To be found in most parts of the country, it is collected in autumn after Frost Descent and dried in the sun.

Taste and Property: Bitter and sweet, and cold.
Attributive Meridian: Lung and liver meridians.
Actions and Indications:

(1) To dispel wind-heat. Indicated for exterior syndrome due to wind-heat, for which it is often combined with Flos Chrysanthemi, Herba Menthae and Fructus Forsythiae. It can also purge lung heat and relieve cough, and is indicated for cough due to heat and dryness in the lung.

(2) To purge heat from the liver and improve vision. Indications: (a) Exterior syndrome due to wind-heat and upward disturbance of liver fire, marked by redness, swelling and pain in the eyes as well as headache. For such cases, Chrysanthemi and Semen Cassiae are often used together with it. (b) Upward disturbance by hyperactive liver *yang*, marked by headache and vertigo. For such cases, Chrysanthemi, Ramulus Uncariae cum Uncis and Concha Ostreae are often added.

Dosage: 5-10 g.

Flos Chrysanthemi(菊花 *ju hua*)

Flos Chrysanthemi is the capitulum of the perennial herb Chrysanthemum morifolium Ramat. of Compositae. Mainly produced in Zhejiang, Anhui, Henan and Jiangsu provinces, it is collected in late autumn and early winter, dried in the shade or by baking, or else fumigated and steamed and then dried in the sun.

Taste and Property: Sweet and bitter, and slightly cold.
Attributive Meridian: Lung and liver meridians.
Actions and Indications:

(1) To dispel wind-heat. It is indicated for exterior syndrome due to wind-heat. In treating such cases, it is often used in combination with Folium Mori, Herba Menthae and Fructus Forsythiae.

(2) To purge heat from the liver and improve vision. Indications: (a) Redness, swelling and pain in the eyes, for which it is often used with Semen Cassiae and Folium Mori. (b) Upward disturbance of hyperactive liver *yang*, marked by headache and vertigo, for which it is combined with Folium Mori, Ramulus Uncariae cum Uncis and Concha Ostreae.

Additionally, it purges heat and eliminates toxicins, and so is used to cure carbuncle and abscess due to toxic heat. For such cases, fresh leaves of Chrysanthemi can be pounded into a paste and applied externally.

Dosage: 5-10 g.
Remarks: Flos Chrysanthemi is generally classified as yellow or white. The yellow is used to dispel wind-heat, the white is used to eliminate liver heat and improve eyesight. Both Folium Mori and Flos Chrysanthemi can dispel wind and heat, purge heat from the liver and improve vision, and so they are often used together. Yet, Folium Mori can purge heat from the lung and relieve cough, and it is often used for cough due to lung heat and dryness; Flos Chrysanthemi is more effective in purging heat from the liver, improving vision and removing toxicins.

Radix Puerariae(葛根 *ge gen*)

Radix Puerariae is the root of the perennial trailing plant Pueraria lobata (Willd.) Ohwi, or P. thomsonii Benth. of Leguminosae. Mainly produced in Henan, Hunan, Zhejiang and Sichuan provinces, it is collected in autumn and winter, cut into pieces and dried in the sun.

Taste and Property: Sweet, acrid and bland.
Attributive Meridian: Spleen and stomach meridians.
Actions and Indications:

(1) Diaphoretic and antipyretic. It is indicated for exterior syndrome due to either wind-cold or wind-heat. It is particularly effective in treating stiffness in the neck and back. In cases due to wind-cold, it is prescribed together with Herba Ephedrae and Ramulus Cinnamomi; and in cases due to wind-heat, it is often used together with Radix Bupleuri and Radix Scutellariae.

(2) To promote the eruption of rashes. It is indicated for the early stage of infantile measles when the eruptions are insufficient. For its action in relieving exterior syndrome and fever, promoting fluid secretion, relieving thirst and stopping diarrhea, it is especially suitable for measles accompanied by fever, thirst, or diarrhea, and incomplete eruptions.

(3) To raise *yang* and prevent diarrhea. It is indicated for diarrhea due to spleen weakness, for which it is often prescribed together with drugs that strengthen the spleen, such as Radix Codonopsis Pilosulae and Rhizoma Atractylodis Macrocephalae. For diarrhea and dysentery due to heat accompanied by exterior syndrome, it can be used with Rhizoma Coptidis and Radix Scutellariae.

Dosage: 5-10 g. It is used raw for relieving exterior syndrome, promoting rash eruption and promoting fluid secretion. To prevent diarrhea, it is baked with wet coatings.
Remarks: Radix Puerariae is characterized by its ability to lift and float. In addition to relieving exterior syndrome, reducing fever and promoting eruptions, it can promote fluid secretion and lift *yang* to stop thirst and diarrhea. It can be therefore applied for fever and thirst in febrile diseases and fever in diarrhea and dysentery. Moreover, it is effective in relieving the stiffness of the neck and back in exterior syndromes. It has also been proved effective for stiff neck and back due to hypertension.

Radix Bupleuri(柴胡 *chai hu*)

Radix Bupleuri refers to the root or entire plant of the perennial herb Bupleurum chinense DC. , or B. scorzonerifolium Willd. of Umbelliferae. The former is mainly produced in Liaoning, Gansu, Hebei and Henan provinces; the latter is mainly produced in Hubei, Jiangsu and Sichuan provinces. It is collected in spring and autumn and dried in the sun.

Taste and Property: Bitter and acrid, and slightly cold.
Attributive Meridian: Liver and gallbladder meridians.
Actions and Indications:

(1) To relieve exterior syndrome and subdue fever. It is indicated for fever from exterior syndrome, and is especially important for Shaoyang syndrome marked by alternate chills and fever. For such cases, it is often prescribed with Radix Scutellariae, as in Decoction of Bupleuri for Regulating Shaoyang. It can also be used in the treatment of malaria.

(2) To soothe the liver and relieve *qi* stagnation. It is indicated for liver *qi* stagnation that gives rise to fullness in the chest and epigastrium, distensive intercostal and hypochondriac pain, masses in the breast and irregular menstruation. In such cases, it is often used with Radix Angelicae Sinensis and Radix Paeoniae Alba, as in *Xiaoyao* Powder.

(3) To lift *qi* of the middle *jiao. It is indicated for gastroptosis, prolapse of the anus and uterus due to the prolapse of qi* of the middle *jiao*. For such cases, it is combined with Rhizoma Cimicifugae and Radix Astragali.

Dosage: 3-10 g,
Remarks: Radix Bupleuri differs from other drugs that eliminate toxicins in that it enters the liver and gallbladder meridians, reduces heat in the Shaoyang Meridian, soothe the liver and relieve liver *qi* stagnation. It is therefore a major drug for Shaoyang syndrome accompanied by alternate chills and fever as well as *qi* stagnation. Besides, it is frequently used in cases due to prolapse of *qi* of the middle *jiao* owing to its ability to lift *yang*.

Rhizoma Cimicifugae(升麻 *sheng ma*)

Rhizoma Cimicifugae refers to the dried root of the perennial herb Cimicifuga heracleifolia Kom. , or C. Dahurica (Turcz.) Maxim. , and C. foetida L. of Ranunculaceae. The former two are mainly produced in Liaoning and Heilongjiang provinces, the latter mainly in Shanxi and Sichuan. It is collected in autumn and dried in the sun.

Taste and Property: Sweet and acrid, and slightly cold.
Attributive Meridian: Lung, spleen and stomach meridians.
Actions and Indications:

(1) To relieve exterior syndrome and promote rash eruption. It is indicated for measles at the early stage when the eruptions are not complete. Here, it is often used with Radix Puerariae.

(2) To purge heat and eliminate toxicins. Indications: (a) Hyperactive stomach fire accompanied by headache, fetid ulcers in the gums or ulcers in the tongue and mouth, as

well as congested and sore throat. For such cases, it is often prescribed with Gypsum Fibrosum and Rhizoma Coptidis. (b) Boils and ulcers, erysipelas in the face. For such diseases, it is often combined with Fructus Forsythiae and Radix Isatidis.

(3) To lift *qi* of the middle *jiao*. It is often prescribed with Radix Bupleuri and Radix Astragali for the prolapse of the middle *jiao qi*.

Dosage: 3-10 g. Used raw for relieving exterior syndrome, promoting rash eruptions, purging heat and eliminating toxicins; used stir-baked with honey as an adjuvant to lift *qi* of the middle *jiao*.

Remarks: Rhizoma Cimicifugae possesses strong ascending and dispelling properties, and it is effective in promoting rash eruption and lifting *yang*. In addition, it can also purge heat and toxicins, and is often used for hyperactive stomach fire, boils and ulcers.

Table 2. Actions of the Drugs for Relieving Exterior Syndrome

Division	Drug	Similarities	Differences
Drugs for Dispelling Wind-Cold	Herba Ephedrae	Inducing perspiration and dispelling cold	Promoting dispersing function of the lung and relieving asthma, promoting water metabolism and relieving edema
	Ramulus Cinnamomi		Eliminating cold from the *qi* system, warming up meridians and removing stagnation of *yang qi*
	Folium Perillae	Dispelling wind-cold and regulating the spleen and stomach	Removing stagnation of *qi* of spleen and stomach, relieving restlessness of the fetus
	Rhizoma Zingiberis Recens		Warming the middle *jiao*, stopping vomiting, eliminating toxins
	Herba Elsholtziae		Eliminating summer-heat and dampness, promoting water metabolism and relieving edema
	Herba Schizonepetae	Eliminating wind and relieving exterior syndrome	Promoting rash eruptions, stopping bleeding after being stir-baked to carbonized
	Radix Ledebouriellae		Essential drug for eliminating wind; moistening drug among the drugs for eliminating wind
	Rhizoma seu Radix Notopterygii		Dispelling cold, drying dampness
	Radix Angelicae Dahuricae		Good for treating diseases in the head and face
	Fructus Xanthii	Dispelling wind-cold and removing obstruction from the nose	Eliminating wind and dampness
	Flos Magnoliae		

Division	Drug	Similarities	Differences
Drugs for Dispelling Wind-Heat	Herba Menthae	Dispelling wind-heat; facilitating the throat; promoting eruptions	Fairly strong effect of dispersing and dispelling; clearing heat from the head and eye
	Fructus Arctii		Weaker effect of dispelling and dispersing; clearing heat and toxins
	Periostracum Cicadae		Relieving hoarseness of voice, and spasms and convulsions; relieving itching by eliminating wind; relieving eye nebulae
	Semen Sojae Preparatum		Relieving exterior syndrome; relieving restlessness of the mind
	Folium Mori	Dispelling wind and heat; clearing heat from the liver, brightening eyes	Clearing heat from the lung and relieving cough
	Flos Chrysanthemi		Fairly strong effect of clearing heat from the liver and facilitating the eye; clearing heat and eliminating toxins
	Radix Puerariae	Diaphoretic and subduing fever; lifting *yang*	Relieving stiffness of the nape and back; promoting secretion of fluids and relieving thirst; promoting eruptions
	Radix Bupleuri		Subduing heat in the Shaoyang meridians, regulating the liver and relieving stagnation of *qi* of the liver
	Rhizoma Cimicifugae		Promoting eruptions; clearing heat and toxins

Note: Drugs such as Herba Asari, Radix Angelicae Pubescentis and Herba Agastaches also relieve exterior syndrome. They are discussed in other chapters and sections of this book.

CHAPTER FIVE
DRUGS FOR ELIMINATING HEAT

Drugs that mainly purge heat from the interior are known as *qing re yao*.

In heat syndrome, there is a difference between exterior and interior heat, and excess and deficiency heat. Drugs for purging heat are mainly indicated for interior and excess heat syndromes, and some are also used for deficiency heat syndrome. In line with their action, they can be classified into the following four categories:

(1) Drugs for eliminating and purging heat and fire (*qing re xie huo yao*). Their major actions are: (a) Purging internal heat arising from exogenous pathogenic factors. These drugs are often used for excess heat syndromes of the *qi* system, which are marked by persistent high fever as seen in febrile diseases, restlessness and thirst; (b) Purging endogenous fire, i.e., fire in the *zang-fu* organs. They are often used to treat cases due to hyperactive fire in the lung, heart, stomach, liver and kidney. Moreover, some of the drugs for purging fire, fairly cold and bitter, not only purge heat, but also dry dampness. They are often prescribed in such dampness-heat syndromes as marked by diarrhea, dysentery, jaundice and exudative boils; thus they are also known as drugs for purging heat and overcoming pathogenic dampness.

(2) Drugs for eliminating heat and toxicins (*qing re jie du yao*). They are often prescribed for febrile diseases, in which the toxic heat is intensive, as well as for such surgical diseases as carbuncles and boils. Some can also relieve poisoning from snake and insect bites.

(3) Drugs for eliminating heat and cooling blood (*qing re liang xue yao*). Able to purge heat from the *xue* (blood) system, these drugs are often used for febrile diseases marked by persistent high fever, deep red tongue, coma, petechiae and echymoses, in which the pathogenic factors have entered the *ying* and *xue* systems, as well as for hematemesis and epistaxis due to excessive heat in the blood, as in diseases caused by endogenous factors. Some also nourish *yin*, and so can be applied for *yin* deficiency syndromes.

(4) Drugs for eliminating deficiency heat (*qing xu re yao*). These are mainly applied for heat syndrome due to *yin* deficiency, such as the late stage of febrile diseases, in which the body fluid is consumed by heat, leading to fever during the night and chills in the morning, and also hectic fever due to *yin* deficiency, as seen in some chronic diseases.

This is only a general classification. Some drugs can purge heat of different types. For example, Rhizoma Coptidis purges fire and eliminates toxicins; Cortex Moutan Radicis cools the blood and purges fire; and Herba Artemisiae Annuae purges both deficiency heat and excess heat.

In applying drugs that purge heat, it is necessary to match or combine them with other drugs in accordance with the specific conditions of different diseases. For example, in cases of high fever accompanied with unconsciousness, they are used in combination with drugs for promoting resuscitation; for cases in which excessive heat stirs up wind and gives rise to convulsions, they are prescribed with drugs for purging liver heat and calming wind; for cases in which pathogenic heat is not yet eliminated while the antipathogenic *qi* has already become deficient, they are used with drugs that strengthen the antipathogenic *qi*; for cases in which *yin* is injured, they are combined with drugs for nourishing *yin*; and in cases of *qi* deficiency, they are used with drugs that replenish *qi*.

Improper use of drugs for purging heat may cause damage to *yang qi* of the spleen and stomach and result in such side effects as poor appetite, nausea, epigastric pain, diarrhea, etc. Moreover, these drugs are contraindicated for syndromes with false heat and true cold, so as to avoid possible serious damage to *yang*. Overuse of the bitter and cold drugs that purge heat and dry dampness may damage *yin* fluid; whereas sweet, cold and moistening drugs for promoting fluid secretion may also generate dampness. Attention should be given to this point in applying drugs for purging heat.

Section 1
Drugs for Eliminating Heat and Purging Fire

Gypsum Fibrosum(石膏 *shi gao*)

Gypsum Fibrosum refers to calcium sulfate mineral anhydrite that contains $Ca(SO_4)\cdot 2H_2O$. It is mainly produced in Hubei, Anhui, Sichuan and Gansu provinces. It can be mined any time with foreign matters removed.

Taste and Property: Acrid and bitter, and cold.
Attributive Meridian: Lung and stomach meridians.
Actions and Indications:

(1) To purge heat and fire, mainly excess lung and stomach heat. It is indicated for: (a) Febrile diseases involving the *qi* system, with high fever, restlessness, severe thirst, profuse sweating, and bounding and large pulse. For such cases, it is used as the main drug in combination with Rhizoma Anemarrhenae and Radix Glycyrrhizae, as in White Tiger Decoction. If both the *qi* and *xue* systems are damaged by heat, exhibiting high fever, echymoses and petechiae, it is used with Radix Rehmanniae, Radix Scrophulariae and Cortex Moutan Radicis. (b) Excess lung heat, with cough, asthma and fever. For such cases, it is combined with Herba Ephedrae and Semen Armeniacae Amarum, as in Decoction of Ephedrae, Armeniacae Amarum, Glycyrrhizae and Gypsum Fibrosum. (c) Headache and toothache due to the flare-ups of stomach fire. For such cases, it is often prescribed with Rhizoma Anemarrhenae, Radix Rehmanniae and Radix Achyranthis Bidentatae.

(2) To purge heat, promote granulation and heal ulcers. It is indicated for lingering

boils, ulcers, eczema and burns. In such cases, it is calcined, crushed and ground into fine powder for external use.

Dosage and Preparation: 15-60 g normally, and 120 g for heavy doses; raw for oral intake, and calcined for external use in a moderate amount.

Remarks: As Gypsum Fibrosum can purge excess heat from the lung and stomach, it can be used as the main drug in the treatment of exogenous febrile diseases in which the *qi* system is affected by pathogenic factors, resulting in high fever, restlessness and thirst; or cough due to heat in the lung; or diseases caused by the upward disturbance of stomach fire. Excessive heat leads to restlessness, and fluid consumption to thirst with a strong desire to drink. Since this drug is effective in purging heat and purging fire, it can relieve restlessness and quench thirst.

Rhizoma Anemarrhenae(知母 *zhi mu*)

Rhizoma Anemarrhenae refers to the root of the perennial herb Anemarrhena asphodeloides Bge. of Liliaceae. Mainly produced in Hebei, Shanxi and the northeastern China provinces, it is dug and collected in spring and autumn, and dried in the sun with the fibrous roots and foreign matters removed.

Taste and Property: Bitter and sweet, and cold.

Attributive Meridian: Lung, stomach and kidney meridians.

Actions and Indications:

(1) To purge heat and fire, especially heat in the lung and stomach. Indications: (a) Febrile diseases involving the *qi* system accompanied by high fever and restlessness. For such cases, it is often used with Gypsum Fibrosum, as in White Tiger Decoction. (b) Cough due to lung heat with expectoration of yellow sticky sputum. It can also nourish *yin* and moisten dryness and be prescribed for dry cough due to *yin* deficiency. For both kinds of cough, it can be combined with Bulbus Fritillariae Cirrhosae.

(2) To subdue fire through nourishing *yin*. It is indicated for the insufficient kidney *yin* which gives rise to hyperactive fire as manifested by hectic fever, nocturnal emission and night sweating. Here, it is often combined with Cortex Phellodendri to form recipes for nourishing kidney *yin*.

(3) To promote fluid secretion and moisten dryness. It is indicated for: (a) Stomach heat with thirst, especially in diabetes. For such cases, it is often used with Radix Trichosanthis and Radix Ophiopogonis. (b) Constipation due to fluid consumption in febrile diseases. For such cases, it is often used with Radix Rehmanniae, Radix Scrophulariae and Radix Ophiopogonis.

Dosage and Preparation: 6-12 g; used raw in general, stir-baked with salty water for nourishing *yin* and suppressing fire.

Remarks: Because it is bitter, sweet, cold and moistening, Rhizoma Anemarrhenae not only clears excess heat from the lung and stomach, but also nourishes *yin*, promotes fluid secretion and moistens dryness; thus it is indicated for both excess and deficiency heat syndromes. This distinguishes it from Gypsum Fibrosum, which mainly purges excess heat from the lung and stomach.

Rhizoma Phragmitis(芦根 *lu gen*)

Rhizoma Phragmitis is the root of the perennial plant Phragmites communis Trin. of Gramineae. To be found in all parts of China, it can be collected any time throughout the year. It is dried in the sun, or used fresh, in the latter form to better effect.

Taste and Property: Sweet, and cold.
Attributive Meridian: Lung and stomach meridians.
Actions and Indications:

(1) To purge heat from the lung. It is indicated for cough due to lung heat accompanied by yellow sticky sputum, pulmonary abscess and cough with expectoration of purulent sputum. For such cases, it is often prescribed with drugs for purging heat from the lung and resolving phlegm, such as Radix Scutellariae, Herba Houttuyniae and Radix Platycodi.

(2) To purge heat and promote the generation of fluid. It is indicated for consumption of fluid by febrile diseases, marked by irritability, feverishness and thirst. Here, it is often combined with Gypsum Fibrosum, Radix Ophiopogonis and Radix Trichosanthis. If fluid consumption is severe, the drug can be mixed with Fructus Pyri, Rhizoma Nelumbinis, Radix Ophiopogonis and Cormus Heleocharis Dulcis. Together, they are pounded into a juice for oral intake.

It can also be used for vomiting caused by stomach heat. For such a case, it can either be decocted singly for frequent drinking or used with Rhizoma Zingiberis Recens and Caulis Bambusae in Taeniam to produce a decoction.

Dosage: 15-30 g. Better used fresh in doubled dosage.
Remarks: Rhizoma Phragmitis is sweet in taste and cold; it is effective in purging heat from the lung and stomach and promoting fluid secretion. It is sweet but not greasy and can promote fluid secretion without causing undesired retention of pathogenic factors. It is therefore often used to treat febrile diseases in which the pathogenic factors have permitted the *wei* (defensive) and *qi* systems, or thirst due to too much fluid consumption in the later stage of a febrile disease. However, it is usually as an adjuvant for its mild effect.

Radix Trichosanthis(天花粉 *tian hua fen*)

Radix Trichosanthis refers to the dried root of the perennial herb or vine Trichosanthes Kirilowii Maxim., or T. japonica Regel of Cucurbitaceae. Mainly produced in Henan, Jiangsu, Shandong and Anhui provinces, it is collected in autumn and winter, then washed with skin removed, cut into pieces and dried in the sun or by baking.

Synonym: *Gua lou gen.*
Taste and Property: Sweet, sour and slightly bitter, and cold.
Attributive Meridian: Lung and stomach meridians.

Actions and Indications:

(1) To purge heat and promote fluid secretion. It is indicated for febrile diseases with fluid consumption and thirst, as well as diabetes. When fluid is consumed by excessive heat, it can be combined with Gypsum Fibrosum and Rhizoma Phragmitis. In cases of *yin* deficiency, it can be used in combination with Radix Adenophorae and Radix Ophiopogonis.

(2) To relieve swelling and discharge pus. It is used to treat carbuncles and boils caused by toxic heat to relieve swelling in unruptured carbuncles and boils and discharge pus in ruptured ones. It can be taken orally or ground into a powder and applied externally.

It can also moisten the lung and relieve cough, and is prescribed for cough due to heat and dryness in the lung.

Dosage: 10-15 g.

Remarks: Both Radix Trichosanthis and Rhizoma Phragmitis can purge heat and promote fluid secretion. They are both indicated for diseases due to attack of the *qi* system by pathogenic heat, fluid consumption, and thirst. But, the latter's ability to purge heat is stronger than the former; the former's ability to promote fluid secretion is stronger than the latter; and the former also relieves swelling and discharges pus, and is frequently used to treat surgical diseases.

Rhizoma Coptidis(黄连 *huang lian*)

Rhizoma Coptidis refers to the rhizome of the perennial herb Coptidis chinensis Franch., C. deltoidea C. Y. Cheng et Hsiao, or C. teetoides C. Y. Cheng of Ranunculaceae. Mainly produced in Sichuan and Yunnan provinces, it is collected in autumn and dried with the fibrous roots and foreign matters removed.

Taste and Property: Bitter, and cold.

Attributive Meridian: Heart, liver, stomach and large intestine meridians.

Actions and Indications:

(1) To purge heat and fire, especially fire in the heart, stomach and liver meridians. Indicated for: (a) Febrile diseases with excessive heat in the Heart Meridian accompanied by high fever, restlessness, coma and delirium; miscellaneous diseases with hyperactive heart fire accompanied by restlessness, insomnia, and ulcers of the tongue and mouth. For such cases, it is often used with Fructus Gardeniae to enhance the effect of purging fire. In cases of excessive endogenous heart fire which causes extravasation of blood, it is often used with Radix et Rhizoma Rhei and Radix Scutellariae to purge fire and stop bleeding, as in Decoction for Purging Stomach Fire. (b) Vomiting due to stomach heat, epigastric fullness and distention. For such cases, it is combined with Folium Perillae and Rhizoma Pinelliae to pacify the stomach and reduce heat. In cases of attack of the stomach by liver fire with intercostal and hypochondriac distensive pain, vomiting and acid regurgitation, it is combined with Fructus Evodiae to purge heat and pacify the liver and stomach, as in *Zoujin* Pill. (c) Hyperactive liver fire accompanied by congestion, swelling and soreness of

the eye. For such cases, it can either be taken orally or decocted for external use as eye drops.

(2) To purge heat and eliminate pathogenic dampness. It is indicated for: (a) Febrile diseases due to dampness and summer-heat accompanied by heat accumulation in the interior, which is marked by fever, epigastric fullness and distention, nausea, vomiting and yellow greasy tongue coating. For such cases, it is often used with drugs for dissolving dampness, such as Cortex Magnoliae Officinalis and Fructus Amomi Rotundus. (b) Diarrhea and dysentery due to dampness-heat. For such cases, it is often prescribed together with Radix Aucklandiae, as in Pill of Aucklandiae and Coptidis. If the diarrhea or dysentery is complicated by fever, it is used with Radix Puerariae.

(3) To purge heat and relieve toxicins. It is indicated for boils and ulcers due to toxic heat. In such a case, it is used in combination with Radix Scutellariae and Fructus Forsythiae. It can also be ground into a powder for external use.

Dosage and Preparation: 2-6 g. In cases of severe toxic heat, the dosage can be 9-12 g. Generally, it is used raw. For vomiting, it is mixed and baked with ginger juice. For heat in the upper body, it is baked with wine. A moderate dosage is prescribed for external use.

Remarks: Rhizoma Coptidis is quite bitter and cold. Overdose or long-term administration may impair normal stomach function and give rise to poor appetite or even nausea and vomiting, thus care should be taken. Since it is dry and tends to consume body fluid, in cases of hyperactive fire consuming body fluid, it should be used in combination with drugs that nourish *yin* to avoid possible damage to fluid.

Radix Scutellariae(黄芩 *huang qin*)

Radix Scutellariae is the root of the perennial herb Scutellaria baicalensis Georgi of Labiatae. Mainly produced in Hebei, Shanxi and Shandong provinces as well as the Inner Mongolia Autonomous Region, it is collected in spring and autumn, first dried in the sun with the fibrous root and foreign matters removed; the rough root skin is then removed by bumping, and it is again dried in the sun.

Taste and Property: Bitter, and cold.
Attributive Meridian: Lung, liver, gallbladder, heart and large intestine meridians.
Actions and Indications:

(1) To purge heat and purge fire from the heart, lung, liver and gallbladder meridians. Indicated for: (a) Febrile diseases accompanied by high fever, coma, hematemesis and epistaxis due to heat in the blood that leads to extravasation; For such cases, it is often used with Rhizoma Coptidis. (b) Cough due to lung heat accompanied by yellow thick sputum. Here, it is often combined with Cortex Mori Radicis and Rhizoma Anemarrhenae. (c) Headache and congested eye due to the flare-ups of liver fire, for which it is often used with Spica Prunellae and Flos Chrysanthemi. (d) Alternate chills and fever in Shaoyang syndrome, for which it is often used with Radix Bupleuri.

(2) To purge heat and eliminate dampness. Indications: (a) Fever, and stuffiness in

the chest in diseases caused by dampness and summer-heat, in which it is often combined with Rhizoma Coptidis and drugs for dissolving dampness. (b) Diarrhea and dysentery due to dampness-heat. For such diseases, it is often combined with Rhizoma Coptidis and Radix Paeoniae Alba.

(3) To purge heat and toxicins. It is indicated for boils and ulcers due to toxic heat, for which it is used in combination with Rhizoma Coptidis and Fructus Gardeniae.

It can also eliminate heat and appease the fetus, and it is indicated for restlessness of the fetus due to excessive heat.

Dosage and Preparation: 5-10 g. Stir-baked with wine for purging heat in the upper body.

Cortex Phellodendri (黄柏 *huang bai*)

Cortex Phellodendri refers to the bark (with cork removed) of the deciduous tree Phellodendron chinense Schneid, or P. amurense Rupr. of Rutaceae. The former is known as *chuan huang bai*, mainly produced in Sichuan and Guizhou provinces; and the latter is commonly known as *guan huang bai*, mainly produced in northeastern and northern China. The bark is peeled off around the Qingming Festival in early April, dried in the sun with the rough coverings removed and flattened out.

Taste and Property: Bitter, and cold.

Attributive Meridian: Kidney, urinary bladder and large intestine meridians.

Actions and Indications:

(1) To purge heat and purge fire, especially kidney fire. It is indicated for hectic fever, night sweating and seminal emission due to insufficient kidney *yin* that leads to hyperactive fire. For such cases, it is often prescribed with Rhizoma Anemarrhenae and Radix Rehmanniae Preparata to nourish *yin* and suppress fire.

(2) To purge heat and eliminate dampness. Indications: (a) Dampness-heat syndrome of the lower *jiao*, manifesting dribbling and painful urination, morbid pinkish leukorrhea, swelling and pain of the pudenda, swelling and pain or weakness in the feet and knees as well as wet boils on the lower body. Here, it is often used with Rhizoma Atractylodis, as in Powder of Phellodendri and Atractylodis. (b) Jaundice due to dampness-heat, in which it is often combined with Herba Artemisiae Scopariae and Fructus Gardeniae. (c) Dysentery due to dampness-heat, in which it is combined with Rhizoma Coptidis and Radix Pulsatillae.

(3) To purge heat and toxicins. Indicated for boils and ulcers due to toxic heat; in such cases it is often used with Rhizoma Coptidis and Radix Scutellariae.

Dosage and Preparation: 5-10 g. Stir-baked with salty water to purge fire in the lower *jiao*.

Remarks: Rhizoma Coptidis, Radix Scutellariae and Cortex Phellodendri are all bitter and cold, and all purge heat, eliminate dampness, purge fire and eliminate toxicins; all can be applied in combination with each other clinically. However, each of them has its own strong point: Coptidis is especially effective in purging fire from the heart and stomach, Scutellariae in purging heat from the lung and gallbladder, and Phellodendri in purging fire from the kidney and heat from the lower *jiao*.

Fructus Gardeniae(栀子 *zhi zi*)

Fructus Gardeniae refers to the ripe fruit of the evergreen shrub plant Gardenia jasminoides Ellis of Rubiaceae. Mainly produced in Zhejiang, Jiangxi, Hunan and Fujian provinces, it is collected between September to November when the fruit is ripe and turns red or orange. It is lightly steamed or boiled and dried with foreign matter removed.

Synonym: *Shan zhi*.
Taste and Property: Bitter, and cold.
Attributive Meridian: Heart, liver and gallbladder meridians.
Actions and Indications:

(1) To purge heat and purge fire and eliminate toxicins. Indications: (a) Febrile diseases involving the *qi* system, with such manifestations as fever, stuffiness in the chest and restlessness; in such cases, it is often prescribed with Semen Sojae Preparatum, as in Decoction of Gardeniae and Sojae Preparatum, to purge heat and relieve restlessness. In cases of excessive toxic heat with high fever, restlessness, coma and delirium, it is used in combination with Rhizoma Coptidis and Radix Scutellariae to strengthen the elimination of heat, fire and toxicins. (b) Flare-up of liver fire with such manifestations as congestion and pain in the eyes. For such cases, it is used with Flos Chrysanthemi and Radix Gentianae. (c) Carbuncles, swellings, boils and ulcers, for which it is prescribed with Rhizoma Coptidis and Fructus Forsythiae.

(2) To cool the blood and stop bleeding. Indicated for hematemesis, epistaxis and hematuria due to heat in the blood leading to extravasation, in such cases it is often used with Radix Rehmanniae, Rhizoma Imperatae and Cortex Moutan Radicis to strengthen the effect. It can also be applied externally for traumatic bleeding and epistaxis.

(3) To eliminate heat and dampness. Indications: (a) Jaundice due to dampness-heat, in which it is often used with Herba Artemisiae Scopariae and Radix et Rhizoma Rhei, as in Decoction of Artemisiae Scopariae. (b) Diseases of the urinary system due to dampness-heat, with dribbling urination, dysuria and painful urination, as well as hematuria; in such cases it is used together with Caulis Akebiae and Talcum.

The powder of raw Fructus Gardeniae can be mixed with water or vinegar and applied externally in the treatment of sprains and contusions.

Dosage and Preparation: 5-10 g, used either raw or stir-baked. To stop bleeding, it is stir-baked until carbonized.

Radix Gentianae(龙胆草 *long dan cao*)

Radix Gentianae refers to the root or rhizome of the perennial herb Gentiana manshurica Kitag., G. scabra Bge., and G. triflora Pall. of Gentianaceae. Mainly produced in northeastern China, it is collected in spring and autumn, washed clean and dried.

Taste and Property: Bitter, and cold.
Attributive Meridian: Liver and gallbladder meridians.
Actions and Indications:

(1) To purge excess fire in the liver and gallbladder. Indications: (a) Headache, congestion, swelling and pain of the eyes, stabbing pain in the chest and hypochondrium, tinnitus, swelling and pain in the ears due to excess fire in the liver and gallbladder. For such cases, it is often prescribed with Fructus Gardeniae, Radix Bupleuri and Radix Rehmanniae, as in Decoction of Gentianae for Purging Liver Fire. (b) High fever and convulsion due to excessive heat in the Liver Meridian in febrile diseases; in such cases it is often used with drugs for purging heat and toxicins, as well as Ramulus Uncariae cum Uncis and Bombyx Batryticatus.

(2) To purge heat from the lower *jiao*. It is indicated for dampness-heat syndrome in the lower *jiao* with dribbling, difficult and painful urination, swelling and pain of the testis and scrotum, leukorrhagia and eczema in the lower body. For such cases, it is often used in combination with drugs that eliminates heat and dampness, such as Semen Plantaginis and Caulis Akebiae.

It is also effective for jaundice due to dampness-heat.

Dosage: 3-6 g.

Spica Prunellae(夏枯草 *xia ku cao*)

Spica Prunellae is the spike of the perennial herb Prunella vulgaris L. of Labiatae. Collected in summer and dried in the sun, it is produced in most places of China, but mainly in Jiangsu, Anhui and Henan provinces.

Synonym: *Xia ku hua*, *bang tou cao*.
Taste and Property: Bitter and acrid, and cold.
Attributive Meridian: Liver and gallbladder meridians.
Actions and Indications:

(1) To purge liver fire. It is indicated for flare-up of liver fire with such symptoms as congestion , swelling and pain in the eye, pain in the eyeball, headache and vertigo. For such cases, it is often used with Flos Chrysanthemi, Semen Cassiae and Radix Scutellariae.

(2) To dispel stagnant phlegm-fire which gives rise to scrofula, soft and movable nodules and goiter. In such cases, it can be used either singly as a decoction or extract for oral use, or in a compound prescription together with Bulbus Fritillariae, Cirrhosae and Concha Ostreae, and drugs to resolve phlegm and soften hard masses, such as Thallus Eckloniae and Sargassum.

Dosage and Preparation: 10-15 g. In most cases, it is applied as a decoction, and occasionally also taken as an extract.

Remarks: Fructus Gardeniae, Radix Gentianae and Spica Prunellae are all bitter and cold, and purge fire from the liver and gallbladder. The difference is that Gardeniae not only purges fire in the *qi* system and purges heat in the *xue* system, but also purges heat and toxicins, promotes urination and eliminates dampness-heat; Gentianae is intensely bitter and cold, is more effective in suppressing excess fire in the liver and gallbladder as well as purging dampness-heat from the lower *jiao*; and Prunellae dispels stagnant phlegm-fire and is frequently used in the treatment of goiter and scrofula.

Semen Cassiae(决明子 *jue ming zi*)

Semen Cassiae refers to the mature seed of the annual herb Cassia obtusifolia L., or C. tora L. of Leguminosae. Mainly produced in Jiangsu, Anhui, Sichuan provinces and the Guangxi Zhuang Autonomous Region, it is collected in autumn when the fruit is ripe, and dried in the sun with foreign matters removed.

Synonym: *Cao jue ming*.
Taste and Property: Bitter and sweet, and slightly cold.
Attributive Meridian: Liver and large intestine meridians.
Actions and Indications:

(1) To purge liver heat and benefit the eye. Indications: (a) Hyperactive liver *yang* that leads to headache and vertigo. For such cases, it is often used with Ramulus Uncariae cum Uncis and Concha Ostreae. (b) Flare-up of liver fire that gives rises to congestion, swelling and pain in the eye. For such cases, it is often combined with Flos Chrysanthemi and Spica Prunellae.

(2) To moisten the intestine and relax the bowels. It is indicated for constipation due to accumulated heat and dryness in the intestine. In such cases, it can either be prepared as a kind of tea, or stir-baked and decocted for oral use.

Dosage: 10-15 g.

Radix Sophorae Flavescentis(苦参 *ku shen*)

Radix Sophorae Flavescentis is the root of the sub-shrub Sophora flavescens Ait. of Leguminosae. To be found in all parts of China, it is collected in spring and autumn, washed clean, cut into pieces and dried in the sun with the root top and rootlets removed.

Taste and Property: Bitter, and cold.
Attributive Meridian: Large intestine, liver and kidney meridians.
Actions and Indications:

(1) To purge heat and dry dampness. It is effective for diarrhea and dysentery due to dampness-heat; used either singly for decoction, or else in combination with Radix Aucklandiae and Radix Glycyrrhizae, as in Pill of Aucklandiae and Sophorae Flavescentis. For hematochezia, it can be combined with Radix Sanguisorbae and Fructus Sophorae.

(2) To expel parasites and relieve itching. Indications: (a) Skin diseases, such as exudative boils, scabies, tinea and leprosy. For such cases, it can be decocted for either oral use or external application. (b) Leukorrhagia and pruritus vulvae (as in trichomonous vaginitis), in which it can be applied externally alone or in combination with Fructus Cni-

dii.

It also promotes urination and is effective for jaundice due to dampness-heat and dysuria.

Dosage and Preparation: 5-10 g in decoction for oral use; and a proper amount in decoction for external application.

Precaution: This drug is incompatible with Rhizoma et Radix Veratri.

Remarks: Radix Sophorae Flavescentis has an intense bitter taste and is fairly cold, its ability to purge heat and dry dampness is similar to that of Radix Scutellariae and Rhizoma Coptidis. Yet, it is unique in promoting urination and eliminating parasites. For its strong bitter taste and cold property, a large dosage should be avoided to prevent any possible damage to stomach function.

Section 2
Drugs for Eliminating Heat and Toxicins

Flos Lonicerae(金银花 *jin yin hua*)

Flos Lonicerae is the bud or early flower of the semi-evergreen twining shrub Lonicera japonica Thunb., or L. hypoglauca Miq. and other plants of the same genus of Carprifoliaceae. Mainly produced in Henan and Shandong provinces, it is collected in early summer before it blossoms, dried or smoked with sulfur and then dried.

Synonym: *Yin hua*, *shuang hua*, *er bao hua*, *ren dong hua*.

Taste and Property: Sweet, and cold.

Attributive Meridian: Lung and stomach meridians.

Actions and Indications:

Clearing away heat and toxicins. Indications: (a) Exogenous febrile diseases, in which the lung and the *wei* systems are affected by pathogenic factors, with such manifestations as fever, cough, sore throat and thirst. In such cases, it is used with drugs for relieving exterior syndrome and purging heat, such as Herba Schizonepetae, Herba Menthae, Fructus Arctii and Fructus Forsythiae, as in Powder of Lonicerae and Forsythiae. For cases in which the *qi*, *ying* and *xue* systems are all affected, it is used in accordance with symptoms. (b) Carbuncles or swellings due to toxic heat. In such cases, it is applied either singly or in combination with Herba Taraxaci, Herba Violae and Fructus Forsythiae to enhance the elimination of heat and toxicins. (c) Dysentery with bloody discharge due to toxic heat, for which it can be either applied singly in concentrated decoction for frequent drinking, or else combined with Rhizoma Coptidis, Radix Pulsatillae and Radix Paeoniae Rubra.

It can also purge summer-heat and is indicated for restlessness and thirst with this cause.

Dosage and Preparation: 10-15 g, up to 60 g for cases with severe toxic heat. Extract can be made from the drug by distillation, and it can be taken as a drink in summer to purge summer-heat and eliminate toxicins in cases of carbuncles and boils.

APPENDIX:

Caulis Lonicerae (忍冬藤 *ren dong teng*)

Also known as *yin hua teng*, it is the stem and leaf of Lonicera japonica. Its property, taste and efficacy are similar to those of Flos Lonicerae, though a weaker action. Mainly indicated for carbuncles and swellings due to toxic heat, it can also purge pathogenic heat from the meridians and is indicated for *bi*-syndrome due to wind, dampness and heat. The dosage is 15-60 g.

Fructus Forsythiae(连翘 *lian qiao*)

Fructus Forsythiae is the fruit of the deciduous shrublet Forsythia suspensa (Thunb.) Vahl of Oleaceae. Mainly produced in Shanxi, Henan, Shaanxi and Shandong provinces, it is collected before White Dew (a solar term between the Limit of Heat and the Autumnal Equinox) when the fruit ripens. It is steamed and dried in the sun while retaining its still green color. Hence, it also known as *qing qiao* (green plant of Fructus Forsythiae). If collected before Cold Dew (between the Autumnal Equinox and the Frost's Descent) when the fruit is completely ripened, and dried in the sun. This is called *lao qiao* (old plant of Fructus Forsythiae). Its seed is called *lian qiao xin*.

Taste and Property: Bitter, and cold.

Attributive Meridian: Heart and gallbladder meridians.

Actions and Indications:

To purge heat and toxicins, it is effective in treating carbuncles and stagnation. Indications: (a) Exogenous febrile diseases in which the lung and the *wei* systems are affected by pathogenic factors. For such cases, it is often combined with Flos Lonicerae, Herba Menthae and Fructus Arctii. As it can purge pathogenic heat from the Heart Meridian, it is also indicated for febrile diseases involving the Heart Meridian with such manifestations as fever, irritability, delirium and skin eruptions. For such cases, it often used with Radix Rehmanniae, Cortex Moutan Radicis and Rhizoma Coptidis. (b) Carbuncles and swellings due to toxic heat. For such cases, it is often combined with Lonicerae and Herba Taraxaci. Since it can relieve carbuncles and hard masses, so it is often used with Bulbus Fritillariae Cirrhosae, Radix Scrophulariae and Spica Prunellae to treat scrofula and masses due to phlegm.

Dosage: 5-15 g.

Remarks: Both Lonicerae and Forsythiae are effective in purging heat and toxicins; they are frequently used for febrile diseases, boils and ulcers due to toxic heat. However, Lonicerae is also frequently used to cure dysentery with blood discharge due to toxic heat, and to purge summer-heat; while Forsythiae, owing to its ability to purge heart fire and relieve irritability and fever, is also frequently used for attack of the pericardium by pathogenic heat, which often results in coma and delirium. For such cases, Semen Forsythiae would be more effective.

Herba Taraxaci(蒲公英 *pu gong ying*)

Herba Taraxaci refers to the whole plant of the perennial herb Taraxacum mongolicum Hand. -Mazz. , and other plants of the same genus of compositae. To be found in all parts of China, it is collected in the period between spring to autumn when it begins blooming, washed clean and dried in the sun, or applied fresh shortly after collection.

Synonym: *Huang hua di ding.*
Taste and Property: Bitter and sweet, and cold.
Attributive Meridian: Liver and stomach meridians.
Actions and Indications:

To purge heat and toxicins. It is indicated for carbuncles and swellings due to toxic heat, especially mastitis. It can be applied singly for oral intake or pound fresh into a paste to be applied externally on the affected site. In a compound formula, it is often combined with other drugs for purging heat and toxicins, such as Flos Lonicerae and Herba Violae. It is also effective for such internal abscesses as appendicitis and pulmonary abscess.

It can also eliminate heat and dampness, and is indicated for stranguria and jaundice due to dampness-heat.

Dosage and Preparation: 10-30 g, which should be doubled when used fresh; the dosage for external application should be moderate.

Herba Violae(紫花地丁 *zi hua di ding*)

Herba Violae refers to the whole plant of the perennial herb Viola yedoensis Makino of Violaceae. Produced in the lower reaches of the Yangtze River and southern China, it is collected between summer and autumn and dried in the sun, or used fresh.

Taste and Property: Bitter and acrid, and cold.
Attributive Meridian: Heart and liver meridians.
Actions and Indications:

Effective in purging heat and toxicins, it is indicated for carbuncles, swellings, deep-rooted boils and ulcers due to toxic heat. It can be made into a decoction for oral intake or pound fresh into a paste to be applied externally on the affected site, or prescribed together with Herba Taraxaci, Flos Lonicerae, Fructus Forsythiae and Flos Chrysanthemi Indici.

The drug can also be used to treat snakebites.

Dosage and Preparation: 10-30 g, which should be doubled if used fresh; a moderate dosage for external application.

Remarks: Both Taraxaci and Violae can purge heat and toxicins and treat carbuncles and swellings, and they are often used in combination. But the former is especially effective in treating mastitis for its ability to dispel stagnation and relieve hard masses. It is also effective in eliminating heat and dampness. The latter is more effective in purging heat and toxicins, and is particularly suitable for deep-rooted boils and snakebites.

Folium Isatidis(大青叶 *da qing ye*)

Folium Isatidis is the leaf of the biennial herb Isatis indigotica Fort of Cruciferae. Mainly produced in eastern, central south, northwestern and northeastern China, most of the drug is cultivated. It is collected at two or three separate occasions in summer and autumn, and dried in the sun with foreign matter removed.

Taste and Property: Bitter, and cold.
Attributive Meridian: Heart and stomach meridians.
Actions and Indications:

To purge heat and toxicins, cool blood and relieve macula. It is indicated for: (a) Febrile diseases with persistent high fever or affection of the *ying* and *xue* systems by pathogenic factors, with such manifestations as coma, delirium, skin eruptions, hematemesis and epistaxis. For such cases, it can be combined with other drugs for eliminating heat and toxicins and drugs for cooling blood. (b) Sore throat, aphthae, erysipelas and carbuncles due to toxic heat. In such cases, it can be used either singly or combined with other drugs for purging heat and toxicins.
Dosage: 10-30 g.

APPENDIX:

Radix Isatidis(板兰根 *ban lan gen*)

Radix Isatidis is the root of Isatis indigotica Fort. It has similar property, taste, efficacy and indications as Folium Isatidis, and the method of administration is also the same. The dosage is 10-15 g.

Indigo Naturalis(青黛 *qing dai*)

Indigo Naturalis is a dry blue powder or mass prepared from the leaves or peduncles of Baphicacanthus cusia (Nees) Bremek. of Acanthaceae, Indigofera suffruticosa Mill. of Leguminosae, Polygonum tinctorium Ait. of Polygonaceae, or Isatis indigotica Fort. of Cruciferae. It is mainly produced in Fujian, Yunnan, Jiangsu and Anhui provinces.

Synonym: *Dian hua.*
Taste and Property: Salty, and cold.
Attributive Meridian: Liver meridian.
Actions and Indications:

(1) To purge heat and toxicins. It is indicated for eczema, erysipelas, sore throat and aphthae. For such cases, it is often combined with Cortex Phellodendri and Rhizoma Coptidis in powder form for external use.

(2) To cool the blood and stop bleeding, and remove macula. Indications: (a) Hematemesis and epistaxis due to heat in blood. In such cases, it can be applied either singly

or in combination with the powder of Concha Meretricis, as in Powder of Indigo Naturalis and Concha Meretricis. (b) Febrile diseases with skin eruptions, in which it is used with other drugs for purging heat and toxicins and cooling the blood.

The drug also purges liver heat and treat epilepsy in infants.

Dosage and Preparation: 1.5-3 g. As it is easily soluble in water, and it is advisable to prepare it into pills or powder for oral administration. The dosage for external application should be decided according to actual needs, and it should be applied in the form of powder or paste.

Herba Andrographitis(穿心莲 *chuan xin lian*)

This refers to the aerial part of the annual herb Andrographis paniculata (Burm. f.) Nees of Acanthaceae. Cultivated in southern, southeastern and southwestern China, it is collected in early autumn when the stem and leaves are growing luxuriantly, and dried in the sun.

Synonym: *Yi jian xi, lan he lian.*
Taste and Property: Bitter, and cold.
Attributive Meridian: Lung, stomach and large intestine meridians.
Actions and Indications:

To purge heat and toxicins. Indications: (a) Febrile diseases, cough due to lung heat, pulmonary abscess and sore throat. For such cases, it can be applied either singly or in combination with other drugs in accordance to symptoms and signs. (b) Diarrhea and dysentery due to dampness-heat and stranguria due to heat. For such cases, it is applied either singly or in combination with other drugs for treating diarrhea, dysentery and stranguria. (c) Carbuncles and swellings due to toxic heat and snakebites. For such cases, it can be made into a decoction for oral intake, or ground into a powder for external application, or pound the fresh herb into a paste for external application to the affected site.

Dosage and Preparation: 5-10 g for decoction, and 1-1.5 g for powder to be taken orally. For external application, the dosage should be decided according to specific needs.

Precaution: This drug is extremely bitter, and can cause vomiting if used as decoction. It would be better to grind it into a powder and made into capsules for oral intake. Overdose and long-term administration should be avoided to prevent possible damage to stomach *qi*.

Herba Houttuyniae(鱼腥草 *yu xing cao*)

Herba Houttuyniae refers to the whole plant of the perennial herb Houttuynia cordate Thunb. of Saururaceae. Produced in areas south of the Yangtze River, it is collected in summer when the plant is growing luxuriantly and with abundant flowers, and dried in the shade.

Synonym: *Ji cai.*
Taste and Property: Acrid, and slightly cold.

Attributive Meridian: Lung meridian.
Actions and Indications:

To purge heat, eliminate toxicins and relieve carbuncles and swellings. Indications: (a) Cough due to lung heat, expectoration of purulent sputum in pulmonary abscess. For such cases, it is used with Radix Platycodi and Rhizoma Phragmitis. (b) Carbuncles and swellings, hemorrhoids, rectal prolapse with redness and swelling due to toxic heat, and eczema. For such cases, it is either decocted for oral use or pound into a paste for external application.

It can also promote urination and relieve stranguria, and is indicated for stranguria due to dampness-heat.

Dosage and Preparation: 10-30 g for decoction. As it contains volatile oil and so it is not advisable to be decocted for a long time. The dosage for external use should be decided in line with actual needs.

Remarks: This drug has a fishy smell, hence its name *yu xing cao* (fishy smell herb). For its effects in purging heat and toxicins, and relieving carbuncles and abscesses, it is indicated for both internal and external abscesses. Nowadays, it is an important drug often used to treat pulmonary abscess caused by accumulation of phlegm and heat in the lung.

Rhizoma Belamcandae(射干 *she gan*)

Rhizoma Belamcandae is the rhizome of Belamcanda chinensis (L.) DC. of Iridaceae. Mainly produced in Hubei, Henan, Jiangsu and Anhui provinces, it is collected in early spring and late autumn, washed clean and dried in the sun with the fibrous roots removed.

Taste and Property: Bitter, and cold.
Attributive Meridian: Lung meridian.
Actions and Indications:

(1) To purge heat and toxicins, and soothe the throat. It is indicated for sore throat due to phlegm-heat in the lung. For such cases, it can be pounded into a juice that is to be held in the mouth near the throat, or used together with Radix Scutellariae, Radix Platycodi and Radix Glycyrrhizae to produce a decoction.

(2) To eliminate heat and phlegm. It is indicated for productive cough and dyspnea. If phlegm is due to lung heat, it is used in combination with Fructus Trichosanthis and Bulbus Fritillariae Cirrhosae. And if due to cold, it is used with Herba Ephedrae, Herba Asari and Rhizoma Pinelliae.

Dosage: 5-10 g.

Radix Sophorae Tonkinensis(山豆根 *shan dou gen*)

Radix Sophorae Tonkinensis refers to the root and rhizome of Sophora tonkinensis Gapnep. of Leguminosae. Mainly produced in Guangdong, Jiangxi and Guizhou provinces and the Guangxi Zhuang Autonomous Region, it is collected in autumn, washed clean and dried in the sun.

Synonym: *Guang dou gen.*
Taste and Property: Bitter, and cold.
Attributive Meridian: Lung meridian.
Actions and Indications:

To purge heat and toxicins, and soothe the throat. It is indicated for sore throat, especially that due to accumulation of toxic heat. It can be administered singly in oral decoction or held in the mouth near the throat. It can also be combined with Rhizoma Belamcandae, Radix Scrophulariae and Radix Isatidis.

Dosage: 3-10 g.
Remarks: This drug has fairly strong a purgative effect for its bitter taste and cold property, and is especially effective for sore throat due to accumulated toxic heat. If sore throat is caused by affection of the lung by wind and heat, the treatment should aim at dispelling wind and heat. Here, it is not advisable to apply this drug too early, to prevent the pathogenic factors from being inhibited and becoming lingering.

Herba Portulacae(马齿苋 *ma chi xian*)

Herba Portulacae is the whole plant of the annual fleshy herb Portulaca oleracea L. of Portulacaceae. Produced in all parts of the country, it is collected in summer and autumn, washed clean, slightly soaked in boiling water or steamed, and dried in the sun; or else used fresh.

Synonym: *Ma chi cai, jiang ban cai.*
Taste and Property: Sour, and cold.
Attributive Meridian: Large intestine meridian.
Actions and Indications:

To purge heat and toxicins. Indications: (a) Diarrhea and dysentery due to dampness-heat, for which it can be applied singly and prescribed in large dosage for oral decoction, or combined with Rhizoma Coptidis and Radix Pulsatillae. (b) Carbuncles and abscesses due to toxic heat, and eczema. It can be decocted for oral intake or pounded into a paste for external application. To treat eczema, it can be decocted for washing or wet compress.

Dosage: 30-60 g, doubled if used fresh; moderate amount for external use.
Remarks: This drug is fairly effective for acute diarrhea or dysentery due to dampness-heat. But, the dosage should be large and the treatment should be given thoroughly until the condition is cured. As it is mild and produces hardly any side effects, people often eat it as a vegetable. Frequent eating of this herb in the right season produces a prophylactic effect for diarrhea or dysentery.

Radix Pulsatillae(白头翁 *bai tou weng*)

Radix Pulsatillae is the root of the perennial herb Pulsatilla chinensis (Bge.) Regel of Ranunculaceae. Distributed in northern and northeastern China as well as Jiangsu and Anhui provinces, it is collected in spring and autumn, washed clean and dried in the sun with the aerial part removed.

Taste and Property: Bitter, and cold.
Attributive Meridian: Large intestine meridian.
Actions and Indications:

To purge heat and toxicins, and cool blood. It is indicated for dysentery due to toxic heat with red and white mucus or blood in the stool. For such cases, it is often used with Rhizoma Coptidis, Cortex Phellodendri and Cortex Fraxini, as in Decoction of Pulsatillae, to enhance the effect of purging heat and toxicins. The drug can also be applied singly. Modern research shows that this drug is also effective in treating bacillary and amebic dysentery.

It is also effective in treating carbuncles, swellings and scrofula.

Dosage and Preparation: 6-15 g, and up to 30 g. In addition to oral decoction, it can also be used as an enema.

Cortex Fraxini(秦皮 *qin pi*)

Cortex Fraxini refers to the bark of the branch or stem of the deciduous tree Fraxinus rhynchophylla Hance, F. chinensis Roxb., or other plants of the same genus of Oleaceae. Mainly distributed in Shaanxi, Hebei, Henan, Shanxi, Liaoning and Jilin provinces, it is peeled off and collected in spring and autumn, and dried in the sun.

Taste and Property: Bitter, and cold.
Attributive Meridian: Large intestine and liver meridians.
Actions and Indications:

(1) To purge heat and toxicins, and eliminate dampness. It is indicated for diarrhea and dysentery due to dampness-heat, and leukorrhagia. In treating dysentery, it is combined with Radix Pulsatillae; in treating leukorrhagia, with Cortex Ailanthi and Cortex Phellodendri.

(2) To purge liver heat and improve eyesight. It is indicated for congestion, swelling and pain of the eyes due to liver heat. For such cases, it is used singly to produce a decoction that is either taken orally or used to wash the eyes.

Dosage: 5-10 g.

Caulis Sargentodoxae(红藤 *hong teng*)

Caulis Sargentodoxae refers to the viny stem of the deciduous climbing shrub Sargentodoxa cuneta (Oliv.) Rehd. et Wils. of Lardizabalaceae. Mainly produced in Hubei, Sichuan, Jiangxi, Henan and Jiangsu provinces, it is collected in autumn and winter, then cut into segments with the branches removed, and dried.

Synonym: *Da xue teng, da huo xue.*
Taste and Property: Bitter, and mild.

Attributive Meridian: Large intestine and liver meridians.
Actions and Indications:

(1) To purge heat and toxicins, and relieve carbuncles and swelling. It is used with Flos Lonicerae, Fructus Forsythiae and Cortex Moutan Radicis to treat appendicitis, as in Decoction of Sargentodoxae.

(2) To activate blood circulation and remove blood stagnation. It is particularly effective for amenorrhea due to blood stagnation, contusions and sprains.
Dosage: 15-30 g.

Herba Patriniae(败酱 *bai jiang*)

Herba Patriniae refers to the whole plant of the perennial herb Patrinia scabiosaefolia Fisch., or P. villosa Juss. of Valerianaceae. Distributed throughout the country, it is collected in summer before the flower blooms, partially dried in the sun, tied into bundles, and dried in the shade.

Taste and Property: Acrid and bitter, and slightly cold.
Attributive Meridian: Large intestine and liver meridians.
Actions and Indications:

(1) To purge heat and toxicins, and promote pus discharge. It is particularly effective for appendicitis with formation of abscess, in which it is usually used in combination with Semen Coicis and Radix Aconiti Lateralis Preparata, as in Powder of Coicis, Aconiti Lateralis and Patriniae, recorded in *Synopsis of the Golden Cabinet*. For appendicitis without abscess, it is combined with other drugs for purging heat and toxicins and activating blood circulation, such as Caulis Sargentodoxae, Radix et Rhizoma Rhei and Cortex Moutan Radicis.

(2) To activate blood circulation and remove stasis. It is indicated for postpartum abdominal pain due to blood stasis. For such cases, it is often used with drugs for activating *qi* and blood circulation. It can also be applied singly and prepared into an oral decoction.
Dosage: 5-10 g.

Section 3
Drugs for Eliminating Heat and Cooling Blood

Cornu Rhinocerotis(犀角 *xi jiao*)

Cornu Rhinocerotis refers to the horn of rhinoceros of Rhinocerotidae. It is divided into two kinds: Siam horn and *Guang* horn. Siam horn is Asian, cut from Rhinoceros unicornis L., R. sondaicus Desmarest, or R. sumatrensis (Fischer). *Guang* horn is African, from R. bicornis L. and R. simus Barchell. Siam horn is mainly produced in India, Nepal, Burma, Thailand, Malaysia and Indonesia; *Guang* horn is mainly produced in East and Southeast Africa. The horn is cut when the rhinoceros has been caught.

Taste and Property: Bitter and salty, and cold.
Attributive Meridian: Heart and liver meridians.
Actions and Indications:

To purge heat, cool the blood, eliminate toxicins and relieve convulsion. Indications: (a) Hematemesis and epistaxis due to heat in the blood which leads to extravasation and maculation; For such cases, it is often combined with Radix Rehmanniae, Cortex Moutan Radicis and Radix Paeoniae Rubra, as in Decoction of Cornu Rhinocerotis and Rehmanniae. (b) Febrile diseases involving the *xue* system with such manifestations as high fever, coma and convulsion. For such cases, it is often used with large doses of drugs that eliminate heat and toxicins and prepared into pills for emergencies, as in Bolus of Calculus Bovis for Resurrection and Bolus of Precious Drugs.

Dosage and Preparation: 1.5-6 g. It is first filed into fine powder and taken with boiled water, or applied as an ingredient in pills and powders.

Precaution: This drug is incompatible with Radix Aconiti and Radix Aconiti Kusnezoffii. For pregnant women, it should be used with great care.

Remarks: Cornu Rhinocerotis has a powerful effect in purging heat, cooling the blood and eliminating toxicins. It is an important drug for treating diseases due to heat in the blood. It is valuable for its limited resources. Therefore, it is used when it is absolutely necessary.

APPENDIX:

Cornu Bubali(水牛角 *shui niu jiao*)

Cornu Bubali is the horn of Bubalus bubalis L. of Bovidae. Bitter, salty and cold, it has similar effects to that of Cornu Rhinocerotis in purging heat, cooling the blood, eliminating toxicins, tranquilizing the mind and relieving convulsion. The dosage should be large, 15-30 g in general. If to be used in a decoction, it should be boiled first before other ingredients are added. It can also be filed into fine powder and taken with boiled water directly.

Radix Rehmanniae(生地黄 *sheng di huang*)

Radix Rehmanniae is the fresh or dried tuberous root of the perennial herb Rehmannia glutinosa Libosch. of Scrophulariaceae. Mainly distributed in Henan and Zhejiang provinces, that produced in Henan is known as *huai di huang* which is better in quality. It is collected in autumn. If covered with sandy earth and stored fresh, it is known as *xian sheng di* (fresh Radix Rehmanniae). If *xian sheng di* is washed, baked with mild heat until it turns black and kneaded into round shape, it becomes *gan di huang*, conventionally known as *sheng di*.

Taste and Property: Sweet and bitter, and cold.
Attributive Meridian: Heart, liver and kidney meridians.
Actions and Indications:

(1) To purge heat and cool the blood. It is indicated for febrile diseases involving the

ying and *xue* systems accompanied by fever, red tongue, thirst, and maculation, and also for hematemesis, epistaxis and hematuria due to heat in the blood leading to extravasation. For such cases, it is often prescribed in combination with Cortex Moutan Radicis, Radix Paeoniae Rubra and Radix Scrophulariae to purge heat from the *ying* system and cool the blood.

(2) To nourish *yin* and promote fluid secretion. It is indicated for *yin* deficiency syndrome leading to internal heat, such as damage of *yin* in febrile diseases, exhibiting diabetes, sore throat, hectic fever, lumbago and seminal emission, and constipation caused by fluid consumption. For such cases, it is often used with Radix Scrophulariae, Radix Ophiopogonis and Rhizoma Anemarrhenae to nourish *yin*, eliminate heat and promote fluid secretion.

Dosage: 10-30 g, doubled if used fresh.

Precaution: The drug is contraindicated for patients with spleen deficiency and excessive dampness.

Remarks: There is a difference between fresh and dried Radix Rehmanniae. The former is good at purging heat and cooling the blood, and is especially indicated for febrile diseases involving the *ying* and *xue* systems. The latter is more often used clinically to nourish *yin*, and is indicated for *yin* deficiency that leads to internal heat.

Radix Scrophulariae(玄参 *xuan shen*)

Radix Scrophulariae is the root of the perennial herb Scrophularia ningpoensis Hemsl. of Scrophulariaceae. Mostly cultivated, it is mainly produced in Zhejiang, Sichuan and Hubei provinces. It is gathered in winter, partially dried in the sun with the stem, leaves and foreign matter removed, piled up for three to four days and dried in the sun again. This procedure is repeated until it is entirely dried.

Synonym: *Yuan shen*, *hei shen*.

Taste and Property: Sweet, bitter and salty, and cold.

Attributive Meridian: Lung, stomach and kidney meridians.

Actions and Indications:

To nourish *yin*, purge fire and eliminate toxicins. Indications: (a) Febrile diseases involving the *ying* and *xue* systems, thirst due to the consumption of *yin*, and eruptive diseases. For such cases, it is combined with Radix Rehmanniae, Radix Paeoniae Rubra and Cortex Moutan Radicis. For damage to *yin* in febrile diseases and constipation due to fluid consumption, it is used with Radix Rehmanniae and Radix Ophiopogonis. (b) Sore throat. This drug is frequently used to treat disorders of the throat, as witnessed in exterior syndrome due to wind-heat, or hyperactive fire and *yin* deficiency. For cases due to exogenous wind-heat, it is combined with Herba Menthae and Fructus Arctii; for cases due to *yin* deficiency that leads to hyperactive fire, it is used with Radix Rehmanniae, Radix Ophiopogonis and Cortex Lycii Radicis. (c) Scrofula, in which it is used with Bulbus Fritillariae Cirrhosae and Concha Ostreae, as in Pill for Resolving Scrofula.

Dosage: 10-15 g, up to 30 g.

Remarks: Both Radix Scrophulariae and Radix Rehmanniae can purge heat and nourish *yin*. The former is particularly effective in purging fire and eliminating toxicins, and is frequently used in treating sore throat and scrofula; the latter is more effective in nourishing *yin* and blood, it is more often used in cases of *yin* and blood deficiency.

Cortex Moutan Radicis(牡丹皮 *mu dan pi*)

Cortex Moutan Radicis is the root bark of deciduous shrublet Paeonia suffruticosa Andr. of Ranunculaceae. Mainly distributed in Anhui, Sichuan, Gansu and Shaanxi provinces, the root is dug in autumn, the rootlets are removed and the bark is peeled, and then it is dried in the sun.

Taste and Property: Bitter and acrid, and cold.
Attributive Meridian: Heart and liver meridians.
Actions and Indications:

(1) To purge heat and cool the blood. It is indicated for febrile diseases involving the *ying* and *xue* systems with such manifestations as high fever, deep-red tongue, skin eruptions, hematemesis and epistaxis due to extravasation caused by heat in the blood. To treat such diseases, it can be used with Cornu Rhinocerotis, Radix Rehmanniae and Radix Paeoniae Rubra, as in Decoction of Cornu Rhinocerotis and Rehmanniae. It can also be used in cases of attack of the *xue* system by pathogenic heat, manifested as night fever and hectic fever without sweating. For such cases, it is combined with Herba Artemisiae Annuae, Rhizoma Anemarrhenae and Carapax Trionycis.

(2) To activate blood circulation and remove stagnation or masses. It is indicated for amenorrhea, dysmenorrhea, hard or soft masses in the abdomen, contusions and sprain, especially those due to heat accumulation and blood stagnation. For such cases, it is often used with drugs that activate blood circulation, such as Radix Angelicae Sinensis, Radix Paeoniae Rubra and Semen Persicae. To cure appendicitis, it is often prescribed with Radix et Rhizoma Rhei and Semen Benincasae.

This drug can also purge liver fire, and it is indicated for diseases in which stagnant liver *qi* turns into fire. For such diseases, it is often used in combination with Fructus Gardeniae, as in modified *Xiaoyao* Powder.

Dosage and Preparation: 5-10 g. Generally, it is used crude. For bleeding, it is charred.
Precaution: For pregnant women, it should be used with great care.

Radix Paeoniae Rubra(赤芍 *chi shao*)

Radix Paeoniae Rubra is the root of the perennial plant Paeonia lactiflora Pall., or P. veitcnii Lynch of Ranunculaceae. Mainly produced in the Inner Mongolia Autonomous Region, Sichuan Province and northeastern China, it is collected in spring and autumn, and dried in the sun with the rhizome, fibrous roots and foreign matters removed.

Taste and Property: Bitter, and slightly cold.

Attributive Meridian: Liver meridian.

Actions and Indications:

(1) To purge heat and cool the blood. It is Indicated for febrile diseases involving the *ying* and *xue* systems marked by fever, deep-red tongue and skin eruptions, or hematemesis and epistaxis due to heat in the blood that leads to extravasation. For such cases, it is often combined with other drugs that purge heat and cool the blood, such as Radix Rehmanniae and Cortex Moutan Radicis.

(2) To activate blood circulation and remove blood stagnation. It is indicated for amenorrhea due to blood stagnation, contusions and sprains. In such cases, it is often used with drugs that activate blood circulation, such as Radix Angelicae Sinensis and Flos Carthami. It is also effective for carbuncles, for which it is combined with drugs that purge heat and eliminate toxicins.

It is also used to cure redness, pain and swelling of the eyes due to flare-ups of liver fire for its action of purging liver fire.

Dosage: 5-15 g.

Precaution: This drug is incompatible with Rhizoma et Radix Veratri.

Remarks: Both Radix Paeoniae Rubra and Cortex Moutan Radicis can purge heat and cool the blood, and are indicated for diseases caused by heat in the blood and blood stagnation. But the latter produces a better effect in purging heat and cooling the blood, while the former is more effective in activating blood circulation and removing blood stagnation, it has a weaker action in cooling the blood.

Radix Arnebiae seu Lithospermi(紫草 *zi cao*)

Radix Arnebiae seu Lithospermi refers to the root of the perennial herb Arnebia euchroma (Royle) Johnst., or Lithospermum erythrorhizon Sieb. et Zucc. of Boraginaceae. The former is known as *ruan* (soft) *zi cao* and is mainly produced in Xinjiang and Tibet; the latter is known as *ying* (hard) *zi cao* and is mainly distributed in Heilongjiang, Liaoning and Jilin provinces. It is collected in spring and autumn and dried with foreign matters removed.

Taste and Property: Sweet and salty, and cold.

Attributive Meridian: Heart and liver meridians.

Actions and Indications:

To cool the blood, activate blood circulation, remove toxicins and promote skin eruptions. It is indicated for measles due to excessive toxic heat in the *xue* system with incomplete eruptions, and for febrile diseases with purplish dark eruptions. It also moistens and lubricates the intestine and promotes bowel movements, and is especially indicated for constipation due to excessive toxic heat. In such cases, it is often used with Radix Paeoniae Rubra and Periostracum Cicadae.

It can be prepared into a plaster for external use in treating wet boils and scalds.

Dosage: 3-10 g.

Precaution: It is contraindicated for measles with plenty of fresh red eruptions, and for diarrhea.

Section 4
Drugs for Eliminating Deficiency Heat

Herba Artemisiae Annuae(青蒿 *qing hao*)

Herba Artemisiae Annuae is the aerial part of the annual herb Artemisia annua L. of Compositae. Distributed throughout the country, it is cut and collected in summer when the branches and leaves are growing luxuriantly and before it blossoms, and dried in the shade with the tough stems removed.

Taste and Property: Bitter, and cold.
Attributive Meridian: Liver and gallbladder meridians.
Actions and Indications:

(1) To purge deficiency heat. It is indicated for late stages of febrile diseases when pathogenic factors affect *yin*, causing night fever, for chronic diseases with fever due to *yin* deficiency, and hectic fever. In such cases, it is used with such drugs as Carapax Trionycis, Cortex Moutan Radicis, Radix Rehmanniae and Rhizoma Anemarrhenae.

(2) To purge heat from the Shaoyang meridians. It is indicated for Shaoyang diseases with alternate chills and fever, in which fever is predominant. For such cases, it is often used with Radix Scutellariae, Caulis Bambusae in Taeniam and Rhizoma Pinelliae.

(3) To purge summer-heat. It is indicated for summer-heat syndrome, and summer fever in children, for which it is often prescribed with Talcum and Flos Lonicerae.

(4) To treat malaria, including malignant malaria. For such cases, it is used fresh in a large dosage and mixed with water to produce a juice for oral use, or the dried drug is boiled into a decoction for oral administration. Now, some tablets and injections are made from the drug for convenience of clinical application.

It is also used to cure pruritus due to heat in blood.

Dosage and Preparation: 10-15 g. For malaria, it is 20-40 g. If used fresh, the dosage should be doubled. Decoct no longer than five minutes.

Remarks: Herba Artemisiae Annuae is bitter and cold, and is fairly effective in purging deficiency and excess heat. It is aromatic, and so can also eliminate dampness and treat heat syndrome complicated by dampness.

This drug has been used in the treatment of malaria since ancient times. Through recent scientific research, an antimalarial ingredient, artemisinine, has been extracted from this drug. It has been applied in several thousand cases of tertian malaria, malignant malaria, cerebral malaria and those patients with chloroquine tolerance. The results show that it is more effective than chloroquine and other antimalarial drugs, with the advantages of low toxicity and quick result.

Radix Cynanchi Atrati(白薇 *bai wei*)

Radix Cynanchi Atrati is the root and rhizome of Cynanchum atratum Bge. , or C. Versicolor Bge. of Asclepiadaceae. It is collected in spring and autumn, washed and dried.

Taste and Property: Bitter and salty, and cold.
Attributive Meridian: Liver meridian.
Actions and Indications:

To purge both excess and deficiency heat and cool the blood. It is indicated for febrile diseases involving the *ying* and *xue* systems accompanied by persistent fever, as well as for *yin* deficiency leading to endogenous heat or postpartum deficiency heat. Related drugs can be prescribed together with it in line with the types of heat. For febrile diseases involving the *ying* and *xue* systems, it is combined with Radix Rehmanniae and Herba Artemisiae Annuae; for cases of endogenous heat due to *yin* deficiency, it is used with Cortex Lycii Radicis, Rhizoma Anemarrhenae and Radix Rehmanniae.

It has also a diuretic effect and is indicated for stranguria due to heat and stranguria accompanied by hematuria.

Dosage: 5-10 g.

Cortex Lycii Radicis(地骨皮 *di gu pi*)

Cortex Lycii Radicis is the root bark of the deciduous shrub Lycium chinense Mill. , or L. barbarum L. of Solanaceae. Distributed throughout the country, it is collected in early spring or late autumn, washed, and dried in the sun with the bark peeled off.

Taste and Property: Sweet, and cold.
Attributive Meridian: Lung and kidney meridians.
Actions and Indications:

(1) To purge deficiency heat. It is indicated for fever due to *yin* deficiency with such manifestations as hectic fever and night sweating. For such cases, it is often used with Herba Artemisiae Annuae and Rhizoma Anemarrhenae.

(2) To purge lung fire. It is indicated for cough, asthma and hemoptysis due to lung heat. For such cases, it is combined with Cortex Mori Radicis and Radix Glycyrrhizae, as in Powder for Expelling Lung Heat.

It also cools the blood and stops bleeding, and is indicated for extravasation due to heat. Additionally, it relieves thirst and is indicated for diabetes.

Dosage: 5-15 g.

Radix Stellariae(银柴胡 *yin chai hu*)

Radix Stellariae is the root of the perennial herb Stellaria dichotoma L. var. lanceolata Bge. of Caryophyllaceae. Mainly produced in Shaanxi and Gansu provinces, and the Inner Mongolia and Ningxia Hui autonomous regions, it is collected in spring when it is going to sprout, or in late autumn when the stem and leaves withered, and then dried in the sun with the fibrous roots and foreign matter removed.

Taste and Property: Sweet, and slightly cold.
Attributive Meridian: Kidney meridian.
Actions and Indications:

To purge deficiency heat. It is indicated for fever due to *yin* deficiency manifested as hectic fever and night sweating. It is often used in combination with Herba Artemisiae Annuae, Cortex Lycii Radicis, Carapax Trionycis and Radix Rehmanniae to nourish *yin* and eliminate heat.

It can also be applied in treating infantile fever caused due to malnutrition.
Dosage: 5-10 g.

Table 3. Actions of Drugs for Clearing Heat

Division	Drug	Similarities	Differences
Drugs for Clearing Heat and Purging Fire	Gypsum Fibrosum	Clearing heat of excess type from the lung and stomach	Calcined for external use, clearing heat, promoting granulation and astringing ulcers
	Rhizoma Anemarrhenae		Nourishing *yin* and suppressing fire, moistening dryness
	Rhizoma Phragmitis	Clearing heat and promoting the secretion of body fluid	It is stronger than Radix Trichosanthis in the effect of clearing heat
	Radix Trichosanthis		Stronger than Rhizoma Thragmitis in the effect of promoting secretion of body fluid; also relieves swelling and discharges pus
	Rhizoma Coptidis	Clearing heat and purging fire, clearing heat and relieving toxic materials and clearing heat and drying dampness	Purging fire mainly from the heart, stomach and liver
	Radix Scutellariae		Clearing heat mainly from the lung and Shaoyang Meridian, also relieving restlessness of the fetus
	Cortex Phellodendri		Purging fire mainly from the kidney and clearing dampness-heat mainly from the lower *jiao*
	Fructus Gardeniae	Purging fire from the liver and gallbladder	Cooling blood, eliminating toxic materials and dampness
	Radix Gentianae		Strong effect of purging excess fire from the liver and gallbladder; also clearing heat from the lower *jiao*
	Spica Prunellae		Dispelling stagnation and retention of phlegm-fire giving rise to scrofula, nodules and goiter
	Semen Cassiae		Moistening intestine and relaxing bowels
	Radix Sophorae Flavescentis	Clearing heat and drying dampness	Eliminating parasites and relieving itching

Division	Drug	Similarities	Differences
Drugs for Clearing Heat and Toxic Materials	Flos Lonicerae	Clearing heat and toxic materials; relieving carbuncles and hard masses	Clearing summer-heat
	Fructus Forsythiae		Purging heart fire
	Herba Taraxaci		Especially good for relieving mastitis; eliminating heat and dampness
	Herba Violae		Effective for relieving deep-rooted carbuncles and boils
	Folium Isatidis, Radix Isatidis	Clearing heat and toxic materials; cooling blood and relieving skin eruptions	Usually applied in decoction
	Indigo Naturalis		Good effect in cooling blood and stopping bleeding; clearing heat from the liver; usually applied in forms of pill and powder
	Herba Andrographitis	Clearing heat and toxic materials; especially heat from the lung	Extremely bitter and cold; strong effect of clearing heat and relieving toxic materials
	Herba Houttuyniae		Effective for lung abscess
	Rhizoma Belamcandae		Benefiting the throat; resolving phlegm
	Radix Sophorae Tonkinensis		Benefiting the throat
	Herba Portulacae	Clearing heat and toxic materials; effective for diarrhea and dysentery	Treating carbuncles and masses, and eczema
	Radix Pulsatillae		Cooling blood; especially indicated for dysentery with blood due to toxic heat
	Cortex Fraxini		Clearing heat from the liver and improving the eye sight

Division	Drug	Similarities	Differences
Drugs for Clearing Heat and Toxic Materials	Caulis Sargentodoxae	Clearing heat and toxic materials; activating blood circulation; treating lung abscess	
	Herba Patriniae		Discharging pus
Drugs for Clearing Heat and Cooling Blood	Cornu Rhinocerotis	Clearing heat and cooling blood	Eliminating toxic materials, calming the mind and convulsion
	Radix Rehmanniae		Nourishing *yin*, promoting secretion of body fluid
	Radix Scrophulariae		Nourishing *yin*, purging fire, relieving toxic materials, effective for disorders of throat
	Cortex Moutan Radicis		Activating blood circulation; purging fire from the liver
	Radix Paeoniae Rubra		Activating blood circulation; purging fire from the liver
	Radix Arnebiae seu Lithospermi		Eliminating toxic materials and promoting skin eruptions
Drugs for Clearing Deficiency Heat	Herba Artemisiae Annuae	Clearing heat of deficiency type	Clearing heat from the Shaoyang meridian; clearing summer-heat; good for malaria
	Radix Cynanchi Atrati		Cooling blood
	Cortex Lycii Radicis		Clearing heat from the lung
	Radix Stellariae		Also treating fever due to infantile malnutrition

Note: In other chapters or sections, the drugs which also have the effect of clearing heat are: Calculus Bovis, Cornu Saigae Tataricae, Talcum, Radix Gentianae Macrophyllae and Radix et Rhizoma Rhei.

CHAPTER SIX

CATHARTICS (DRUGS FOR PURGATION)

Drugs that can cause diarrhea or lubricate the intestinal tract and promote bowel movement are known as cathartics (*xie xia yao*).

Cathartics promote and facilitate defecation, remove intestinal stasis, accumulated fluid, phlegm or other harmful substances, and some also purge excess heat. They are indicated for interior excess syndromes, such as constipation, intestinal stasis, the accumulation of excess heat, edema, and fluid and phlegm retention. According to their actions and indications, they are divided into three categories: potent purgatives (for strong purgation), lubricant purgatives (for mild purgation), and drastic purgatives (for eliminating retained water).

(1) Potent purgatives (*gong xia yao*): Most are bitter, cold and powerful in promoting defecation and purging fire. They are indicated for retention of excess heat in the intestines marked by constipation, the initial stages of dysentery due to heat accumulated in the large intestine, abdominal pain due to worm stasis and upward disturbance of excess fire that gives rise to headache, redness of the eyes, swelling and pain of the gums. They are often combined with drugs that promote *qi* circulation to enhance the purgative effect. For constipation due to accumulated heat, it is often prescribed together with drugs that purge heat and purge fire. For constipation due to interior excess syndrome in patients with weak constitution, it is often applied in combination with tonic drugs.

(2) Lubricant purgatives (*run xia yao*): Such drugs are sweet and mild, and most are seeds or kernels of oily plants. They moisten and lubricate the large intestine and make it easier to discharge waste matter from the bowels. They are indicated for intestinal dryness due to blood loss and fluid depletion which gives rise to constipation. For such cases, they are combined with drugs that nourish the blood or *yin*. In cases complicated by *qi* stagnation, they are combined with drugs that activate *qi* circulation.

(3) Drastic purgatives (*jun xia zhu shui yao*): Most are bitter and cold, toxic and drastic in action. They can cause copious watery discharge from the bowels; some also have a diuretic effect and can relieve water retention through bowel movements and urination. These drugs are indicated for edema, pleural effusion and ascites. Drugs in this category, however, are likely to cause damage to the antipathogenic *qi*, and so they should be combined with tonic drugs. Attention should be given to their processing, dosage, use and contraindications.

Great care should be taken in prescribing potent and drastic purgatives to old patients, women who are pregnant, or during menstruation, or just after childbirth, as well as patients with weak constitution due to long-term illness.

Section 1
Potent Purgatives

Radix et Rhizoma Rhei(大黄 *da huang*)

Radix et Rhizoma Rhei is the root and rhizome of the perennial herb Rheum palmatum L., R. tanguticum Masim. ex Balf., or R. officinale Baill. of Polygonaceae. The former two are mainly produced in Qinghai, Gansu and Sichuan provinces; and the last is mainly distributed in Sichuan and Hubei provinces. It is collected in late autumn when the stem and leaves are withered, or in the next spring before it sprouts, cut into sections or segments, and dried in the shade or by baking with the fibrous roots removed and the cortex scraped off.

Synonym: *Jiang jun, chuan jun, jin wen.*
Taste and Property: Bitter, and cold.
Attributive Meridian: Stomach, large intestine, heart and liver meridians.
Actions and Indications:

(1) To remove stasis. It is indicated for constipation due to intestinal stasis, especially that due to the accumulation of heat; this is owing to its bitter taste and cold property. For febrile diseases with constipation, high fever, coma and delirium, it is combined with Natrii Sulfas, Fructus Aurantii Immaturus and Cortex Magnoliae Officinalis, as in Decoction for Potent Purgation, to enhance the purgative effect. For constipation due to cold retention, it is used with Radix Aconiti Lateralis Preparata and Rhizoma Zingiberis, both of which warm the interior. It can also be used at the initial stage of dysentery when the accumulated dampness-heat obstructs the intestinal tract.

(2) To purge fire and eliminate toxicity. Indications: (a) Hematemesis and epistaxis due to heat in the blood, and redness of the eyes, headache, sore throat, and swelling and pain of the teeth and gums due to flare-up of fire. For such cases, it is often used with Rhizoma Coptidis and Radix Scutellariae, both of which purge fire, as in Decoction for Purging Stomach Fire. (b) Carbuncles due to toxic heat, erysipelas and scalds. For such cases, it can be taken orally or applied externally.

(3) To activate blood circulation and remove stasis. It is indicated for diseases due to blood stasis, such as amenorrhea, contusions and sprains, abdominal lumps or masses, and pain due to blood stasis. For such cases, it is often used with other drugs that activate blood circulation and remove blood stasis, such as Radix Angelicae Sinensis, Radix Paeoniae Rubra, Semen Persicae and Flos Carthami.

It can also eliminate dampness-heat, and is indicated for jaundice and stranguria due to this factor.

Dosage and Preparation: 3-12 g in decoction. The dosage for external application should be decided according to actual needs. Can be used crude, or baked with adjuvants, or stir-baked. The crude drug is a powerful purgative. When used in decoctions, it should be added later or just soaked in hot water, since prolonged decocting would reduce its purgative effect. If prepared, it has a weaker purgative effect but is still good at activating blood circulation, and is indicated for cases of blood stagnation for which drastic purgation is not suitable. If stir-baked until carbonized, it is indicated for cases of bleeding.

Precaution: It is contraindicated for or should be used with great care in women during pregnancy, menstruation and lactation.

Remarks: It promotes bowel movements and purges fire, and is thus an important drug for constipation due to accumulated heat. Its indications, however, are not confined to relieving constipation. It is also indicated for some other excess-heat syndromes marked by persistent fever, or for headache, redness of the eyes and sore throat due to upward disturbance of heat and fire; or for bleeding in the upper body due to hyperactive heat and fire. For such cases, no matter whether there is constipation or not, the drug can be used to make the heat going down through its purgative action.

Natrii Sulfas(芒硝 *mang xiao*)

Natrii Sulfas refers to the crystal obtained from processing sulfate mineral. It contains mainly sodium sulfate $Na_2(SO_4) \cdot 10\ H_2O$ and is mainly distributed in alkaline-soil areas of Hebei, Henan, Shandong, Jiangsu and Anhui provinces. The natural mirabilite is first boiled, dissolved and filtered, with soil and indissoluble foreign matter removed. The filtrate is cooled down and crystallized. The product at this stage is known as *pu xiao* or *pi xiao* (crystals of mirabilite). If it is boiled together with radish and filtered. Then the supernatant liquid is poured out and the remains are left to cool down and crystallize, Natrii Sulfas is obtained. If Natrii sulfas is dehydrated by airing in the shade and turns into white powders, it is called Natrii Sulfas Exsiccatus.

Taste and Property: Salty and bitter, and cold.

Attributive Meridian: Stomach and large intestine meridians.

Actions and Indications:

(1) To promote purgation and soften hard masses. It is indicated for constipation due to accumulated excess heat. For such cases, it is used with Radix et Rhizoma Rhei to enhance the purgative effect.

The drug can also be applied externally to soften hard masses, and is indicated for mastitis and galactostasis during ablactation.

(2) To purge heat and fire. Indicated for sore throat, aphthae, redness and swelling and pain of the eyes due to heat and fire. Here, it is often used with Borax, Borneolum Syntheticum and Indigo Naturalis, all of which are ground into powder for external use, or dissolved in water as eye drops.

Dosage and Preparation: 5-12 g. Taken orally with medicinal juice or warm water. The dosage for external use should be decided according to needs.

Precaution: Great care should be taken when prescribing it for pregnant women.

Remarks: *Pu xiao*, *mang xiao* and Natrii Sulfas Exsiccatus have basically the same effect. *Pu xiao* contains foreign matter and is usually applied externally; *mang xiao* has been purified and is usually prescribed for oral administration; Natrii Sulfas Exsiccatus has been dehydrated and can be prescribed for oral or external use in treating buccal and ophthalmic diseases.

Both Natrii Sulfas and Radix et Rhizoma Rhei promote purgation and purge heat. But the former is salty and cold, and is more effective in softening hard masses, while the latter is bitter and cold, and is effective at purging fire, eliminating toxicins and removing stagnation.

Folium Sennae(番泻叶 *fan xie ye*)

Folium Sennae refers to the leaves of the herb-like shrub Cassia angustifolia Vahl, or C. acutifolia Delile of Leguminosae. Mainly produced in India and Egypt, it is also cultivated in China's Hainan and Yunnan provinces. It is usually picked in September and dried in the sun with foreign matter removed.

Taste and Property: Sweet and bitter, and cold.
Attributive Meridian: Large intestine meridian.
Actions and Indications:

To promote purgation and remove stasis. It is indicated for constipation due to stasis, or habitual constipation. It is usually applied alone. Sometimes, it is used with Fructus Aurantii Immaturus and Cortex Magnoliae Officinalis to enhance the purgative effect.

Dosage and Preparation: 1.5-3 g for mild purgation; 5-10 g for strong purgation. Soak in hot water for five minutes, then take orally. When applied in decoction, it should be added later.

Precaution: Great care should be taken when prescribing it for pregnant women.

Remarks: The drug is good at promoting bowel movements and is easy to use; clinically, it is frequently used for constipation due to stasis, habitual constipation and postpartum constipation. It can also be used to clear the intestinal tract for X-ray diagnosis. If it is used in a small dosage, it usually takes four to six hours to soften or loose the stool. If a large dosage is used, it will cause diarrhea. In some rare cases, it may produce such undesirable side effects as nausea, vomiting and abdominal pain. If such a situation occurs, the drug can be combined with drugs that activate *qi* circulation and pacify the middle *jiao*, such as Radix Aucklandiae and Herba Agastaches.

Section 2
Lubricant Purgatives

Fructus Cannabis(大麻仁 *da ma ren*)

Fructus Cannabis is the ripe fruit of the annual herb Cannabis sativa L. of Moraceae. Distributed in most parts of China, the whole plant is cut in autumn when the fruits are ripe; the fruits are knocked off and dried in the sun.

Synonym: *Huo ma ren*, *ma zi ren*.
Taste and Property: Sweet, and mild.
Attributive Meridian: Spleen and large intestine meridians.
Actions and Indications:

To lubricate the intestine and promote bowel movements. It is indicated for constipation due to intestinal dryness in senile and debilitated patients as well as puerperants, fluid depletion and blood deficiency. For such cases, it is often prescribed with Semen Pruni and Semen Trichosanthis. For cases accompanied by gastro-intestinal dryness and heat, it is used with Radix et Rhizoma Rhei and Fructus Aurantii Immaturus, as in Bolus of Cannabis.

Dosage and Preparation: 10-15 g. Crushed and decocted for oral administration, or applied as bolus and powder.

Semen Pruni(郁李仁 *yu li ren*)

Semen Pruni refers to the ripe seed of the deciduous shrub Prunus humilis Bge. , or P. Japonica Thunb. of Rosaceae. Mainly produced in Liaoning, Henan and Hebei provinces, as well as the Inner Mongolia Autonomous Region, it is collected in autumn when the fruit is ripe, with the shell removed. The seeds are dried in the sun.

Taste and Property: Acrid, bitter and sweet, and mild.
Attributive Meridian: Large intestine and small intestine meridians.
Actions and Indications:

(1) To lubricate the intestines and relax the bowels. It is indicated for constipation due to intestinal dryness, in which it is often used with Fructus Cannabis, Semen Biotae and Semen Armeniacae Amarum, as in Pill of Five Seeds, to strengthen the effect of lubricating the intestines.

(2) To promote water metabolism and relieve edema. It is indicated for edema with abdominal distention, difficult urination and defecation. Here, it is often prescribed with Semen Coicis and Exocarpium Benincasae to promote water metabolism and relieve edema.

Dosage and Preparation: 3-10 g. Crushed.
Remarks: Both Semen Pruni and Fructus Cannabis lubricate the intestines and relax the bowels, and are indicated for constipation due to intestinal dryness, as witnessed in cases of general debility after diseases, and in pregnant and postpartum women. However, Semen Pruni has a stronger effect than Fructus Cannabis, and it is also diuretic.

Section 3
Drastic Purgatives

Radix Kansui(甘遂 *gan sui*)

Radix Kansui refers to the tuberous root of the perennial herb Euphorbia kansui T. N. Liou ex T. P. Wang of Euphorbiaceae. Mainly produced in Shaanxi, Shanxi and

Henan provinces, it is collected in spring before the plant begins to blossom, or in late autumn when the stem and leaves are withered, and dried in the sun with the cortex knocked off.

Taste and Property: Bitter and cold, and toxic.
Attributive Meridian: Lung, kidney and large intestine meridians.
Actions and Indications:

To promote the excretion of fluid and water. It is indicated for edema with abdominal distention (such as ascites in hepatocirrhosis), and phlegm and fluid retention in the chest and hypochondrium (such as in exudative pleurisy), with such manifestations as dyspnea, short breath, difficult urination and defecation. For such cases, it is used either singly or in combination with Radix Euphorbiae Pekinensis and Flos Genkwa; they are ground into powder and taken orally with Decoction of Jujubae.

It relieves swelling and removes stasis, and is indicated for carbuncles, for which it is ground into powder for external application.

Dosage and Preparation: Since the active ingredient of the drug is not water soluble, it is advisable to apply it in the form of pill or powder. The dosage is 0. 5-1 g. To reduce its toxicity, it can be prepared with vinegar. The dosage for external application should be decided according to actual needs.

Precaution: It is contraindicated for debilitated patients and pregnant women. It is incompatible with Radix Glycyrrhizae.

Radix Euphorbiae Pekinensis(大戟 *da ji*)

Radix Euphorbiae Pekinensis is the root of the perennial herbaceous plant Euphorbia pekinensis Rupr. of Euphorbiaceae, or Knoxia Valerianoides Thorel. et pitard of Rubiaceae. The former is mainly produced in Jiangsu Province, the latter in Guangdong and Yunnan provinces as well as the Guangxi Zhuang Autonomous Region. Both are collected in spring before they sprout, or in autumn when the stem and leaves are withered. With the remnant stem and fibrous roots removed, they are washed clean and dried in the sun.

Taste and Property: Better and cold, and toxic.
Attributive Meridian: Lung, kidney and large intestine meridians.
Actions and Indications:

To promote the excretion of water and phlegm. It is indicated for hydrothorax and ascites, in which it is used either singly or together with Kansui and Flos Genkwa. For a case accompanied by dragging and wandering pain and numbness of the limbs due to phlegm, fluid and dampness retention in the meridians, tendons and muscles, it is used with Kansui and Semen Sinapis Albae, as in Pill for Treating Phlegm Syndrome.

It can also be used to treat boils, ulcers and carbuncles, for which it is used with Pseudobulbus Cremastrae Appendiculatae and Realgar, as in *Zijin* Troche, to relieve toxins, swelling and masses.

Dosage and Preparation: 1. 5-3 g in decoction and 0. 5-1 g for pill or powder. Boiled or stir-baked with vinegar to reduce its toxicity.

Precaution: The drug is contraindicated for debilitated patients and pregnant women. It is incompatible with Radix Glycyrrhizae.

Remarks: There are two kinds of the drug: Radix Euphorbiae Pekinensis of Euphorbiaceae and Radix Knoxiae of Rubiaceae; the latter is more widely used. Both possess the effect to promote fluid excretion, but the former has a stronger purgative effect and toxicity than the latter.

Flos Genkwa(芫花 *yuan hua*)

Flos Genkwa refers to the flower bud of the deciduous shrub plant Daphne genkwa Sieb. et Zucc. of Thymelaeaceae. Mainly produced in Anhui, Jiangsu, Zhejiang, Sichuan and Shandong provinces, it is collected in spring before the flower buds open, and dried in the shade.

Taste and Property: Acrid and bitter, and warm and toxic.

Attributive Meridian: Lung, kidney and large intestine meridians.

Actions and Indications:

To promote fluid and phlegm excretion. The drug is often used with Radix Kansui and Radix Euphorbiae Pekinensis to cure hydrothorax and ascites. It is especially effective for hydrothorax.

External application kills parasites, and is indicated for tinea capitis and scalp boils. For such cases, it is ground into fine powder together with Realgar and mixed with lard.

Dosage and Preparation: 1.5-3 g in decoction; 0.6-1 g for pills or powder. To be stir-baked or boiled with vinegar to reduce the toxicity.

Precaution: It is contraindicated for debilitated patients and pregnant women, and incompatible with Radix Glycyrrhizae.

Remarks: Radix Kansui, Radix Euphorbiae Pekinensis and Flos Genkwa are all toxic, and thus may cause continuous diarrhea accompanied by relief of water retention. They are drastic, with such strong side effects as nausea, vomiting and abdominal pain, and may bring damage to the antipathogenic *qi*. They should, therefore, be applied with caution. In treating ascites, they are especially indicated for patients with a large amount of retained water, who fail to respond to diuretics or other regimens and whose antipathogenic *qi* is not yet greatly damaged. Drugs for strengthening antipathogenic *qi* can be used together with them in order to purge and reinforce simultaneously and to avoid damage to the antipathogenic *qi*. It is contraindicated for patients with very weak constitution, severe heart disease, peptic ulcer and bleeding, as well as pregnant women.

Semen Pharbitidis(牵牛子 *qian niu zi*)

Semen Pharbitidis refers to the ripe seed of the annual herbaceous climber Pharbitis nil (L.) Choisy, or P. purpurea (L.) Voigt of Convolvulaceae. Distributed throughout China, the plant is cut in autumn when the fruit is ripe but the shell not yet cracked. The seeds are knocked off and dried in the sun with foreign matter removed.

Synonym: *Hei bai chou*, *er chou*.
Taste and Property: Bitter and acrid, cold and toxic.
Attributive Meridian: Lung, kidney and large intestine meridians.
Actions and Indications:

(1) To promote purgation and excretion of water. It is effective for edema, ascites, difficult urination and defecation. It can either be applied singly and ground into powder for oral administration, or used with Radix et Rhizoma Rhei and Radix Kansui to enhance the purgative and hydragogue effects.

(2) To relieve stasis. It is indicated for food stasis and constipation. For such cases, it can be applied singly and ground into powder and taken with ginger juice.

(3) To eliminate parasites, such as roundworms and tapeworms. It is indicated for abdominal pain caused by worm stasis. In such cases, the worms are killed and expelled through purgation. If it is combined with Semen Arecae, as in Pill of Pharbitidis and Arecae, a better anthelmintic effect can be achieved.

Dosage and Preparation: 3-10 g. Pound into pieces and decoct; 1.5-3 g in powder form. It can be used either crude or stir-baked; the latter is mild.

Precaution: It is contraindicated for pregnant women and should be applied for debilitated patients with caution.

Remarks: For its different colors, the drug has different names, i.e., *hei chou* (black) and *bai chou* (white). In fact, there is not much difference in efficacy, and at present they are not separated in clinical application, and are generally referred to in prescriptions as *hei bai chou*. Although it produces a weaker purgative action than Radix Kansui and Radix Euphorbiae Pekinensis, it is toxic and has drastic effect and should be applied with caution. Furthermore, its indications vary with the dosage: A small dosage relieves food stasis and promote defecation, while a large dosage promotes water and phlegm excretion.

Table 4. Actions of the Cathartics

Division	Drug	Similarities	Differences
Potent purgatives	Radix et Rhizoma Rhei	Promoting purgation and removing stasis	Purging fire, eliminating toxic materials activating blood circulation and removing stagnation of blood
	Natrii Sulfas		Softening hard masses and purging fire
	Folium Sennae		
Lubricant Purgatives	Fructus Cannabis	Lubricating intestines, and promoting bowel movement	
	Semen Pruni		Facilitating excretion of water, relieving edema
Drastic Purgatives	Radix Kansui	Toxic; drastic purgative; promoting excretion of water	Toxic: most powerful in promoting excretion of water
	Radix Euphorbiae Pekinensis		Radix Knoxiae is less toxic and weaker in the effect of promoting excretion of water
	Flos Genkwa		Especially effective for hydrothorax; external use for eliminating worms (e. g. ringworm of scalp)
	Semen Pharbitidis		Facilitating excretion of water, removing food stasis, killing roundworms

Note: Other drugs with lubricant effect include Mel, Radix Polygoni Multiflori, Radix Angelicae Sinensis, Herba Cistanches, Semen Armeniacae Amarum, Semen Persicae, Semen Biotae, Semen Cassiae and Semen Trichosanthis.

CHAPTER SEVEN

DRUGS FOR ELIMINATING WIND-DAMPNESS

Drugs that eliminate wind-dampness and relieve pain are known as drugs for eliminating wind-dampness (*qu feng shi yao*).

Most such drugs are acrid and bitter and warm or cool; can eliminate wind-dampness from the muscles, tendons and meridians; and some ease the tendons, remove obstruction from collaterals and relieve pain; some nourish the liver and kidney and strengthen the muscles and bones. They are indicated for *bi*-syndrome with such manifestations as arthralgia, ankylosis and muscle spasms, and some are also indicated for flaccidity of the lower limbs and hemiplegia.

Pathogenic factors causing *bi*-syndrome include wind, dampness, cold and heat. Therefore, it is necessary to apply the right drugs for the right diseases, i. e. , drugs for eliminating wind should be applied for cases with predominant wind; drugs for eliminating dampness should be given for cases caused by pathogenic dampness; drugs for eliminating cold should be used for cases caused by excessive cold; and drugs for eliminating heat should be administered for cases due to excessive heat. For cases marked by the obstruction of the meridians by wind and dampness as well as *qi* and blood stagnation, drugs that activate blood circulation and remove obstruction from the meridians and drugs of insect origin that eliminate lingering pathogenic factors and relieve pain should be applied accordingly. For chronic *bi*-syndrome with deficiency of both *qi* and blood, tonics that replenish *qi* and blood should be added. For chronic cases with weak tendons and bones, drugs that nourish the kidney and strengthen the tendons, muscles and bones should be prescribed.

Radix Angelicae Pubescentis(独活 *du huo*)

Radix Angelicae Pubescentis refers to the root of the perennial herb Angelicae pubescens Maxim. f. biserrata Shan et Yuan of Umbelliferae. Mainly produced in Hubei and Sichuan provinces, it is collected in early spring or late autumn, and then baked dry on a slow fire or dried in the sun with fibrous roots removed.

Taste and Property: Acrid and bitter, and warm.
Attributive Meridian: Liver, kidney and urinary bladder meridians.
Actions and Indications:

To eliminate wind-dampness and kill pain. It is indicated for *bi*-syndrome due to wind, cold and dampness, especially cases in which the lower body is affected. For such cases, it is often used with Ramulus Taxilli and Radix Achyranthis Bidentatae.

This drug can also dispel wind and cold, and is indicated for exterior syndrome due to wind and cold. For cases with excessive dampness, headache and severe pain in the limbs, it is often combined with Rhizoma seu Radix Notopterygii, Radix Ledebouriellae and Rhizoma Chuanxiong.

Dosage: 5-10 g.

Remarks: Both Rhizoma seu Radix Notopterygii and Radix Angelicae Pubescentis eliminate wind-dampness and kill pain. The former is dry and strong, and is especially effective for promoting perspiration and relieving exterior syndrome; it is usually used to treat *bi*-syndromes with pain due to wind, cold and dampness in the upper part of the body. The latter is mild and is not as strong as the former in inducing perspiration; it is usually used in treating *bi*-syndromes with pain due to wind, cold and dampness in the lower part of the body. For cases with pain in the whole body, they can be applied together.

Radix Clematidis(威灵仙 *wei ling xian*)

Radix Clematidis is the root and rhizome of the perennial climbing shrub Clematis chinensis Osbeck, or the herbaceous plant C. hexapetala Pall. of Ranunculaceae. The former is mainly produced in Jiangsu, Anhui and Zhejiang provinces, and the latter in northeastern and northern China, as well as Shandong and Jiangsu provinces. It is collected in autumn and dried in the sun with soil removed.

Taste and Property: Acrid, and warm.

Attributive Meridian: Liver meridian.

Actions and Indications:

(1) To eliminate wind-dampness, remove obstruction in the meridians and kill pain. It is indicated for *bi*-syndrome due to wind-dampness with numbness of the limbs, ankylosis, and soreness and pain of the tendons, muscles and bones. Here, it is often combined with Rhizoma seu Radix Notopterygii, Radix Angelicae Pubescentis, Radix Achyranthis Bidentatae and Radix Gentianae Macrophyllae.

(2) To remove bones. Indicated for cases with fish bone stuck in the throat, for which it is decocted, held in mouth and swallowed slowly. It can be mixed with vinegar or granulated sugar.

Dosage: 5-10 g; and 30 g for cases if bones are stuck in the throat.

Radix Stephaniae Tetrandrae(防己 *fang ji*)

Radix Stephaniae Tetrandrae refers to the root of the perennial woody liana Stephania tetrandra S. Moore of Menispermaceae, or the perennial climbing herbaceous plant Aristolochia fangchi Y. C. Wu ex L. D. Chou et S. M. Hwang of Aristolochiaceae. In traditional Chinese medicine, the term for the former is *han fang ji*, which is mainly produced in Zhejiang, Anhui, Jiangxi and Hubei provinces; that for the latter is *mu fang ji*, which is produced in Guangdong Province and the Guangxi Zhuang Autonomous Region. Both are collected in autumn, washed clean, cut into segments and dried in the sun.

Taste and Property: Bitter and acrid, and cold.
Attributive Meridian: Urinary bladder and kidney meridians.
Actions and Indications:

(1) To eliminate wind-dampness. It is indicated for *bi*-syndrome due to wind-dampness. For such cases, it is often used with Radix Ledebouriellae, Rhizoma seu Radix Notopterygii and Radix Angelicae Pubescentis. If cold-dampness is predominant, it is combined with Radix Aconiti and Ramulus Cinnamomi to dispel cold and kill pain. If dampness-heat predominates, it is used with Talcum, Semen Coicis and Fructus Forsythiae to eliminate heat and dampness.

(2) To promote water metabolism and relieve swelling. It is indicated for edema. For patients with symptoms of exterior deficiency, such as sweating, aversion to wind and superficial pulse, it is combined with Radix Astragali, Rhizoma Atractylodis Macrocephalae and Radix Glycyrrhizae to benefit *qi*, promote water metabolism and relieve edema.
Dosage: 5-10 g.
Remarks: Both Radix Aristolochia Fangchi and Radix Stephaniae Tetrandrae eliminate wind-dampness and promote water metabolism. The former is particularly effective in eliminating wind-dampness and stopping pain, the latter in promoting water metabolism and relieving edema. Both are bitter and cold, and likely injure the antipathogenic *qi*. They are contraindicated for patients with poor appetite and *yin* deficiency and those without pathogenic dampness in the interior.

Radix Gentianae Macrophyllae(秦艽 *qin jiao*)

Radix Gentianae Macrophyllae is the root of the perennial herb Gentiana macrophylla Pall., G. straminea Maxim., or plants of the same genus of Gentianaceae. Mainly produced in Gansu, Shaanxi, Qinghai and Hebei provinces, it is collected in spring and autumn, dried in the sun with soil removed.

Taste and Property: Bitter and acrid, and mild.
Attributive Meridian: Stomach, liver and gallbladder meridians.
Actions and Indications:

(1) To eliminate wind-dampness and kill pain. It is indicated for *bi*-syndrome due to wind-dampness with spasms in the limbs because of the predominance of either cold or heat. For cases with predominant cold, it is used with Rhizoma seu Radix Notopterygii, Radix Angelicae Pubescentis and Ramulus Cinnamomi; for those with predominant heat, it is used with Radix Stephaniae Tetrandrae and Caulis Lonicerae.

(2) To subdue deficiency heat. It is indicated for fever due to *yin* deficiency and hectic fever, in which it is often used with Carapax Trionycis, Rhizoma Anemarrhenae and Cortex Lycii Radicis to nourish *yin* and subdue heat.

(3) To remove dampness by diuresis and relieve jaundice. It is indicated for jaundice due to dampness-heat. For such cases, it is combined with Herba Artemisiae Scopariae,

Poria and Rhizoma Alismatis to eliminate dampness and heat.

Dosage: 5-10 g.

Remarks: Radix Gentianae Macrophyllae not only eliminates wind-dampness but also removes dampness-heat and subdues deficiency heat. It is indicated for fever caused by *bi*-syndrome, jaundice due to dampness-heat, as well as hectic fever due to *yin* deficiency. Unlike most drugs for eliminating wind-dampness, which are acrid and dry, Radix Gentianae Macrophyllae lubricates the intestines; overdose may result in loose stools. It is contraindicated for cases with spleen deficiency and diarrhea.

Fructus Chaenomelis(木瓜 *mu gua*)

Fructus Chaenomelis refers to the ripe fruit of the deciduous shrub Chaenomeles speciosa (Sweet) Nakai of Rosaceae. Mainly produced in Anhui, Hubei, Zhejiang, Sichuan and Yunnan provinces, it is collected in summer and autumn when the fruit turns greenish yellow, cut vertically and dried in the sun.

Taste and Property: Sour, and warm.

Attributive Meridian: Liver and spleen meridians.

Actions and Indications:

(1) To ease the tendons. It is indicated for *bi*-syndrome due to wind-dampness with spasms in the tendons and muscles. For such cases, it is combined with Olibanum and Myrrha. If pathogenic dampness is predominant, it is used with Semen Coicis and Radix Achyranthis Bidentatae.

(2) To eliminate dampness and pacify the stomach. It is indicated for summer-heat-dampness syndrome manifested as vomiting, diarrhea, abdominal pain and muscular spasm (such as gastrocnemius spasm in cases of acute gastroenteritis). In such cases, it is combined with Herba Agastaches, Cortex Magnoliae Officinalis and Rhizoma Pinelliae.

It also promotes digestion, and is indicated for dyspepsia.

Dosage and Preparation: 5-10 g. To treat *bi*-syndrome, it is prepared as medicinal wine for oral administration.

Remarks: Fructus Chaenomelis is good for easing the tendons and muscles. Not only can it be applied for *bi*-syndrome with spasms in the tendons and muscles, but also spasms in the gastrocnemius muscle due to such factors as blood deficiency, cold retention, or vomiting and diarrhea.

Ramulus Taxilli(桑寄生 *sang ji sheng*)

Ramulus Taxilli refers to the foliferous branch of Taxillus chinensis (DC.) Danser (*sang ji sheng*) and Viscum coloratum (Komar.) Nakai (*hu ji sheng*) of Loranthacear. The former is produced mainly in Guangdong Province and the Guangxi Zhuang Autonomous Region, the latter in Hebei, Liaoning, Jilin and Anhui provinces. They are gathered from winter to spring, and dried in the sun.

Taste and Property: Bitter, and mild.
Attributive Meridian: Liver and kidney meridians.
Actions and Indications:

(1) To eliminate wind-dampness, nourish the liver and kidney and strengthen the tendons, muscles and bones. It is indicated for *bi*-syndrome or liver and kidney deficiency exhibiting soreness and pain in the lumbar region and knee joints, flaccidity of the lower limbs and ankylosis. For such cases, it is often combined with Radix Angelicae Pubescentis, Cortex Eucommiae, Radix Dipsaci and Radix Achyranthis Bidentatae.

(2) To appease the fetus or prevent abortion. It is indicated for lumbago, restlessness of the fetus and uterine bleeding during pregnancy due to liver and kidney deficiency or dysfunction of the Chong and Ren Meridians. For such cases, it is often used with Dipsaci, Eucommiae and Colla Corii Asini.

Dosage: 10-15 g.

Cortex Acanthopanacis(五加皮 *wu jia pi*)

Cortex Acanthopanacis refers to the root cortex of the deciduous shrub Acanthopanax gracilistylus W. W. Smith of Araliaceae. It is conventionally known as *nan wu jia pi*, and mainly produced in Shanxi, Zhejiang and Hubei provinces. Another species is the root cortex of the woody vine Periploca sepium Bge. of Asclepiadaceae, known as *bei wu jia pi* or *xiang jia pi*, and produced mainly in Shanxi, Hebei, Shaanxi and Gansu provinces. Both are collected in spring and autumn, and dried in the sun with the root cortex peeled off.

Taste and Property: Acrid, and warm.
Attributive Meridian: Liver and kidney meridians.
Actions and Indications:

To eliminate wind-dampness and strengthen the tendons, muscles and bones. It is indicated for *bi*-syndrome due to wind-dampness and spasms of the tendons and muscles, in which it is often combined with Rhizoma seu Radix Notopterygii, Radix Angelicae Pubescentis and Radix Clematidis to eliminate wind-dampness and stop pain. For chronic *bi*-syndrome accompanied by liver and kidney insufficiency marked by soreness and pain in the lumbar region and knee joints, and flaccidity of the lower limbs, it is often prescribed with Fructus Chaenomelis, Radix Achyranthis Bidentatae, Cortex Eucommiae and Radix Dipsaci to nourish the liver and kidney and strengthen the tendons, muscles and bones.

It also facilitates excretion of dampness, and is indicated for edema and dysuria, for which it is combined with Poria and Pericarpium Arecae.

Dosage and Preparation: 5-10 g. It can be soaked in alcoholic liquor for oral administration.

Remarks: The two varieties of this drug originate from plants of different families, and their efficacy is also a little different. *Nan wu jia pi* is especially good for eliminating wind-dampness and strengthening the tendons, muscles and bones; and *bei wu jia pi* is more effective in removing dampness through diuresis and relieving edema. Moreover, *bei wu jia pi* is poisonous and its dosage should not be large.

Os Tigris(虎骨 *hu gu*)

Os Tigris refers to the bone of the vertebrate tiger Panthera tigris L. of Felidae. This type of tiger mainly lives in the big mountains in northeastern and southern China. After it was shot or captured, the flesh and muscles attached to the bones are removed, and the bones are sawed into segments, dried in the shade, and then stir-baked until yellow with heated sands or baked until crispy with edible oil.

Taste and Property: Acrid, and warm.
Attributive Meridian: Liver and kidney meridians.
Actions and Indications:

To dispel wind, relieve pain and strengthen the tendons and bones. It is effective in treating *bi*-syndrome due to wind-dampness marked by wandering arthralgia, spasms of the limbs and ankylosis, or flaccidity of lower limbs due to liver and kidney deficiency. For *bi*-syndrome due to wind-dampness, it is often prescribed together with other drugs that dispel wind-dampness. Together, they are made into a medicinal wine. For flaccidity of the lower limbs, it combined with drugs that nourish the liver and kidney, as in *Huqian* Pill.

Dosage and Preparation: 5-10 g. Usually prepared as medicinal wine or pills, and occasionally decoction.

Remarks: This drug is fairly effective for *bi*-syndrome and flaccidity of the lower limbs. But, it is in short supply as measures have been adopted to protect the tigers which are nearly on the verge of extinction.

Agkistrodon seu Bungarus(白花蛇 *bai hua she*)

The drug is actually of two kinds: The big one is called *qi she* and it refers to the dried body of Agkistrodon acutus (Guenther) of Crotalidae, which is mainly found in Zhejiang, Jiangxi and Fujian provinces. The small one is called *jin qian bai hua she* and it is the dried body of the young snake of Bungarus multicinctus Blyth of Elapididae, which is mainly distributed in Guangdong Province and the Guangxi Zhuang Autonomous Region. Both the snakes are captured in summer, coiled up and dried or baked on fire with the belly cut open and the internal organs removed. The belly is held open with bamboo sticks.

Taste and Property: Sweet and salty, warm and toxic.
Attributive Meridian: Liver meridian.
Actions and Indications:

(1) To dispel wind and remove obstruction in the meridians. It is indicated for stubborn cases of *bi*-syndrome due to wind-dampness marked by numbness of the limbs and muscular spasms. For such cases, it is often combined with Rhizoma seu Radix Notopterygii, Radix Ledebouriellae, Radix Angelicae Sinensis and Radix Paeoniae Rubra to eliminate wind and activate blood circulation. For chronic cases of apoplexy and hemiplegia, it is often used with Radix Astragali, Ramulus Cinnamomi and Angelicae Sinensis to nourish *qi* and blood, dispel wind and release the obstruction in the meridians.

(2) To relieve spasms. It is indicated for infantile convulsion and tetanus. For such cases, it is combined with Zaocys and Scolopendra.

It also cures leprosy, scrofula and serious cases of tinea and sores.

Dosage and Preparation: Agkistrodon: 3-10 g in decoction; and 1-1. 5 g in powder. Bungarus: 0. 5-1 g in powder. Both can be prepared as medicinal wine for oral administration.

Remarks: The drug recorded in ancient medical literature actually refers to Agkistrodon and Bungarus. They are similar in efficacy and are used similarly. But the latter is more powerful and used in a comparatively small dosage. Since they have different sources, they should be written clearly as Agkistrodon or Bungarus in prescriptions to avoid possible mistakes in dispensation.

APPENDIX:

Zaocys(乌梢蛇 *wu shao she*)

Zaocys refers to the dried body of Zaocys dhumnades (Cantor) of Colubridae, with the internal organs removed. It is sweet and not poisonous. It is similar to Agkistrodon seu Bungarus in efficacy, but less powerful. Dosage: 5-10 g in decoction, and 2-3 g in powder.

Table 5. Actions of Drugs for Eliminating Wind-Dampness

Drug	Similarities	Differences
Radix Angelicae Pubescentis	Warm in property, eliminating wind and dampness	Especially effective for *bi*-syndrome in the lower part of the body
Radix Clematidis		Effective for cases of (fish) bones getting stuck in throat
Radix Stephaniae Tetrandrae	Cold in property, eliminating wind and dampness	Facilitating water excretion and relieving edema
Radix Gentianae Macrophyllae		Subduing heat of deficiency type and relieving jaundice
Fructus Chaenomelis		Effective for easing tendons and muscles, also dissolving dampness and pacifying stomach
Ramulus Taxilli	Eliminating wind-dampness, strengthening tendons, muslces and bones	Relieving restlessness of the fetus
Cortex Acanthopanacis		Facilitating excretion of water and relieving edema
Os Tigris		Powerful in eliminating wind and stopping pain
Agkistrodon seu Bungarus		Powerful in eliminating wind and clearing away obstruction from collaterals, relieving spasms and convulsions

Note: Other drugs that eliminate wind-dampness include Rhizoma seu Radix Notopterygii, Radix Ledebouriellae, Herba Asari, Radix Aconiti and Rhizoma Atractylodis. They are discussed elsewhere in this book.

CHAPTER EIGHT
AROMATIC DRUGS FOR DISPELLING DAMPNESS

Drugs that are aromatic and dispel dampness and promote the transformative and transporting functions of the spleen are known as aromatic drugs for dispelling dampness (*fang xiang hua shi yao*).

The spleen prefers dryness and dislikes dampness. Dampness retained in the middle *jiao* impairs the splenic and gastric functions. The aromatic drugs for dispelling dampness are acrid, warm and dry, and work to activate *qi* circulation, dispel dampness and strengthen splenic and gastric functions. They are mainly indicated for cases with dampness retention in the middle *jiao* exhibiting distention and fullness in the epigastrium and abdomen, nausea, vomiting, anorexia, sticky and greasy sensation in the mouth, a heavy feeling in the limbs, loose stools and thick greasy tongue coating. The drugs are also indicated for dampness-warm and summer-heat-dampness syndromes.

Dampness may be either cold-dampness or dampness-heat, so drugs for dispelling dampness should be combined with other drugs in line with the nature of the dampness. For cases with cold-dampness, drugs that warm the interior should be applied with them; for those with dampness-heat, drugs that eliminate heat and remove dampness should be used. Since dampness is characterized by stickiness and stagnation, activated *qi* circulation can help dispel it. Drugs for dispelling dampness are therefore often combined with drugs that activate *qi* circulation. Weakness of the spleen may result in formation of dampness, and so in cases of excessive dampness due to spleen deficiency, they are combined with drugs that nourish the spleen.

Such drugs are mostly warm and dry and likely injure *yin*. They should therefore be prescribed with caution to patients with *yin* deficiency. Since they are aromatic and contain volatile oil, it is not advisable to decoct them for a long time.

Rhizoma Atractylodis(苍术 *cang zhu*)

Rhizoma Atractylodis is the rhizome of the perennial herb Atractylodes lancea (Thunb.) DC., or A. chinensis (DC.) koidz. of Compositae. The former is mainly produced in Jiangsu, Hubei and Henan provinces, the latter in Hebei and Liaoning provinces as well as the Inner Mongolia Autonomous Region. Both are collected in spring and autumn, and dried in the sun with soils and fibrous roots removed.

Taste and Property: Acrid and bitter, and warm.

Attributive Meridian: Spleen and stomach meridians.

Actions and Indications:

(1) To dry pathogenic dampness and strengthen the spleen. It is indicated for dampness retention in the middle *jiao* (spleen and stomach), with such manifestations as epigastric and abdominal distention and stuffiness, anorexia, loose stools, and white and greasy tongue coating. For such cases, it is often used with Cortex Magnoliae Officinalis and Pericarpium Citri Reticulatae, as in Powder for Regulating Stomach Function, to activate *qi* circulation and eliminate dampness. It is also indicated for cases with retained phlegm and edema due to excessive spleen dampness.

(2) To eliminate wind-dampness. It is indicated for *bi*-syndrome due to wind-dampness, particularly cases in which dampness is predominant. For its diaphoretic effect, it is also indicated for exterior syndrome accompanied by general achiness. For such cases, it is usually applied with Rhizoma seu Radix Notopterygii and Radix Ledebouriellae. For cases with dampness-heat retention in the lower *jiao*, manifested as redness, swelling, pain and weakness in the lower limbs, it is combined with Cortex Phellodendri, as in Powder of Phellodendri and Atractylodis.

It also improves eyesight, and is indicated for night blindness. For such a case, it is taken together with cooked pig and sheep liver.

Dosage and Preparation: 3-10 g. Either used crude or stir-baked.

Remarks: This drug is acrid and bitter, and warm and dry. It can eliminate wind-dampness from the exterior and dispel dampness from the middle *jiao*. If combined with Cotex Phellodendri, it can purge heat and remove dampness, and is good for dampness-heat retention in the lower *jiao*. It is therefore important for treating dampness syndromes, no matter whether the exterior or interior, the upper or the lower part of the body is involved.

Cortex Magnoliae Officinalis(厚朴 *hou po*)

Cortex Magnoliae Officinalis refers to the bark of the deciduous tree Magnolia officinalis Rehd. et Wils. , or M. officinalis Rehd. et Wils. var. blioba Rehd. et Wils. of Magnoliaceae. Mainly produced in Sichuan, Hubei and Zhejiang provinces, the bark is peeled off in summer, piled up in the shade, evaporated, and finally dried in the sun.

Synonym: *Chuan po*.

Taste and Property: Bitter and acrid, and warm.

Attributive Meridian: Spleen, stomach and lung meridians.

Actions and Indications:

(1) To activate *qi* circulation, eliminate dampness and relieve stasis. Indications: (a) Blocked *qi* circulation by dampness in the middle *jiao* giving rise to epigastric and abdominal distention and fullness. For such cases, it is often used with Rhizoma Atractylodis and Pericarpium Citri Reticulatae to help activate *qi* circulation and dispel dampness. If cold-dampness is predominant, it should be combined with drugs that warm yang, such as Rhizoma Zingiberis and Radix Aconiti Lateralis Preparata. (b) Constipation due to intestinal

stasis, manifested as epigastric and abdominal distention and fullness, for which it is often prescribed with Radix et Rhizoma Rhei and Fructus Aurantii Immaturus to activate *qi* circulation, relieve intestinal stasis and promote bowel movements.

(2) To check the abnormal ascent of *qi* and relieve dyspnea. It is indicated for dyspneic cough with profuse sputum, stuffiness in the chest, thick and sticky tongue coating due to the accumulation of phlegm-dampness in the lung and the abnormal ascent of lung *qi*. Here, it is combined with Semen Armeniacae Amarum and Rhizoma Pinelliae to restore the normal descent of *qi*, resolve phlegm and relieve dyspnea.

Dosage and Preparation: 3-10 g. Prepared with ginger juice.

Remarks: The drug is bitter and acrid, and warm and dry. It is especially effective at activating *qi* circulation and eliminating dampness. It is particularly indicated for epigastric and abdominal distention and fullness due to dampness, stasis or pathogenic cold that blocks *qi* passages, since it has a rather powerful action in activating *qi* circulation and drying dampness, and relieve stasis and warm the middle *jiao*. But its activation of *qi* is rather drastic, and any improper use may consume *qi*; for epigastric and abdominal distention and fullness due to *qi* deficiency, its dosage therefore should be small. In such cases, it should combined with drugs that replenish *qi*, such as Radix Ginseng and Radix Codonopsis Pilosulae.

Herba Agastaches(霍香 *huo xiang*)

Herba Agastaches refers to the stem and leaves of the perennial herb Pogostemon cablin (Blanco) Benth, or Agastache rugosa (fisch. et Mey.) O. Ktze of Labiatae. The former is mainly produced in Guangdong Province, and the latter in most parts of China. It is cut and collected in summer and autumn when the stem and leaves are growing luxuriantly and dried in the sun. It can also be used fresh.

Taste and Property: Acrid, and slightly warm.

Attributive Meridian: Spleen and stomach meridians.

Actions and Indications:

(1) To dispel dampness and summer-heat. Indications: (a) Retention of dampness in the middle *jiao* marked by epigastric stuffiness, anorexia, nausea, vomiting, loose stools, general lassitude and heaviness in the limbs, and white greasy tongue coating. Here, it is often combined with Rhizoma Atractylodis and Cortex Magnoliae Officinalis. (b) Summer-heat-dampness syndrome manifested as chills, fever, headache, vomiting and diarrhea. For such cases, it is often prescribed together with Folium Perillae, Rhizoma Pinelliae and Magnoliae Officinalis.

(2) To stop vomiting, especially that due to dampness. It can also be applied for other kinds of vomiting, including morning sickness, in combination with other drugs.

Dosage: 3-10 g, doubled if used fresh.

Herba Eupatorii(佩兰 *pei lan*)

Herba Eupatorii is the aerial part of the perennial herb Eupatorium fortunei Turcz. of Compositae. Mainly produced in Jiangsu, Jiangxi, Hebei and Guangdong provinces, it is harvested twice in summer and autumn, cut into sections and dried in the sun. It can also be used fresh.

Taste and Property: Acrid, and mild.
Attributive Meridian: Spleen and stomach meridians.
Actions and Indications:

To dispel dampness and summer-heat. Indications: (a) Retention of dampness in the middle *jiao*, marked by epigastric and abdominal stuffiness, anorexia, nausea, vomiting, white greasy tongue coating or sweetish and greasy sensation in the mouth. Here, it is often used with Herba Agastaches to help dispel dampness. (b) Summer-heat-dampness syndrome or the early stages of dampness syndrome, manifested as chills, fever, distention in the head, epigastric stuffiness, stickiness in the mouth and anorexia; for this it is often combined with Agastaches, Cortex Magnoliae Officinalis, Rhizoma Pinelliae and Folium Nelumbinis.
Dosage: 3-10 g, doubled if used fresh.
Remarks: This herb is effective in dispelling dampness and summer-heat. The fresh herb is even more effective. It is similar to Agastaches, and they are often used together. But Agastaches is acrid and warm and can relieve exterior syndrome and stop vomiting, Herba Eupatorii is mild, mainly used to dispel dampness and harmonize the middle *jiao*.

Fructus Amomi(砂仁 *sha ren*)

Fructus Amomi is the dried fruit of the perennial herb Amomum villosum Lour., or A. xanthioides Wall. of Zingiberaceae. The former is mainly produced in Guangdong Province, the latter Southeast Asian countries, such as Vietnam, Indonesia and Kampuchea. Both are collected in July and August when the fruit is ripe, dried in the sun or baked until dry over a slow fire.

Taste and Property: Acrid, and warm.
Attributive Meridian: Spleen, stomach and kidney meridians.
Actions and Indications:

(1) To activate *qi* circulation and dispel dampness. It is indicated for epigastric and abdominal distention and fullness, anorexia, nausea, vomiting, abdominal pain and diarrhea due to dampness retained in the middle *jiao* or stagnant spleen and stomach qi. For such cases, it is often used with Radix Aucklandiae and Pericarpium Citri Reticulatae. In cases of dampness retention due to spleen deficiency, it is prescribed with drugs that strengthen the spleen, such as Radix Codonopsis Pilosulae and Rhizoma Atractylodis Macrocephalae.

(2) To ease the fetus. It is indicated for morning sickness and restlessness of the fetus. For such cases, it is often used with Atractylodis Macrocephalae, Fructus Aurantii and Caulis Perillae to strengthen the spleen, activate *qi* circulation and ease the fetus.

Dosage and Preparation: 2-5 g. To be used in decoction, it should be pounded into pieces first and then decocted.

Fructus Amomi Rotundus(白豆蔻 *bai dou kou*)

Fructus Amomi Rotundus refers to the dried fruit of the perennial herb Amomum cardamomum L. of Zingiberaceae. Mainly produced in Vietnam and Thailand, it has been cultivated in Guangdong and Yunnan provinces of China. It is collected in autumn when the fruit is ripe, and dried in the sun. The seeds are known as Semen Amomi Rotundus.

Taste and Property: Acrid, and warm.
Attributive Meridian: Spleen, stomach and lung meridians.
Actions and Indications:

(1) To activate *qi* circulation and dispel dampness. Indications: (a) Retention of dampness in the middle *jiao*. For such cases, it is often used with Rhizoma Atractylodis, Cortex Magnoliae Officinalis and Pericarpium Citri Reticulatae. (b) The early stages of dampness-warm syndrome, marked by stuffiness in the chest, poor appetite, greasy tongue coating and soft pulse; here it is often combined with Semen Armeniacae Amarum, Yiren Semen Coicis and Medulla Tetrapanacis, as in Three Seeds Decoction.

(2) To pacify the stomach and stop vomiting. It is indicated for vomiting due to cold and dampness retained in the middle *jiao*. For such cases, it is often used with Rhizoma Pinelliae and Rhizoma Zingiberis Recens. For vomiting in infants after breast feeding due to stomach cold, it is ground into fine powder together with Fructus Amomi and Radix Glycyrrhizae for oral feeding.

Dosage and Preparation: 3-5 g. Pounded into pieces and then decocted.
Remarks: Both Fructus Amomi and Semen Amomi Rotundus activate *qi* circulation, dispel dampness and strengthen the stomach. But the former is particularly indicated for diseases of the middle *jiao* and the lower *jiao*, such as diarrhea due to cold and restlessness of the fetus; the latter is indicated for such middle and upper *jiao* diseases as the early stages of dampness-warm syndrome and vomiting due to pathogenic dampness.

Fructus Tsaoko(草果 *cao guo*)

Fructus Tsaoko is the ripe fruit of the perennial herb Amomum tsao-ko Crevost et Lemaire of Zingiberaceae. Mainly produced in Yunnan and Guizhou provinces as well as the Guangxi Zhuang Autonomous Region, it is collected in autumn when the fruit is ripe, and dried in the sun.

Taste and Property: Acrid, and warm.
Attributive Meridian: Spleen and stomach meridians.
Actions and Indications:

(1) To warm the middle *jiao* and eliminate dampness. It is indicated for retention of cold and dampness in the middle *jiao*, marked by epigastric and abdominal stuffiness and

fullness, anorexia, and white, thick and turbid greasy tongue coating. Here, it is combined with Rhizoma Atractylodis, Cortex Magnoliae Officinalis and Pericarpium Citri Reticulatae.

(2) To check malarial attack. It is indicated for malaria with predominant phlegm and dampness, for which it is often used with Radix Dichroae, Semen Arecae and Cortex Magnoliae Officinalis.

Dosage and Preparation: 3-6 g. Stir-baked until blackish yellow, with the shell of the fruit removed. Prescribed as stewed Tsaoko.

Remarks: This drug is acrid, warm and rather dry, and is mainly used for cold-dampness syndromes, as well as malaria with predominant dampness.

Table 6. Actions of Drugs for Dispelling Dampness

Drug	Similarities	Differences
Rhizoma Atractylodis	Strong effect of drying dampness	Drying dampness, strengthening spleen, eliminating wind-dampness
Cortex Magnoliae Officinalis		Activating *qi* circulation, relieving stasis, relieving epigastric and abdominal stuffiness, restoring normal descending of *qi* and relieving dyspnea
Herba Agastaches	Dispelling dampness and relieving summer-heat syndrome	
Herba Eupatorii		Of mild property; with no effect of checking vomiting
Fructus Amomi	Activating *qi* circulation; dispelling dampness	Warming up middle *jiao* and treating diarrhea due to cold; easing the fetus
Fructus Amomi Rotundus		Effective for dispelling dampness in middle and upper *jiao*, early stage of dampness-warm syndrome, vomiting due to dampness
Fructus Tsaoko		Effective mainly for warming up middle *jiao* and drying dampness, and for checking malaria as well

Note: In other chapters or sections, some other drugs that dispel dampness are discussed, such as Herba Elsholtziae, Rhizoma Acori Graminei and Rhizoma Atractylodis Macrocephalae.

CHAPTER NINE
DIURETICS

Drugs that promote urination and help eliminate dampness are known as diuretics (*li shui shen shi yao*).

Most diuretics are sweet or bland and slightly cold, or bitter and cold. They can increase the volume of urine, facilitate urination and eliminate water and dampness, and are indicated for water and dampness retention, dysuria, edema, ascites, phlegm retention, stranguria, jaundice and dampness-warm syndrome. Drugs that are sweet or bland and slightly cold are called "bland drugs for promoting diuresis"; drugs that are bitter and cold are called "drugs for purging heat and promoting diuresis"; and drugs frequently used in treating stranguria are known as "diuretics for relieving stranguria."

Diuretics should be prescribed selectively and used in combination with other related drugs. For example, for sudden onset of edema accompanied by exterior syndrome, they are combined with drugs that relieve exterior syndrome and promote the lung's dispersive function; for chronic edema accompanied by spleen and kidney *yang* deficiency, they are used together with drugs that warm and nourish the spleen and kidney; for stranguria with predominant dampness-heat, they are combined with drugs that purge heat; for stranguria complicated by hematuria due to excessive heat that has injured the blood vessels, they are prescribed together with drugs that cool the blood and stop bleeding.

Diuretics are likely to consume fluid, and should be prescribed with caution to patients who have shown the lack of body fluid due to *yin* deficiency.

Poria(茯苓 *fu ling*)

Poria is the sclerotium of the fungus Poria cocos (Schw.) Wolf of Polyporaceae, a parasite usually found at the root of pine tree. Mainly produced in Anhui, Yunnan, Hubei and Sichuan provinces, it is usually collected from July to September. It is piled up and let to evaporate, then spread out to dry in the shade; this process is repeated several times until it is completely dry. The fresh fungus may also be cut into pieces and dried in the shade.

Taste and Property: Sweet and bland, and mild.
Attributive Meridian: Heart, spleen and kidney meridians.
Actions and Indications:

(1) To promote diuresis and remove dampness. It is indicated for dysuria and edema

due to water and dampness retention, and fluid-retention syndrome. Since it strengthens the spleen, it is especially indicated for spleen deficiency that leads to excessive dampness. For such cases, it is often combined with Ramulus Cinnamomi, Rhizoma Atractylodis Macrocephalae and Rhizoma Alismatis. For a case complicated by dampness-heat, it is used with Semen Plantaginis and Caulis Akebiae.

(2) To strengthen the spleen. Indicated for spleen deficiency marked by general lassitude and heaviness in the limbs, poor appetite and loose stools. For such cases, it is often used with drugs that nourish the spleen, such as Radix Codonopsis Pilosulae and Atractylodis Macrocephalae, as in Four Mild Drugs Decoction.

(3) To calm the mind. Indicated for restlessness, palpitation and insomnia, for which it is often combined with Semen Ziziphi Spinosae and Radix Polygalae to calm the heart and mind.

Dosage and Preparation: 10-15 g. To calm the mind, it can be mixed with Cinnabaris in decoction, and prescribed as Poria-Cinnabaris.

Remarks: In the past, Poria was divided into several kinds whose application was slightly different. Those with white inner layers are called Poria Alba, and are mainly indicated for strengthening the spleen; those with light red outer layers are called Poria Rubra, effective for eliminating dampness; and those through which the fine fibrous roots of the pine tree have grown are called Lignum Pini Poriaferum, mainly effective for calming the mind. The cortex of the sclerotium is called Exo-Poria, and is mainly effective for promoting diuresis and relieving edema. Now, Poria Alba and Poria Rubra are no longer separated, and both are called Poria.

Polyporus Umbellatus(猪苓 *zhu ling*)

Polyporus Umbellatus is the sclerotium of the fungus Polyporus umbellatus (Pers.) Fries of Polyporaceae. Growing as a parasite on the rotten roots of Betula, Quercus, Acer and Salix trees, it is mainly produced in Shaanxi, Henan and Shanxi provinces. It is collected in spring, washed and dried in the shade, then cut into slices for medical use.

Taste and Property: Sweet and bland, and slightly cold.

Attributive Meridian: Kidney and urinary bladder meridians.

Actions and Indications:

To eliminate water and dampness. It is indicated for dysuria, edema, stranguria and leukorrhagia due to water and dampness retention. For such cases, it is often combined with Poria and Rhizoma Alismatis.

Dosage: 5-10 g.

Rhizoma Alismatis(泽泻 *ze xie*)

Rhizoma Alismatis is the tuber of the perennial marsh plant Alisma orientalis (Sam.) Juzep. of Alismataceae. Mainly produced in Fujian, Sichuan and Jiangxi provinces, it is collected in winter, washed, and dried by baking over a slow fire with the fibrous roots and coarse skin removed.

Taste and Property: Sweet, and cold.
Attributive Meridian: Kidney and urinary bladder meridians.
Actions and Indications:

To promote diuresis, excrete dampness and purge heat. It is indicated for dysuria, edema, stuffiness and fullness in the epigastrium and abdomen, loose stools, stranguria and leukorrhagia due to water and dampness retention. For such cases, it is often combined with Poria and Polyporus Umbellatus to enhance the effect. For vertigo due to retained phlegm and fluid, it is prescribed together with Rhizoma Atractylodis Macrocephalae, as in Decoction of Alismatis.

Dosage: 5-10 g.

Remarks: Poria, Polyporus Umbellatus and Rhizoma Alismatis are all sweet and bland, and work to excrete dampness; they are indicated for water and dampness retention. But Poria is mild, and can strengthen the spleen and calm the mind; the latter two have a stronger effect, but do not affect the spleen and mind.

Semen Coicis(薏苡仁 *yi yi ren*)

Semen Coicis refers to the ripe seed of the perennial herb Coix lacryma-Jobi L. var. ma-yuen (Roman.) Stapf of Gramineae. Produced in most places of China, the aerial part is cut in autumn when the fruit is ripe, the fruit is knocked off, and then dried in the sun with the shell removed.

Synonym: *Yi mi, yi ren, mi ren.*
Taste and Property: Sweet and bland, and slightly cold.
Attributive Meridian: Spleen, stomach and lung meridians.
Actions and Indications:

(1) To excrete water and dampness. Indicated for dysuria, edema and beriberi due to water and dampness retention, for which it is often used with Poria and Rhizoma Alismatis.

(2) To strengthen the spleen and stop diarrhea. It is indicated for diarrhea due to spleen deficiency. For such cases, it is often combined with Radix Codonopsis Pilosulae, Rhizoma Atractylodis Macrocephalae and Poria to strengthen the spleen, excrete pathogenic dampness and stop diarrhea.

(3) To eliminate pathogenic dampness and relieve *bi*-syndrome. Indicated for *bi*-syndrome with predominant dampness, marked by heaviness and soreness of the body as well as spasms and stiffness of the tendons and muscles; it is often used with Radix Stephaniae Tetrandrae, Fructus Chaenomelis and Cortex Acanthopanacis to eliminate dampness and ease the tendons and muscles.

(4) To purge heat and discharge pus. Indications: (a) Pulmonary abscess, for which it is combined with Rhizoma Phragmitis, Semen Persicae and Semen Benincasae, as in Decoction of Phragmitis. (b) Appendicitis with abscess, here it is often used with Herba Pa-

triniae and Caulis Sargentodoxae.

Dosage and Preparation: 15-30 g. Stir-baked to strengthen the spleen, and used in crude form for other purposes.

Remarks: Semen Coicis possesses similar effects as Poria. Yet, it also eliminates dampness, relieves *bi*-syndrome, purges heat and discharges pus, and is often used to treat *bi*-syndrome due to dampness, as well as pulmonary abscess and appendicitis.

This drug is mild, and in treating chronic diseases it should be in a large dosage for a longer time. In addition to being prepared as decoction, pills and powder, it can be made into thick soup or cooked with non-glutinous rice as a porridge, which is good for diet therapy.

Semen Plantaginis(车前子 *che qian zi*)

Semen Plantaginis is the seed of the perennial herb Plantago asiatica L., or P. depressa Willd. of Plantaginaceae. To be found throughout China, it is gathered in summer and autumn when the seed is ripe, and dried in the sun.

Taste and Property: Sweet, and cold.

Attributive Meridian: Kidney, liver and lung meridians.

Actions and Indications:

(1) To purge heat and excrete dampness. It is indicated for dysuria, edema and stranguria, especially those due to dampness-heat. For stranguria due to heat, it is often used with Caulis Akebiae and Talcum. Since it excretes water and dampness, separates the clear fluid from the turbid and stops diarrhea, it is also indicated for diarrhea due to dampness and summer-heat, for which it is used alone as a powder or combined with Talcum.

(2) To strengthen the liver and improve eyesight. It is indicated for redness, swelling and pain in the eyes due to flare-up of liver fire. For such cases, it is often used with Spica Prunellae, Flos Chrysanthemi and Semen Cassiae to purge liver fire. It is also indicated for hypertension due to flare-up of liver fire.

(3) To purge heat from the lung and remove phlegm. It is indicated for cough with copious sputum due to excessive heat in the lung; here it is often combined with Semen Armeniacae Amarum, Radix Platycodi and Radix Peucedani to eliminate phlegm and stop cough.

Dosage and Preparation: 5-10 g. Wrapped in a piece of cloth and decocted.

Remarks: Sweet, bland and cold, the drug can excrete dampness and purge heat, mainly heat in the kidney, liver and lung meridians. It purges dampness-heat in the lower *jiao*, liver fire and lung heat.

Talcum(滑石 *hua shi*)

Talcum is a mineral of silicate, composed mainly of hydrous magnesium silicate $Mg_3[Si_4O_{10}](OH)_2$. Mainly distributed in Shandong, Jiangxi, Jiangsu and Shaanxi provinces, it can be mined at any time of the year, with soil and foreign matter (or stones) removed.

Taste and Property: Sweet, and cold.
Attributive Meridian: Stomach and urinary bladder meridians.
Actions and Indications:

(1) To purge heat and excrete dampness. It is indicated for stranguria due to dampness-heat, marked by dribbling and painful urination, for which it is often combined with Caulis Akebiae and Semen Plantaginis.

(2) To purge summer-heat. It is indicated for summer-heat syndrome complicated by dampness and marked by fever, restlessness and thirst, dysuria or diarrhea. For such cases, it is often used with Radix Glycyrrhizae, as in Six-to-One Powder.

This drug also purges heat and dampness when used externally, and is indicated for skin diseases, such as eczema and miliaria.

Dosage and Preparation: 10-15 g. Ground into powder in water, and decocted by wrapping it in a piece of cloth. The dosage for external application should be decided in line with actual needs.

Caulis Akebiae(木通 *mu tong*)

Caulis Akebiae refers to the stem of the twining vine Aristolochia manshuriensis Kom. of Aristolochiaceae, or the stem of the evergreen climbing shrub Clematis armandii Franch. of Ranunculaceae, or the stem of C. montan Buch. Ham. They are of the same genus. The first one is mainly produced in Jilin, Heilongjiang and Liaoning provinces, and the latter two in Sichuan. They are collected in spring and autumn, and dried in the sun with the coarse cortex removed.

Taste and Property: Bitter, and cold.
Attributive Meridian: Heart, small intestine and urinary bladder meridians.
Actions and Indications:

(1) To purge heat and dampness. It is indicated for stranguria due to dampness-heat, marked by scanty and dark yellow urine, as well as dribbling and painful urination. For such cases, it is often combined with Semen Plantaginis and Talcum.

(2) To purge heart fire. It is indicated for aphthae, restlessness and dark yellow urine due to hyperactive heart fire. Here, it is often combined with Radix Rehmanniae and Radix Glycyrrhizae.

(3) To promote lactation. It is indicated for galactostasis after childbirth. For such cases, it is used with Squama Manitis and Semen Vaccariae.

Dosage: 3-6 g.
Precaution: For pregnant women, it should be applied with caution.
Remarks: There are different kinds of Caulis Akebiae, and Caulis Aristolochia Manshuriensis is the one most commonly used at present. The drug is rather bitter and cold, and purges heart fire. Ancient physicians pointed out that a large dose of the drug may consume the primordial *qi* of the human body. Modern medical literature also has reported

that Caulis Aristolochia Manshuriensis, used in large dosage, may cause renal failure, and so attention should be paid to limiting its dosage.

Medulla Tetrapanacis(通草 *tong cao*)

Medulla Tetrapanacis is the pith of the shrub Tetrapanax paphriferus (Hook. I.) K. Koch of Araliaceae. Mainly produced in Yunnan, Guizhou and Sichuan provinces as well as the Guangxi Zhuang Autonomous Region, the stem is collected in autumn and cut into segments, and then the pith is taken out when it is still fresh, straightened and dried in the sun, and finally processed into thin slices.

Taste and Property: Sweet and bland, and slightly cold.
Attributive Meridian: Lung and stomach meridians.
Actions and Indications:

(1) To purge heat and eliminate dampness. It is indicated for stranguria due to dampness-heat marked by scanty and dark yellow urine, and dribbling and painful urination; here it is used with Talcum and Semen Plantaginis.

(2) To promote lactation. It is indicated for postpartum hypogalactia or galactostasis. For such cases, it is often combined with Squama Manitis in decoction, or cooked with pigs' trotters.

Dosage: 2-5 g.
Remarks: Caulis Akebiae and Medulla Tetrapanacis have different names in ancient and modern times. What is now *mu tong* was known as *tong cao* in ancient medical books, while *tong cao* was called *tong tuo mu*. One should be aware of this difference and not confuse one with the other. In terms of efficacy, both drugs can purge heat, eliminate dampness and promote lactation. But the former is bitter and cold, and is effective at purging heart fire; the latter is bland, and is good for excreting dampness, but weak at purging heat.

Herba Lysimachiae(金钱草 *jin qian cao*)

Herba Lysimachiae refers to the whole plant of Lysimachia christinae Hance of Primulaceae. Distributed in all provinces to the south of the Yangtze River, it is collected in May, cut into sections and dried in the sun, with foreign matter removed.

Synonym: *Da jin qian cao*, *shen xian dui zuo cao*.
Taste and Property: Sweet and bland, and slightly cold.
Attributive Meridian: Liver, gallbladder, kidney and urinary bladder meridians.
Actions and Indications:

(1) To remove dampness and expel stones. It is indicated for stranguria due to dampness-heat or urinary stones. For such cases, it is used alone in a large dosage for daily decoction, or else combined with Spora Lygodii and Endothelium Corneum Gigeriae Galli.

(2) To remove dampness and relieve jaundice. It is indicated for jaundice due to

dampness-heat; here it is prescribed with Herba Artemisiae Scopariae and Fructus Gardeniae. It can also be used to treat hepatic and cholecystic calculus.

It also purges heat and eliminates toxicins, and is effective in treating carbuncles and poisonous snakebites.

Dosage: 30-60 g, doubled if used fresh.

Remarks: For its effect in expelling stones, this drug is frequently used to treat hepatic, cholecystic and urinary stones. To achieve the desired results, it is usually used in large dosage and administered for a long time.

Herba Lysimachiae covers many varieties and are used for different purposes in different areas. Apart from Lysimachia christinae Hance of Primulaceae discussed above, there are Glechoma Longituba (Nakai) Kupr. of Labiatae, Desmodium styracifolium (Osbeck) Merr. of Leguminosae, and Hydrocotyle sibthorpioides Lam. var batrachium (Hance) Hand-Mazz. of Umbelliferae.

Spora Lygodii(海金沙 *hai jin sha*)

Spora Lygodii are ripe spores of the perennial climbing fern Lygodium Japonicum (Thunb.) SW. of Schizaeaceae. Mainly produced in Guangdong, Zhejiang, Hunan, Hubei and Shaanxi provinces, the vines with leaves are cut in autumn when the spores are ripe but not yet fallen off, dried in the sun and finally have the spores rubbed or knocked off and collected.

Taste and Property: Sweet, and cold.

Attributive Meridian: Urinary bladder meridian.

Actions and Indications:

To purge heat, excrete dampness and expel calculi. It is indicated for edema and stranguria due to dampness-heat, especially due to urinary stones. Here, it is often used with Herba Lysimachiae and Folium Pyrrosiae to enhance the effect.

Dosage and Preparation: 6-12 g, wrapped in a piece of cloth and decocted.

Folium Pyrrosiae(石韦 *shi wei*)

Folium Pyrrosiae is the leaf of the perennial herb Pyrrosia sheareri (Bak.) Ching, P. petiolosa (Christ) Ching, or P. lingua (Thunb.) Farwell of Polypodiaceae. It grows wild everywhere in China, but mainly in Zhejiang, Jiangsu, Hubei, Hunan and Hebei provinces. It can be gathered in any season of the year, washed clean, then dried in the sun.

Taste and Property: Bitter, and slightly cold.

Attributive Meridian: Lung and urinary bladder meridians.

Actions and Indications:

(1) To purge heat and excrete dampness. It is indicated for dampness-heat in the urinary bladder, marked by scanty dark red urine, dribbling, difficult and painful urination

and even hematuria. For such cases, it is often combined with Spora Lygodii, Talcum and Rhizoma Imperatae. For stranguria due to urinary stones, it is used with Spora Lygodii, Herba Lysimachiae and Endothelium Corneum Gigeriae Galli.

(2) To resolve phlegm and relieve cough. It is indicated for productive cough and dyspnea, for which it is used alone or combined with other drugs that relieves cough and dyspnea.

This drug also stops bleeding and is indicated for hematemesis, epistaxis and metrorrhagia.

Dosage: 5-10 g.

Rhizoma Dioscoreae Septemlobae(萆薢 *bi xie*)

Rhizoma Dioscoreae Septemlobae refers to the rhizome and tuber of the perennial trailing plant Dioscorea hypoglauca palibin., or D. septemloba Thunb. of Dioscoreaceae. Mainly produced in Zhejiang and Hubei provinces, it is collected in autumn and winter, cut into pieces and dried in the sun with the fibrous roots removed.

Taste and Property: Bitter, and mild.

Attributive Meridian: Liver, stomach and urinary bladder meridians.

Actions and Indications:

(1) To eliminate dampness and turbidity. It is indicated for stranguria complicated by chyluria and marked by turbid urine. For such cases, it is often used with Rhizoma Acori Graminei, as in Decoction of Dioscoreae Septemlobae for Clearing Turbid Urine. It can also be used to treat leukorrhagia.

(2) To eliminate wind-dampness. It is indicated for *bi*-syndrome with predominant dampness, marked by soreness, heaviness and pain in the lower back and knee joints; here it is often combined with Semen Coicis, Rhizoma Atractylodis and Fructus Chaenomelis.

Dosage: 10-15 g.

Remarks: This drug is particularly good for eliminating dampness. First, it can excrete dampness and separate the clear from the turbid, and is indicated for stranguria complicated by chyluria. Second, it eliminates wind-dampness, and is indicated for *bi*-syndrome with predominant dampness.

Herba Artemisiae Scopariae(茵陈蒿 *yin chen hao*)

Herba Artemisiae Scopariae refers to the spire of the perennial plant Artemisia capillaris Thunb., or A. scoparia Waldst. et Kit. of Compositae. To be found in most places of China, but produced mainly in Shaanxi, Shanxi and Anhui provinces, it is cut and collected in spring when the spire is about 10 centimeters high, and dried in the sun.

Taste and Property: Bitter, and slightly cold.

Attributive Meridian: Spleen, stomach, liver and gallbladder meridians.

Actions and Indications:

To purge heat, eliminate pathogenic dampness and relieve jaundice. It is indicated for jaundice. For *yang*-type jaundice due to dampness-heat marked by a bright yellow skin and sclera, fever and scant urination, it is combined with Fructus Gardeniae and Radix et Rhizoma Rhei, as in Decoction of Artemisiae Scopariae. For *yin*-type jaundice due to cold-dampness and marked by a dim yellowish skin and sclera, poor appetite and epigastric fullness, listlessness and aversion to cold, it is used with Radix Aconiti Lateralis Preparata and Rhizoma Zingiberis, as in Decoction of Artemisiae Scopariae for Treating *Yang* Exhaustion.

Since it eliminates dampness-heat, it can also be applied either orally or externally to treat wet boils and pruritus.

Dosage: 10-30 g.

Table 7. Actions of Diuretics

Drug	Similarities	Differences
Poria	Of bland taste, facilitating urination and excreting dampness, indicated for dysuria and edema	Strengthening spleen and calming the mind
Polyporous Umbellatus		Strong effect of facilitating urination
Rhizoma Alismatis		Strong effect of facilitating urination; indicated for vertigo due to retention of phlegm
Semen Coicis		Strengthening spleen, relieving *bi*-syndrome due to dampness, clearing heat and discharging pus
Semen Plantaginis	Of sweet taste, clearing heat and dampness and indicated for stranguria due to dampness-heat	Clearing heat from the liver and the lung
Talcum		Clearing summer-heat; external use for clearing heat and dampness in skin diseases
Caulis Akebiae	Clearing heat and dampness indicated for stranguria due to dampness-heat and for promoting lactation	Bitter and cold; purging fire from the heart
Medulla Tetrapanacis		Bland in taste and slightly cold; weak effect of clearing heat
Herba Lysimachiae	Excreting dampness, relieving stranguria, especially those due to dampness-heat or presence of calculi	Treating calculosis of various types and relieving jaundice
Spora Lygodii		Mainly indicated for stranguria
Folium Pyrrosiae		Resolving phlegm and relieving cough
Rhizoma Dioscoreae Septemlobae		Excreting dampness and turbidity, and indicated for stranguria complicated by chyluria; and eliminating wind-dampness
Herba Artemisiae Scopariae		Excreting dampness; important drug for relieving jaundice

CHAPTER TEN
DRUGS FOR WARMING THE INTERIOR

Drugs that warm the interior, dispel internal cold, and are indicated for interior cold syndrome are known as drugs for warming the interior (*wen li yao*).

These drugs are acrid and hot, and can warm the middle *jiao*, strengthen spleen and stomach functions, dispel cold and relieve pain. Some also warm and invigorate *yang*, and restore depleted *yang*. They are indicated for various interior cold syndromes that can be classified into two categories: attack by pathogenic cold and stagnation of spleen and stomach *yang qi*, marked by cold and pain in the epigastrium and abdomen, vomiting and diarrhea; and weakness of *yang qi* and excessive accumulation of cold in the interior, marked by aversion to cold, cold limbs, pallor, increased volume of clear urine, pale tongue with white coating, deep and thready pulse, or collapse of *yang* due to profuse sweating, marked by cold limbs and faint pulse.

These drugs can be combined with others in line with the specific conditions of the patients. For attack of the interior by exogenous cold accompanied by exterior syndrome, they are combined with drugs that relieve exterior syndrome; for cold retention and *qi* stagnation, they are combined with drugs that activate *qi*; for cold and dampness retention in the spleen, they are used with drugs that strengthen the spleen and dispel dampness; for spleen and kidney *yang* deficiency, they are combined with drugs that benefit *qi* and nourish the kidney; and for exhaustion of *yang* and depletion of *qi*, they are prescribed with drugs that replenish the primordial *qi*.

Drugs for warming the interior, acrid, and hot and dry, are likely to consume body fluid, and so they are contraindicated or should be used with caution for heat syndromes, *yin* deficiency syndromes and pregnant women.

Radix Aconiti Lateralis Preparata(附子 *fu zi*)

Radix Aconiti Lateralis Preparata is the lateral root of Aconitum carmichaeli Debx. of Ranunculaceae. Mainly produced in Sichuan and also cultivated in Hubei and Hunan provinces, it is collected between the Summer Solstice to Slight Heat. With the fibrous roots removed, it is washed clean and soaked in bittern and finally processed into *yan fu zi* (salted aconite), *hei shun pian* (black slices of aconite) and *bai fu pian* (white slices of aconite) according to different requirements.

Taste and Property: Acrid, and hot and toxic.

Attributive Meridian: Heart, spleen and kidney meridians.

Actions and Indications:

(1) To restore depleted *yang*. It is indicated for *yang* exhaustion syndrome marked by cold limbs, pallor, cold sweating and faint pulse. For such cases, it is often combined with Radix Ginseng, as in Decoction of Ginseng and Aconiti Lateralis, or else with Rhizoma Zingiberis and Radix Glycyrrhizae, as in Decoction for Treating *Yang* Exhaustion, to restore *yang*, replenish *qi* and rescue the patient from collapse.

(2) To warm *yang*. (a) To warm kidney *yang*. Indicated for kidney *yang* insufficiency marked by weakness, cold and pain in the lumbar region and knees, contraction in the lower abdomen, frequent urination or dysuria, edema, or impotence. In such cases, it is often combined with Cortex Cinnamomi, Radix Rehmanniae Preparata and Fructus Corni, as in Pill of Eight Ingredients Containing Cinnamomi and Aconiti Lateralis. (b) To warm spleen *yang*. Indicated for cases of deficiency cold in the spleen and stomach, marked by epigastric pain, watery vomiting, borborygmus, abdominal pain, loose stools and cold limbs. For such cases, it is often used with Radix Codonopsis Pilosulae, Rhizoma Atractylodis Macrocephalae and Rhizoma Zingiberis, as in Pill of Aconiti Lateralis for Regulating the Middle *Jiao*. (c) To warm heart *yang*. Indicated for heart *yang* deficiency marked by palpitation, shortness of breath, stuffiness and pain in the chest and heart region, cyanosis in the lips and nails, aversion to cold, cold limbs, pallor, and thready and weak pulse. For such cases, it is often used with Ginseng or Codonopsis Pilosulae and Ramulus Cinnamomi.

It is also indicated for spontaneous sweating due to *yang* deficiency in the surface, for which it is often combined with Ramulus Cinnamomi and Radix Astragali.

(3) To dispel cold and relieve pain. It is indicated for epigastric and abdominal pain due to cold and for *bi*-syndrome due to cold and dampness. For such cases, Ramulus Cinnamomi and Atractylodis Macrocephalae are often added.

Dosage and Preparation: 3-15 g. Prepared and then applied as a decoction. If used in large dosage, it should be decocted first for 30-60 minutes to reduce the toxicity.

Precaution: Never used for pregnant women.

APPENDIXES:

(1) **Radix Aconiti**(川乌头 *chuan wu tou*)

The root of Aconitum carmichaeli Debx. of Ranunculaceae, it is acrid, and hot and toxic. It enters the heart, liver and spleen meridians.

It eliminates wind and dampness, dispels cold and relieves pain, and is indicated for *bi*-syndrome due to cold and dampness, cold pain in the heart and abdominal region, lingering headache (head-wind syndrome), and migraine and pain caused by traumatic injuries. The recommended dosage is 3-9 g, which should be decocted first for 30-60 minutes to reduce the toxicity. It is contraindicated for pregnant women, and incompatible with Rhizoma Pinelliae, Fructus Trichosanthis, Bulbus Fritillariae, Cirrhosae Rhizoma Bletillae and Radix Ampelopsis.

(2) **Radix Aconiti Kusnezoffiae**(草乌头 *cao wu tou*)

It is the root of Aconitum Kusnezoffii Reichb. of Ranunculaceae. Its taste, property, actions, indications and contraindications are similar to those of Radix Aconiti. But it is more toxic. The recommended dosage is 1.5-4.5 g.

Remarks: Radix Aconiti Lateralis Preparata, acrid, hot and toxic, with a remarkable ability to warm *yang* and dispel cold, is indicated for various kinds of *yang* deficiency syndromes and pains due to excessive cold. It is essential for treating cases of exhaustion of *yang*. Its clinical indications are: faint and thready or deep and slow pulse, pale flabby tongue with thin white or white greasy coating, absence of thirst, cold limbs and aversion to cold, soreness and cold in the lumbus and knees, loose stools and increased volume of clear urine. As the drug is toxic, doctors should pay attention to its usage, dosage and contraindications.

Radix Aconiti and Radix Aconiti Kusnezoffiae are stronger than Radix Aconiti Lateralis Preparata in relieving pain, but milder in warming *yang*. Both of them, especially the latter, are very poisonous, and should be prescribed with caution.

Rhizoma Zingiberis(干姜 *gan jiang*)

Rhizoma Zingiberis is the dried rhizome of the perennial plant Zingiber officinale (Willd.) Rosc. of Zingiberaceae. Grown in most parts of China, particularly Sichuan and Guizhou provinces, it is harvested in winter, washed and dried in the sun or baked until dry, with the stem, leaves and fibrous roots removed.

Taste and Property: Acrid, and hot.
Attributive Meridian: Spleen, stomach, heart and lung meridians.
Actions and Indications:

(1) To warm the middle *jiao*. It is indicated for either excess or deficiency cold syndrome of the spleen and stomach, with symptoms of cold and pain in the epigastrium and abdomen, vomiting and diarrhea. It can be used alone or combined with Radix Codonopsis Pilosulae, Rhizoma Atractylodis Macrocephalae and Radix Glycyrrhizae, as in Decoction for Regulating the Middle *Jiao*. For vomiting due to stomach cold, it is often combined with Rhizoma Pinelliae.

(2) To restore *yang*. Indicated for *yang* exhaustion syndrome. It is used with Radix Aconiti Lateralis Preparata to help restore *yang*, prevent collapse and reduce the toxicity of Radix Aconiti Lateralis Preparata.

(3) To warm the lung and resolve phlegm and accumulated fluid. It is indicated for cases due to accumulation of cold phlegm and fluid in the lung, marked by cough, dyspnea, aversion to cold, cold in the back, and profuse and dilute sputum. For such cases, it is often combined with Herba Asari and Fructus Schisandrae.

(4) To warm the meridians and stop bleeding. It is indicated to hematemesis, hematochezia and metrorrhagia due to deficiency and cold; here, Terra Flava Usta, Folium Artemisiae Argyi and Colla Corii Asini are often added.

Dosage and Preparation: 3-10 g. Usually used crude, and for hemorrhage due to deficiency and cold, it is baked until black (Rhizoma Zingiberis Preparata).

Precaution: For pregnant women, it should be applied with caution.
Remarks: Rhizoma Zingiberis Recens, Rhizoma Zingiberis and Rhizoma Zingiberis Preparata can all warm the middle *jiao*. But Zingiberis Recens is acrid and warm, and mainly used to dispel wind and cold; Rhizoma Zingiberis, acrid and hot, is good for warming the middle *jiao* and restoring exhausted *yang*; and Zingiberis Preparata, bitter and warm, is mainly used to warm the meridians and stop bleeding.

Cortex Cinnamomi(肉桂 *rou gui*)

Cortex Cinnamomi refers to the bark of the stem and main branches of the evergreen tree Cinnamomum cassia Presl. of Lauraceae. The bark with the epidermis removed is known as *gui xin*, and the bark from the main branches or the stem of the young tree is known as *guan gui*. It is mainly produced in Guangdong Province and the Guangxi Zhuang Autonomous Region. The bark is cut open apart before the Great Heat (12th solar term) and cut off from the tree after the Beginning of Autumn (13th solar term) with cork scraped off.

Taste and Property: Acrid and sweet, and hot.
Attributive Meridian: Kidney, spleen heart and liver meridians.
Actions and Indications:

(1) To warm kidney *yang*. Indications: (a) Insufficient kidney *yang* leading to the decline of fire of the life gate, marked by soreness and weakness of the lumbar region and knee joints, aversion to cold, cold limbs, frequent urination and impotence. For such cases, it is often combined with Radix Aconiti Lateralis Preparata, Radix Rehmanniae Preparata and Fructus Corni. (b) Deficiency cold in the lower *jiao* and upward floating of asthenic *yang*, manifested as flushed face, sore throat with a purplish color and cold lower limbs; for which it is often used with Cortex Cinnamomi to "conduct the fire back to its source." (c) Kidney dysfunction in receiving *qi*, marked by dyspnea with difficulty to lie flat, cold limbs and sweating on the forehead; for this it is often combined with Radix Aconiti Lateralis Preparata, Lignum Aquilariae Resinatum and Fructus Schisandrae to warm the kidney and enhance kidney function.

(2) To dispel cold, reopen the meridians and relieve pain. Indications: (a) Stomachache and abdominal pain due to spleen and stomach deficiency cold, lower abdominal pain and hernia pain due to cold retained in the liver meridian, and dysmenorrhea. (b) *Bi*-syndrome and lumbago due to cold and dampness.

It promotes the production of *qi* and blood and is frequently used in recipes to replenish *qi* and blood. It is also indicated for unruptured or unhealed festers.
Dosage and Preparation: 2-5 g in decoction and decocted later; or 1-2 g in powder. As *guan gui* is milder, its dosage can be increased accordingly.
Precaution: Contraindicated for patients with *yin* deficiency, interior heat and extravasation of blood due to heat in the blood, as well as pregnant women.
Remarks: Ramulus Cinnamomi and Cortex Cinnamomi are derived from the same plant, and both dispel cold and warm the meridians. The former tends to go up and is mainly

used to dispel cold and relieve exterior syndrome; the latter is mainly used to warm the interior and treat disorders of the lower *jiao*.

Cortex Cinnamomi, Rhizoma Zingiberis and Radix Aconiti Lateralis Preparata are all acrid and hot, and serve to warm *yang*. They are often combined. Cortex Cinnamomi warms the kidney and meridians and dispels cold from the blood system; Rhizoma Zingiberis warms the spleen, and also resolves phlegm and fluid and stops bleeding; and Radix Aconiti Lateralis Preparata warms *yang* of the whole body, and is especially good for restoring exhausted *yang* and preventing collapse. Attention should be paid to their special indications.

Fructus Evodiae(吴茱萸 *wu zhu yu*)

Fructus Evodiae is the mature fruit of the deciduous shrub or tree Evodia rutaecarpa (Juss.) Benth., or other plants of the same genus of Rutaceae. Mainly produced in Sichuan, Yunnan, Guizhou and Hunan provinces, it is collected in the period from August to November when the fruit is nearly ripe but not yet cracked, and dried in the sun or under low temperature, with the branches, leaves and foreign matter removed.

Taste and Property: Acrid and bitter, hot and slightly toxic.
Attributive Meridian: Liver, spleen and stomach meridians.
Actions and Indications:

(1) To dispel cold and relieve pain. It is indicated for stomachache, abdominal pain, hernia pain and pain in beriberi due to accumulation of cold. For such cases, it is combined with other drugs that dispel cold and relieve pain. For stomachache due to cold, it is used with Rhizoma Zingiberis and Semen Alpiniae Katsumadai; for abdominal pain due to cold, it is combined with Ramulus Cinnamomi and Herba Asari; for hernia pain due to cold, it is combined with Radix Linderae and Fructus Foeniculi; and for beriberi with pain, it is prescribed together with Fructus Chaenomelis and Semen Arecae.

(2) To suppress the adverse upward flow of *qi* and relieve vomiting. It is indicated for vomiting and acid regurgitation. For cases caused by cold in the stomach, it is combined with Rhizoma Zingiberis to warm the middle *jiao* and dispel cold; for cases with a bitter taste in the mouth and hypochondriac pain due to stagnant liver *qi* that turns into fire affecting the stomach, it is often used with Rhizoma Coptidis, as in *Zuojin* Pill.

The drug is also effective in treating headache and frothy vomiting due to deficiency cold in the middle *jiao* and upward displacement of liver *qi* associated with cold and turbidity; this is because it can warm the middle *jiao*, dispel cold, suppress the adverse upward flow of *qi* and relieve vomiting. Besides, it can also be used to treat diarrhea due to cold and dampness.

Dosage and Preparation: 1.5-5 g. Soaked in the decoction of Radix Glycyrrhizae before use.

Precaution: The drug is acrid, hot and dry, and likely to produce fire and consume body fluid. It is, therefore, not advisable for prolonged use. In addition, it is contraindicated for patients with *yin* deficiency due to internal heat.

Herba Asari(细辛 *xi xin*)

Herba Asari refers to the whole plant of the perennial herb Asarum heterotropoides Fr. var. mandshuricum (Maxim.) Kitag, or A. siebolbii Miq. of Aristolochiaceae. The former is mainly produced in Liaoning, Jilin and Heilongjiang provinces; the latter in Shaanxi province. It is collected in summer and dried in the shade.

Taste and Property: Acrid, and warm.
Attributive Meridian: Lung and kidney meridians.
Actions and Indications:

(1) To eliminate wind, dispel cold and relieve pain. It is indicated for *bi*-syndrome, headache, toothache and abdominal pain, especially pain due to cold. For *bi*-syndrome due to cold and dampness, it is used with Radix Angelicae Pubescentis and Radix Aconiti to relieve pain; for headache due to wind and cold, it is prescribed together with Rhizoma seu Radix Notopterygii, Radix Ledebouriellae and Rhizoma Chuanxiong to eliminate wind and stop pain; for toothache, it is used alone as a decoction for gargling, or combined with Radix Angelicae Dahuricae; and for cases complicated by heat syndrome, it is combined with Gypsum Fibrosum.

For exterior syndrome with predominant cold, marked by severe headache and general achiness, it can be added to acrid-warm prescriptions for relieving exterior syndrome in order to help dispel cold and relieve pain. For exterior syndrome in a *yang* deficient constitution, marked by severe chills, slight fever and deep pulse, it is used in combination with Herba Ephedrae and Radix Aconiti Lateralis Preparata, as in Decoction of Ephedrae, Aconiti Lateralis and Asari, to promote *yang* and relieve exterior syndrome.

(2) To warm the lung and resolve accumulated fluid. It is indicated for retention of cold and fluid in the lung, marked by cough and dyspnea with expectoration of profuse and dilute sputum; here it is combined with Ephedrae, Rhizoma Zingiberis and Fructus Schisandrae.

(3) To relieve nasal obstruction. It is indicated for sinusitis (including chronic rhinitis and paranasal sinusitis), marked by headache, nasal obstruction and clear nasal discharge. For such cases, it is often combined with Radix Angelicae Dahuricae, Herba Menthae and Flos Magnoliae.

Dosage: 1-3 g.
Precaution: It is incompatible with Rhizoma et Radix Veratri.
Remarks: Since Herba Asari has a strong acrid and aromatic flavor and dispersive action, it is contraindicated for patients with profuse sweating due to *qi* deficiency, headache due to *yin* deficiency leading to hyperactive *yang*, and cough due to deficient *yin* and lung heat. Large dosage should be avoided.

Pericarpium Zanthoxyli(花椒 *hua jiao*)

Pericarpium Zanthoxyli refers to the pericarp of the shrub or tree Zanthoxylum schinifolium Sieb. et Zucc., or Z. bungeanum Maxim. of Rutaceae. Mainly produced in Sichuan, Henan, Shaanxi and Shandong provinces, it is collected in autumn when the fruit gets cracked, and dried in the sun.

Synonym: *Chuan jiao, shu jiao.*
Taste and Property: Acrid, and hot.
Attributive Meridian: Spleen and stomach meridians.
Actions and Indications:

(1) To warm the middle *jiao* and relieve pain. It is indicated for epigastric and abdominal pain due to deficiency cold in the middle *jiao*, for which it is often combined with Rhizoma Zingiberis and Radix Codonopsis Pilosulae.

(2) Anthelminthic. It is indicated for ascariasis with abdominal pain, or vomiting of ascarids. For such cases, it is often combined with Fructus Mume.

Dosage: 2-5 g.

Rhizoma Alpiniae Officinarum(高良姜 *gao liang jiang*)

Rhizoma Alpiniae Officinarum is the rhizome of the perennial herb Alpinia officinarum Hance of Zingiberaceae. Produced in Guangdong, Taiwan and Yunnan provinces, as well as the Guangxi Zhuang Autonomous Region, it is collected in late summer and early autumn, then dried in the sun.

Taste and Property: Acrid, and warm.
Attributive Meridian: Spleen and stomach meridians.
Actions and Indications:

To warm the middle *jiao* and relieve pain. It is indicated for cold retained in the middle *jiao*, marked by epigastric and abdominal pain, vomiting and diarrhea. For epigastric pain due to stomach cold, it is often used with Rhizoma Cyperi, as in Pill of Alpiniae Officinarum and Cyperi; for abdominal cold pain and diarrhea, it is used with Cortex Cinnamomi and Cortex Magnoliae Officinalis; and for vomiting due to cold in the stomach, it is often combined with Rhizoma Pinelliae and Rhizoma Zingiberis Recens.

Dosage: 3-10 g.

Flos Caryophylli(丁香 *ding xiang*)

Flos Caryophylli refers to the flower bud of the evergreen tree Eugenia caryophyllata Thunb. of Myrtaceae. Mainly produced in Southwest Africa and Southeast Asia, and also cultivated in Guangdong Province of China, it is usually gathered from September to March of the next year when the flower bud turns red. With the pedicel removed, it is then dried in the sun.

Taste and Property: Acrid, and warm.
Attributive Meridian: Spleen, stomach and kidney meridians.

Actions and Indications:

(1) To warm the middle *jiao* and suppress the adverse rise of *qi*. It is indicated for hiccup due to cold in the stomach. For such cases, it is often used with Calyx Kaki, Radix Ginseng and Rhizoma Zingiberis Recens, as in Powder of Caryophylli and Kaki. It can also be used to treat stomachache and vomiting due to cold.

(2) To warm the kidney and promote *yang*. It is indicated for insufficient kidney *yang* that leads to impotence and lower abdominal cold pain; here it is often prescribed together with Radix Morindae Officinalis and Herba Cistanches.

Dosage: 2-5 g.

Precaution: The drug is incompatible with Radix Curcumae.

Remarks: Flos Caryophylli is an important drug for the treatment of hiccup due to cold in the stomach, and also vomiting due to stomach cold and epigastric and abdominal pain due to cold. The crude drug is divided into two kinds: its flower bud is called Flos Caryophylli, with a stronger fragrant smell and action; its fruit is called Fructus Caryophylli, with a milder fragrant smell and action. The former is more frequently used in clinical practice.

Fructus Foeniculi(小茴香 *xiao hui xiang*)

Fructus Foeniculi is the fruit of the perennial plant Foeniculum vulgare Mill. of Umbelliferae. Cultivated in various parts of China, the whole plant is cut and collected in late summer and early autumn when the fruit is ripe and dried in the sun. Finally, the fruit is knocked off and kept for use.

Taste and Property: Acrid, and warm.

Attributive Meridian: Liver, spleen and stomach meridians.

Actions and Indications:

(1) To dispel cold and relieve pain. It is indicated for hernia pain due to cold and weighted pain in the testis, for which it is often combined with Semen Citri Reticulatae, Semen Litchi and Radix Linderae.

(2) To regulate *qi* circulation and pacify the stomach. It is indicated for epigastric and abdominal distention and pain, vomiting and anorexia. For such cases, it is often used with Rhizoma Zingiberis and Radix Aucklandiae.

Dosage: 3-8 g.

Table 8. Actions of Drugs for Warming the Interior

Drug	Similarities	Differences
Radix Aconiti Lateralis Praeparata	Dispel cold, relieve pain and warm *yang*	To warm *yang* of the whole body; important drug of restoring the depleted *yang*
Rhizoma Zingiberis		To warm spleen mainly and lung as well, warm meridians and stop bleeding; adjuvant for restoring the depleted *yang*
Cortex Cinnamomi		To warm the kidney *yang* mainly, and dispel cold from the *xue* system as well
Fructus Evodiae	Dispel cold and relieve pain	To lower the adverse *qi*, relieve vomiting and acid regurgitation; treat *Jueyin* headache
Herba Asari		To dispel wind and cold in the exterior; and resolve accumulated fluids and remove nasal obstruction
Pericarpium Zanthoxyli		To warm mainly spleen and stomach and expel ascarid
Rhizoma Alpiniae Officinarum		To warm spleen and stomach
Flos Caryophylli		To lower the adverse *qi* and treat hiccup due to cold in stomach
Fructus Foeniculi		Good for treating hernia pain

Note: Other sections deal with additional drugs that warm the interior, such as Ramulus Cinnamomi, Rhizoma Zingiberis Recens and Folium Artemisiae Argyi.

CHAPTER ELEVEN
DRUGS FOR REGULATING *QI*

Drugs that regulate *qi*, promote the free flow of *qi* and relieve *qi* stagnation are known as drugs for regulating *qi* (*li qi yao*).

Most of these drugs are acrid, warm and aromatic, and can invigorate *qi* circulation, relieve symptoms of the middle *jiao*, relieve *qi* stagnation, stop pain, suppress the adverse rise of *qi*, strengthen the spleen and harmonize the stomach. They are indicated for spleen and stomach *qi* stagnation marked by epigastric and abdominal distensive pain and poor appetite; liver *qi* stagnation marked by hypochondriac pain; the adverse rise of stomach *qi* marked by nausea, vomiting, belching and hiccup; and the adverse rise of lung *qi* marked by cough and dyspnea.

Qi stagnation and the adverse rise of *qi* can be divided into four types: cold, heat, deficiency and excess, and drugs that regulate *qi* should be prescribed together with other drugs in line with the different conditions. For instance, for *qi* stagnation accompanied by cold retention, drugs that regulate *qi* are combined with drugs that warm the interior; for stagnant *qi* that turns into fire, they are used with drugs for purging heat; for *qi* stagnation complicated by phlegm and dampness retention, they are combined with drugs that resolve phlegm and remove dampness; for stagnation of both *qi* and blood, they are used with drugs that activate blood circulation; for *qi* stagnation due to food stasis, they are used with digestives; for cases due to spleen and stomach deficiency, they are combined with drugs that strengthen the spleen and replenish *qi*.

Drugs for regulating *qi* are usually warm and dry, and likely consume *qi* and *yin*. And so attention should be paid to their application.

Pericarpium Citri Reticulatae(橘皮 *ju pi*)

Pericarpium Citri Reticulatae is the peel of the mature fruit of the evergreen tree Citrus reticulata Blanco and its cultivated species of Rutaceae. Mainly produced in Guangdong, Fujian and Zhejiang provinces, the fruit ripens in autumn, and the peel is kept and dried in the sun or in the shade.

Synonym: *Chen pi*, *xin hui pi*, *guang pi*.
Taste and Property: Acrid and bitter, and warm.
Attributive Meridian: Spleen and lung meridians.
Actions and Indications:

(1) To invigorate *qi* circulation, strengthen the spleen and pacify the stomach. It is indicated for spleen and stomach *qi* stagnation, marked by epigastric and abdominal distensive pain, dyspepsia, anorexia, nausea and vomiting. For such cases, it is often combined with other drugs that regulate *qi* circulation, such as Radix Aucklandiae and Fructus Amomi. For patients with spleen deficiency, it is used with Radix Codonopsis Pilosulae, Rhizoma Atractylodis Macrocephalae, etc. For vomiting, it is used with Rhizoma Pinelliae and Rhizoma Zingiberis Recens.

(2) To eliminate dampness and resolve phlegm. It is indicated for dampness and phlegm retention marked by cough, stuffiness in the chest and expectoration of copious white sputum. Here, it is often combined with Rhizoma Pinelliae and Poria, as in *Erchen* Decoction, to dry dampness and resolve phlegm.

Dosage: 5-10 g.

APPENDIX:

Exocarpium Citri Rubrum(橘红 *ju hong*)

It is the exocarp of the immature Citrus grandis Blanco of Rutaceae. It is bitter, acrid and warm, and invigorates *qi* circulation and relieves stagnation in the middle *jiao*, eliminates dampness and resolves phlegm. It is indicated for spleen and stomach *qi* stagnation, as well as cough with profuse expectoration of sputum and stuffiness in the chest. The dosage is 3-10 g.

Pericarpium Citri Reticulatae Viride(青皮 *qing pi*)

Pericarpium Citri Reticulatae Viride is the green exocarp of the immature fruit of the evergreen tree Citrus reticulata Blanco, or its cultivated species. It is collected in the May-June period, washed and dried in the sun. The big ones are first boiled in water, then dried in the sun with the pulp removed.

Taste and Property: Bitter and acrid, and warm.

Attributive Meridian: Liver and stomach meridians.

Actions and Indications:

(1) To remove *qi* stagnation and disperse liver *qi*. It is indicated for liver *qi* stagnation with such symptoms as hypochondriac distention and pain, or lump and distensive pain in the breast. For such cases, it is often used with Radix Bupleuri and Rhizoma Cyperi. For hernia pain, it is used with Fructus Foeniculi and Fructus Toosendan.

(2) To remove food stasis. It is indicated for dyspepsia, for which it is combined with Fructus Crataegi and Fructus Hordei Germinatus.

Dosage: 5-10 g.

Remarks: Both Pericarpium Citri Reticulatae and Pericarpium Citri Reticulatae Viride refer to the exocarp of the mandarin orange; they are different in maturity and action. The former mainly regulates spleen and stomach *qi*, resolves phlegm and eliminates dampness; the latter removes *qi* stagnation and relieves food stasis, and is better at invigorating *qi* circulation.

Fructus Aurantii Immaturus(枳实 *zhi shi*)

Fructus Aurantii Immaturus is the immature fruit of the evergreen tree Citrus aurantium L. and its cultivated species C. sinensis Osbeck of Rutaceae. Mainly produced in Jiangsu, Zhejiang, Sichuan, Jiangxi and Fujian provinces, it is collected in July and August, crosscut into two halves, and dried in the sun and then finally cut into smaller pieces.

Taste and Property: Bitter and acrid, and slightly cold.
Attributive Meridian: Spleen, stomach and large intestine meridians.
Actions and Indications:

(1) To remove stagnant *qi* and relieve food stasis. It is indicated for gastrointestinal stasis. To this end, it is often combined with digestives, such as Fructus Crataegi and Massa Medicata Fermentata. For patients with spleen and stomach deficiency, marked by dyspepsia, it is combined with Rhizoma Atractylodis Macrocephalae, as in Pill of Aurantii Immaturus and Atractylodis Macrocephalae. For patients with constipation, it is used with Radix et Rhizoma Rhei.

(2) To resolve phlegm and relieve fullness and stuffiness. It is indicated for obstruction of the *qi* passages by phlegm and turbidity, leading to stuffiness and fullness in the chest and epigastrium. For such cases, it is often combined with Rhizoma Pinelliae and Pericarpium Citri Reticulatae. For patients with phlegm heat, it may be used with Rhizoma Coptidis and Fructus Trichosanthis. It can also be prescribed for chest *bi*-syndrome due to the *qi* obstruction.

It is also indicated for gastroptosis, rectal prolapse and hysteroptosis; here it is combined with Radix Astragali and Rhizoma Cimicifugae.
Dosage: 3-10 g.

APPENDIX:
Fructus Aurantii(枳壳 *zhi ke*)

It is the mature fruit of Citrus aurantium. L. and its cultivated species, with the pulp removed. Its taste, property and action are similar to and milder than Fructus Aurantii Immaturus. It can invigorate *qi* circulation and relieve stagnancy in the middle *jiao*. It is often used to treat epigastric and abdominal distention and pain, and poor appetite. The recommended dosage is 3-10 g. It is used either crude or after baking.

Remarks: Fructus Aurantii Immaturus and Fructus Aurantii are derived from the same plant but different in maturity. Both invigorate *qi* circulation. However, the former is stronger than the latter, and more often used to relieve gastrointestinal stasis; the latter is often used to remove stagnancy in the middle *jiao*.

Fructus Citri(香橼 *xiang yuan*)

Fructus Citri is the fruit of Citrus medica L. , or C. Wilsonii Tanaka, an evergreen tree of Rutaceae. Mainly produced in Jiangsu, Zhejiang and Guangdong provinces as well as the Guangxi Zhuang Autonomous Region, it is collected in September and October when the fruit is ripe, cut into thin pieces and dried in the sun.

Taste and Property: Acrid and slightly bitter, sour and warm.
Attributive Meridian: Liver, spleen and lung meridians.
Actions and Indications:

(1) To invigorate *qi* circulation. It is indicated for stagnation of liver, spleen and stomach *qi*, marked by hypochondriac, epigastric and abdominal distention and pain, belching and poor appetite; here it is often combined with other drugs that regulate *qi*, such as Rhizoma Cyperi and Radix Aucklandiae.

(2) To resolve phlegm. It is often used with Rhizoma Pinelliae and Poria to cure productive cough.

Dosage: 5-10 g.

APPENDIX:

Fructus Citri Sarcodactylis(佛手 *fo shou*)

It is the fruit of Citrus medica L. var. sarcodactylis Swingle, an evergreen tree or shrub of Rutaceae. It is acrid, bitter and warm. With similar actions and indications as Fructus Citri, i. e. , to invigorate *qi* circulation and resolve phlegm. It is indicated for syndromes of liver and spleen *qi* stagnation, and cough with expectoration of profuse sputum. The recommended dosage is 5-10 g.

Remarks: Pericarpium Citri Reticulatae, Pericarpium Citri Reticulatae Viride, Exocarpium Citri Rubrum, Fructus Aurantii Immaturus, Fructus Aurantii, Fructus Citri and Fructus Citri Sarcodactylis are fruits or exocarp of orange, the tangerine, or other citrus of the same genius. They all invigorate *qi* circulation and resolve phlegm, and are mainly indicated for liver and spleen *qi* stagnation, and cough with expectoration of profuse sputum. Generally, the immature ones, such as Citri Reticulatae Viride and Aurantii Immaturus, are stronger. The mature ones, such as Citri Reticulata and Aurantii, are milder.

Radix Aucklandiae(木香 *mu xiang*)

Radix Aucklandiae refers to the root of the perennial herb Aucklandia lappa Decne. of Compositae. Mainly produced in Yunnan Province, it is collected in autumn and winter, with foreign matter and fibrous roots removed, then cut into segments. The large ones are cut again vertically into pieces and dried, and the rough outer covering is removed.

Taste and Property: Acrid and bitter, and warm.
Attributive Meridian: Spleen, stomach and large intestine meridians.
Actions and Indications:

To invigorate *qi* circulation and stop pain, and particularly to remove *qi* stagnation in the spleen, stomach and large intestine. Indications: (a) Spleen and stomach *qi* stagnation, marked by epigastric and abdominal distention and pain, and anorexia. For such cases, it is often combined with Fructus Amomi and Pericarpium Citri Reticulatae to intensify the invigoration of *qi*. For spleen deficiency with impaired transforming and transporting functions leading to anorexia, abdominal distention and diarrhea, it is used with Radix Codonopsis Pilosulae and Rhizoma Atractylodis Macrocephalae to regulate *qi* circulation and strengthen the spleen. (b) Diarrhea and dysentery due to dampness-heat and *qi* stagnation in the large intestine, marked by abdominal pain and tenesmus. For such cases, it is often combined with Rhizoma Coptidis, as in Pill of Aucklandiae and Coptidis, to invigorate *qi*, stop pain, purge heat and eliminate dampness.

Dosage and Preparation: 3-10 g; used crude to invigorate *qi* circulation, and burnt to relieve diarrhea. Do not decoct for a long time.

Rhizoma Cyperi(香附 *xiang fu*)

Rhizoma Cyperi is the rhizome of the perennial herb Cyperus rotundus L. of Cyperaceae. Mainly produced in Guangdong, Henan, Sichuan and Shandong provinces, it is collected in autumn, slightly cooked in boiling water or steamed with the fine fibrous root burnt and then dried in the sun, or else dried in the sun just after the fibrous roots have been burnt.

Taste and Property: Acrid and slightly bitter, and mild.

Attributive Meridian: Liver meridian.

Actions and Indications:

(1) To invigorate *qi* circulation and appease the liver. It is indicated for liver *qi* stagnation marked by distention and pain in the hypochondrium, epigastrium and abdomen. For such cases, it is often combined with Radix Bupleuri and Fructus Aurantii to regulate liver *qi*. For cases accompanied by heat, it is prescribed together with Fructus Gardeniae to purge heat. For those marked by cold, it is used with Rhizoma Alpiniae Officinarum, as in Pill of Alpiniae Officinarum and Cyperi, to promote the free flow of liver *qi* and dispel cold.

(2) To regulate menstruation and stop pain. It is indicated for liver *qi* stagnation, and irregular menstruation with premenstrual distention and pain in the breasts, hypochondriac and lower abdominal pain. For such cases, it is often combined with Radix Bupleuri, Radix Angelicae Sinensis and Rhizoma Chuanxiong to appease the liver, invigorate *qi* circulation and harmonize the *qi* and blood.

Dosage and Preparation: 5-10 g; used either in crude form or baked with vinegar.

Radix Linderae(乌药 *wu yao*)

Radix Linderae is the root of the evergreen shrub or tree Lindera strychnifolia (Sieb. et Zucc.) Vill. of Lauraceae. Mainly produced in Zhejiang, Anhui and Jiangxi provinces, the root is collected in August, washed, cut into thin pieces and dried in the sun.

Taste and Property: Acrid, and warm.
Attributive Meridian: Spleen, kidney and urinary bladder meridians.
Actions and Indications:

To invigorate *qi* circulation, dispel cold and kill pain. It is indicated for epigastric and abdominal distention and pain, and dysmenorrhea. For such cases, it is often combined with other drugs that regulate *qi* and relieve pain, such as Rhizoma Cyperi and Radix Aucklandiae. For hernia pain, it is prescribed with Fructus Foeniculi and Fructus Toosendan.

It also warms the kidney, dispels cold and eliminates cold from the urinary bladder, and is therefore indicated for deficiency cold in the lower *jiao*, marked by frequent urination and enuresis; here it is often combined with Fructus Alpiniae Oxyphyllae and Rhizoma Dioscoreae, as in Pill for Decreasing Urination.

Dosage: 5-10 g.
Remarks: Radix Aucklandiae, Rhizoma Cyperi and Radix Linderae all invigorate *qi* circulation and stop pain. They are often used in combination. However, Radix Aucklandiae, warm and dry, can invigorate *qi* stagnation in the spleen, stomach and large intestine, and is indicated for epigastric and abdominal distention and pain, diarrhea and dysentery with tenesmus. Rhizoma Cyperi promotes and regulates the flow of liver *qi* and regulates menstruation, and is indicated for syndromes of liver *qi* stagnation; and it is important for gynecological diseases. Radix Linderae, which dispels cold and enters the lower *jiao*, can be applied for cold retention in the urinary bladder, which is manifested as frequent urination, urgent urination and distention and pain in the lower abdomen.

Lignum Aquilariae Resinatum(沉香 *chen xiang*)

Lignum Aquilariae Resinatum is the wood with black resin of the evergreen tree Aquilaria agallocha Roxb., or A. sinensis (Lour.) Gilg. of Thymelaeaceae. The former is mainly produced in India and Malaysia and also cultivated in Taiwan and Guangdong provinces as well as the Guangxi Zhuang Autonomous Region of China; the latter is mainly produced in Hainan Province. It can be cut and collected any time of the year, the resinous wood is taken and dried in the shade.

Taste and Property: Acrid and bitter, and warm.
Attributive Meridian: Spleen, stomach and kidney meridians.
Actions and Indications:

(1) To invigorate *qi* circulation and kill pain. It is indicated for epigastric and abdominal pain due to *qi* stagnation. For such cases, it is often combined with Radix Aucklandiae and Radix Linderae.

(2) To suppress the adverse rise of *qi* and stop vomiting. It is indicated for hiccup and vomiting due to stomach cold. For such diseases, it is often used with Fructus Amomi Rotundus and Flos Caryophylli.

(3) To suppress the adverse rise of *qi* and relieve dyspnea. It is indicated for dyspnea

and excess phlegm syndrome. Here, it is combined with Semen Lepidii seu Descurainiae, Semen Armeniacae Amarum and Rhizoma Pinelliae. For impaired kidney function in receiving *qi*, it is used with Radix Rehmanniae Preparata and Fructus Psoraleae.

Dosage and Preparation: 1-3 g, decocted later; 0. 5-1. 5 g in powder form and taken with boiled water.

Remarks: This drug is good at invigorating *qi* circulation and relieving pain, especially cases due to the adverse rise of lung and stomach *qi*. It is often applied in treating hiccup, vomiting and dyspnea. Since it can warm the kidney and help it receive *qi*, it is often used to cure dyspnea due to kidney failure in receiving *qi*.

Lignum Aquilariae Resinatum can be prepared as a decoction, long decoction results in loss of fragrance, and so it is better to be taken as powder.

Rhizoma Corydalis(延胡索 *yan hu suo*)

Rhizoma Corydalis is the tuber of the perennial herb Corydalis turtschaninovii Bess. f. yanhusuo Y. H. chou et C. C. Hsu of Papaveraceae. Mainly produced in Zhejiang and Hebei provinces, it is collected after the Beginning of Summer. Having the seedlings and fibrous roots removed, it is washed clean, cooked in boiling water until its interior turns yellow, and then dried in the sun.

Synonym: *Xuan hu suo*, *yuan hu suo*.

Taste and Property: Acrid and bitter, and warm.

Attributive Meridian: Heart, liver and spleen meridians.

Actions and Indications:

To invigorate *qi* and blood circulation and relieve pain. It is indicated for various kinds of pain caused by *qi* and blood stagnation, such as epigastric pain, hypochondriac pain, hernia pain, dysmenorrhea and pain due to traumatic injuries. It can be prescribed either alone or with other drugs according to the specific symptoms. For patients with *qi* stagnation, it is combined with Rhizoma Cyperi, Pericarpium Citri Reticulatae Viride and Radix Aucklandiae; for cases due to blood stasis, it is used with Semen Persicae and Flos Carthami; for cases due to heat, it is combined with Fructus Toosendan; and for cases due to cold, it is used with Rhizoma Alpiniae Officinarum and Cortex Cinnamomi.

Dosage and Preparation: 3-10 g in decoction; and 1. 5-3. 0 g in powder; used either crude or baked with vinegar.

Remarks: Rhizoma Corydalis invigorates *qi* and blood circulation, and relieves pain, and is indicated for various kinds of pain due to *qi* and blood stagnation.

Fructus Toosendan(川楝子 *chuan lian zi*)

Fructus Toosendan refers to the mature fruit of the deciduous tree Melia toosendan Sieb. et Zucc. of Meliaceae. Mainly produced in Sichuan Province, it is collected in winter when the fruit is ripe, and dried in the sun.

Synonym: *Lian shi*, *jin lian zi*, *ku lian zi*.
Taste and Property: Bitter and cold, and slightly toxic.
Attributive Meridian: Liver meridian.
Actions and Indications:

(1) To invigorate *qi* circulation and relieve pain. It is indicated for hypochondriac, epigastric and abdominal pain due to liver and stomach *qi* stagnation, especially cases of a heat nature. For such cases, it is often combined with Rhizoma Corydalis, as in Powder of Toosendan. For hernia pain, it is used with Fructus Foeniculi and Pericarpium Citri Reticulatae Viride.

(2) Anthelminthic. Indications: (a) Abdominal pain due to helminthiasis, for which it is combined with Semen Arecae and Fructus Quisqualis. (b) Tinea capitis, for which it is ground into fine powder and mixed with lard or sesame oil for external application.
Dosage: 5-10 g. A moderate amount for external application.

Bulbus Allii Macrostemi(薤白 *xie bai*)

Bulbus Allii Macrostemi is the underground bulb of the perennial herb of Allium macrostemon Bge. of Liliaceae. Mainly produced in Jiangsu and Zhejiang provinces, it is collected in summer and autumn, washed clean with the fibrous roots removed, steamed or soaked in boiling water, and then dried in the sun.

Taste and Property: Acrid and bitter, and warm.
Attributive Meridian: Lung, stomach and large intestine meridians.
Actions and Indications:

To activate *qi* flow and invigorate stagnant *yang*. It is indicated for chest *bi*-syndrome due to obstruction of the chest by phlegm and turbidity and stagnant *yang qi*, marked by stuffiness and pain in the chest and shortness of breath. For such cases, it is often combined with Fructus Trichosanthis and Rhizoma Pinelliae. For cases accompanied by blood stagnation, it is used with drugs that activates blood circulation, such as Rhizoma Chuanxiong, Flos Carthami and Radix Salviae Miltiorrhizae.

It is also indicated for dysentery with tenesmus.
Dosage: 5-10 g.

Table 9. Actions of Drugs for Regulating *Qi*

Drug	Similarities	Differences
Pericarpium Citri Reticulatae	To activate circulation of *qi* and resolve phlegm	To activate stagnated *qi* circulation of spleen and stomach; dry dampness and resolve phlegm
Pericarpium Citri Reticulatae Viride		To promote flow of liver *qi*, remove stagnation of *qi*, and remove stagnancy
Fructus Aurantii Immaturus		To remove stagnation of *qi* and stasis; to resolve phlegm and relieve fullness and stuffiness
Fructus Aurantii		To activate circulation of *qi* and alleviate stagnation in the middle *jiao*
Fructus Citri		To activate the stagnated *qi* circulation of liver, spleen and stomach
Radix Aucklandiae	To activate circulation of *qi* and relieve pain	To activate mainly the stagnated *qi* circulation of the spleen, stomach and large intestine
Rhizoma Cyperi		To promote the flow of liver *qi* and regulate the menstruation; an important drug for women's diseases
Radix Linderae		With the action of entering the lower *jiao*, it is applied in treating lower abdominal pain and frequent urination
Lignum Aquilariae Resinatum		To lower the adverse *qi*, relieve dyspnea, vomiting and hiccup
Rhizoma Corydalis		To activate circulation of *qi* and blood, used in pain due to stagnated *qi* and blood
Fructus Toosendan		To activate circulation of liver *qi*, used in pain especially of heat nature, used as anthelminthic
Bulbus Allii Macrostemi		To activate the stagnated *yang qi*, mainly used in treating chest *bi*-syndrome

Note: Other sections discuss additional drugs that activate 1qi0 circulation. They include Folium Perillae, Cortex Magnoliae Officinalis, Fructus Amomi, Fructus Amomi Rotundus, Flos Caryophylli, Rhizoma Chuanxiong, Olibanum, Myrrha, Radix Curcumae, Rhizoma Zedoariae, Semen Raphani, Semen Arecae and Pericarpium Arecae.

CHAPTER TWELVE
DIGESTIVES

Drugs that promote digestion and help remove food stasis are known as digestives (*xiao shi yao*). They are mainly indicated for diseases due to food stasis, manifested as distention and fullness in the epigastrium and abdomen, anorexia, belching, acid regurgitation, nausea and vomiting, and disorders of defecation, along with dyspepsia and poor appetite due to spleen and stomach deficiency.

Food stasis usually leads to *qi* stagnation, and since activating *qi* circulation help digestion, digestives are usually combined with drugs that activate *qi* circulation. In cases of food stasis accompanied by constipation, digestives are combined with purgatives; for dyspepsia due to spleen and stomach deficiency, they are used together with drugs that strengthen these organs; for cases complicated by cold, they are prescribed together with drugs that warm the interior; for cases with dampness, they are combined with drugs that remove dampness; and for cases due to heat derived from pathogens, they are used with drugs that eliminate heat.

Fructus Crataegi(山楂 *shan zha*)

Fructus Crataegi refers to the mature fruit of the deciduous tree or shrub Crataegus pinnatifida Bge. var. major N. E. Br., C. pinnatifida Bge., or C. cuneata Sieb. et Zucc. of Rosaceae. The former two are planted mainly in Shandong, Hebei, Henan and Liaoning provinces, and the latter mainly in Jiangsu, Zhejiang, Yunnan and Sichuan provinces. It is collected in autumn when the fruit is ripe. The former are cut into slices and dried, and the latter bathed in boiling water and dried afterwards, or dried directly.

Taste and Property: Sour and sweet, and slightly warm.
Attributive Meridian: Spleen, stomach and liver meridians.
Actions and Indications:

(1) To improve digestion and eliminate food stasis. It is indicated for food stasis, especially that caused by meat. Here, it is used either alone or in combination with Massa Medicata Fermentata, Fructus Hordei Germinatus and Semen Raphani. It is also indicated for diarrhea and dysentery complicated by food stasis.

(2) To invigorate blood circulation and remove stasis. It is indicated for postpartum abdominal pain, lochiostasis and dysmenorrhea due to blood stasis, for which it can be used either alone and prepared into a decoction and taken with granulated sugar, or in

combination with Radix Angelicae Sinensis, Rhizoma Chuanxiong and Herba Leonuri. It can also be applied for abdominal masses, as in hepatomegaly and splenomegaly.

Dosage and Preparation: 5-10 g; baked and charred to improve digestion, and used in crude form to remove blood stasis.

Massa Fermentata Medicinalis(神曲 *shen qu*)

Massa Fermentata Medicinalis refers to the fermented mixture of flour and certain drugs. The flour and bran, Semen Armeniacae Amarum (pounded), Semen Phaseoli (powder) and the juice from fresh Herba Artemisae Annuae, Herba Polygoni Hydropiperis and Herba Xanthii are mixed and made into small bricks, put in a basket and covered with flax leaves, kept warm and ferment for about one week until the hyphae grows out (with yellow coating), and finally dried in the sun.

Synonym: *Liu qu*, *liu shen qu*.

Taste and Property: Sweet and acrid, and warm.

Attributive Meridian: Spleen and stomach meridians.

Actions and Indications:

To promote digestion and regulate the stomach. It is indicated for indigestion and food stasis, especially that caused by rice and flour, which leads to epigastric and abdominal distention and stuffiness, foul belching and anorexia, as well as for food stasis complicated by diarrhea and dysentery. For such cases, it is often used with Fructus Crataegi and Semen Raphani.

Massa Fermentata Medicinalis is usually added to pills containing minerals that are difficult to digest and absorb, decocted into paste and prepared into pills. One example is Pill of Magnetitum and Cinnabaris, in which it is used as the excipient to promote digestion.

Dosage: 6-12 g.

Fructus Hordei Germinatus(麦芽 *mai ya*)

Fructus Hordei Germinatus is the dried germinated ripe fruit of the annual plant Hordeum vulgare L. of Gramineae. The fruits are soaked in water and kept under appropriate temperature and humidity until the plumules grow to a length of about 0. 5 cm. It is then taken out and dried in the sun or baked dry in mild temperature.

Taste and Property: Sweet, and mild.

Attributive Meridian: Spleen and stomach meridians.

Actions and Indications:

(1) To promote digestion. Indicated for indigestion and food stasis, especially that caused by rice and flour. For such cases, it is often combined with Fructus Oryzae Germinatus and Massa Fermentata Medicinalis. For poor appetite due to spleen dysfunction, it is often used with drugs that replenish *qi* and strengthen the spleen, such as Radix

Codonopsis Pilosulae and Rhizoma Atractylodis Macrocephalae. It is also indicated for milk indigestion in infants.

(2) To inhibit milk secretion. It is used for cessation of milk secretion in women after breast feeding, or for distensive pain in the breasts due to excessive accumulation of milk, for which it is used alone and in crude form in large dosage and prepared into oral decoction.

Dosage: 10-15 g; and 60-90 g for cessation of milk secretion.

Precaution: Contraindicated for women during breast feeding.

Fructus Oryzae Germinatus(谷芽 *gu ya*)

Fructus Oryzae Germinatus is the dried germinated fruit of the annual herb Oryza sativa L. of Gramineae. First, they are soaked in water, kept under appropriate temperature and humidity until the plumules grow to a length of about 1 cm., then taken out and dried in the sun.

Synonym: *Dao ya.*

Taste and Property: Sweet, and mild.

Attributive Meridian: Spleen and stomach meridians.

Actions and Indications:

To promote digestion and strengthen the spleen. Indicated for indigestion and food stasis. Its action is similar to Fructus Hordei Germinatus but milder; the two are often used in combination to enhance the digestive effect. For spleen and stomach deficiency marked by poor appetite and indigestion, it is often combined with Rhizoma Atractylodis Macrocephalae, Radix Glycyrrhizae Preparata and Fructus Amomi, as in *Gushen* Pill, to strengthen spleen function.

Dosage: 10-15 g.

Semen Raphani(莱服子 *lai fu zi*)

Semen Raphani is the mature seed of the annual or biennial plant Raphanus sativus L. of Cruciferae. Cultivated in most parts of China, the whole plant is cut in summer and autumn when the seeds are ripe and dried in the sun, then the seeds are rubbed out and dried again, with foreign matter removed.

Synonym: *Luo bo zi.*

Taste and Property: Acrid and sweet, and mild.

Attributive Meridian: Spleen, stomach and lung meridians.

Actions and Indications:

(1) To promote digestion and relieve distention. It is indicated for food stasis and *qi* stagnation marked by epigastric and abdominal distention and fullness, belching, acid regurgitation, unsmooth bowel movements or diarrhea. Here, it is often used in combination with Massa Fermentata Medicinalis, Fructus Crataegi and Pericarpium Citri Reticulatae,

as in Pill for Promoting Digestion, to promote digestion, invigorate *qi* circulation and remove stagnation. Nowadays, it is applied for severe abdominal distention and pain as well as constipation (as seen in simple intestinal obstruction). For such cases, it is often combined with Radix et Rhizoma Rhei, Natrii Sulfas, Fructus Aurantii Immaturus and Cortex Magnoliae Officinalis.

(2) To suppress the adverse rise of *qi* and resolve phlegm. It is indicated for accumulation of phlegm and obstruction of *qi* circulation, marked by cough, dyspnea and expectoration of abundant sputum. For such cases, it is often prescribed along with Semen Sinapis Albae and Fructus Perillae, as in Decoction Containing Three Kinds of Seed for the Aged, to suppress the adverse rise of *qi*, resolve phlegm, and relieve cough and dyspnea.

Dosage and Preparation: 5-10 g; used crude or after baking.

Remarks: In addition to promoting digestion, Semen Raphani is good for invigorating *qi* circulation, and is indicated for distention and fullness due to stagnant *qi*, especially abdominal distention due to food stasis and *qi* stagnation. It can also suppress the adverse rise of lung *qi* and resolve phlegm and turbidity, and is often applied when accumulated phlegm obstructs *qi* and impaired the descending function of the lung, leading to dyspneic cough with copious sputum. But since it can consume *qi*, it should be applied with caution in cases of *qi* deficiency.

Endothelium Corneum Gigeriae Galli(鸡内金 *ji nei jin*)

Endothelium Corneum Gigeriae Galli is the dried membrane of the gizzard of the Gallus domesticus Brisson of Phasianidae. When the chicken is slaughtered, the gizzard is cut open, the lining membrane is peeled off, washed clean and dried in the sun.

Synonym: *Ji zhun pi*.

Taste and Property: Sweet, and mild.

Attributive Meridian: Spleen, stomach, kidney and urinary bladder meridians.

Actions and Indications:

(1) To be used as a digestive. It is effective in treating dyspepsia, food stasis and infantile malnutrition, for which it is used either alone or in combination with Fructus Hordei Germinatus and Massa Fermentata Medicinalis. For spleen dysfunction in transformation and transportation marked by loss of appetite, it is combined with drugs that invigorate the spleen, such as Radix Codonopsis Pilosulae and Rhizoma Atractylodis Macrocephalae.

(2) To be used as an astringent. It is effective in treating enuresis and frequent urination, for which it is often used with Ootheca Mantidis and Concha Osthrae. For nocturnal emission, it is often combined with Semen Cuscutae, Semen Euryales and Semen Nelumbinis. For this purpose, it can also be used singly and prepared into a powder.

It also removes stones, and is indicated for urinary calculus and biliary calculus.

Dosage: 5-10 g in decoction, and 1.5-3 g in powder.

Table 10. Actions of the Digestives

Drug	Similarities	Differences
Fructus Crataegi	To promote digestion and strengthen the stomach	Good for relieving meat indigestion; to remove blood stasis
Massa Fermentata Medicinalis		To relieve rice and flour food indigestion
Fructus Hordei Germinatus		To relieve rice and flour food indigestion and to inhibit milk secretion
Fructus Oryzae Germinatus		To relieve rice and flour food indigestion
Semen Raphani		To activate *qi* circulation, relieve distention; lower the adverse *qi* and resolve phlegm
Endothelium Corneum Gigeriae Galli		Strong effect in promoting digestion; and to astringe the kidney essence, relieve enuresis and remove calculi

Note: Other sections discuss additional drugs that promote digestion, such as Cortex Magnoliae Officinalis, Fructus Aurantii Immaturus, Pericarpium Citri Reticulatae Viride, Rhizoma Zedoariae and Semen Arecae.

CHAPTER THIRTEEN
ANTHELMINTICS

Drugs that expel or kill intestinal worms are known as anthelmintics (*qu chong yao*). They are mainly used to kill or expel such intestinal parasitoses as ascariasis, ancylostomiasis, oxyuriasis, taeniasis and fasciolopsis, with symptoms of abdominal distensive pain around the umbilicus, loss of appetite, or polyorexia and paroxia, pruritus of the anus, ear and nose, and sallow complexion and emaciation.

One or several anthelmintics are applied depending on the parasites, the patient's constitution and the accompanying symptoms. Certain other drugs are also added. For example, for patients with constipation and strong constitution, purgatives are added to help expel the parasites; for those with spleen and stomach deficiency, add drugs that strengthen the spleen and stomach so that the parasites are expelled but the organs remain uninjured; for cases accompanied by dyspepsia, digestives are added; for cases of cold retention, drugs that warm the interior are added; and for protracted diseases accompanied by weak constitution, tonics can be prescribed first and anthelmintics later, or both applied at the same time. For cases of ascariasis with severe abdominal pain, first apply drugs that calm the ascarids to relieve the colic, and give anthelmintics afterwards when the pain is relieved.

Generally, anthelmintics are used in larger dosages and they should be taken empty-stomached so that the drugs can directly act on the parasites to achieve better effects. Toxic anthelmintics should be applied with caution for pregnant women, asthenic and senile patients. During the application of anthelmintics, attention should be paid to personal hygiene so as to prevent superinfection.

Fructus Quisqualis(使君子 *shi jun zi*)

Fructus Quisqualis is the mature fruit of the vine-like shrub Quisqualis indica L. of Combretaceae. Mainly produced in Sichuan and Guangdong provinces as well as the Guangxi Zhuang Autonomous Region, it is collected in autumn when the epidermis turns purplish black, and dried in the sun.

Taste and Property: Sweet, and warm.
Attributive Meridian: Spleen, stomach and large intestine meridians.
Actions and Indications:

To expel parasites and strengthen the spleen. It is indicated for ascariasis and infantile malnutrition. For such cases, it can be used either alone or else combined with Cortex Meliae and Semen Arecae to enhance the anthelmintic effect. For infantile malnutrition complicated by serious parasitosis, manifested as sallow complexion, emaciation, abdominal distention and loose stools, it is often used with Semen Arecae, Endothelium Corneum Gigeriae Galli, Radix Codonopsis Pilosulae and Rhizoma Atractylodis Macrocephalae to expel worms, remove stasis and improve spleen and stomach functions.

Dosage and Preparation: 6-10 g; pounded into pieces and prepared into decoction; or with the pulp stir-baked and taken directly. The dosage for children should vary with age, i. e. one piece for one year of age and 20 at the maximum.

Precaution: Overdose or long-term administration of the drug with hot tea may cause hiccup, vomiting and dizziness; this can be relieved after a period of suspension, or by frequent doses of Flos Caryophylli Decoction.

Cortex Meliae(苦楝皮 *ku lian pi*)

Cortex Meliae refers to the bark of the root or stem of the tree Melia azedarach L. and M. toosendan Sieb. et Zucc. of Meliaceae. Produced in most places of China, it is collected in spring and autumn, and dried in the sun with the brownish epidermis scraped off.

Taste and Property: Bitter and cold, and toxic.

Attributive Meridian: Spleen, stomach and liver meridians.

Actions and Indications:

To expel parasites. It is indicated for ascariasis, oxyuriasis, ancylostomiasis and vaginal trichomoniasis. It can be administered either alone or together with Semen Arecae and Fructus Evodiae; For vaginal trichomoniasis, it is combined with Fructus Cnidii to produce a decoction for external washing, or else prepared into a suppository.

This drug can also be used to treat tinea capitis and scabies; here it is prepared into a decoction for external washing or ground into a powder that is mixed with lard for external application.

Dosage and Preparation: 10-15 g, or 15-30 g (fresh), prepared into decoction. Moderate amount for external application.

Precaution: This drug is toxic, and overdosage should be avoided. It should be applied with care for patients with liver disorders.

Remarks: Both Fructus Quisqualis and Cortex Meliae are frequently used as anthelmintics. The former has a sweet taste and can strengthen the spleen; it is less toxic and has fewer side effects, and is suitable for children. The latter has strong anthelmintic action (the fresh root cortex is even stronger); it is strongly toxic and produces more side effects. Overdosage may cause dizziness, headache, somnolence, nausea and abdominal pain. In severe cases, it may cause visceral hemorrhage, toxic hepatitis, mental derangement and visual disturbance, and even death. Special attention should be paid to these adverse effects.

Semen Arecae(槟榔 *bing lang*)

Semen Arecae is the mature seed of the evergreen tree Areca catechu L. of Palmae. Produced mainly in Guangdong, Hainan, Yunnan, Fujian and Taiwan provinces and the Guangxi Zhuang Autonomous Region, it is collected in winter and spring when the fruit is ripe. Having the exocarp removed, the seeds are taken out and dried in the sun.

Synonym: *Hai nan zi*, *da fu zi*.
Taste and Property: Bitter and acrid, and warm.
Attributive Meridian: Spleen, stomach and large intestine meridians.
Actions and Indications:

(1) To expel parasites. Indicated for various intestinal parasitoses, such as teniasis, fasciolopsis, ascariasis and oxyuriasis, especially the former two. Since its mild laxative action helps expel the worms, it can be used alone and prepared into powder for oral administration. If combined with Semen Cucurbitae, it would produce a better effect in expelling tapeworms.

(2) To promote *qi* circulation and relieve stagnation. It is indicated for food stasis and *qi* stagnation, manifested as epigastric and abdominal distention and pain, foul belching and acid regurgitation, dyschezia or dysentery with abdominal pain and tenesmus. Here, it is often combined with Radix Aucklandiae and Fructus Aurantii Immatures.

(3) To activate *qi* circulation and promote diuresis. Indicated for edema of the excess type and abdominal distention due to stagnant *qi*. For such cases, it is often used with Cortex Magnoliae Officinalis, Rhizoma Atractylodis Macrocephalae and Rhizoma Alismatis.

Dosage: 6-15 g; and 60-100 g for anthelmintic purposes.

APPENDIX:

Pericarpium Arecae(大腹皮 *da fu pi*)

This is the pericarp of Areca catechu (Palmae). Acrid and slightly warm, it is effective in activating *qi* circulation, removing stagnation and promoting diuresis, and is indicated for *qi* and dampness stagnation exhibiting such symptoms of epigastric and abdominal distention and fullness, edema and beriberi. The usual dosage is 5-10 g.

Remarks: Semen Arecae is not only effective in expelling worms but also in activating *qi* circulation, removing stagnation and promoting diuresis; it is often applied in treating food stagnation, abdominal distention, dysentery and edema. The dosage should vary accordingly.

Semen Cucurbitae(南瓜子 *nan gua zi*)

Semen Cucurbitae refers to the seed of Cucurbita moschata Duch. of Cucurbitaceae. Cultivated in most parts of China, it is collected between summer and autumn when the fruit is ripe. The seeds are washed clean and dried in the sun.

Taste and Property: Sweet, and warm.
Attributive Meridian: Large intestine meridian.
Actions and Indications:

To be used as an anthelmintic. It is indicated for teniasis and ascariasis, especially the former. For such cases, it is used with Semen Arecae to enhance the effect.

Dosage and Preparation: 30-60 g; and 120 g in a single-drug prescription. Prepared into decoction or ground (together with shells) into powder for oral administration.

Gemma Agrimoniae(鹤草芽 *he cao ya*)

Gemma Agrimoniae is the winter bud of the perennial herb Agrimonia pilosa Ledeb. of Rosaceae. It is collected in winter and early spring and dried in the sun or under low temperature.

Taste and Property: Bitter, astringent and cool.
Attributive Meridian: Large intestine meridian.
Actions and Indications:

To kill parasites. It is indicated for teniasis. This drug is a new anthelmintic effective for expelling and killing tapeworms, which are usually discharged 5-6 hours after its application. External local application can also treat vaginal trichomoniasis.

Dosage and Preparation: 30 g for adults; for children, the dosage is calculated at the rate of 0.7-0.8 g for per kilogram of body weight. Ground into fine powder and taken once in the morning when the stomach is empty.

Precaution: This drug is difficult to dissolve in water, so it is not advisable to be prescribed as a decoction.

Omphalia(雷丸 *lei wan*)

Omphalia is the dried sclerotium of the fungus Omphalia lapidescens Schroet. of Tricholomataceae, which grows as a parasite on the bamboo roots. Produced mainly in Sichuan, Guizhou and Yunnan provinces as well as the Guangxi Zhuang Autonomous Region, it is collected in autumn by digging out the sclerotium on the morbid bamboo (with withered and yellow leaves), and dried in the sun.

Taste and Property: Bitter, cold and slightly toxic.
Attributive Meridian: Stomach and large intestine meridians.
Actions and Indications:

To kill parasites. Indicated for such intestinal parasitoses as teniasis, ancylostomiasis and ascariasis, especially the former two. It can be used either alone or in combination with Semen Arecae and Fructus Quisqualis.

Dosage and Preparation: 15-20 g; ground into powder, taken with cold boiled water, 2-3 times a day for three successive days.

Remarks: The active ingredients will be destroyed at high temperature, so it is not advisable to prepare it as a decoction.

Fructus Carpesii(鹤虱 *he shi*)

Fructus Carpesii is the fruit of the perennial plant Carpesium abrotanoides L. of Compositae, which is distributed mainly in Henan, Shanxi, Shaanxi and Gansu provinces; or the fruit of the biennial plant Daucus carota L. of Umbelliferae, which is known as Fructus Carotae and produced mainly in Jiangsu, Zhejiang, Anhui and Sichuan provinces. Both are collected in autumn when they are ripe.

Taste and Property: Bitter and acrid, mild and slightly toxic.
Attributive Meridian: Spleen, stomach and large intestine meridians.
Actions and Indications:

To kill parasites. Indicated for such intestinal parasitoses as ascariasis, oxyuriasis and teniasis. For such cases, it is combined with Fructus Quisqualis, Fructus Meliae and Semen Arecae.
Dosage: 10-15 g.

Semen Torreyae(榧子 *fei zi*)

Semen Torreyae refers to the mature seed of the evergreen tree Torreya grandis Fort. of Taxaceae. Produced mainly in Zhejiang, Anhui, Jiangsu and Hubei provinces, the fruit is collected in autumn when it ripens. Having the fleshy exocarp removed, the seeds are taken out and dried in the sun.

Taste and Property: Sweet, and mild.
Attributive Meridian: Stomach, large intestine and lung meridians.
Actions and Indications:

To expel parasites. Indicated for such intestinal parasitoses as ascariasis, teniasis, ancylostomiasis, fasciolopsis and oxyuriasis, for which it is often combined with Semen Arecae, Fructus Carpesii and Fructus Evodiae. It is an effective and safe anthelmintic for its fat content that acts as a laxative to help expel intestinal parasites.

This drug can be used to cure cough due to lung dryness as it can moisten the lung.
Dosage and Preparation: 10-15 g, prepared as decoction. It can also be stir-baked for eating directly.

Rhizoma Dryopteris Crassirhizomae(贯众 *guan zhong*)

Rhizoma Dryopteris Crassirhizomae refers to the rhizome and petiole base of the perennial herb Dryopteris crassirhizoma Nakai. of Dryopteridaceae, Lunathyrium acrostichoides (Sw.) Ching of Lunathyriaceae, Woodwardia unigemmata (Makino) Nakai. of Woodwardiae, and Osmunda japonica Thunb. of Osmundaceae. The first is produced mainly in northeastern China, the second mainly in northern and central China, the third in eastern and southern China, and the last mainly in Henan Province and eastern China. Regardless of the species, it is collected in autumn and sun-baked dry, with the fibrous roots and part of the petiole removed.

Taste and Property: Bitter, and slightly cold and toxic.
Attributive Meridian: Liver and spleen meridians.
Actions and Indications:

(1) To kill parasites. Indicated for such intestinal parasitoses as oxyuriasis, teniasis, ancylostomiasis and ascariasis. For such cases, it is often combined with other anthelmintics to achieve better effects.

(2) To eliminate heat and toxicity. It is indicated for common cold due to wind-heat, and for eruptive febrile diseases and mumps. For such diseases, it is often used with Flos Lonicerae, Fructus Forsythiae, Folium Isatidis and other drugs with similar action.

(3) To stop bleeding. Indicated for hematemesis, epistaxis, hematochezia and metrorrhagia, especially those caused by extravasation due to heat in the blood. It can be prescribed either alone or else in combination with other hemostatics.

Dosage and Preparation: 10-15 g; usually used crude; charred by stir-baking for hemostatic treatment.

Table 11. Actions of the Anthelmintics

Drug	Similarities	Differences
Fructus Quisqualis	To expel and kill the intestinal parasites	To treat ascariasis
Cortex Meliae		To treat ascariasis and vaginal trichomoniasis
Semen Arecae		To treat teniasis and fasciolopsis, activate *qi* circulation, remove stagnancy and promote diuresis
Semen Cucurbitae		Mainly to treat teniasis
Gemma Agrimoniae		To treat teniasis and vaginal trichomoniasis
Omphalia		To treat teniasis, ancylostomiasis and ascariasis
Fructus Carpesii		To treat ascariasis, ancylostomiasis, etc.
Semen Torreyae		To treat ascariasis, ancylostomiasis, fasciolopsis, etc.
Rhizoma Dryopteris Crassirhizomae		To treat various intestinal parasitoses, clear heat and toxic materials, and stop bleeding

Note: Other sections discuss more drugs that also have anthelmintic action, such as Semen Pharbitidis, Pericarpium Zanthoxyli, Fructus Toosendan, and Fructus Mume.

CHAPTER FOURTEEN
HEMOSTATICS

Drugs that stop bleeding are known as hemostatics (*zhi xue yao*). They are indicated for various kinds of internal and external bleeding, such as hemoptysis, hematemesis, hematochezia, hematuria, metrorrhagia and traumatic hemorrhage.

Hemostatics are classified into those that cool the blood; those that astringe the blood; those that remove blood stasis; and those that warm the meridians. They are selectively applied and combined with other drugs to achieve satisfactory therapeutic results. For instance, in cases of bleeding due to heat in the blood, they are used together with drugs that eliminate heat and cool the blood; in cases complicated by deficient *yin* and hyperactive *yang*, they are prescribed along with drugs that replenish *yin* and purge fire; in cases of incessant bleeding due to blood stagnation, they are combined with drugs that invigorate *qi* and blood circulation; and in cases due to deficiency cold, they are used in combination with drugs that warm *yang*, replenish *qi* and strengthen the spleen. As for massive blood loss that causes *qi* deficiency and collapse, hemostatics used alone cannot produce a quick result, and powerful tonics for replenishing primordial *qi* should be prescribed first to replenish *qi* and prevent *qi* collapse.

For some hemostatics, stir-baking and charring can enhance the hemostatic effect; others should never be charred.

Since improper use of hemostatics for cooling and astringing the blood promotes blood stasis, such drugs should not be used alone in cases of bleeding accompanied by blood stagnation.

Herba seu Radix Cirsii Japonici(大蓟 *da ji*)

Herba seu Radix Cirsii Japonici refers to the aerial part or the root of the perennial plant Cirsium japonicum DC. of Compositae. To be found in most parts of China, the part above the ground is cut and collected in summer when the flowers are in full bloom, and dried in the sun; the root is dug in autumn and dried in the sun.

Taste and Property: Sweet and bitter, and cool.
Attributive Meridian: Heart and liver meridians.
Actions and Indications:

(1) To cool the blood and check bleeding. Indicated for bleeding due to heat in the blood, such as hematemesis, epistaxis, metrorrhagia and hematuria. It can be applied

alone or in combination with other hemostatics.

(2) To eliminate toxicity and cure carbuncles. Indicated for pulmonary abscess due to the accumulation of toxic heat in the lung. It can be taken orally, or else applied externally after pounding the fresh herb into pieces.

Dosage and Preparation: 10-15 g; used crude or charred. If the fresh herb is used, the dosage should be 30-60 g, prepared as a decoction or pounded into juice for oral administration.

Herba Cephalanoploris(小蓟 *xiao ji*)

Herba Cephalanoploris is the aerial part of the perennial herb Cephalanoplos segetum (Bge.) Kitam. of Compositae. To be found in most parts of China, it is collected in summer when the flowers are in blossom, washed clean and dried in the sun.

Taste and Property: Sweet, and cool.

Attributive Meridian: Heart and liver meridians.

Actions and Indications:

(1) To cool the blood and stop bleeding. Indicated for bleeding due to heat in the blood, such as hematemesis, hemoptysis, epistaxis, metrorrhagia, and especially hematuria. Here it is often combined with Pollen Typhae, Caulis Akebiae, Talcum and Radix Rehmanniae, as in Decoction of Cephalanoploris.

(2) To eliminate toxicity and relieve carbuncles. It is indicated for carbuncles due to toxic heat, for which it can be prepared into a decoction for oral administration, or else the fresh herb is pounded into pieces for external application.

Dosage and Preparation: 10-15 g; used either crude or charred. If used fresh, the dosage should be 30-60 g, prepared as a decoction or pounded into juice for oral administration.

Remarks: Both Herba seu Radix Cirsii Japonici and Herba Cephalanoploris cool the blood and stop bleeding, eliminate toxicity and relieve carbuncles; but the former is stronger than the latter.

Radix Sanguisorbae(地榆 *di yu*)

Radix Sanguisorbae is the root of the perennial plant Sanguisorba officinalis L. of Rosaceae. Produced mainly in Jiangsu, Zhejiang, Shandong and Hebei provinces, it is collected in spring and autumn, washed and dried in the sun.

Taste and Property: Bitter and sour, and slightly cold.

Attributive Meridian: Liver, stomach and large intestine meridians.

Actions and Indications:

(1) To cool blood and stop bleeding. It is indicated for bleeding due to heat in the blood, especially bleeding in the lower part of the body, such as hematochezia, hemorrhoids, hematuria and metrorrhagia. For such cases, it is combined with other related drugs in line with the specific conditions.

(2) To eliminate toxicity and promote the healing of skin diseases. It is indicated for scald, eczema and skin infections. For scald, it is prepared into fine powder and mixed with sesame oil for external application, or mixed with the powder of Radix et Rhizoma Rhei. For eczema and skin infections, the fresh herb is prepared as a decoction for wet compress, or the dried drug is made into a powder for external application.

This drug is also indicated for dysentery due to dampness-heat, especially cases with bloody stools.

Dosage and Preparation: 10-15 g; used in crude form or charred. Moderate dosage for external application.

Radix Boehmeriae(苎麻根 *zhu ma gen*)

Radix Boehmeriae is the root and rhizome of the perennial herb Boehmeria nivea (L.) Gaud. of Urticaceae. Produced mainly in Jiangsu, Shandong and Shaanxi provinces, it is collected in winter and spring, washed and dried in the sun.

Taste and Property: Sweet, and cold.
Attributive Meridian: Heart and liver meridians.
Actions and Indications:

(1) To cool the blood and stop bleeding. It is indicated for bleeding due to heat in the blood system, such as hemoptysis, hematemesis, metrorrhagia and purpura. For such cases, it can be used alone or combined with other drugs according to accompanying symptoms.

(2) To prevent miscarriage. It is indicated for threatened abortion with vaginal bleeding. For such cases, it can be used alone or combined with Radix Rehmanniae Preparata, Colla Corii Asini and Folium Artemisiae Argyi. For cases due to heat in the fetus, it is used with Radix Scutellariae.

(3) To eliminate toxicity and relieve carbuncles. It is indicated for carbuncles due to toxic heat. For such cases, the fresh root of the plant is pounded into pieces for external application. For erysipelas, the drug is prepared into a decoction for use as a topical lotion.

Dosage: 10-30 g. Moderate amount for external use.
Remarks: The root, stem and leaves of the plant can all stop bleeding, and the root is most frequently used. This drug is important for preventing miscarriage, and frequently applied to pregnant women suffering from restlessness of the fetus and incessant vaginal bleeding.

Folium Callicarpae Pedunculatae(紫珠 *zi zhu*)

Folium Callicarpae Pedunculatae refers to the leaf of the herb Callicarpa pedunculata R. Br. of Verbenaceae. Produced mainly in southern China, it is collected in summer and autumn when the leaves are luxuriant, and dried afterwards.

Taste and Property: Bitter, and cold.
Attributive Meridian: Liver meridian.
Actions and Indications:

(1) To cool the blood and stop bleeding. It is indicated for various kinds of internal and external bleeding, for which it is used either alone or combined with other related drugs. For bleeding due to trauma, it is prepared into powder, the fresh leaves are pounded into a paste for external application, or else it is made into a solution in which antiseptic gauze is soaked as a compress.

(2) To purge heat and toxicity. It is indicated for scald and skin infections, in which it is prepared into a powder for external application or made into a solution for wet dressing, and at the same time prepared into a decoction for oral administration.

Dosage and Preparation: 15-30 g in decoction; 2-3 g in powder. Moderate amount for external use.

Remarks: Folium Callicarpae Pedunculatae was originally a drug for purging heat and toxicity, and indicated for carbuncles and furuncles, snakebites and insect-stings. It has been used as a hemostatic agent only in modern times. It can be prepared into decoction, powder, juice and injection for hemoptysis, hematemesis, epistaxis, gingival bleeding, hematuria, hematochezia, metrorrhagia, trauma and oozing of blood from surgical incisions. For scalds, it controls infection, reduces the oozing of blood and promotes healing.

Rhizoma Imperatae(白茅根 *bai mao gen*)

Rhizoma Imperatae is the rhizome of the perennial herb Imperata cylindrica Beauv. var. major (Nees.) C. E. Hubb. of Gramineae. Produced in most places of China, it can be collected in any season, but its rhizome is dug out in winter and spring, washed and dried in the sun.

Taste and Property: Sweet, and cold.
Attributive Meridian: Lung, stomach and kidney meridians.
Actions and Indications:

(1) To cool the blood and stop bleeding. Indicated for bleeding due to heat in the blood, as in hematemesis, epistaxis and hematuria. For such cases, it can be used either alone or in combination with other hemostatics.

(2) To purge heat and promote diuresis. It is indicated for dysuria, stranguria due to heat, and edema. For such cases, it can be prescribed either alone or in combination with such diuretics as Herba Plantaginis.

This drug also purges heat from the lung and stomach, and is indicated for polydipsia in febrile diseases, vomiting due to heat in the stomach and cough caused by heat in the lung.

Dosage: 15-30 g, and 30-60 g if used fresh. The fresh is more effective.

Remarks: Both Rhizoma Imperatae and Rhizoma Phargmitis can purge heat from the lung and stomach. The former is more effective in cooling the blood and stopping bleeding, and mainly enters the blood system, while the latter purges heat, purges fire and promotes the secretion of fluid, and mainly enters the *qi* system.

Flos Sophorae(槐花 *huai hua*)

Flos Sophorae is the flower bud of the deciduous tree Sophora japonica L. of Leguminosae. Produced in most parts of China, it is collected in summer when the flower is going to bloom, and dried in the sun as soon as possible.

Synonym: *Huai mi*.
Taste and Property: Bitter, and slightly cold.
Attributive Meridian: Liver and large intestine meridians.
Actions and Indications:

(1) To cool the blood and stop bleeding. It is indicated for metrorrhagia, hemoptysis and epistaxis, hematochezia and hemorrhoids. For such cases, it is combined with Herba Schizonepetae, Cacumen Biotae and Fructus Aurantii, as in Powder of Flos Sophorae.

(2) To purge heat and pacify the liver. It is indicated for the flare-up of liver fire, marked by headache and flushed eyes. Now, it is also often used in treating hypertension. It can be prepared alone into a decoction to be drunk as tea, or in combination with Spica Prunellae, Flos Chrysanthemi and Radix Scutellariae.

Dosage and Preparation: 10-15 g; usually used in crude form, and charred to stop bleeding.

APPENDIX:

Fructus Sophorae(槐角 *huai jiao*)

It is the bean-like fruit of Sophora Japonica. Its taste, property and action are similar to those of Flos Sophorae. It is indicated for hematochezia and hemorrhoids, as well as headache and flushed eyes due to the flare-up of liver fire. The recommended dosage is 10-15 g. Used with care for pregnant women.

Remarks: Both Flos Sophorae and Fructus Sophorae cool the blood and stop bleeding, and are often employed to treat hemorrhoids and hematochezia. But Flos Sophorae is more effective in stopping bleeding, and Fructus Sophorae is more effective in purging liver fire and lubricating the intestines, and it is particularly effective for hemorrhoids with constipation and bleeding.

Cacumen Biotae(侧柏叶 *ce bai ye*)

Cacumen Biotae is the young twig and leaf of the evergreen tree Biota orientalis (L.) Endl. of Cupressaceae. Cultivated throughout China, the twigs and leaves can be gathered at any season of the year. They are cut off, dried in the shade and cut into segments.

Taste and Property: Bitter, astringent and slightly cold.
Attributive Meridian: Lung, liver and large intestine meridians.

Actions and Indications:

To cool the blood and stop bleeding. Indicated for bleeding due to heat in the blood, such as in hematemesis, hemoptysis, epistaxis, hematochezia, hematuria and metrorrhagia. For such cases, it can be used either alone to prepare into a powder for oral administration, or combined with the fresh herbs of Radix Rehmanniae, Folium Artemisiae Argyi and Folium Nelumbinis, as in Bolus of Four Fresh Drugs. For bleeding due to deficiency cold, it is combined with drugs that warm the meridians and stop bleeding, such as Rhizoma Zingiberis Preparata and Artemisiae Argyi, as in Decoction of Biotae.

This drug also resolves phlegm and relieves cough with expectoration of copious sputum due to lung heat.

Dosage and Preparation: 5-15 g; used either in crude form or charred.

Herba Agrimoniae(仙鹤草 *xian he cao*)

Herba Agrimoniae is the whole plant of the perennial herb Agrimonia pilosa Ledeb. of Rosaceae. Produced mainly in Zhejiang, Jiangsu and Hubei provinces, it is cut and collected between summer and autumn when the stem and leaves are luxuriant and the flowers are not yet in blossom, and dried in the sun.

Taste and Property: Bitter, astringent and mild.
Attributive Meridian: Lung, liver and spleen meridians.
Actions and Indications:

To stop bleeding by arresting secretion. It is indicated for various kinds of bleeding, such as hematemesis, hemoptysis, epistaxis, hematuria and metrorrhagia. For such cases, it is used alone or combined with other related drugs in line with the accompanying symptoms. The extraction from this drug can be prepared into tablets and injections that are frequently applied for various kinds of bleeding. In recent years, it has been made into hemostatic powder for bleeding after trauma and surgery.

This drug also removes food stasis, diarrhea and dysentery.

Dosage: 10-30 g.

Rhizoma Bletillae(白及 *bai ji*)

Rhizoma Bletillae is the tuber of the perennial herb Bletilla striata (Thunb.) Reichb. f. of Orchidaceae. Mainly produced in Guizhou, Sichuan and Zhejiang provinces, it is collected in autumn and winter, washed, steamed until the white color at its center disappears, and dried in the sun with its coarse outer coverings cracked off.

Taste and Property: Bitter and sweet, and astringent and slightly cold.
Attributive Meridian: Lung and stomach meridians.
Actions and Indications:

(1) To stop bleeding by astriction. It is indicated for bleeding in the lung and stomach, for which it is used alone to produce a decoction for oral use with rice soap. If com-

bined with the powder of Radix Notoginseng, the hemostatic effect is enhanced. For stomachache with acid regurgitation and hematemesis, it can be combined with Os Sepiae and prepared into powder, as in Powder of Os Sepiae and Bletillae. For bleeding due to trauma, it is ground into powder for external application.

(2) To relieve swelling and promote tissue regeneration. Indicated for carbuncles, boils and abscesses (whether ruptured or not), rhagadia of the skin of the hand and foot, and anal fissure. Used mainly for external application.

Dosage and Preparation: 5-10 g in decoction, and 2-5 g in powder. Moderate amount for external use.

Precaution: The drug is sticky and astringent, and is an important hemostatic and styptic agent for pulmonary and gastric bleeding. Recent pharmacological research shows that it has an inhibitory effect on tubercle bacilli, and so is indicated for pulmonary tuberculosis with or without bleeding.

Vagina Trichycarpi Carbonisatus(棕榈炭 *zong lu tan*)

Vagina Trichycarpi Carbonisatus refers to the palm fiber of the petiolar sheath of the evergreen tree Trachycarpus wagnerianus Becc. of Palmaceae. Mainly produced in Guangdong, Fujian and Hainan provinces, it is cut and collected around the Winter Solstice, put in an airtight container and charred for medical use.

Taste and Property: Bitter, astringent and mild.

Attributive Meridian: Lung, liver and large intestine meridians.

Actions and Indications:

To stop bleeding by astriction. Indicated for various kinds of bleeding without blood stagnation. It is used either alone or in combination with other hemostatics. For bleeding due to heat in the blood, it is combined with Cacumen Biotae, Rhizoma Imperatae and Cortex Moutan Radicis; for uterine bleeding due to hypofunction of the Chong and Ren meridians, it is combined with Radix Astragali, Os Sepiae and Radix Rubiae.

Dosage: 5-10 g in decoction, and 1-1.5 g in powder.

Radix Notoginseng(三七 *san qi*)

Radix Notoginseng is the root of the perennial herb Panax notoginseng (Burk.) F. H. Chen of Araliaceae. Produced mainly in Yunnan Province and the Guangxi Zhuang Autonomous Region, it is collected at the end of summer and the beginning of autumn before its flowers bloom, or else in winter after the seeds mature. The root that has grown for over three years is dug and collected, with foreign matter, the fine rootlets and stem base are removed; it is then partially dried in the sun, rubbed and kneaded repeatedly before being dried again in the sun.

Synonym: *Ren shen san qi, shen san qi, tian qi and dian qi.*

Taste and Property: Sweet and slightly bitter, and warm.

Attributive Meridian: Liver and stomach meridians.
Actions and Indications:

(1) To remove stagnant blood and stop bleeding. It is indicated for various kinds of bleeding, such as hematemesis, hemoptysis, epistaxis, hematochezia and metrorrhagia. Since it can remove blood stagnation without retaining stagnant blood during hemostasis, it is especially indicated for bleeding with retention of blood stasis. For such cases, it is used either alone and prepared into powder for oral use, or combined with Ophicalcitum and Crinis Carbonisatus. For gastric ulcer with hematemesis and hematochezia, it is often combined with Rhizoma Bletillae and Os Sepiae. For bleeding due to trauma, it is ground into powder for external application.

(2) To remove stagnant blood and relieve pain. Indicated for trauma, swelling and pain due to stagnant blood, for which it is used either alone or in combination with drugs that regulate *qi* and blood circulation. Recent research has proved that powder made of the drug alone, or powder of the drug combined along with Succinum and Radix Ginseng is fairly effective in treating coronary heart diseases and angina pectoris.

Dosage and Preparation: 1-3 g in powder for oral administration.

Radix Rubiae(茜草 *qian cao*)

Radix Rubiae is the root and rhizome of the perennial ivy-like plant Rubia cordifolia L. of Rubiaceae. Produced in most places of China, and mainly in Shaanxi, Hebei, Henan and Shandong provinces, it is collected in spring and autumn, and dried in the sun with foreign matters removed (but not be washed).

Synonym: *Ru lu*, *xue jian chou*.
Taste and Property: Bitter, and cold.
Attributive Meridian: Liver meridian.
Actions and Indications:

(1) To cool the blood and stop bleeding. Indicated for bleeding, as in hematemesis, hemoptysis, epistaxis, hematochezia, hematuria and metrorrhagia, particularly bleeding due to heat in the blood as well as bleeding with blood stagnation. For such cases, it is combined with Herba seu Radix Cirsii Japonici, Herba Cephalanoploris and Cortex Moutan Radicis.

(2) To activate blood circulation and promote menstruation. Indications: (a) Amenorrhea due to blood stagnation, for which it is combined with Semen Persicae, Flos Carthami, Radix Angelicae Sinensis and Radix Paeoniae Rubra. (b) Trauma and *bi*-syndrome due to wind-dampness, for which it is used alone and prepared as a decoction with equal amount of wine and water, or else combined with other drugs that activate blood circulation and remove stagnation in the meridians.

Dosage and Preparation: 10-15 g. Charred for hemostasis, and used crude for promoting menstruation.

Pollen Typhae(蒲黄 *pu huang*)

Pollen Typhae is the pollen of the hydrophyte herb Typha angustifolia L., or T. orientalis Presl. and other plants of Typhaceae. Produced mainly in Jiangsu, Zhejiang, Anhui and Shandong provinces, the yellow male spikes at the upper part of the flower cylinder of the cat-tail are collected in summer when the flower is going to bloom, dried in the sun, husked with a roller and sieved until the fine powder-like substance remains.

Taste and Property: Sweet, and mild.
Attributive Meridian: Liver meridian.
Actions and Indications:

(1) To stop bleeding. Indicated for bleeding, as in hematemesis, hemoptysis, hematochezia, and metrorrhagia. For such cases, it is combined with other related drugs. It also promotes diuresis, and is indicated for stranguria complicated by hematuria, for which it is often used with Herba Cephalanoploris.

(2) To remove blood stasis. Indicated for epigastric and abdominal pain, dysmenorrhea and postpartum abdominal pain caused by blood stagnation. Here, it is often combined with Faeces Trogopterorum, as in Powder for Dissipating Blood Stasis.

Dosage and Preparation: 5-10 g, wrapped for decoction. Baked for hemostasis, and crude for removing blood stagnation.

Crinis Carbonisatus(血余炭 *xue yu tan*)

Crinis Carbonisatus refers to the carbonized human hair. The hair is collected, with foreign matter removed, washed with washing soda, dried in the sun, kept in an airtight container and calcined, then cooled and ground into powder for medical use.

Taste and Property: Bitter, and mild.
Attributive Meridian: Liver and stomach meridians.
Actions and Indications:

To remove blood stasis and stop bleeding. Indicated for bleeding, as in hematemesis, epistaxis, hematochezia and metrorrhagia. For metrorrhagia, it is often combined with Vagina Trichycarpi Carbonisatus. For bleeding due to trauma, it is ground into powder for external use.

This drug also promotes diuresis and is proved effective for stranguria complicated by hematuria or stranguria due to heat.

Dosage: 5-10 g in decoction, and 1-3 g in powder.

Folium Artemisiae Argyi(艾叶 *ai ye*)

Folium Artemisiae Argyi refers to the leaf of the perennial herb Artemisia argyi Levl. et Vant. of Compositae. Produced in most places of the country, it is collected between spring and summer when the flower is not yet in bloom, then dried in the sun or in the shade.

Taste and Property: Bitter and acrid, and warm.
Attributive Meridian: Liver, spleen and kidney meridians.
Actions and Indications:

(1) To warm the meridians and stop bleeding. Indicated for bleeding due to deficiency cold, especially metrorrhagia and menorrhagia. Since it prevents miscarriage, it can be used to cure vaginal bleeding during pregnancy, for which it is often combined with Colla Corii Asini and Radix Rehmanniae. It can also be prescribed with the fresh Cacumen Biotae, Folium Nelumbinis, Radix Rehmanniae, as in Bolus of Four Fresh Drugs, for bleeding due to heat in blood.

(2) To dispel cold and relieve pain. It is indicated for deficiency cold in the lower *jiao*, such as abdominal cold pain in cases of protracted dysentery and dysmenorrhea, and infertility due to cold retained in the uterus. For such cases, it can be combined with Rhizoma Cyperi, Radix Angelicae Sinensis and Cortex Cinnamomi, as in Pill of Artemisiae Argyi and Cyperi for Warming the Uterus.

This drug can also be prepared into a decoction for external washing in cases of eczema and skin pruritus. It can also warm the meridians and activate *qi* and blood circulation when pounded into wool and made into moxa cones or moxa sticks to be applied on acupuncture points. It is indispensable for moxibustion therapy.

Dosage and Preparation: 3-10 g; charred for hemostasis, and used crude for other purposes. Moderate amount for external use.

Remarks: Folium Artemisiae Argyi is an important drug frequently used for gynecological diseases. Its indications are mainly deficiency and cold syndromes in the lower *jiao*, such as irregular menstruation, cold and pain in the lower abdomen, infertility due to cold in the uterus, metrorrhagia, leukorrhagia and vaginal bleeding during pregnancy.

Modern research has proved that the volatile oil of the drug has antitussive, expectorant and antiasmmatic effects, and can be applied for dyspneic and productive cough.

Table 12. Actions of Hemostatics

Drug	Similarities	Differences
Herba seu Radix Cirsii Japonici, Herba Cephalanoploris	To cool the blood and arrest bleeding; relieve toxic heat and treat carbuncle and ulcer	Used in various kinds of bleeding syndromes
Radix Sanguisorbae		Frequently used in hematochezia and metrorrhagia; can treat dysentery and burns
Radix Boehmeriae		To prevent abortion to ensure a successful gestation
Folium Callicarpae Pedunculatae		To treat burns

Drug	Similarities	Differences
Rhizoma Imperatae	To cool the blood and arrest bleeding	To clear heat and promote diuresis; clear heat from the lung and stomach
Flos Sophorae		To clear heat and pacify the liver
Cacumen Biotae		To resolve phlegm and relieve cough
Herba Agrimoniae	Hemostatic and styptic	To remove food stagnancy
Rhizoma Bletillae		Used mainly in bleeding of the lung and stomach; external use for relieving swelling and promoting tissue regeneration
Vagina Trichycarpi Carbonisatus		Used in various kinds of bleeding, especially metrorrhagia
Radix Notoginseng	To remove stagnated blood and arrest bleeding	Strong hemostatic effect; important drug for pain due to stagnated blood
Radix Rubiae		To activate blood circulation and promote menstruation
Pollen Typhae		Diuretic; often used in stranguria with hematuria; treat abdominal pain due to stagnation of blood
Crinis Carbonisatus		Diuretic; to treat stranguria with hematuria and stranguria due to heat
Folium Artemisiae Argyi		To warm meridians and arrest bleeding, to dispel cold and relieve pain

Note: Additional hemostatic drugs dealt in other sections of the book include Spica Schizonepetae Carbonisatus, Indigo Naturalis, Fructus Gardeniae, Cornu Rhinocerotis, Radix Rehmanniae, Cortex Moutan Radicis, Radix et Rhizoma Rhei, Rhizoma Zingiberis Preparata, Rhizoma Dryopteris Crassirhizomae, Colla Corii Asini, and Herba Ecliptae.

CHAPTER FIFTEEN

DRUGS FOR ACTIVATING BLOOD CIRCULATION AND REMOVING BLOOD STASIS

Drugs that activate blood flow and eliminate blood stagnation are known as *huo xue hua yu yao*; those with potent effect are known as *po xue yao* or *zhu yu yao*.

Drugs of this kind promote blood circulation, dispel stagnant blood, relieve pain, restore menstrual flow and relieve swelling. They are indicated for various kinds of diseases caused by blood stagnation or impeded blood circulation, such as pain in the chest, epigastrium and hypochondrium, masses in the abdomen, dysmenorrhea, amenorrhea, postpartum abdominal pain, trauma, rheumatic pain, carbuncles and ulcers.

Since smooth *qi* circulation can activate blood flow and *qi* stagnation causes blood stagnation, drugs that activate blood circulation and remove blood stasis are often combined with drugs that activate *qi*, so as to enhance their effects. In addition, they are combined with other related drugs according to different conditions. For instance, for blood stasis due to retained cold, they are combined with drugs that warm the interior; for carbuncles and ulcers due to toxic heat, they are prescribed together with drugs that eliminate heat and toxicity; for *bi*-syndrome due to wind and dampness, they are used with drugs that expel wind and dampness; for masses in the abdomen, they are combined with drugs that soften and resolve hard masses; and for patients with blood stasis and weak constitution, they are prescribed together with drugs that replenish *qi* and nourish blood.

Drugs for activating blood circulation and removing blood stasis should be applied with caution; they are contraindicated for menorrhagia and amenorrhea due to blood deficiency but without blood stasis, as well as for pregnant women.

Rhizoma Chuanxiong(川芎 *chuan xiong*)

Rhizoma Chuanxiong is the rhizome of the perennial herb Ligusticum chuanxiong Hort. of Umbelliferae. Produced mainly in Sichuan Province, it is dug and collected in summer when the nodes of the stem become very prominent and appear purplish. Having foreign matter and the fibrous roots removed, it is aired in the sun, and then baked dry.

Synonym: *Xiong qiong*.
Taste and Property: Acrid, and warm.
Attributive Meridian: Liver, gallbladder and pericardium meridians.
Actions and Indications:

(1) To activate *qi* and blood circulation. Indicated for various kinds of pain due to *qi* and blood stagnation: (a) Irregular menstruation, dysmenorrhea, amenorrhea and postpartum abdominal pain, for which it is used with Radix Angelicae Sinensis, Radix Paeoniae Rubra, Rhizoma Cyperi and Flos Carthami to invigorate *qi* and blood circulation, regulate menstruation and relieve pain. (b) *Bi*-syndrome in the chest, epigastric and hypochondriac stabbing pain, for which it is often combined with Radix Salviae Miltiorrhizae, Rhizoma Corydalis, Radix Bupleuri and Radix Curcumae to activate blood circulation, relieve pain and appease the liver and stomach. (c) Masses in the abdomen, numbness of the limbs, trauma and skin infections, for which it is combined with related drugs according to the concrete conditions.

(2) To eliminate wind and relieve pain. It is indicated for headache due to wind, and *bi*-syndrome due to wind-dampness. For headache due to wind-cold, it is used with Rhizoma seu Radix Notopterygii, Radix Angelicae Dahuricae and Herba Asari to dispel wind and cold; for headache due to wind-heat, it is combined with Flos Chrysanthemi, Gypsum Fibrosum and Bombyx Batryticatus to dispel wind and purge heat; and for headache due to blood deficiency, it is used with Angelicae Sinensis and Radix Paeoniae Alba to nourish the blood and eliminate wind.

Dosage: 3-10 g.

Precaution: Rhizoma Chuanxiong, acrid, warm and dispersing, invigorates *qi* and blood circulation, and regulates *qi* and activates the blood at the same time; it is especially effective for various kinds of pain caused by *qi* and blood stagnation, such as epigastric pain, hypochondriac pain, chest pain, dysmenorrhea, postpartum abdominal pain and rheumatic pain. Since it is good at eliminating wind and relieving pain, it is also an important drug for the treatment of all kinds of headache, such as that due to wind-cold, wind-heat, blood stasis and blood deficiency.

Olibanum(乳香 *ru xiang*)

Olibanum is the resin exuded from the bark of the small tree Boswellia carterii Birdw. of Burseraceae. Produced mainly in Somalia, Ethiopia, Turkey and Libya, it is collected in spring and summer, particularly in spring. The bark is cut from below, and the resin exudes from the cuts and condenses into masses several days later.

Synonym: *Xun lu xiang*.

Taste and Property: Acrid and bitter, and warm.

Attributive Meridian: Heart, liver and spleen meridians.

Actions and Indications:

(1) To promote blood and *qi* circulation and relieve pain. For its marked analgesic effect, it is frequently used for syndromes due to *qi* and blood stagnation. Indications: (a) Pain in the chest and abdomen (such as chest *bi*-syndrome with cardiac pain, stomachache and dysmenorrhea), and abdominal masses. For such cases, it is often combined with Myrrha, Radix Curcumae, Faeces Trogopterori and Pollen Typhae. (b) Trauma with blood stasis, for which it is used with Myrrha, Flos Carthami, Moschus and Borneolum

Syntheticum, as in Seven *Li* Powder; it can be used orally, or ground into a powder and paste for external application. (c) Rheumatic pain and muscle spasms, for which it is combined with Rhizoma seu Radix Notopterygii, Radix Angelicae Pubescentis, Radix Aconiti Kusnezoffii and Rhizoma Chuanxiong to dispel wind-cold, activate blood circulation, and ease the tendons and muscles.

(2) To relieve swelling and promote tissue regeneration. It is indicated for carbuncles at the initial stage, with local redness, swelling and pain. For such cases, it is often prescribed together with Flos Lonicerae, Radix Trichosanthis and Radix Paeoniae Rubra. For carbuncles that have ruptured and are unhealed, it is used with Myrrha to produce a powder for external application, as in Powder of Olibanum and Myrrha, to remove rotten tissues and promote granulation.

Dosage and Preparation: 3-10 g, defatted by baking. For external application, a moderate amount of the drug is ground into powder and prepared into paste.

Precaution: Contraindicated for pregnant women.

APPENDIX:

Myrrha(没药 *mo yao*)

Myrrha refers to the resin obtained from the bark of the shrub or tree Commiphora myrrha Engl. , or Balsamodendron ehrenbergianum Berg. of Burseraceae. Its taste and property, action and indications are similar to that of Olibanum, and the two are often used together. The recommended dosage is 3-10 g. It should be defatted by baking. The dosage for external application is modified according to actual needs. The drug is contraindicated for pregnant women.

Remarks: Both Olibanum and Myrrha are acrid and strongly aromatic, and can promote blood circulation, activate *qi* circulation, relieve pain and swelling, and promote granulation. With a remarkable analgesic effect, they are *qi*-regulating agents among drugs that activate blood circulation, and are effective for various syndromes due to *qi* and blood stagnation. They are often used together and widely applied in treating internal, gynecological, and especially traumatological and surgical disorders. Their difference lies in that Olibanum can also ease the tendons and muscles, while Myrrha is better at activating blood circulation and removing blood stasis.

Radix Curcumae(郁金 *yu jin*)

Radix Curcumae refers to the root tuber of the perennial herb Curcuma aromatica Salisb. , C. kwangsiensis S. Lee et C. F. Liang, C. longa L. , or C. zedoaria Rosc. of Zingiberaceae. Produced mainly in Sichuan and Zhejiang provinces, and the Guangxi Zhuang Autonomous Region, it is dug out in autumn and winter when the plant withers. Having the fibrous roots and foreign matter removed, the root tuber is washed, fully cooked in boiling water, taken out and dried in the sun, and then cut into slices.

Taste and Property: Acrid and bitter, and cool.

Attributive Meridian: Heart, liver and gallbladder meridians.

Actions and Indications:

(1) To invigorate *qi* and blood circulation. It is indicated for syndromes caused by *qi* and blood stagnation; because it regulates liver function, it is especially indicated for hypochondriac pain. For such cases, it is often combined with Radix Bupleuri, Fructus Aurantii, Rhizoma Cyperi and Rhizoma Chuanxiong.

(2) To facilitate gallbladder function and relieve jaundice. Indications: (a) Jaundice due to dampness-heat, for which it is often combined with Herba Artemisiae Scopariae, Radix et Rhizoma Rhei and Fructus Gardeniae. (b) Cholelithiasis, for which it is often used with Herba Lysimachiae and Artemisiae Scopariae.

(3) To resolve phlegm and relieve depression. Indications: (a) Manic-depressive psychosis, for which it is often combined with Alumen, as in Pill of Alumen and Lysimachiae. (b) Coma and delirium in acute febrile diseases due to the obstruction of the heart by phlegm-heat. For such cases, it is often combined with Rhizoma Acori Graminei, Succus Bambusae and Gardeniae.

It also cools blood, and is indicated for hematemesis, epistaxis and hematuria caused by blood-heat or complicated by *qi* and blood stagnation.

Dosage: 5-10 g.

Precaution: Radix Curcumae is incompatible with Flos Caryophylli.

Rhizoma Zedoariae(莪术 *e zhu*)

Rhizoma Zedoariae is the rhizome of the perennial herb Curcuma zedoaria Rosc., C. aromatica Salisb., or C. kwangsiensis S. Lee et C. F. Liang of Zingiberaceae. Produced mainly in the Guangxi Zhuang Autonomous Region as well as Zhejiang and Sichuan provinces, it is dug in autumn and winter, and steamed and then dried in the sun with foreign matter removed.

Synonym: *Peng e zhu.*

Taste and Property: Bitter and acrid, and warm.

Attributive Meridian: Liver and spleen meridians.

Actions and Indications:

(1) To break up blood stasis and activate blood circulation. It is indicated for amenorrhea, postpartum pain and traumatic pain due to *qi* and blood stagnation. For such cases, it is often combined with Rhizoma Sparganii and Rhizoma Chuanxiong to break up blood stasis, invigorate *qi* circulation and remove blood stagnation. For *qi* and blood stagnation associated with weak constitution, it is combined with Radix Codonopsis Pilosulae, Radix Astragali and Radix Angelicae Sinensis to replenish *qi* and at the same time avoid possible damage to the antipathogenic *qi*.

(2) To activate *qi* circulation and promote digestion. It is indicated for dyspepsia and *qi* stagnation marked by distention and pain in the epigastrium and abdomen. For these cases, it is often combined with Radix Aucklandiae, Fructus Aurantii Immaturus and Semen Arecae to promote *qi* circulation and digestion.

Dosage and Preparation: 6-10 g; prepared with vinegar.
Precaution: Contraindicated for pregnant women.

Rhizoma Sparganii(三棱 *san leng*)

Rhizoma Sparganii is the tuber of the perennial herb Sparganium stoloniferum Buch.-Ham. of Sparganiaceae. Produced mainly in Jiangsu, Henan and Shandong provinces, it is collected in winter and spring, washed clean, and dried in the sun with the outer skin peeled off.

Synonym: *Jing san leng.*
Taste and Property: Bitter and acrid, and mild.
Attributive Meridian: Liver and spleen meridians.
Actions and Indications:

To break up blood stasis, invigorate *qi* circulation and remove food stagnation. It is indicated for abdominal mass, cardiac and abdominal pain, hypochondriac distention and pain and amenorrhea due to *qi* and blood stagnation, and postpartum abdominal pain due to blood stasis and food stagnation. For such cases, it is often combined with Rhizoma Zedoariae.
Dosage and Preparation: 5-10 g; baked with vinegar.
Precaution: Contraindicated for pregnant women.
Remarks: Both Rhizoma Zedoariae and Rhizoma Sparganii are frequently used for treatment of abdominal masses, and they are often combined clinically. However, the former is better at activating *qi* circulation, and the latter at eliminating blood stasis.

Radix Salviae Miltiorrhizae(丹参 *dan shen*)

Radix Salviae Miltiorrhizae refers to the root and rhizome of the perennial herb Salvia miltiorrhiza Bge. of Labiatae. Produced in most places of China and mainly in Jiangsu, Anhui, Hebei and Sichuan provinces, it is collected in autumn, washed clean and dried in the sun.

Synonym: *Zi dan shen*, *hong gen.*
Taste and Property: Bitter, and slightly cold.
Attributive Meridian: Heart and liver meridians.
Actions and Indications:

(1) To activate blood circulation and remove blood stasis. It is indicated for syndromes due to blood stasis or retarded blood circulation: (a) Irregular menstruation, dysmenorrhea, amenorrhea, postpartum abdominal pain due to blood stagnation. For such cases, it is used either alone and prepared into powder for oral administration with wine, or else combined with other drugs that activate blood circulation and nourish blood. (b) Stabbing pain in the chest, epigastric and abdominal pain, for which it is often combined with Rhizoma Chuanxiong. (c) Abdominal masses, *bi*-syndrome and carbuncles, for

which it is used in combination with other drugs according to the concrete symptoms.

(2) To calm the mind. Indicated for febrile diseases that damage the *ying* system with symptom of restlessness; or palpitation and insomnia due to insufficient heart blood. Here it is often combined with drugs that purge heat from the heart and nourish the blood, such as Radix Rehmanniae, Rhizoma Coptidis, Semen Ziziphi Spinosae and Radix Angelicae Sinensis.

It also cools the blood and is often used in prescriptions for purging heat and cooling the blood, in the treatment of acute febrile diseases marked by affection of the *ying* and *xue* systems by pathogenic heat.

Dosage: 5-15 g.

Precaution: It is incompatible with Rhizoma et Radix Veratri.

Remarks: This drug is widely used, and is effective for various syndromes due to blood stasis by activating blood circulation and removing blood stasis; it is especially important for gynecological diseases. It is cold, and is particularly good for cases due to blood heat and blood stasis. Modern clinical research shows that it can be applied to treat coronary heart diseases and angina pectoris, cerebral vascular accidents, hepatomegaly and splenomegaly. For such cases, it has fairly good therapeutic effect in alleviating pain, reducing attacks, preventing cerebral thrombosis, promoting the recovery of the paralyzed limbs and reducing the abnormal enlargement of the liver and spleen.

Rhizoma Polygoni Cuspidati(虎杖 *hu zhang*)

Rhizoma Polygoni Cuspidati is the rhizome and root of the perennial herb Polygonum cuspidatum Sieb. et Zucc. of Polygonaceae. Produced in central and southern China, mainly in Jiangsu, Shandong, Jiangxi, Henan and Sichuan provinces, it is collected in spring and autumn, washed clean, cut into sections or thick slices, and dried in the sun with the fibrous roots removed.

Synonym: *Yin yang lian*, *da ye she zong guan*, *ban gen*.

Taste and Property: Bitter, and slightly cold.

Attributive Meridian: Liver, gallbladder and lung meridians.

Actions and Indications:

(1) To activate blood circulation and restore normal menstruation. Indications: (a) Amenorrhea, dysmenorrhea, trauma and abdominal masses due to blood stasis, for which it is often combined with other drugs that activate blood circulation and remove blood stasis, such as Radix Achyranthis Bidentatae, Radix Angelicae Sinensis, Radix Salviae Miltiorrhizae and Flos Carthami. (b) Rheumatic pain, for which it is used alone in the form of decoction, or soaked in wine for oral administration. It can also be prescribed along with other drugs for dispelling wind-dampness, such as Radix Stephaniae Tetrandrae and Radix Gentianae Macrophyllae.

(2) To eliminate dampness and relieve jaundice. It is indicated for cases due to dampness-heat, such as jaundice, stranguria and leukorrhagia. For jaundice, it is often combined with drugs that purge heat and dispel dampness, such as Herba Artemisia Scopari-

ae, Fructus Gardeniae and Herba Lysimachiae. It can also be used to treat cholelithiasis and urinary lithiasis.

(3) To purge heat and toxins. Indications: (a) Scalds, for which it is ground into fine powder and mixed with sesame oil or strong tea for external application, or else decocted until concentrated and applied as a wet dressing several times a day to prevent the scab from getting dry and cracked. (b) Cough due to lung heat, for which it is often combined with Cortex Mori Radicis and Radix Scutellariae.

This drug can also be used to treat carbuncles and poisonous snakebites.

Dosage: 10-30 g.

Herba Leonuri(益母草 *yi mu cao*)

Herba Leonuri is the aerial part of the annual or biennial herb Leonurus heterophyllus Sweet of Labiatae. Produced in most places of China, the part above the ground is collected and dried in the sun in summer when the stem and leaves grow luxuriant and before or when the flowers just start to bloom.

Synonym: *Chong wei*.

Taste and Property: Acrid and slightly bitter, and mildly cold.

Attributive Meridian: Heart, liver and kidney meridians.

Actions and Indications:

(1) To invigorate blood circulation and restore normal menstruation. Indicated for syndromes due to blood stagnation, such as irregular menstruation, dysmenorrhea, amenorrhea, difficult labor, postpartum abdominal pain, abdominal masses and trauma; here it is used either alone or combined with drugs that activate blood circulation, such as Radix Angelicae Sinensis, Rhizoma Chuanxiong and Rhizoma Cyperi.

(2) To promote diuresis. It is indicated for dysuria and edema, for which it is combined with Semen Plantagini and Rhizoma Imperatae to strengthen the promotion of diuresis and relief of edema.

It also purges heat and toxins, and is applied to treat dysentery and carbuncles.

Dosage and Preparation: 10-30 g, or 60 g when used alone; prepared into decoction or extract.

Remarks: This drug mainly enters the heart and liver meridians and the blood system. Since it is good at activating blood circulation and restoring normal menstruation, it is frequently applied in gynecological and obstetric diseases. It also promotes diuresis. Modern research shows that it is also effective in treating acute and chronic nephritis, particularly the acute.

Semen Persicae(桃仁 *tao ren*)

Semen Persicae is the mature seed of the deciduous small tree Prunus persica (L.) Batsch, or P. davidiana (Carr.) Frach. of Rosaceae. Produced in most parts of China and mainly in Sichuan, Shaanxi, Hebei, Shandong and Guizhou provinces, the mature fruit is collected in September; the pulp is removed, the shell broken and the kernel taken out and dried in the sun.

Taste and Property: Bitter and sweet, and mild.
Attributive Meridian: Heart, liver and large intestine meridians.
Actions and Indications:

(1) To invigorate blood circulation and remove blood stasis. It is indicated for disorders due to blood stasis, such as amenorrhea, dysmenorrhea, postpartum abdominal pain and trauma. For such cases, it is often combined with Radix Angelicae Sinensis, Rhizoma Chuanxiong and Flos Carthami. Its effect in removing blood stasis will be strengthened if it is combined with Radix et Rhizoma Rhei, as in Decoction of Persicae for Purgation. It can also be used along with drugs that purge heat and toxins to treat pulmonary abscess and acute appendicitis.

(2) To lubricate the intestines. It is indicated for constipation due to dryness in the intestine; often used with Fructus Cannabis, Semen Pruni, Semen Trichosanthis and Radix Angelicae Sinensis.

It also relieves cough and dyspnea.

Dosage: 6-10 g.
Precaution: Contraindicated for pregnant women.

Flos Carthami(红花 *hong hua*)

Flos Carthami refers to the tubular flower of the annual herb Carthamus tinctorius L. of Compositae. Mainly cultivated in Henan, Zhejiang, Sichuan and Jiangsu provinces, its flower blooms in summer, and when the petals turn from yellow to bright red, the flower is collected and dried in the shade.

Synonym: *Hong lan hua.*
Taste and Property: Acrid, and warm.
Attributive Meridian: Heart and liver meridians.
Actions and Indications:

To invigorate blood circulation, remove blood stasis and restore normal menstruation. Indicated for amenorrhea, dysmenorrhea, postpartum abdominal pain, abdominal masses, trauma, pain in the limbs, carbuncles and abscess due to blood stasis. For such cases, it is often combined with other drugs that activate blood circulation and remove blood stasis, such as Semen Persicae, Radix Angelicae Sinensis and Radix Paeoniae Rubra.

Dosage: 3-10 g.
Precaution: Contraindicated for pregnant women.
Remarks: Flos Carthami is frequently used to activate blood circulation and remove blood stasis, and is indicated for various kinds of disorders due to blood stasis. Ancient physicians considered it a drug which, "if applied in large dosage, breaks up the blood stasis, and in small amount nourishes the blood."

Faeces Trogopterorum(五灵脂 *wu ling zhi*)

Faeces Trogopterorum is the dried faeces of Trogopterus xanthipes Milne-Edwards of Petauristidae. Mainly found in Hebei and Shanxi provinces, it can be collected any time of the year, and dried in the sun with foreign matter removed.

Taste and Property: Bitter and sweet, and warm.
Attributive Meridian: Liver meridian.
Actions and Indications:

(1) To invigorate blood circulation and relieve pain. It is indicated for amenorrhea, dysmenorrhea, postpartum lochiostasis, stomachache, chest and abdominal pain due to blood stagnation. For such cases, it is often used along with Pollen Typhae, as in Powder for Dissipating Blood Stasis.

(2) To remove blood stasis and stop bleeding. It is indicated for bleeding complicated by blood stasis, such as metrorrhagia and menorrhagia accompanied by purplish blood clots and abdominal pain; it is combined with other drugs that remove blood stasis and stop bleeding, such as Radix Notoginseng, Cortex Moutan Radicis and Radix Paeoniae Rubra.

Besides, this drug is also used in the treatment of bites by poisonous snakes, scorpions and centipedes. Here it is often prescribed along with Realgar and the two are prepared into powder together for both oral and external application.

Dosage and Preparation: 6-10 g, and moderate amount for external use; used in crude form to activate blood circulation and stir-baked to check bleeding.
Precaution: Contraindicated for pregnant women; and incompatible with Radix Ginseng.
Remarks: Faeces Trogopterorum, good at activating blood circulation and relieving pain, is an important drug for removing blood stasis and relieving pains; and is frequently used not only in gynecological diseases but also in pain due to blood stasis, such as stomachache, chest pain, hypochondriac pain and pain in the limbs. In recent years, it has been used with other drugs that activate *qi* and blood circulation to treat coronary heart diseases and angina pectoris.

Radix Achyranthis Bidentatae(牛膝 *niu xi*)

Radix Achyranthis Bidentatae is the root of the perennial plant Achyranthes bidentata Bl. (huai niu xi), or Cyathula officinalis Kuan (chuan niu xi) of Amaranthaceae. The former is produced mainly in Henan Province and the latter in Sichuan Province. Both are dug in winter, washed clean and dried in the sun.

Taste and Property: Bitter and sour, and mild.
Attributive Meridian: Liver and kidney meridians.
Actions and Indications:

(1) To invigorate blood circulation and restore normal menstruation. Indicated for ir-

regular menstruation, dysmenorrhea, amenorrhea and postpartum abdominal pain due to blood stasis; here it is often combined with other drugs that activate blood circulation and remove blood stasis, such as Semen Persicae, Flos Carthami, Radix Angelicae Sinensis and Rhizoma Chuanxiong.

(2) To relieve rigidity of the joints and strengthen the lumbar region and the knees. Indicated for lumbago with sore knees and weak lower limbs. For those cases due to kidney insufficiency, it is often used with Cortex Eucommiae, Radix Rehmanniae Preparata and Radix Dipsaci to strengthen the kidney as well as the bones and muscles; for cases of *bi*-syndrome due to wind and dampness, it is often prescribed with Radix Angelica Pubescentis, Cortex Acanthopanacis and Radix Clematidis to eliminate wind and dampness and strengthen the muscles and bones; and for cases of weak foot and knee joints accompanied by redness, swelling and pain due to the downward attack of dampness-heat, it is combined with Rhizoma Atractylodis, Cortex Phellodendri and Semen Coicis, as in Pill of Four Wonderful Ingredients, to eliminate dampness-heat.

(3) To promote diuresis and relieve stranguria. It is particularly effective for stranguria due to heat, stranguria complicated by hematuria and stranguria due to urinary stones. For such cases, it is often combined with Herba Dianthi and Talcum.

(4) To guide the fire (blood) downwards. It is indicated for disorders due to fire (heat) in the upper part of the body: (a) Headache and vertigo due to hyperactive liver *yang*, for which it is often prescribed along with Haematitum, Os Draconis, Concha Ostreae and Radix Paeoniae Alba to ease the liver and pacify *yang*. (b) Aphthae, swelling and pain in the gums due to the upward disturbance of stomach fire. For such cases, it is often combined with Gypsum Fibrosum, Rhizoma Anemarrhenae and Radix Ophiopogonis, as in Jade Maid Decoction, to purge heat, replenish *yin* and suppress fire. (c) Extravasation marked by hematemesis and epistaxis due to the adverse flow of *qi*, fire and blood-heat. For such cases, it is often combined with Rhizoma Imperatae and Fructus Gardeniae to guide the blood downwards, cool blood and stop bleeding.

Dosage: 6-15 g.

Precaution: Contraindicated for pregnant women and patients with metrorrhagia, seminal emission, and diarrhea due to spleen deficiency.

Remarks: This drug tends to flow downwards and works to: (a) activate blood circulation and restore normal menstruation, and is often employed for diseases in the lower part of the body, such as sore and weak lumbar region and knee joints, swelling and redness of the feet and knees, as well as various kinds of stranguria; (b) suppress the flare-ups of fire, and is used for diseases in the upper part of the body due to fire and heat.

Moreover, Achyranthis Bidentatae (*huai niu xi*) is more often used to strengthen the lumbus and knees, while Radix Cyathulae (*chuan niu xi*) is frequently used to activate blood circulation and remove blood stasis.

Squama Manitis(穿山甲 *chuan shan jia*)

Squama Manitis refers to the scales of the vertebrate pangolin Manis pentadactyla L. of Manidae. To be found mainly in the Guangxi Zhuang Autonomous Region and Guangdong, Guizhou and Yunnan provinces, the animal can be caught at any time of the year; it is then slaughtered and its crust is taken and bathed in boiling water, then the scales are collected and dried in the sun. (The animal is now listed as an endangered species under state protection.)

Taste and Property: Salty, and slightly cold.
Attributive Meridian: Liver and stomach meridians.
Actions and Indications:

(1) To activate blood circulation and restore normal menstruation. Indicated for amenorrhea due to blood stagnation, abdominal masses and rheumatic pain. Normally, it is combined with Radix Angelicae Sinensis, Radix Paeoniae Rubra and Flos Carthami; for abdominal masses, it is used with Rhizoma Sparganii and Rhizoma Zedoariae.

(2) To promote lactation. It is indicated for insufficient lactation in puerperants, and is used either alone or combined with Semen Vaccariae.

(3) To relieve swelling and discharge pus. It is indicated for carbuncles and unruptured abscess, for which it is often combined with Spina Gleditsiae, Flos Lonicerae, Olibanum and Myrrha.

Dosage and Preparation: 3-10 g, stir-baked with sand until it becomes loose; or 1-1.5 g in powder.
Precaution: Contraindicated for pregnant women and patients with ruptured carbuncles and abscess.

Eupolyphaga seu Steleophaga(地鳖虫 *di bie chong*)

Eupolyphaga seu Steleophaga is the dried body of the female insect Eupolyphaga sinensis Walker, or Steleophaga Plancyi (Boleny) of Corydiidae. Produced mainly in Jiangsu, Zhejiang, Henan and Hebei provinces, the insect is either wild or artificially raised, caught in summer and autumn, killed in boiling water and dried in the sun.

Synonym: *Zhe chong, tu bie chong, tu yuan.*
Taste and Property: Salty, and cold and slightly toxic.
Attributive Meridian: Liver meridian.
Actions and Indications:

(1) To break up and remove blood stasis. Indicated for blood stagnation that leads to amenorrhea, stagnation occurring after childbirth, and abdominal masses; here it is often used with Radix et Rhizoma Rhei and Semen Persicae, as in Decoction for Discharging Blood Stasis.

(2) To promote the regeneration of tissues and reunion of fractured bones. It is indicated for trauma, soft tissue injury, fracture, swelling and pain due to stagnant blood, for which it is often combined with Rhizoma Drynariae, Olibanum, Myrrha and Flos Carthami. The dried insect is ground into powder and taken with rice wine, or else the living insect is pounded into pieces and mixed with rice wine; the juice is taken orally and the residue applied externally.

Dosage and Preparation: 6-16 g in decoction, and 1-1. 5 g in powder, to be taken with rice wine.
Precaution: Contraindicated for pregnant women.

Hirudo(水蛭 *shui zhi*)

Hirudo is the body of the annelid Whitmania pigra Whitman, W. acranulata Whitman or Hirude nipponica Whitman of Hirudinidae. To be found in most parts of China, it is caught in summer and autumn, killed in boiling water and dried in the sun or under low temperature.

Synonym: *Ma huang*.
Taste and Property: Salty, bitter and mild; and slightly toxic.
Attributive Meridian: Liver meridian.
Actions and Indications:

To break up and remove blood stasis. It is indicated for amenorrhea due to blood stagnation, abdominal masses and trauma. For such cases, it is often used with Rhizoma Sparganii and Rhizoma Zedoariae; and drugs that nourish blood, such as Radix Rehmanniae, Radix Angelicae Sinensis and Radix Paeoniae Alba, are often added to prevent injury to the antipathogenic *qi*.
Precaution: Contraindicated for pregnant women.
Remarks: Both Eupolyphaga seu Steleophaga and Hirudo are drugs that vigorously break up and remove blood stasis, and are indicated for amenorrhea and abdominal masses caused by severe blood stagnation. As they can easily cause damage to the antipathogenic *qi*, in cases with evident excessive pathogenic factors and complicated by deficient antipathogenic *qi*, they should be prescribed simultaneously along with drugs that replenish *qi*, or used after measures have been taken to strengthen the antipathogenic *qi*. The difference between the two lies in that Eupolyphaga seu Steleophaga is more effective in promoting the regeneration of tissues and the reunion of fractured bones, and Hirudo is good at breaking up and removing blood stasis.

Table 13. Actions of Drugs for Activating Blood Circulation and Removing Blood Stasis

Drug	Similarities	Differences
Rhizoma Chuanxiong	To activate the circulation of blood and *qi*, with good effect in relieving pain	To dispel wind and relieve pain; an important drug for headache
Olibanum, Myrrha		A commonly used drug for diseases in surgery and traumatology
Radix Curcumae		To regulate functions of the liver and gallbladder; resolve phlegm

Drug	Similarities	Differences
Rhizoma Zedoariae	To break up blood stasis, activate circulation of qi; remove food stagnancy	More effective for promoting *qi* circulation
Rhizoma Sparganii		More effective for removing blood stasis
Radix Salviae Mithorrhizae	To activate blood circulation and remove blood stasis	Major drug for activating blood circulation and removing blood stasis; to calm mind
Rhizoma Polygoni Cuspidati		To eliminate dampness and relieve jaundice; clear heat and relieve toxin
Herba Leonuri		To promote diuresis and relieve edema
Semen Persicae		To lubricate intestines and relieve constipation
Flos Carthami		Used in small dosage for nourishing the blood while used in large dosage for breaking up blood stasis
Faeces Trogopterorum		To relieve pain and used in pain due to blood stagnation; relieve intoxication by poisonous snake and insects
Radix Achyranthis Bidentatae		With the property of going downwardly it can strengthen the lumbus and kness, treat stranguria and ensure the downward flow of fire (blood)
Squama Manitis		Emmenagogue and galactagogue; relieve swelling and carbuncle and discharge pus
Eupolyphaga seu Steleophaga	To break up and remove blood stasis	To promote tissue regeneration and reunion of fractured bones
Hirudo		Strong effect in removing blood stasis

Note: Other sections deal with additional drugs that activate blood circulation and remove blood stasis, such as Radix et Rhizoma Rhei, Ramulus Cinnamomi, Cortex Moutan Radicis, Radix Paeoniae Rubra, Radix Notoginseng, Radix Rubiae Pollen Typhae, Rhizoma Corydalis, Radix Angelicae Sinensis and Fructus Crataegi.

CHAPTER SIXTEEN

EXPECTORANTS, ANTITUSSIVES AND DYSPNEA-RELIEVING DRUGS

Drugs that resolve phlegm, and relieve cough and dyspnea are known as expectorants, antitussives or dyspnea-relieving drugs. Some act mainly to resolve phlegm, and others mainly to relieve cough and dyspnea; they are divided into expectorants and drugs that relieve cough and dyspnea, which are discussed separately.

Drugs that resolve phlegm are used mainly to treat diseases caused by phlegm. Phlegm is both a pathological product and a causative factor of diseases, and there are many kinds of diseases and syndromes caused by phlegm. The most commonly seen ones are: retention of phlegm in the lung marked by cough, dyspnea and expectoration of copious sputum; phlegm blocking the lucid *yang*, leading to heaviness in the head and vertigo; phlegm attacking the heart, resulting in unconsciousness and manic-depressive psychosis; and phlegm affecting the meridians, leading to goiter, scrofula, subcutaneous nodule, multiple abscess, phlegmon, or numbness of the limbs and hemiplegia. Drugs that resolve phlegm can be applied for the above diseases and syndromes. But since their properties are different, some warm and dry, and some cool and moistening, and since the disorders caused by phlegm may manifest cold, dampness, heat or dryness, these drugs should be selected accordingly. For instance, drugs that are warm and dry are often used for disorders due to cold-phlegm and dampness-phlegm, while cool and moistening drugs are often used for syndromes due to heat-phlegm and dryness-phlegm. Some are especially effective for resolving phlegm and softening hard masses, and are mainly used for goiter and scrofula.

Drugs that relieve cough and dyspnea are either warm or cool and have different actions, such as promoting the dispersive role of the lung, eliminating fire from the lung, purging lung heat, restoring the normal descent of lung *qi* and resolve phlegm, through which cough and dyspnea are relieved.

Although drugs that resolve phlegm and those that relieve cough and dyspnea are discussed separately, cough, dyspnea and phlegm are closely related to each other. Generally speaking, cough and dyspnea are often complicated by phlegm, and phlegm retained in the lung usually results in cough and dyspnea. Therefore, drugs that relieve cough and dyspnea are often combined with those that resolve phlegm.

Copious phlegm, cough and dyspnea may occur in nearly all diseases due to either internal damage or exogenous affection. When using drugs that resolve phlegm and relieve cough and dyspnea, other related drugs should be combined. For cases characterized by heat, drugs that purge heat are added; for cold, they are used with drugs that warm the interior; for spleen deficiency and excessive dampness, they should be combined with drugs that strengthen the spleen and resolve dampness; for deficient lung *yin*, they are prescribed along with drugs that replenish *yin* and purge heat from the lung; for cases complicated by the exterior syndrome, they are combined with drugs that relieve exterior syndrome; and for cases complicated by endogenous wind, they are used with drugs that eliminate wind. Besides, retained phlegm often leads to *qi* stagnation, and so the drugs that resolve phlegm are usually combined with drugs that activate *qi*.

Moreover, warm and dry drugs that resolve phlegm and relieve cough and dyspnea are contraindicated for cases with consumption of *yin* and bleeding, and cool and moistening drugs are contraindicated for syndromes due to cold-phlegm and dampness-phlegm.

Section 1
Drugs for Resolving Phlegm

Rhizoma Pinelliae(半夏 *ban xia*)

Rhizoma Pinelliae is the tuber of the perennial herb Pinellia ternata (Thunb.) Breit. of Araceae. Distributed in most parts of China, but mainly in Sichuan, Hubei, Jiangsu and Anhui provinces, it is collected in the July-September period, washed, and dried in the sun with the outer epidermis and fibrous roots removed.

Taste and Property: Acrid and warm, and toxic.
Attributive Meridian: Spleen, stomach and lung meridians.
Actions and Indications:

(1) To remove dampness and resolve phlegm. It is indicated for syndrome due to dampness and phlegm marked by stuffiness in the chest, for which it is often used with Pericarpium Citri Reticulatae and Poria, as in *Erchen* Decoction. For cases accompanied by cold syndrome marked by expectoration of copious dilute sputum, it is combined with Rhizoma Zingiberis and Herba Asari. For cases accompanied by heat syndrome marked by yellow sputum, it is prescribed along with Radix Scutellariae and Caulis Bambusae in Taeniam.

(2) To suppress the adverse rise of *qi* and stop vomiting. It is indicated for vomiting due to phlegm retention, stomach heat and stomach *qi* deficiency. For vomiting due to phlegm retention, it is combined with Rhizoma Zingiberis Recens; for vomiting due to stomach heat, it is used with Rhizoma Coptidis; and for vomiting due to stomach *qi* deficiency, it is used with Radix Codonopsis Pilosulae. This drug can also be used to treat stuffiness and fullness in the chest and epigastrium due to phlegm retention and *qi* stagnation.

It also relieves swelling and pain when applied externally, and is indicated for carbuncles and poisonous snakebites, for which the fresh herb is ground into powder for external application.

Dosage and Preparation: 5-10 g, stir-baked with ginger decoction for oral administration;

moderate amount for external application, used either fresh or prepared.

Precaution: Contraindicated for dry cough due to *yin* deficiency and cases with expectoration of blood-tinged sputum. It is incompatible with Radix Aconiti.

Rhizoma Arisaematis(天南星 *tian nan xing*)

Rhizoma Arisaematis is the spherical tuber of the perennial plant Arisaema erubescens (Wall.) Schott., A. heterophyllum Bl., or A. amurense Maxim. of Araceae. A. erubescens is mainly produced in Henan, Hebei and Sichuan provinces, A. heterophyllum mainly in Jiangsu and Zhejiang provinces, and A. amurense mainly in northeastern China. They are all collected in autumn and winter, and dried in the sun with the fibrous roots and outer epidermis removed.

Taste and Property: Bitter and acrid, and warm and toxic.

Attributive Meridian: Liver and spleen meridians.

Actions and Indications:

(1) To eliminate dampness and resolve phlegm. It is indicated for dampness-phlegm syndrome marked by cough with copious sputum and stuffiness in the chest. For such cases, it is often combined with Radix Pinelliae, Pericarpium Citri Reticulatae and Fructus Aurantii Immaturus, as in Decoction for Eliminating Phlegm.

(2) To eliminate wind and relieve convulsion. Indications: (a) Vertigo due to wind-phlegm, apoplexy associated with deviation of the mouth and eye and hemiplegia, and epilepsy due to retention of phlegm. For such cases, it is often combined with Pinelliae and Rhizoma Gastrodiae. (b) Tetanus, for which it is usually used with Radix Ledebouriellae, Rhizoma Gastrodiae and Rhizoma Typhonii, as in *Yuzhen* Powder for Tetanus, which can be taken orally and applied externally.

External use of this drug can relieve swelling and pain, and is indicated for carbuncles and poisonous snakebites. For such cases, it is ground into powder.

Dosage and Preparation: 3-10 g; prepared with ginger decoction for oral administration. Moderate amount for external use, fresh or prepared.

Precaution: Contraindicated for patients with *yin* deficiency; used with caution for pregnant women.

APPENDIX:

Arisaema cum Bile (胆南星 *dan nan xing*)

It refers to the fine powder of Rhizoma Arisaematis prepared with the biles of ox, sheep or pig, or the fermented mixture of the powdered herb and bile. Bitter and slightly acrid and cool, it purges heat, resolves phlegm, eliminates wind and relieves convulsion, and is indicated for apoplexy, infantile convulsion, epilepsy, vertigo, and cough due to phlegm and heat. The recommended dosage is 3-10 g.

Remarks: Radix Pinelliae and Rhizoma Arisaematis are plants of the same family, and both are acrid, warm and toxic; they are effective in eliminating dampness and phlegm, and in relieving swelling and pain if applied externally. However, Radix Pinelliae is particularly good for suppressing the adverse rise of *qi* and relieving vomiting, and it is important for vomiting and epigastric fullness and stuffiness; Rhizoma Arisaematis is more effective in eliminating wind and relieving convulsion, and is frequently used to treat apoplexy with accumulated phlegm, hemiplegia, vertigo and tetanus.

Arisaema cum Bile is different from Rhizoma Arisaematis. Since bile is cold and moistening, the warm action of Rhizoma Arisaematis turns into a cold one, and its drying effect is reduced; Arisaema cum Bile is therefore frequently used for syndromes due to wind-phlegm and heat-phlegm.

Semen Sinapis Albae(白芥子 *bai jie zi*)

Semen Sinapis Albae is the annual or biennial herb Sinapis alba L. or Brassica juncea (L.) Czern. et Coss. of Cruciferae. Cultivated in all places of China and mainly produced in Anhui and Henan provinces, the whole plant is cut at the end of summer or the beginning of autumn when the seed is ripe, then dried in the sun; the seeds are knocked off for medical use.

Taste and Property: Acrid, and warm.
Attributive Meridian: Lung meridian.
Actions and Indications:

(1) To resolve phlegm and regulate *qi* circulation. Indications: (a) Retention of cold phlegm in the lung, marked by cough and dyspnea, expectoration of profuse sputum and stuffiness in the chest, for which it is often combined with Semen Perillae and Semen Raphani, as in Decoction Containing Three Kinds of Seeds for the Aged, to suppress the adverse rise of *qi* and resolve phlegm. (b) Retention of phlegm and fluid in the chest and hypochondrium, marked by cough, dyspnea, chest fullness and hypochondriac pain as seen in hydrothorax, or else for retention of phlegm in the meridians, marked by painful joints and numb limbs; here it is used with Radix Kansui and Radix Euphorbiae, as in Pill for Treating Phlegm Syndrome, to resolve phlegm and eliminate excessive fluid.

(2) To purge lung heat and remove nodules. It is indicated for multiple abscesses and *yin* boils, for which it is often combined with Herba Ephedrae, Cortex Cinnamomi, Rhizoma Zingiberis Preparata and Radix Rehmmaniae Preparata, as in Decoction for Warming *Yang*, to warm yang, dispel cold, resolve phlegm and remove stagnation. It can also be ground into powder and mixed with vinegar for external application.

Dosage: 3-6 g. Moderate amount for external application.
Precaution: Contraindicated for protracted cough leading to lung deficiency and deficient *yin* and hyperactive *yang*. Its external application may cause blisters on the skin, and it is not advisable for patients with skin allergy.
Remarks: Semen Sinapis Albae, acrid, warm and dispersive, is good for resolving phlegm, regulating *qi* circulation and removing obstruction in the meridians. It is indicated for cough and dyspnea due to cold-phlegm, and also for retention of phlegm in the chest, hypochondrium and meridians. Since it has a strong acrid taste, warm nature and powerful dispersive action, it is likely to consume *qi* and promote fire, and is contraindicated for pa-

tients with deficiency of lung *qi* and *yin*, as well as excessive lung heat.

Radix Platycodi(桔梗 *jie geng*)

Radix Platycodi is the root of the perennial herb Platycodon grandiflorum (Jacq.) A. DC. of Campanulaceae. Mainly produced in Jiangsu, Anhui, Henan and Hebei provinces, it is collected in spring and autumn, with that collected in autumn being of better quality. The sprouts and stems are removed, washed clean, and it is then dried in the sun with the cork scraped off.

Taste and Property: Bitter and acrid, and slightly warm.
Attributive Meridian: Lung meridian.
Actions and Indications:

(1) To promote the dispersive function of the lung and resolve phlegm. Indicated for productive cough or difficult expectoration of sputum due to either cold or heat in the lung. For such cases, it is often combined with Semen Armeniacae Amarum and Radix Glycyrrhizae. For cases associated with exterior syndrome, it is combined with drugs that relieve exterior syndrome.

(2) To promote the dispersive function of the lung and ease the throat. Indicated for sore throat and hoarseness of voice, especially cases caused by exogenous pathogenic wind and impaired pulmonary function. For such cases, it is often combined with Radix Glycyrrhizae, as in Decoction of Platycodi. Other drugs may be added accordingly for cases due to wind-cold and wind-heat.

(3) To discharge pus. It is indicated for pulmonary abscess with expectoration of purulent sputum, for which it is used with Herba Houttuyniae, Semen Coicis and Semen Benincasae.

Dosage: 3-10 g; for pulmonary abscess, the dosage can be increased.
Precaution: Contraindicated for patients with cough due to *yin* deficiency and hemoptysis.
Remarks: Radix Platycodi acts on the *qi* system of the lung meridian. It promotes the dispersive function of the lung, dispels pathogenic factors from the lung, resolves phlegm and eases the throat. It is indicated for affection of the lung by exogenous pathogenic factors, either cold or hot in nature, with the symptoms of productive cough, sore throat and hoarseness. It also discharges pus, and is often prescribed for pulmonary abscess with expectoration of purulent sputum. Generally speaking, its indications include diseases caused by exogenous pathogens or accumulated phlegm-fire in the lung and impaired dispersion. Since "the lung is the upper source of water (metabolism)" and this drug promotes lung dispersion, it can also be used to treat retention of urine.

Flos Inulae(旋复花 *xuan fu hua*)

Flos Inulae is the capitulum of the perennial herb Inula japonica Thunb., or I. britannica L. of Compositae. Produced mainly in Henan, Hebei, Zhejiang and Anhui provinces, the capitulum is picked and gathered in summer and autumn when the flowers are going to bloom, and dried in the sun with stem, leaves and foreign matter removed.

Taste and Property: Bitter, acrid and salty, and slightly warm.
Attributive Meridian: Lung and stomach meridians.
Actions and Indications:

(1) To resolve phlegm and suppress the adverse rise of *qi*. Indicated for syndromes due to retained phlegm and the adverse rise of *qi*, marked by cough and dyspnea with copious sputum and stuffiness in the chest. For such cases, it is often combined with Exocarpium Citri Reticulatae, Semen Armeniacae Amarum and Rhizoma Pinelliae.

(2) To suppress the abnormal ascent of stomach *qi*. Indicated for vomiting and belching, in which it is often used with Haematitum and Pinelliae. For cases of stomach *qi* deficiency, it is used with Radix Ginseng.

Dosage and Preparation: 5-10 g; wrapped with a piece of cloth and decocted to prevent irritation of the throat by the fine hairs of the capitulum.

Remarks: Both Flos Inulae and Radix Platycodi are expectorants frequently used in clinical practice. The former has a descending action and checks the abnormal ascent of lung and stomach *qi*, while the latter has an ascending action and promotes the dispersive function of lung *qi*.

Radix Peucedani(前胡 *qian hu*)

Radix Peucedani is the root of the perennial herb Peucedanum praeruptorum Dunn., or P. decursivum Maxim. of Umbelliferae. Produced mainly in Zhejiang, Hunan, Sichuan, Anhui and Jiangsu provinces, it is dug and collected in winter and spring, washed, then dried in the sun.

Taste and Property: Bitter and acrid, and slightly cold.
Attributive Meridian: Lung meridian.
Actions and Indications:

To suppress the adverse rise of *qi*, resolve phlegm and dispel wind-heat. Indicated for syndromes due to phlegm accumulation in the lung and obstructed descent of lung *qi*, marked by cough, shortness of breath and difficult expectoration of thick sputum. For such cases, it is often combined with Semen Armeniacae Amarum, Semen Perillae and Radix Platycodi to regulate the ascent and descent of *qi*, resolve phlegm and relieve cough. For cough due to exogenous wind-heat, it is combined with Herba Menthae, Platycodi and Fructus Arctii to dispel and eliminate wind and heat, and relieve cough.

Dosage: 5-10 g.

Fructus Trichosanthis(瓜蒌 *gua lou*)

Fructus Trichosanthis is the mature fruit of the perennial herbaceous vine Trichosanthes kirilowii Maxim., or T. rosthornii Harms of Cucurbitaceae. Produced mainly in Shandong, Anhui, Henan, Sichuan and Jiangsu provinces, it is picked and gathered in autumn when the fruit is ripe, hung up and dried by airing. The peel of the fruit is called Pericarpium Trichosanthis, and the seed is called Semen Trichosanthis, and together they are known as Fructus Trichosanthis.

Taste and Property: Sweet, and cold.
Attributive Meridian: Lung and large intestine meridians.
Actions and Indications:

(1) To purge heat, dry dampness and resolve phlegm. It is used to treat syndromes due to lung heat and dryness, marked by cough and difficult expectoration of yellow sticky sputum, for which it is often combined with Bulbus Fritillariae and Rhizoma Anemarrhenae to purge heat and resolve phlegm.

(2) To relieve stagnation and stuffiness in the chest. It is indicated for chest *bi*-syndrome, for which it is often prescribed along with Bulbus Allii Macrostemi and Rhizoma Pinelliae, as in Decoction of Trichosanthis, Allii Macrostemi and Pinelliae, to resolve phlegm and relieve stuffiness and pain in the chest.

(3) To lubricate the intestines and promote bowel movements. Indicated for constipation due to intestinal dryness, for which it is often used with other laxatives, such as Fructus Cannabis and Semen Pruni.

Precaution: Contraindicated for patients with spleen deficiency, and incompatible with Radix Aconiti.

Remarks: Fructus Trichosanthis, sweet and cold, purges heat and resolves dryness and phlegm, and is indicated for syndromes due to heat-phlegm and dryness-phlegm. Clinically, Pericarpium Trichosanthis is particularly effective in resolving phlegm and relieving stuffiness and pain in the chest, and is frequently used to treat cough and chest *bi*-syndrome; Semen Trichosanthis is good at moistening dryness, and frequently used to relieve constipation due to intestinal dryness.

Bulbus Fritillariae(贝母 *bei mu*)

There are two kinds of Bulbus Fritillariae—Bulbus Fritillariae Cirrhosae (*chuan bei mu*) and Bulbus Fritillariae Thunbergii (*zhe bei mu*). The former is the bulb of the perennial herb Fritillaria cirrhosa D. Don, F. unibractaeta Hsiao et K. C. Hsia, F. przewalskii Maxim., or F. delavayi Franch. of Liliaceae. It is produced mainly in Sichuan, Qinghai and Gansu provinces. It is dug and collected in summer and autumn or when the snow has just melted, and dried in the sun or under low temperature with the fibrous roots, the coarse epidermis and foreign matter removed. The latter is the bulb of the perennial herb Fritillaria thunbergii Miq. of Liliaceae. Produced mainly in Zhejiang Province, it is collected in early summer when the plant withers, washed with the outer epidermis rubbed off, mixed with calcined shell (of shellfish) powder and dried; or it is cut into thick pieces when fresh, and dried.

Synonym: *Zhe bei mu* is also called *xiang bei mu*.
Taste and Property: F. Cirrhosae: sweet and bitter, and slightly cold; Bulbus Fritillariae

Thunbergii: bitter and cold.

Attributive Meridian: Lung and heart meridians.

Actions and Indications:

(1) To resolve phlegm and relieve cough. Indicated for cough due to heat-phlegm and cough due to dryness-phlegm. For cough due to accumulated phlegm and fire with expectoration of yellow thick sputum, it is often used with Rhizoma Anemarrhenae, as in Powder of Fritillariae and Anemarrhenae, to purge heat and resolve phlegm. For prolonged cough due to *yin* deficiency with scanty and difficult expectoration, dry throat and red tongue, it is often combined with Fructus Trichosanthis, Radix Adenophorae and Radix Ophiopogonis to moisten the lung and resolve phlegm.

(2) To purge heat and toxins and disperse masses. Indicated for carbuncles due to toxic heat and scrofula. For carbuncles, it is often combined with Flos Lonicerae, Radix Trichosanthis, Fructus Forsythiae and Herba Taraxaci to purge heat and toxins; and for scrofula, it is often used with Radix Scrophulariae and Concha Ostreae to resolve phlegm and hard masses, as in Pill for Resolving Scrofula.

Dosage: 3-10 g in decoction, and 1-2 g in powder.

Precaution: Incompatible with Radix Aconiti.

Remarks: Both Bulbus Fritillariae Cirrhosae and Bulbus Fritillariae Thunbergii can purge heat and resolve heat-phlegm. The former is sweet, bitter and slightly cold, and has a stronger action of moistening the lung, and is indicated for cough due to heat and dryness in the lung and prolonged cough due to *yin* deficiency. The latter is bitter and cold, and is better at purging heat and toxins. There is another sort of *bei mu*, that is the tuber of Bolbostemma paniculatum (Maxim.) Franguet of Cucurbitaceae; it does not belong to the same species. It can only purge heat and toxins, and is used to treat carbuncles due to toxic heat. But it cannot resolve phlegm and relieve cough. It should not be confused with Bulbus Fritillariae Cirrhosae and Bulbus Fritillariae Thunbergii.

Concretio Silicea Bambusae(天竹黄 *tian zhu huang*)

Concretio Silicea Bambusae is the coagulum of the sap excreted from the bites of parasitic wasps and accumulated in the joints of a kind of bamboo (Bambusa textilis McClure of the Gramineae). Produced mainly in Yunnan and Guangdong provinces as well as the Guangxi Zhuang Autonomous Region, it is collected in autumn and winter by splitting the bamboo and dried in the sun.

Synonym: *Zhu huang*.

Taste and Property: Sweet, and cold.

Attributive Meridian: Heart and liver meridians.

Actions and Indications:

To purge heat, resolve phlegm and relieve convulsion. It is indicated for syndromes of the heart and liver meridians due to phlegm-heat. (a) Infantile convulsion due to phlegm-heat accompanied with loss of consciousness, for which it is combined with Ramulus Uncariae cum Uncis, Bombyx Batryticatus and Arisaema cum Bile to purge heat, resolve

phlegm, eliminate wind and relieve convulsion. (b) Febrile diseases or apoplexy due to phlegm-heat attacking the heart, marked by coma and accumulation of phlegm. For such cases, it is often used with Rhizoma Acori Graminei, Radix Curcumae and Arisaema cum Bile to resolve phlegm and restore consciousness.
Dosage and Preparation: 3-10 g in decoction, and 0.6-1 g in powder.

Caulis Bambusae in Taeniam(竹茹 *zhu ru*)

Caulis Bambusae in Taeniam is the middle layer of the culm of the perennial evergreen tree or shrub Bambusa tuldoides Munro, or Phyllostachys nigra var. henonis Stapf of the Gramineae. Produced mainly in the drainage areas of the Yangtze River and southern China, it can be collected any time of the year. The fresh culm is taken with the epidermis removed, and the intermediate layer of greenish color is then made into thready slices and dried in the shade.

Synonym: *Zhu er qing*.
Taste and Property: Sweet, and slightly cold.
Attributive Meridian: Lung and stomach meridians.
Actions and Indications:

(1) To purge heat and resolve phlegm. Indications: (a) Cough due to heat in the lung with yellow, thick and sticky sputum, for which it is often combined with Fructus Trichosanthis and Radix Scutellariae. (2) Restlessness, insomnia and palpitation due to disturbance of the heart by phlegm-heat, for which it is often prescribed along with Rhizoma Pinelliae and Poria.

(2) To purge heat and stop vomiting. Indicated for vomiting due to stomach heat, for which it is often used with Rhizoma Coptidis.
Dosage and Preparation: 5-10 g. Stir-baked with ginger juice to check vomiting.

Succus Bambusae(竹沥 *zhu li*)

Succus Bambusae refers to the excretion from the heated fresh culm of Phyllostachys nigra var. henonis Stapf of the Gramineae. It is obtained by cutting the fresh bamboo culm into segments and baking the middle part on a fire, catching the light yellowish bamboo sap excretion from both ends of the segment in a container.

Synonym: *Zhu you*.
Taste and Property: Sweet, and cold.
Attributive Meridian: Heart, lung and stomach meridians.
Actions and Indications:

To purge heat and resolve phlegm. Indications: (a) Acute febrile diseases with high fever, coma, wheezing sounds in the throat, or apoplexy with coma, profuse expectoration and hemiplegia. It can be taken singly or in combination with drugs that purge heat and restore consciousness. (b) Cough due to heat in the lung with profuse expectoration and shortness of breath, for which it is used with Fructus Trichosanthis and Bulbus Fritillariae.

Dosage and Preparation: 30-60 g; taken either singly or with herbal decoction.

Remarks: Concretio Silicea Bambusae, Caulis Bambusae in Taeniam and Succus Bambusae are all derived from bamboo and have similar actions, such as purging heat and resolving phlegm; they are used for syndromes due to heat-phlegm. But Concretio Silicea Bambusae is particularly good at relieving (infantile) convulsion, Caulis Bambusae in Taeniam at purging heat from the stomach and stopping vomiting, and Succus Bambusae (cold and slippery) at purging heat and resolving phlegm.

Lapis Chloriti Usta(礞石 *meng shi*)

Lapis Chloriti Usta refers to the efflorescent product of chlorite-schist, or mica-schist of metamorphic rock. The former is greenish gray and is thus known as *qing* (green) *meng shi*; it is produced mainly in Sichuan, Hunan and Hubei provinces. The latter is golden yellow and is thus known as *jin* (metal) *meng shi*; it is produced mainly in Henan and Hebei provinces. Conventionally, the former is considered better in quality, and is widely used. With foreign matter and stones removed, it is calcined for medical use.

Taste and Property: Sweet and salty, and mild.

Attributive Meridian: Lung and liver meridians.

Actions and Indications:

To promote expectoration of stubborn phlegm and arrest convulsion. Indicated for phlegm syndrome of the excess and heat types, marked by difficult expectoration of thick and sticky sputum, cough and dyspnea, or stagnant stubborn phlegm in the interior, leading to manic-depressive psychosis and epilepsy; here it is often used with Radix et Rhizoma Rhei, Radix Scutellariae and Lignum Aquilariae Resinatum, as in Pill of Lapis Chloriti Usta for Expelling Phlegm, to purge fire and expel phlegm. It can also be used for infantile convulsion with symptoms of dyspnea due to excessive phlegm obstructing the throat. For such cases, it is made into powder, mixed with Menthae juice and honey for oral administration.

Dosage and Preparation: 10-15 g in decoction, and 1.5-3 g in pills or powder.

Precaution: To be used with caution for pregnant women.

Remarks: Lapis Chloriti Usta is heavy, can expel stubborn phlegm and is indicated for dyspneic cough and manic-depressive psychosis caused by excess syndrome due to stagnant stubborn phlegm. It is often used in combination with Radix et Rhizoma Rhei, especially for cases complicated by constipation. It is contraindicated for cases due to deficient spleen *qi*.

Sargassum(海藻 *hai zao*)

Sargassum is the whole alga Sargassum Pallidum (Turn.) C. Ag., or S. fusiforme (Harv.) Setch. of Sargassaceae. Produced mainly in the coastal areas of Shandong, Zhejiang, Fujian and Guangdong provinces, it is collected in summer, washed clean and dried in the sun with foreign matter removed.

Taste and Property: Bitter and salty, and cold.
Attributive Meridian: Liver and kidney meridians.
Actions and Indications:

To resolve phlegm and soften hard masses. It is indicated for goiter and scrofula, for which it is often combined with Thallus Eckloniae or Thallus Laminariae, Spica Prunellae, Radix Scrophulariae and Bulbus Fritillariae Thunbergii to enhance the effect of resolving phlegm and softening hard masses.

This drug can be applied for swollen testes.
Dosage: 10-15 g.
Precaution: Incompatible with Radix Glycyrrhizae.

Thallus Laminariae seu Eckloniae(昆布 *kun bu*)

Thallus Laminariae seu Eckloniae refers to the thallus of the kelp Laminaria japonica Aresch. , or Ecklonia kurome Okam. of Laminariaceae or Alariaceae. Produced mainly in the coastal areas of Liaoning, Shandong, Zhejiang and Fujian provinces, it is collected in summer and autumn, and dried in the sun.

Taste and Property: Salty, and cold.
Attributive Meridian: Liver and kidney meridians.
Actions and Indications: To resolve phlegm and soften hard masses. It is indicated for goiter, scrofula and swollen testes. For such cases, it is often used with Sargassum.
Dosage: 10-15 g.
Remarks: Both Thallus Eckloniae and Sargassum contain iodine and are effective in treating goiter due to shortage of iodine. It can be taken for a long time.

Section 2
Drugs for Relieving Cough and Dyspnea

Semen Armeniacae Amarum(苦杏仁 *ku xing ren*)

Semen Armeniacae Amarum is the bitter mature seed of the deciduous tree Prunus armeniaca L. var. ansu Maxim. , or P. armeniaca L. of Rosaceae. Produced in most parts of China, it is collected in summer when the fruit is ripe; having the pulp of the fruit and the shell removed, the seed is kept and dried in the sun.

Taste and Property: Bitter and warm, and slightly toxic.
Attributive Meridian: Lung and large intestine meridians.
Actions and Indications:

(1) To relieve cough and dyspnea. For cases due to affection by wind-cold, it is pre-

scribed along with Herba Ephedrae and Radix Glycyrrhizae; for those due to affection by wind-heat, it is used with Herba Menthae and Fructus Arctii; for those due to lung heat, it is used with Gypsum Fibrosum and Radix Scutellariae.

(2) To lubricate the intestines. It is indicated for constipation due to intestinal dryness, for which it is often combined with Fructus Cannabis and Semen Pruni.

Dosage: 5-10 g.

Remarks: There are two kinds of such seeds—the bitter and the sweet. The bitter is more frequently used in medicine, and the sweet is mild, and can moisten the lung; its ability to relieve cough and dyspnea is weaker, and is mainly used for protracted cough due to lung *yin* deficiency.

Radix Stemonae(百部 *bai bu*)

Radix Stemonae is the root of the perennial herb Stemona sessilifolia (Miq) Miq., S. japonica (Bl) Miq. of Stemonaceae. Produced mainly in Jiangsu, Anhui, Hubei and Zhejiang provinces, it is collected in spring before the root gives new sprouts or in autumn when the sprouts wither. With the fibrous roots removed, it is washed clean and slightly bathed in boiling water or steamed until the white color of its center disappears. It is then taken out and dried in the sun.

Taste and Property: Sweet and bitter, and slightly warm.

Attributive Meridian: Lung meridian.

Actions and Indications:

(1) To moisten the lung and relieve cough. Indicated for cough, either acute or chronic, either deficiency or excess type. It can be combined with other drugs in line with the accompanying symptoms. For cough and dyspnea due to attack of the body surface by pathogenic factors, it is used with Spica Schizonepetae and Radix Platycodi; and for chronic cough due to lung *yin* deficiency, it is combined with Radix Ophiopogonis and Radix Adenophorae. It can also be prepared as syrup to cure whooping cough in children.

(2) To kill parasites. Indications: (a) Oxyuriasis, for which 30 g of the drug is decocted into 30 ml. of concentrate for enema every night before sleep (10 days in succession). (b) Pediculosis, for which it is prepared into 20% alcoholic extract or 50% decoction for external application.

Dosage and Preparation: 5-10 g; used either crude or baked with honey. Moderate amount for external application.

Radix Asteris(紫菀 *zi wan*)

Radix Asteris is the root and rhizome of the perennial herb Aster tataricus L. f. of Compositae. Produced mainly in Hebei and Anhui provinces, it is collected in spring and autumn, and dried in the sun with stem and leaves as well as foreign matter removed.

Taste and Property: Acrid and bitter, and slightly warm.

Attributive Meridian: Lung meridian.

Actions and Indications:

To resolve phlegm and relieve cough. It is a drug frequently used to treat cough either due to exterior affection or interior damage and of either a cold or heat nature. For cough due to exterior affection marked by difficult expectoration of profuse sputum, it is often combined with Spica Schizonepetae, Radix Platycodi and Rhizoma Cynanchi; for cough due to *yin* deficiency with expectoration of blood-tinged sputum, it is often prescribed along with Rhizoma Anemarrhenae, Bulbus Fritillariae Cirrhosae and Colla Corii Asini; and for chronic cough, it is often combined with Flos Farfarae and Radix Stemonae.

Dosage and Preparation: 5-10 g; used either crude or baked with honey.

Flos Farfarae(款冬花 *kuan dong hua*)

Flos Farfarae is the bud of the perennial herb Tussilago farfara L. of Compositae. Produced mainly in Shanxi, Gansu, Sichuan and Henan provinces, it is picked and collected in the period around the Winter Solstice, when the flower bud just grows above the ground, and dried in the shade with the pedicel and foreign matter removed.

Taste and Property: Acrid, and warm.

Attributive Meridian: Lung meridian.

Actions and Indications:

To relieve cough and resolve phlegm. With similar actions as Radix Asteris, it can be used to treat various kinds of cough. For cough and dyspnea due to retention of cold or phlegm, it is often prescribed along with Herba Ephedrae and Herba Asari; for cough with blood-tinged sputum, it is combined with Bulbus Lilli; and for chronic cough, it is often used with Radix Asteris.

Dosage and Preparation: 5-10 g; used either crude or baked with honey.

Remarks: Both Radix Asteris and Flos Farfarae are warm and moistening; they can resolve phlegm and relieve cough, and are used to treat various kinds of cough. But Radix Asteris is more effective in resolving phlegm, and Flos Farfarae in relieving cough, and their combination can produce a better therapeutic effect.

Fructus Perillae(苏子 *su zi*)

Fructus Perillae is the fruit of the annual herb Perilla frutescens (L.) Britt. of Labiatae. Produced mainly in Jiangsu, Anhui, Hubei and Henan provinces, it is collected in autumn when the fruit is ripe and dried in the sun.

Taste and Property: Acrid, and warm.

Attributive Meridian: Lung meridian.

Actions and Indications:

To suppress the adverse rise of *qi*, resolve phlegm and relieve cough and dyspnea. Indicated for accumulation of phlegm and the adverse rise of *qi*, marked by cough, dyspnea and fullness and stuffiness in the chest. Here it is often combined with Rhizoma Pinelliae, Pericarpium Citri Reticulatae and Cortex Magnoliae Officinalis, as in Decoction of Perillae for Keeping *Qi* Downwards, to suppress the adverse rise of *qi*, resolve phlegm and relieve cough and dyspnea.

This drug can also be used as a laxative for constipation due to intestinal dryness.

Dosage and Preparation: 5-10 g; slightly baked and pounded into pieces.

Fructus Aristolochiae(马兜铃 *ma dou ling*)

Fructus Aristolochiae is the mature fruit of the perennial twining or creeping slender herb Aristolochia contorta Bge., or A. debilis Sieb et Zuce of Aristolochiaceae. The former is produced mainly in Heilongjiang, Hebei and Shandong provinces, and the latter mainly in Jiangsu, Anhui and Zhejiang provinces. It is gathered in autumn when the green fruit turns yellow and dried in the sun.

Taste and Property: Bitter, and cold.
Attributive Meridian: Lung meridian.
Actions and Indications:

To purge heat from the lung, resolve phlegm and relieve cough and dyspnea. Indicated for productive cough and dyspnea due to lung heat, for which it is prescribed along with Cortex Mori Radicis, Radix Scutellariae, Folium Eriobotryae and Radix Peucedani to enhance the effect of purging lung heat, resolving phlegm and relieving cough and dyspnea.

Dosage and Preparation: 3-10 g; used either crude or baked with honey.

Cortex Mori Radicis(桑白皮 *sang bai pi*)

Cortex Mori Radicis is the root bark of the deciduous tree Morus alba L. of Moraceae. Produced mainly in Jiangsu, Zhejiang and Anhui provinces, the root is dug out in spring and autumn and the yellow-brownish cork is scraped off when it is still fresh, cut vertically in order to obtain the bark, and dried in the sun.

Synonym: *Sang pi*, *sang gen bai pi*.
Taste and Property: Sweet, and cold.
Attributive Meridian: Lung meridian.
Actions and Indications:

(1) To purge lung heat and relieve dyspnea. It is indicated for cough and dyspnea due to lung heat, for which it often combined with Cortex Lycii Radicis, as in Powder for Expelling Lung Heat.

(2) To promote diuresis. Indicated for edema and dysuria, for which it is often prescribed along with Pericarpium Arecae and Poria.

Dosage and Preparation: 5-15 g; used either crude or baked with honey.

Semen Lepidii seu Descurainiae(葶苈子 *ting li zi*)

Semen Lepidii seu Descurainiae is the mature seed of the annual or biennial herb Lepidium apetalum Wild. , or Descurainia sophia (L.) Webb ex prantl of Cruciferae. The former is produced mainly in Hebei and Liaoning provinces as well as the Inner Mongolia Autonomous Region; the latter mainly in Jiangsu, Anhui and Shandong provinces. It is collected in summer when the fruit is ripe, the part above the ground is cut and dried in the sun, and the seeds are knocked off for medical use.

Taste and Property: Acrid and bitter, and cold.
Attributive Meridian: Lung and urinary bladder meridians.
Actions and Indications:

(1) To purge heat from the lung and relieve dyspnea. Indicated for cough and orthopnea with copious sputum and facial puffiness due to retention of phlegm in the lung. For such cases, It is often prescribed along with Fructus Jujubae, as in Decoction of Lepidii seu Descurainiae and Jujube for Purging Lung Heat.

(2) To promote diuresis. Indicated for hydrothorax, ascitis, edema of face, and dysuria; here it is often combined with Radix Stephaniae Tetrandrae, Pericarpium Zanthoxyli and Radix et Rhizoma Rhei, as in Pill of Stephaniae Tetrandrae, Zanthoxyli, Lepidii seu Descurainiae and Rhei, to promote diuresis and relieve edema.

Dosage: 3-10 g.
Remarks: This drug is effective in eliminating fluid from the lung and relieving dyspnea and cough. So, for excessive fluid retained in the lung which leads to cough, orthopnea, facial puffiness and edema, it is usually used as the major remedy. Now, it is frequently used to treat pulmonary heart diseases. For its drastic purgative action, it likely causes damage to stomach *qi*, so it is often combined with Fructus Jujubae to offset this disadvantage.

Table 14. Actions of Expectorants, Antitussives and Dyspnea-Relieving Drugs

Drug	Similarities	Differences
Rhizoma Pinelliae	To dry dampness and resolve phlegm; external use for relieving carbuncle and pain	An important antemetic
Rhizoma Arisaematis		To eliminate wind and relieve convulsion
Semen Sinapis Albae		To resolve phlegm, regulate *qi*, relieve swelling, disperse *qi*, and remove nodules
Radix Platycodi	To resolve phlegm and relieve cough	To disperse the lung *qi*, relieve sore throat, and promote pus discharge
Flos Inulae		To lower the adverse-rising *qi* of the lung and stomach
Radix Peucedani		To dispel wind and heat
Fructus Trichosanthis	To clear heat and resolve phlegm	To relieve stuffiness and pain in the chest; to promote bowel movement
Bulbus Fritillariae		To clear toxic heat, and relieve carbuncle
Concretio Silicea Bambusae		To control convulsion
Caulis Bambusae in Taeniam		To clear heat and stop vomiting
Succus Bambusae		Strong effect for clearing heat and resolving phlegm
Lapis Chloriti Usta		To pull down stubborn phlegm; to arrest convulsion
Sargassum, Thallus Laminariae seu Eckloniae		To resolve phlegm, and soften lumps

Drug	Similarities	Differences
Semen Armeniacae Amarum		To relieve dyspnea, moisturize lung and promote bowel movement
Radix Stemonae		To kill parasites and lice
Radix Asteris, Flos Farfarae	Antitussives	Warm and moistening in nature; expectorant
Fructus Perillae		To descend *qi*; expectorant; to relieve dyspnea
Fructus Aristolochiae		To clear lung heat; to resolve phlegm
Cortex Mori Radicis	To purge the lung, relieve dyspnea and promote diuresis	To clear lung heat particularly
Semen Lepidii seu Descurainiae		To purge excessive fluid in the lung

Note: Other sections discuss additional drugs that have expectorant and antitussive actions and the ability to relieve dyspnea. These include Herba Ephedrae, Herba Asari, Radix Polygalae, Exocarpium Citri Reticulatae, Fructus Schisandrae, Fructus Mume and Semen Raphani.

CHAPTER SEVENTEEN
SEDATIVES

Drugs that calm the mind and allay excitement are known as sedatives (*an shen yao*).

The sedatives are indicated mainly for restlessness of the heart and mind, marked by palpitation, insomnia, dream-disturbed sleep, manic-depressive psychosis and epilepsy. Mineral sedatives, heavy in weight, have a better tranquilizing effect and are conventionally known as "sedatives to calm the mind"; some herbal sedatives possess a nourishing effect and are known as "sedatives to nourish the heart."

Since irritability and restlessness of the heart and mind have different causes, the sedatives should be applied in combination with different drugs. For cases due to hyperactive heart fire, they are used with drugs that purge heart fire; for cases due to heart blood insufficiency, they are combined with drugs that nourish the blood; for cases due to hyperactive liver *yang*, they are used with drugs that ease the liver and pacify *yang*; and for cases due to obstruction of the heart by phlegm, they are prescribed along with drugs that resolve phlegm.

Mineral sedatives, if prepared into pills or powder, are likely to cause damage to stomach *qi* and should be combined with drugs that strengthen the spleen; prolonged use should be avoided. Toxic drugs should be applied with caution.

Cinnabaris(朱砂 *zhu sha*)

Cinnabaris is the sulfide ore of cinnabar, composed mainly of mercuric sulfide. Distributed mainly in Hunan, Sichuan, Guizhou and Yunnan provinces, it can be mined at any time, and the pure ore is selected; foreign matter containing iron is removed with a magnet and other foreign matter is washed away.

Synonym: *Chen sha*, *dan sha*.
Taste and Property: Sweet, and slightly cold and toxic.
Attributive Meridian: Heart meridian.
Actions and Indications:

(1) To tranquilize the heart and mind. Indicated for palpitation, insomnia, manic-depressive psychosis and epilepsy. For cases due to hyperactive heart fire, it is combined with Rhizoma Coptidis; for cases due to insufficient heart blood, it is used with Radix Rehmanniae and Radix Ophiopogonis; for epilepsy, it is combined with Rhizoma Arisaematis.

(2) To remove toxins. It is used externally for skin infections, pharyngitis and aphthae.

It can also be used to coat antiseptic pills.

Dosage and Preparation: 0.3-1 g, to be taken with water; or prepared into pills or powder; or mixed with Poria and Fructus Forsythiae to produce a decoction. Moderate dosage for external application.

Precaution: Overdose and continuous long-term administration should be avoided to prevent mercury poisoning. It should never be calcined, otherwise mercury will be separated out and the drug will become very toxic.

Magnetitum(磁石 *ci shi*)

Magnetitum is magnetic iron ore, composed mainly of Fe_3O_4(ferric oxide). It is mainly distributed in Hebei, Shandong, Liaoning and Jiangsu provinces. Having mined it, foreign matter is removed.

Taste and Property: Salty, and cold.

Attributive Meridian: Liver, heart and kidney meridians.

Actions and Indications:

(1) To tranquilize the heart and calm the mind. Indicated for restlessness of the heart and mind, marked by palpitation, insomnia, irritability, manic-depressive psychosis, for which it is often combined with Cinnabaris, as in Pill of Magnetitum and Cinnabaris, to enhance the sedative effect.

(2) To subdue hyperactive liver *yang*. Indicated for headache, vertigo and tinnitus due to hyperactive liver *yang*, for which it is often used with Os Draconis and Concha Ostreae; and for tinnitus and deafness due to kidney deficiency, it is often combined with drugs that invigorate the kidney, such as Radix Rehmanniae Preparata and Fructus Corni.

(3) To promote the reception of *qi* and relieve dyspnea. Indicated for deficiency-type dyspnea due to impaired renal function, for which it is often combined with drugs that nourish the kidney and promote the reception of *qi*, such as Radix Rehmanniae Preparata, Fructus Schisandrae and Semen Juglandis.

Dosage and Preparation: 15-30 g, pounded into pieces and decocted first (with other ingredients added later), or prepared into pills. Used either in crude form or after calcination.

Os Draconis(龙骨 *long gu*)

Os Draconis refers to the fossilized bone of ancient large mammals, such as the tripletoe horse, rhinoceros, deer, ox and elephant. Distributed mainly in Shanxi, Shaanxi, Gansu, Hebei and Hubei provinces as well as the Inner Mongolia Autonomous Region, it can be mined and collected any time of the year (with official permission). With foreign matter removed, it is kept in a dry place.

Taste and Property: Sweet, and astringent and mild.
Attributive Meridian: Heart, liver and kidney meridians.
Actions and Indications:

(1) To calm the heart and mind. Indicated for restlessness of the heart and mind, leading to insomnia, dream-disturbed sleep, palpitation, epilepsy and manic-depressive psychosis. For such cases, it is often prescribed along with Cinnabaris and Magnetitum.

(2) To subdue hyperactive liver *yang*. Indicated for headache, vertigo and tinnitus due to hyperactive liver *yang*. For such cases, it is often used with Concha Ostreae and Radix Paeoniae Alba.

(3) To induce astringency. Indications: (a) Seminal emission and enuresis, for which it is often combined with Semen Euryales and Stamen Nelumbinis. (b) Spontaneous and night sweating, for which it is often used with Radix Astragali and Concha Ostreae. For prostration due to the collapse of *yang* with symptoms of profuse sweating, cold limbs and feeble pulse, it is often combined with Radix Ginseng, Radix Aconiti Lateralis Preparata and Concha Ostreae to restore the depleted *yang* and prevent collapse. (c) Metrorrhagia and leukorrhagia, for which it is often prescribed along with Os Sepiae and Concha Ostreae to arrest excessive uterine bleeding and vaginal discharge.

Dosage and Preparation: 10-30 g. Crushed into pieces and decocted first (with other ingredients added later). To be used in crude form to calm the mind and pacify the liver, and calcined for astringent effect. Moderate dosage is used for external application.

Remarks: Cinnabaris, Magnetitum and Os Draconis are all mineral drugs heavy in weight and possessing tranquilizing effect for the heart and mind. Cinnabaris is particularly effective in calming the heart and mind; Magnetitum and Os Draconis are good at subduing hyperactive liver *yang*. Moreover, Magnetitum can promote renal function to receive *qi* and relieve dyspnea, and Os Draconis serves as an important astringent.

Semen Ziziphi Spinosae(酸枣仁 *suan zao ren*)

Semen Ziziphi Spinosae is the mature seed of the deciduous shrub or tree Ziziphus spinosa Hu of Rhamnaceae. Produced mainly in Shandong, Hebei and Henan provinces, the mature fruit is gathered in late autumn and early winter, the pulp and testa are removed, and the seeds are collected and dried in the sun.

Taste and Property: Sweet, and mild.
Attributive Meridian: Heart, liver and gallbladder meridians.
Actions and Indications:

(1) To nourish the heart and calm the mind. Indicated for insomnia and palpitation due to fright. For cases of heart and liver blood deficiency, it is combined with Radix Angelicae Sinensis and Radix Paeoniae Alba; for liver deficiency which leads to heat, it is used with Rhizoma Anemarrhenae and Poria; and for hyperactive *yang* due to *yin* deficiency, it is combined with Radix Rehmanniae and Radix Ophiopogonis.

(2) To replenish *yin* and check sweating. Indicated for night sweating due to *yin* deficiency, for which it is used with Concha Ostreae and Fructus Schisandrae.

Dosage: 10-15 g.
Remarks: The pulp is sour and the seed is sweet in taste. The sour taste of this drug as described in ancient medical literature refers to the pulp.

Semen Biotae(柏子仁 *bai zi ren*)

Semen Biotae refers to the mature seed of the evergreen tree Biota orientalis (L.) Endl. of Cupressaceae. Distributed mainly in Shandong, Henan and Hebei provinces, the mature seed is collected in autumn and winter, and dried in the sun with the testa removed.

Taste and Property: Sweet, and mild.
Attributive Meridian: Heart and large intestine meridians.
Actions and Indications:

(1) To nourish the heart and calm the mind. It is indicated for palpitation and insomnia, especially cases due to insufficient heart blood. It is often combined with Semen Ziziphi Spinosae, and with other drugs according to the accompanying symptoms.

(2) To promote bowel movements. Indicated for constipation due to blood deficiency and intestinal dryness, for which it is often combined with Fructus Cannabis and Semen Pruni.

Dosage: 6-12 g.

Radix Polygalae(远志 *yuan zhi*)

Radix Polygalae is the root of the perennial herb Polygala tenuifolia Willd., or P. sibirica L. of Polygalaceae. Produced mainly in Shanxi, Shaanxi and Henan provinces, it is collected in spring and autumn, and dried in the sun with the fibrous roots and foreign matter removed.

Taste and Property: Bitter and acrid, and warm.
Attributive Meridian: Heart and lung meridians.
Actions and Indications:

(1) To calm the heart and mind. Indicated for restlessness of the heart and mind, palpitation due to fright and insomnia, especially cases complicated by phlegm syndrome. For such cases, it is often combined with Semen Biotae and Semen Ziziphi Spinosae.

(2) To resolve phlegm. Indications: (a) Mental disorders or coma due to block of the heart by phlegm, for which it is often prescribed along with Rhizoma Acori Graminei and Radix Curcumae to resolve phlegm and restore consciousness. (b) Cough with difficulty in expectoration, for which it is often used with Radix Platycodi and Radix Asteris to resolve phlegm and relieve cough.

It also relieves carbuncles, abscesses and ulcers, for which it can either be taken orally or applied externally.

Dosage and Preparation: 3-10 g. Moderate amount for external application.

Remarks: Semen Ziziphi Spinosae, Semen Biotae and Radix Polygalae can all tranquilize the mind, and are frequently used for insomnia. Their difference lies in that the former two nourish the heart, and the latter resolves phlegm and is indicated for palpitation caused by fright, insomnia, coma and cough with difficulty in expectoration due to retention of phlegm and turbidity.

Table 15. Actions of Sedative

Drug	Similarities	Differences
Cannabaris	To calm the heart and mind	Toxic; external application for skin infection and aphthae
Magnetitum		To subdue the hyperactivity of liver *yang*, promote *qi* receiving and relieve dyspnea
Os Draconis		To subdue the hyperactivity of liver *yang* and act as an astringent
Semen Ziziphi Spinosae	To nourish the heart and calm the mind	To check sweating
Semen Biotae		To promote bowel movement
Radix Polygalae		To resolve phlegm

Note: Other sections deal with additional tranquilizing drugs, including Poria, Concha Ostreae, Concha Margaritifera Usta and Haematitum.

CHAPTER EIGHTEEN

DRUGS FOR CALMING THE LIVER AND SUPPRESSING WIND

Drugs that subdue hyperactive liver *yang* and suppress liver wind are known as drugs for calming the liver and suppressing wind (*ping gan xi feng yao*).

These drugs subdue *yang*, purge liver heat and arrest convulsion, and are indicated for headache and dizziness due to hyperactive liver *yang* and convulsion due to irritation by liver wind in the interior, as well as for redness of the eyes and nebulae. Drugs derived from shellfish are particularly effective in calming the liver and subduing *yang*, those derived from insects are more effective in stopping convulsion, and some do both.

In clinical practice, these drugs may be used in combination with other drugs. For example, drugs that purge heat are added for cases with wind produced by excessive heat; drugs that resolve phlegm are added for cases complicated by phlegm syndrome; drugs that nourish *yin* are added for cases with the irritation of wind by *yin* deficiency; and drugs that nourish the blood are added for cases with blood deficiency. Hyperactive liver *yang* and irritation of liver wind are frequently associated with palpitation and insomnia, and so sedatives are always applied simultaneously.

Drugs derived from shellfish and minerals are heavy, and their dosages should be large, but some insect drugs are warm, dry and toxic, and their dosage should be small. Cold and cool drugs are not advisable for the treatment of chronic infantile convulsion due to spleen deficiency, and those that are warm and dry should be applied with caution for patients with *yin* and blood deficiency.

Concha Haliotidis(石决明 *shi jue ming*)

Concha Haliotidis is the shell of Haliotis diversicolor Reeve, H. discus hannai Lno, H. ovina Gmelin, or H. gigantea discus Reeve of Haliotidae. To be found mainly in Shandong, Liaoning, Fujian and Taiwan provinces, it is collected in summer and autumn, the flesh is removed, and then it is washed and dried.

Taste and Property: Salty, and slightly cold.
Attributive Meridian: Liver meridian.
Actions and Indications:

(1) To pacify the liver and subdue yang. Indicated for headache and dizziness due to hyperactive liver yang, for which it is often combined with Concha Ostreae, Radix

Rehmanniae, Radix Paeoniae Alba and Flos Chrysanthemi.

(2) To purge liver heat and improve vision. Indicated for nebulae in the eyes, optic atrophy, night blindness and other eye diseases due to liver heat. For such cases, it is used with Chrysanthemi, Flos Eriocauli and Periostracum Cicadae, as well as drugs that nourish the blood, replenish *yin* and purge liver heat according to accompanying symptoms.

Dosage and Preparation: 15-30 g, crushed into pieces and prepared into a decoction (with this drug being decocted first). Used either in crude form or after calcination.

Concha Ostreae(牡蛎 *mu li*)

Concha Ostreae is the shell of Ostrea gigas Thunb., O. taliemwhanensis Crosse, or O. rivularis Gould of Oystreidae. Produced in the coastal areas of China, it can be collected at any time of the year. With the flesh removed, it is washed clean and dried in the sun.

Taste and Property: Salty, and astringent and slightly cold.

Attributive Meridian: Liver, heart and kidney meridians.

Actions and Indications:

(1) To subdue hyperactive liver *yang*. Indicated for dizziness and headache due to hyperactive liver *yang*, for which it is often combined with Concha Haliotidis, Radix Rehmanniae and Flos Chrysanthemi. In late stages of febrile diseases with wind stirred up by *yin* deficiency, it is used with Plastrum, Testudinis and Carapax Trionycis.

(2) To calm the heart and mind. Indicated for restlessness, palpitation, insomnia and dream-disturbed sleep. For such cases, it is often combined with Os Draconis, Semen Ziziphi Spinosae and Semen Biotae.

(3) To induce astringency. Indicated for spontaneous sweating, night sweating, seminal emission, leukorrhagia and metrorrhagia, for which it is often combined with Os Draconis or other drugs according to the accompanying symptoms.

(4) To soften hard lumps. It is indicated for scrofula and subcutaneous nodules, for which it is often used with Bulbus Fritillariae and Radix Scrophulariae, as in Pill for Resolving Scrofula. It can also be used for hepatomegaly and splenomegaly.

This drug can also regulates acid secretion, and is used for gastric gastroxynsis and epigastric pain.

Dosage and Preparation: 10-30 g, crushed into pieces and decocted first. Usually used crude, but after calcination as an astringent.

Remarks: Both Concha Ostreae and Os Draconis can calm the mind and subdue hyperactive liver *yang*, and work as astringents. So they are often used in combination. But the former is better in subduing hyperactive liver *yang* and softening hard lumps, while the latter is more effective in calming the mind and has a stronger astringent effect.

Margarita(珍珠 *zhen zhu*)

Margarita is the abnormal nacreous growth (after being stimulated) formed within Pteria martensii (Dunker) of Pteriidae, Hyriopsis cumingii (Lea), or Cristaria Plicate (Leach) of Unionidae. The marine pearl is produced mainly by the coast in Guangdong, Hainan and Taiwan provinces as well as the Guangxi Zhuang Autonomous Region; the freshwater pearl is produced in all parts of the country. It can be collected at any time of the year.

Taste and Property: Sweet and salty, and cold.
Attributive Meridian: Heart and liver meridians.
Actions and Indications:

(1) To calm the heart and stop convulsion. It is indicated for palpitation due to fright, infantile convulsion and epilepsy, for which it is often combined with Cinnabaris and Arisaema cum Bile.

(2) To purge liver heat and remove nebulae. It is indicated for such eye diseases as redness, nebulae and dryness and pain in the eyes. For such cases, it is often prepared as eyedrops, as in Eyedrop with Eight Ingredients.

(3) To promote granulation. Indicated for unhealed ulceration, such as ulcers in the throat and gums, for which it is often prescribed along with Calculus Bovis as powder to be insufflated onto the lesions.

Dosage and Preparation: 0. 3-1 g, prepared into pills or powder. Moderate amount for external use.

Concha Margaritifera Usta(珍珠母 *zhen zhu mu*)

Concha Margaritifera Usta refers to the shell of Hyriopsis cumingii (Lea) of Unionidae, or Pteria martensii (Dunker) of Pteriidae. Produced in rivers and lakes throughout China and in the coastal areas, it can be collected any time of the year. The shell is boiled in soda water and rinsed with the black outer skin scraped off.

Synonym: *Zhu mu.*
Taste and Property: Salty, and cold.
Attributive Meridian: Liver and heart meridians.
Actions and Indications:

(1) To subdue hyperactive liver *yang*. Indicated for headache, dizziness and blurred vision due to hyperactive liver *yang*, for which it is often prescribed along with Concha Ostreae and Magnetitum.

(2) To calm the heart and mind. Indicated for restlessness, irritability, palpitation and insomnia, for which it is often used with Semen Ziziphi Spinosae and Semen Biotae.

(3) To improve vision. Indicated for blurred vision due to liver deficiency, night blindness or conjunctivitis with photophobia due to liver heat, as well as nebulae in the eyes.

This drug also regulates acid secretion, and is used for epigastric pain due to too much gastric acid.

Dosage and Preparation: 15-30 g; decocted first. Calcined to relieve gastroxynsis and used in crude form for other purposes.
Remarks: Concha Haliotidis, Concha Ostreae and Concha Margaritifera Usta are all derived from shellfish and are salty and cold. They can all subdue hyperactive liver yang. But Concha Haliotidis improves vision by purging liver heat, Concha Ostreae is astringent, and can soften hard lumps, and Concha Margaritifera Usta improves vision and calms the mind.

Haematitum(代赭石 *dai zhe shi*)

Haematitum is a kind of red iron ore composed mainly of ferric oxide. Distributed mainly in Shanxi, Shandong, Guangdong, Henan and Hebei provinces, it is mined and washed to remove foreign matter.

Taste and Property: Bitter, and cold.
Attributive Meridian: Liver, stomach and heart meridians.
Actions and Indications:

(1) To subdue hyperactive liver *yang*. Indicated for headache and dizziness due to the upward disturbance of hyperactive liver *yang*, for which it is often combined with Magnetitum, Radix Achyranthis Bidentatae and Radix Paeoniae Alba.

(2) To make the adversely rising *qi* go downwards. Indications: (a) Vomiting, hiccup and belching due to the adverse rise of stomach *qi*, for which it is often combined with Flos Inulae, Rhizoma Pinelliae and Rhizoma Zingiberis Recens; and for cases complicated by deficiency of the middle *jiao*, Radix Ginseng is added to Decoction of Inulae and Haematitum. (b) Cough and dyspnea due to the adverse rise of lung *qi*. For deficiency cases, it is used with Radix Codonopsis Pilosular and Semen Juglandis; and for excess cases, it is combined with Semen Perillae and Rhizoma Cynanchi Stauntonii.

(3) To calm the heart and mind. Indicated for palpitation and insomnia, for which it is often prescribed along with Os Draconis and Magnetitum.

(4) To stop bleeding. Indicated for hematemesis and epistaxis due to the upward disturbance of *qi*, fire and blood-heat, for which it is often combined with Cortex Moutan Radicis, Fructus Gardeniae and Radix Curcumae to check the abnormal ascent of *qi*, purge fire and stop bleeding.
Dosage and Preparation: 15-30 g in decoction, and 3 g in powder. Used either in crude form or after calcination.
Remarks: Haematitum is heavy and descending, and it is indicated for diseases due to the adverse rise of pathogenic factors. It cures dizziness because of its action in subduing hyperactive liver *yang*; it treats vomiting and hiccup for its action in suppressing the adverse rise of stomach *qi*; it relieve cough and dyspnea for its action in making the abnormally ascending lung *qi* go downwards; and it is effective for hematemesis and epistaxis for its action in checking the abnormal rise of *qi* and fire.

Rhizoma Gastrodiae(天麻 *tian ma*)

Rhizoma Gastrodiae is the tuber of the perennial herb Gastrodia elata Bl. of Orchidaceae. Produced mainly in Sichuan, Guizhou and Yunnan provinces, it is dug and collected in winter and spring (with those collected in winter in better quality); with the epidermis, stem above ground and hyphae removed, it is washed clean, steamed and dried under low temperature.

Taste and Property: Sweet, and mild.
Attributive Meridian: Liver meridian.
Actions and Indications:

(1) To subdue hyperactive liver *yang*. It is indicated for dizziness and headache due to the upward disturbance of hyperactive liver *yang*, for which it is often combined with Ramulus Uncariae cum Uncis and Concha Haliotidis. For upward disturbance of wind-phlegm, it is used with Rhizoma Pinelliae and Rhizoma Atractylodis Macrocephalae; for migraine, it is combined with Rhizoma Chuanxiong.

(2) To relieve convulsion. Indicated for convulsion due to irritation by liver wind, for which it is prescribed along with Cornu Saigae Tataricae and Ramulus Uncariae cum Uncis. For tetanus, it is combined with Rhizoma Arisaematis and Radix Ledebouriellae.

(3) To eliminate wind and remove obstruction in the collaterals. It is indicated for rheumatic pain and numbness of the limbs, for which it is combined with Radix Gentianae Macrophyllae, Rhizoma seu Radix Notopterygii and Radix Achyranthis Bidentatae.

Dosage: 3-10 g in decoction, and 1-1.5 g in powder.

Remarks: This drug is mild, and can subdue hyperactive liver *yang*, eliminate wind and remove obstruction in the collaterals, and is indicated for all kinds of wind syndromes, either cold or heat type or due to internal or external wind. For such cases, it is combined with other drugs according to specific conditions. It is an important drug to treat dizziness.

Cornu Saigae Tataricae(羚羊角 *ling yang jiao*)

Cornu Saigae Tataricae refers to the horn of the vertebrate Saiga tatarica Linnaeus of Bovidae. Produced in the Xinjiang Uygur Autonomous Region and Qinghai Province, the animal can be caught any time of the year (those caught in autumn produce horns of better quality), and the horn is removed with a saw.

Taste and Property: Salty, and cold.
Attributive Meridian: Liver and heart meridians.
Actions and Indications:

(1) To purge liver heat and eliminate wind. Indications: (a) Febrile diseases with wind due to excessive heat, marked by high fever, coma and convulsion of the limbs, as well as apoplexy, epilepsy and eclampsia due to wind agitated by hyperactive *yang*. For such cases, it is often combined with Ramulus Uncariae cum Uncis, Flos Chrysanthemi, Radix Rehmanniae and Rhizoma Coptidis, as in Decoction of Cornu Saigae Tataricae and

Ramulus Uncariae cum Uncis. (b) Headache, dizziness and blurred vision due to upward disturbance of hyperactive liver *yang*, for which it is often prescribed along with Ramulus Uncariae cum Uncis, Rhizoma Gastrodiae and Radix Paeoniae Alba.

(2) To purge liver heat and improve vision. It is indicated for flare-ups of liver fire, marked by redness, swelling and pain or nebulae in the eyes. For such cases, it is often combined with Radix Gentianae, Radix Scutellariae and Concha Haliotidis.

Dosage and Preparation: 0.3-0.5 g in powder, 1-3 g in decoction (cut into slices).

Remarks: Both Cornu Saigae Tataricae and Cornu Rhinocerotis can purge heat. The former acts mainly to pacify the liver and eliminate wind, the latter mainly purges heart fire and cools the blood. For cases with excessive heat that leads to coma, irritability and convulsion, they can be applied together to enhance the effect of purging heat and stopping convulsion.

APPENDIX:

Cornu Naemorhedi(山羊角 *shan yang jiao*)

This refers to the horn of Naemorhedus goral Hardwicke of Bovidae. Its taste, property, action and indication are similar to Cornu Saigae Tataricae, but has a milder effect. The recommended dosage is 10-15 g, cut into slices and prepared into a decoction.

Ramulus Uncariae cum Uncis(钩藤 *gou teng*)

Ramulus Uncariae cum Uncis is the hooked stem and branch of the evergreen woody vine Uncaria rhynchophylla (Miq.) Jacks. of Rubiaceae and other plants of the same genus. Produced mainly in the Guangxi Zhuang Autonomous Region, as well as Guangdong, Hunan, Zhejiang and Jiangxi provinces, it is collected in autumn and winter, and dried in the sun with the leaves removed.

Taste and Property: Sweet, and slightly cold.

Attributive Meridian: Liver meridian.

Actions and Indications:

(1) To purge heat and pacify the liver. Indicated for distention and achiness in the head due to heat in the liver meridian, or dizziness and blurred vision due to an upward disturbance of hyperactive liver yang. In the former case, it is combined with Spica Prunellae and Radix Scutellariae, and in the latter, with Rhizoma Gastrodiae and Concha Haliotidis.

(2) To eliminate wind and stop convulsions. It is indicated for febrile diseases, or convulsion due to liver heat with a stirring-up of wind, especially for infantile convulsion due to fever. For such cases, it is used with Cornu Saigae Tataricae, Rhizoma Gastrodiae and Flos Chrysanthemi.

Dosage and Preparation: 10-15 g, up to 30 g. Decocted later than other ingredients.

Scorpio(全蝎 *quan xie*)

Scorpio is the dried body of Buthus martensii Karsch of Buthidae. Produced mainly in Henan, Shandong, Hubei, Anhui and Jiangsu provinces, it is caught in late spring and early autumn; with foreign matter removed, it is boiled in water or salt water until it becomes stiff and the back grooved, then dried in the shade.

Synonym: *Quan chong.*
Taste and Property: Acrid, and mild and toxic.
Attributive Meridian: Liver meridian.
Actions and Indications:

(1) To eliminate wind and stop convulsions. Indicated for acute and chronic infantile convulsion, tetanus and apoplexy with deviation of the eyes and mouth, for which it is combined with other drugs according to the accompanying symptoms. Scolopendra is added, as in Spasmolytic Powder, to enhance spasmolytic effect; Rhizoma Typhonii and Bombyx Batryticatus are added, as in Powder for Treating Face Distortion, for deviation of the mouth and eyes.

(2) To remove obstruction in the collaterals and relieve pain. It is indicated for stubborn rheumatic pain and migraine, for which it is used alone to produce powder for oral administration or else combined with Scolopendra and Bombyx Batryticatus.

(3) To eliminate toxins and remove masses. It is indicated for skin infections, for which it is usually applied externally, and Fructus Gardeniae and wax can be used together with it to produce a plaster for external application.

Dosage and Preparation: 2-5 g in decoction, or 0.5-1 g in powder for oral administration. Moderate amount for external application. In most cases, the whole insect is applied, and sometimes only the tail since its effect is stronger.

Scolopendra(蜈蚣 *wu gong*)

Scolopendra is the dried body of Scolopendra subspinipes mutilans L. Koch of Scolopendridae. To be found in all parts of China, the insect is caught in spring and summer. With a piece of bamboo slice inserted into the body and tail, it is straightened and dried.

Synonym: *Tian long*, *bai jiao.*
Taste and Property: Acrid, and warm and toxic.
Attributive Meridian: Liver meridian.
Actions and Indications:

(1) To eliminate wind and relieve spasm. Indicated for acute and chronic infantile convulsion, apoplexy, epilepsy and tetanus, for which it is often used with Scorpion and Bombyx Batryticatus.

(2) To remove obstruction in the collaterals and relieve pain. Indicated for wandering rheumatic pain and stubborn migraine. For rheumatic pain, it is often combined with Agkistrodon seu Bungarus, Radix Ledebouriellae, Radix Angelicae Pubescentis and Ramulus Taxilli; and for headache, it is often used with Rhizoma Chuanxiong and Ledebouriellae.

(3) To remove toxins and masses. Indicated for skin infections, scrofula, poisonous snakebites and tinea infection, for which it is usually used externally. However, it can also be taken orally.

Dosage and Preparation: 1-3 g or 1-3 pieces in decoction; and 0. 6-1 g in powder. Moderate amount for external application.

Precaution: Contraindicated for pregnant women.

Bombyx Batryticatus(白僵蚕 *bai jiang can*)

Bombyx Batryticatus is the dried dead larva of silkworm Bombyx mori L. of Moniliaceae after infection or artificial vaccination of Beauveria bassiana before it produces silk. Produced mainly in such sericultural areas as Zhejiang, Jiangsu and Sichuan provinces, the dead silkworms are collected and mixed with lime in order to dehydrate them, then dried in the sun or baked.

Synonym: *Tian chong*.

Taste and Property: Salty and acrid, and mild.

Attributive Meridian: Liver and lung meridians.

Actions and Indications:

(1) To eliminate wind and stop convulsions. Indicated for convulsion due to liver wind and accumulated phlegm-heat, for which it is often combined with Scorpio, Rhizoma Gastrodiae and Arisaema cum Bile. For chronic infantile convulsion due to spleen deficiency, it is often prescribed along with Radix Codonopsis Pilosulae, Rhizoma Atractylodis Macrocephalae and Gastrodiae.

(2) To dispel wind and heat. Indications: (a) Urticaria, for which it is often combined with Herba Menthae and Periostracum Cicadae. (b) Headache due to wind-heat, for which it is often administered with Folium Mori and Flos Chrysanthemi. (c) Sore throat, for which it is often combined with Radix Scrophulariae, Radix Platycodi and Radix Glycyrrhizae.

(3) To resolve phlegm and soften masses. Indicated for scrofula and subcutaneous nodules, for which it is often used with Bulbus Fritillariae, Spica Prunellae and Concha Ostreae.

Dosage: 3-10 g.

Remarks: The infection of Beauveria bassiana in silkworm is very harmful to sericultural production, and so Bombyx Batryticatus is usually produced by artificial vaccination in non-sericultural areas to avoid spread of the disease. The dead infected silkworm chrysalis has an action similar to that of the larva.

Lumbricus(地龙 *di long*)

Lumbricus is the dried body of the annelid Pheretima aspergillum (Perrier), or Allolobophora caliginosa (Saviany) trapezoides (Ant. Duges) of Megascolecedae. The former is produced mainly in Guangdong and Fujian provinces as well as the Guangxi Zhuang

Autonomous Region; the latter is produced in all parts of China. It is caught in the period from spring to autumn, its abdomen is cut, the viscera and foreign matter are removed, and it is then dried in the sun or under low temperature; the latter is suffocated in plant ashes, and the ashes are removed, then dried in the sun or under a low temperature.

Synonym: *Qiu yin*.
Taste and Property: Salty, and cold.
Attributive Meridian: Liver and lung meridians.
Actions and Indications:

(1) To purge heat and eliminate wind. It is indicated for febrile diseases with high fever, irritability and convulsion, or dizziness and headache due to upward disturbance of hyperactive liver *yang*. For such cases, it is used with Ramulus Uncariae cum Uncis, Bombyx Batryticatus and drugs that purge heat.

(2) To remove obstruction in the collaterals. Indications: (a) *Bi*-syndrome due to wind-cold with redness, swelling, hot feeling, pain and impaired movement of the limbs, for which it is combined with Ramulus Mori Caulis Lonicerae and Radix Paeoniae Rubra; for *bi*-syndrome due to cold-dampness with impaired movement, it is prescribed along with Radix Aconiti, Radix Aconiti Kusnezoffii and Radix Arisaemae, as in Bolus for Mildly Activating the Meridians. (b) Apoplexy with hemiplegia, for which it is combined with Radix Astragali, Radix Angelicae Sinensis and Flos Carthami, as in Decoction for Invigorating *Yang*.

(3) To relieve asthma, especially those cases due to heat, for which it is used alone to produce a powder for oral administration, or combined with Herba Ephedrae, Semen Armeniacae Amarum and Gypsum Fibrosum.

Dosage: 5-10 g in decoction, and 1-2 g in powder.
Remarks: Scorpio, Scolopendra, Bombyx Batryticatus and Lumbricus are all common drugs derived from insects for relieving convulsion and removing obstruction in the collaterals. They are indicated for convulsions, rheumatic pain and hemiplegia. Among them, Scorpio and Scolopendra are stronger, but they are toxic and overdose should be avoided. Bombyx Batryticatus dispels wind and heat, and resolves phlegm and masses; and Lumbricus is cold and purges heat and relieves asthma.

Table 16. Actions of Drugs for Calming Liver and Suppressing Wind

Drug	Similarities	Differences
Concha Haliotidis	To subdue the hyperactivity of liver *yang*	To clear liver-heat and improve visual acuity
Concha Ostreae		Sedative; astringent; to soften lumps
Margarita		Tranquilizer to calm convulsion; to remove nebulae; to promote granulation
Concha Margaritifera Usta		Sedative; to improve visual acuity
Haematitum		To lower the adverse-rising *qi*; sedative; hemostatic
Rhizoma Gastrodiae		Anticonvulsive; to eliminate wind and remove obstruction from collaterals
Cornu Saigae Tataricae	To clear liver-heat; eliminate wind and relieve spasm	Powerful action of clearing liver-heat and eliminating wind; to improve visual acuity
Ramulus Uncariae cum Uncis		To pacify liver *yang*
Scorpio	To eliminate wind and relieve convulsion	Toxic; to activate circulation of collaterals and relieve pain; to remove toxic materials and resolve masses
Scolopendra		Toxic; to promote circulation of collaterals and relieve pain; to remove toxic materials and resolve masses
Bombyx Batryticatus		To dispel wind-heat; resolve phlegm and masses
Lumbricus		To clear heat, activate circulation of collaterals, and relieve asthma

Note: Other sections deal with additional drugs that have anticonvulsive action, including Radix Paeoniae Alba, Plastrum Testudinis and Carapax Trionycis

CHAPTER NINETEEN
DRUGS FOR PROMOTING RESUSCITATION

Drugs that open the obstructed "heart orifice" and restore consciousness are known as drugs for promoting resuscitation (*kai qiao yao*), or analeptics.

These drugs are acrid, aromatic and dispersive. They mainly enter the heart meridian and restore consciousness in comatous patients. They are applied for loss of consciousness in febrile diseases, apoplexy, epilepsy and syncope due to heat attacking the pericardium, or phlegm and turbidity obstructing the heart orifice.

The "heart orifice obstruction syndrome" can be of either hot or cold type. Those cases of the heat type are due to obstruction by pathogenic heat, exhibiting fever, flushed face, convulsion, deep red tongue with yellow coating and rapid pulse. Here analeptic drugs are combined with drugs that purge heat and toxins, cool the blood and eliminate wind, thus "resuscitating with cool drugs." Cases of the cold type are usually due to obstruction by pathogenic cold or phlegm-turbidity, manifested as bodily coldness, cyanosis, or rattling in the throat due to phlegm, pale tongue with white coating and slow pulse. For such cases, analeptic drugs are used together with drugs that eliminate cold and activate *qi*, thus "resuscitating with warm drugs."

Analeptics are mostly used for emergency cases. As they have a powerful dispersive action and likely cause damage to the primordial *qi*, they should not be taken for a long time. They are contraindicated for prostration with coma, cold sweating, cold limbs, and faint pulse.

Analeptics are mostly prepared into pills or powder, seldom into decoctions, as their effective substances are volatile and will be lost after being heated.

Moschus(麝香 *she xiang*)

Moschus is the secretion obtained from the musk gland of the grown-up male musk deer Moschus berezovskii Flerov, M. sifanicus Przewalski, or M. moschiferus Linnaeus of Cervidae. Mainly found in Sichuan, Yunnan and Shaanxi provinces as well as the Inner Mongolia and Tibet autonomous regions, it is usually collected in winter and spring. For wild musk deer, the musk gland sac is cut off, the water is absorbed with paper, and then it is dried in the shade. For domestically raised musk deer, the musk is surgically obtained from the musk gland sac and then kept airtight in the shade.

Synonym: *Yuan cun xiang*. The granulated musk, which is of high quality, is conventionally called *dang men zi*.

Taste and Property: Acrid, and warm.

Attributive Meridian: Heart, spleen and liver meridians.

Actions and Indications:

(1) To restore consciousness. It is indicated for coma and convulsion in febrile diseases, apoplexy, syncope due to phlegm and other factors. For such cases, it is often combined with Borneolum Syntheticum to enhance the analeptic effect. For heat-stroke of the excess type, it is usually prescribed along with drugs that purge heat and suppress wind, such as Cornu Rhinocerotis and Calculus Bovis, as in Bolus of Calculus Bovis for Resurrection and Purple Snow Pellet. For cold-stroke of the excess type, it is used with drugs that eliminate cold and activate *qi*, such as Storax, Lignum Aquilariae Resinatum and Flos Caryophylli, as in Pill of Storax.

(2) To activate blood circulation and remove blood stasis. Indicated for carbuncles, trauma and abdominal masses. For such cases, it is usually prepared into pills or powder for oral administration, or into adhesive plaster for external application.

Dosage and Preparation: 0.1-0.15 g, prepared into pills or powder. Moderate amount for external application.

Precaution: Contraindicated for pregnant women. Not advisable to prepare as a decoction.

Remarks: Moschus, with strong aromatic, acrid and dispersive properties, is the major drug for excess-type stroke due to cold or heat. It also activates blood circulation, removes blood stasis, relieves swelling and pain for the treatment of carbuncles, trauma, abdominal masses and rheumatic pain.

Calculus Bovis(牛黄 *niu huang*)

Calculus Bovis is the gallstone (in gallbladder and, less commonly, in the bile ducts) of Bos taurus domesticus Gmelin of Bovidae. It is produced in northwestern and northeastern China as well as Hebei, Henan and Jiangsu provinces. If the gallstone is found when slaughtering an ox, it is taken out and dried in the shade with the biles and the outer thin covering removed.

Synonym: *Xi huang*.

Taste and Property: Bitter and sweet, and cool.

Attributive Meridian: Heart and liver meridians.

Actions and Indications:

(1) To subdue the heart fire and stop convulsion, resolve phlegm and induce resuscitation. Indicated for febrile diseases with high fever, coma and convulsion, and apoplexy with coma and lockjaw, for which it is often combined with drugs that purge heat and toxins and other analeptics, prepared into pills or powder for emergency cases, such as Bolus of Calculus Bovis for Eliminating Heart Fire, Bolus of Calculus Bovis for Resurrection and Bolus of Precious Drugs.

(2) To purge heat and toxins. Indicated for pharyngitis, aphthae and carbuncles due to toxic heat, for which it is used either externally or internally. It may be combined with

Margarita, as in Powder of Margarita and Calculus Bovis, to be insufflated into the throat or applied in the buccal cavity. It is used as the chief ingredient in some oral patent medicines that purge heat and toxins, such as Pill of Calculus Bovis for Detoxification and Pill of Cornu Rhinocerotis and Calculus Bovis.

Dosage and Preparation: 0. 15-0. 3 g, prepared into pills or powder, and never a decoction. Moderate amount for external application.

Precaution: Use with caution for pregnant women.

Remarks: Natural calculus is rare. Now, it is artificially cultivated from ox's bile and pig's bile.

Both Calculus Bovis and Moschus are important analeptics. The former is cool and clears heart fire and resolves phlegm, while the latter is acrid, warm and dispersive. Both are effective in treating carbuncles, abscess, ulcer and boils, Calculus Bovis is more effective in purging heat and toxins, and Moschus is in activating blood circulation and relieving swelling.

Borneolum Syntheticum(冰片 *bing pian*)

Borneolum Syntheticum is obtained from the resin or trunk of Dryobalanops aromatica Gaerin. f. of Dipterocarpaceae, or the organic crystalline compound synthesized from turpentine and camphor, or else the sublimate from the leaves of Blumea balsamifera Dc. of Compositae. The first is mainly produced in Southeast Asia and also China's Hainan Province; the second is now produced in most parts of China, and the last, mainly in Guangdong and Yunnan provinces as well as the Guangxi Zhuang Autonomous Region.

Synonym: *Mei pian*, *long nao xiang*.

Taste and Property: Acrid and bitter, and slightly cold.

Attributive Meridian: Heart meridian.

Actions and Indications:

(1) To restore consciousness. Indicated for febrile diseases and apoplexy marked by coma, for which it produces a similar yet weaker action as Moschus with which it is often used together.

(2) To purge heat and relieve pain. Indicated for various kinds of skin infections, pharyngitis, stomatitis and eye diseases. It is commonly used externally in surgery, traumatology, laryngology and ophthalmology.

Dosage and Preparation: 0. 03-0. 1 g, prepared into pills or powder, but not decoction. Moderate amount for external use.

Precaution: Contraindicated for pregnant women.

Storax(苏合香 *su he xiang*)

Storax is a semi-liquid sticky yellow balsam of Liquidambar orientalis Mill. of Hamamelidaceae. It is produced mainly in Turkey and India, and also cultivated in the Guangxi Zhuang Autonomous Region of China. In early summer, cuts are made on the trunk bark to let the balsam out and flow down on the bark. The bark is peeled off in autumn and balsam is extracted. Then it is dissolved in alcohol and filtered when the alcohol is distilled; the highly refined product of Storax is obtained, and kept airtight in the shade.

Taste and Property: Acrid and sweet, and warm.
Attributive Meridian: Heart and spleen meridians.
Actions and Indications:

To restore consciousness and remove turbidity. Indicated for excess syndrome of stroke due to cold, as in apoplexy and phlegm syncope, as well as for sudden severe pain in the cardiac and abdominal region. It is usually applied in compound prescriptions and often used with Moschus, Flos Caryophylli, Borneolum Syntheticum and Lignum Aquilariae Resinatum, as in Pill of Storax, which is a main formula for excess syndrome of stroke due to cold.

Dosage and Preparation: 0.3-1 g, prepared into pills or bolus.

Remarks: This drug, with strong acrid, warm and dispersive properties, has been used in recent years as the chief ingredient to form the Bolus of Storax for Coronary Heart Diseases together with Lignum Santali Albi, Olibanum, Radix Aristolochiae and Borneolum Syntheticum to relieve angina pectoris. It has also been used together with Borneolum Syntheticum to form Pill of Storax and Borneolum Syntheticum with similar analgesic effect.

Rhizoma Acori Graminei(石菖蒲 *shi chang pu*)

Rhizoma Acori Graminei is the rhizome of the perennial herb Acorus gramineus Soland. of Araceae. Produced mainly in Zhejiang, Jiangsu and Sichuan provinces, it is collected in autumn and dried in the sun with foreign matter and the fibrous roots removed.

Taste and Property: Acrid, and warm.
Attributive Meridian: Heart and spleen meridians.
Actions and Indications:

(1) To resolve phlegm and restore consciousness. Indications: (a) Apoplexy and epilepsy due to phlegm-dampness obstructing the heart, marked by unconsciousness, dementia and thick greasy tongue coating, for which it is often combined with Radix Curcumae, Arisaema cum Bile and Rhizoma Pinelliae. (b) Amnesia, tinnitus and deafness due to retention of phlegm-dampness affecting the ascent of lucid *yang*, for which it is often used with Radix Polygalae, Poria and Arisaema cum Bile.

(2) To resolve dampness and harmonize the middle *jiao*. Indications: (a) Distention and stuffiness in the chest and abdomen, poor appetite and greasy tongue coating due to retained dampness in the middle *jiao*; here it is often combined with Rhizoma Atractylodis, Cortex Magnoliae Officinalis and Fructus Amomi Rotundus. (b) Dysentery with vomiting and loss of appetite, for which it is often prescribed along with Rhizoma Coptidis, Semen Begoniae Laciniatae and Radix Codonopsis Pilosulae, as in Powder for Treat-

ing Dysentery Associated with Loss of Appetite.

Dosage: 5-10 g.

Remarks: The analeptic effect of Rhizoma Acori Graminei is not as strong as that of Moschus and Borneolum Syntheticum, but, it resolves phlegm and dampness and is indicated for phlegm-dampness obstructing the heart with unconsciousness and cases due to dampness retained in the middle *jiao*.

Table 17. Actions of Drugs for Promoting Resuscitation

Drug	Similarities	Differences
Moschus	To promote analepsia	To activate blood flow and remove blood stasis
Calculus Bovis		To clear heart fire; anticonvulsant; anti-inflammatory and detoxicant
Borneolum Syntheticum		External use for clearing heat and relieving pain
Storax		Acrid, warm and dispersing in nature, good for treating collapse with unconsciousness of cold type
Rhizoma Acori Graminei		To resolve dampness and harmonize the middle *jiao*

Note: Other sections deal with additional drugs that have anticonsulsive action, including Radix Paeoniae Alba, Plastrum Testudinis and Carapax Trionycis.

CHAPTER TWENTY
TONICS

Drugs that nourish *qi* and blood as well as *yin* and *yang* insufficiency in order to strengthen the body resistance and relieve deficiency syndromes are known as tonics (*bu xu yao*).

Tonics are indicated for various kinds of deficiency syndromes, i.e., *qi* deficiency, *yang* deficiency, blood deficiency and *yin* deficiency, and they are accordingly divided into four categories.

(1) Tonics for *qi* deficiency are sweet and warm, and strengthen the vital activity, especially the functions of the spleen and lung. They are mainly indicated for cases of spleen *qi* deficiency, marked by poor appetite, loose stool, a weighted sensation and distention in the epigastrium and abdomen, spiritlessness, general lassitude and even edema and rectal prolapse; and for liver *qi* deficiency, marked by disinclination to speak and feeble voice, shortness of breath upon exertion and liability to sweating.

(2) Tonics for *yang* deficiency are warm and hot and can particularly nourish kidney *yang*. They are indicated mainly for cases marked by insufficient kidney *yang*, exhibiting aversion to cold, cold limbs, soreness and pain in the lumbar region and knee joints, increased urination in the night, impotence and premature ejaculation. Some can be applied for dyspnea of the deficiency type due to impaired renal ability to receive *qi*, or diarrhea due to spleen and kidney *yang* deficiency.

(3) Tonics for blood deficiency are mostly sweet and warm. They are indicated for cases marked by deficient heart and liver blood, exhibiting sallow complexion, pale lips and nails, dizziness, blurred vision, palpitation, insomnia and irregular menstruation. Most can replenish *yin* as well, and are indicated for disorders of *yin* deficiency.

(4) Tonics for *yin* deficiency are sweet and cold, and can nourish *yin* fluid, promote fluid production and relieve dryness. They are further classified into tonics for replenishing lung *yin*, stomach *yin*, liver *yin* and kidney *yin*. They are indicated respectively for cases of lung *yin* deficiency marked by dry cough, hemoptysis and dryness in the throat; for cases of stomach *yin* deficiency marked by thirst, gastric upset, acid regurgitation and belching; cases of liver *yin* deficiency marked by dizziness and xerophthalmia; and cases of liver *yin* deficiency marked by lumbargo, seminal emission, afternoon fever, night sweating, and hot feeling in the palms and soles.

Qi, blood, *yin* and *yang* are interdependent, and their insufficiency affects of each other. *Qi* and *yang* deficiency indicates hypofunction of the body's vital activity, and *yang* deficiency is often complicated by *qi* deficiency and vice versa. *Yin* and blood deficiency indicates the consumption of essence, blood and body fluid, and *yin* deficiency may be complicated by blood deficiency and vice versa. Therefore, tonics for *qi* deficiency are often used with those for *yang* deficiency, and so are tonics for blood deficiency and those for *yin* deficiency. In cases of deficiency of both *qi* and blood or deficiency of both *yin* and *yang*, therapies for nourishing both *qi* and blood or both *yin* and *yang* should be applied simultaneously.

Tonics are not advisable for syndromes with excessive pathogenic *qi* when the antipathogenic *qi* is not yet deficient, since improper use of tonics may promote pathogenic *qi* and aggravate the diseases. Where the pathogenic factors have not yet been completely expelled and the antipathogenic *qi* has become deficient, the treatment of eliminating pathogens should be combined with certain tonics to strengthen the antipathogenic *qi*, eliminate pathogenic *qi* and cure the disease. But it is vital to decide which should receive the priority—strengthening the antipathogenic *qi* or eliminating the pathogenic factors.

Sweet and greasy tonics are bad to digestion, and so are not indicated for cases of retention of dampness and turbidity in the middle *jiao* marked by epigastric and abdominal distention and fullness, poor appetite and loose stool. For spleen and stomach deficiency, tonics should be used together with drugs that activate *qi* and invigorate the spleen, so as to avoid damaging the appetite. Most tonics to nourish kidney *yang* are warm and dry, and may consume *yin* and fan up fire; they are not advisable for cases with *yin* deficiency and fire hyperactivity.

Section 1
Tonics for *Qi* Deficiency

Radix Ginseng(人参 *ren shen*)

Radix Ginseng is the root of the perennial plant Panax ginseng C. A. Mey. of Araliaceae. The wild one is called *ye shan shen*, and the cultivated one *yuan shen*. Produced mainly in Jilin, Liaoning and Heilongjiang provinces, the root is dug and collected in autumn. The fresh root, after the subterranean stem and foreign matter are removed, if steamed and dried in the sun or baked, is called *hong shen*; if bathed in boiling water and soaked in sugar water and then dried, it is called *bai shen* or *tang shen*; The fresh root directly dried in the sun is called *sheng shai shen*; the fibrous roots broken during processing are called *shen xu*; and the red ginseng produced in Korea is called *bie zhi shen*.

Taste and Property: Sweet and slightly bitter, and slightly warm.

Attributive Meridian: Heart, spleen and lung meridians.

Actions and Indications:

(1) To replenish the primordial *qi*. It is indicated for collapse due to prostration of primordial *qi*. For such cases, it is used alone to produce a decoction for oral administration to replenish *qi* and rescue the patient from prostration. For cases of decline of *yang qi* with cold limbs, it is combined with Radix Aconiti Lateralis Preparata, as in Decoction of Ginseng and Aconiti Lateralis, to replenish *qi* and restore the depleted *yang*. In cases of

exhaustion of *yin* and *qi* accompanied by profuse sweating and thirst, it is combined with Radix Ophiopogonis and Fructus Schisandrae, as in Powder for Restoring the Pulse, to replenish *qi* and *yin*.

(2) To nourish the spleen and stomach. Indicated for cases of spleen and stomach deficiency marked by general lassitude, poor appetite, epigastric fullness, vomiting and loose stools, it is often combined with Rhizoma Atractylodis Macrocephalae, Poria and Radix Glycyrrhizae Preparata to reinforce the spleen and replenish *qi*.

(3) To invigorate lung *qi*. It is indicated for lung *qi* deficiency marked by rapid and short breathing and feeble voice, for which it is prescribed along with Schisandrae and Radix Astragali to replenish lung *qi*. For long-standing dyspnea due to deficiency of both the lung and kidney, it is combined with Semen Juglandis and Gecko to nourish both the organs, strengthen the renal function in receiving *qi* and relieve dyspnea.

(4) To promote the production of body fluid. Indicated for diabetes, for which it is often used with Radix Rehmanniae and Radix Trichosanthis. For febrile diseases with fluid and *qi* consumption marked by fever, thirst, profuse sweating and feeble pulse, it is combined with Gypsum Fibrosum and Rhizoma Anemarrhenae to replenish *qi*, promote fluid production and purge heat.

It also replenishes *qi* and promotes the generation of blood, and so can be used for palpitation and insomnia due to *qi* and blood insufficiency.

Dosage and Preparation: 3-10 g, decocted alone on a slow fire for oral administration; in larger dosage for emergent cases; or 1-1.5 g as powder which is taken three times a day.

Precaution: Incompatible with Rhizoma et Radix Veratri and antagonistic to Faeces Trogopterorum.

Remarks: Radix Ginseng is the first choice for replenishing primordial *qi*. It is indicated for various types of *qi* deficiency, especially critical cases of *qi* collapse. It is not advisable for patients with strong constitution and absence of deficiency syndrome, since otherwise it may result in *qi* stagnation marked by stuffiness in the chest and abdominal distention. It should not be used in such excess syndromes as exterior syndrome due to exogenous pathogenic factors or accumulated excess heat in the interior, so as to avoid possible retention of the pathogenic factors. For cases of hyperactive pathogenic *qi* and weak antipathogenic *qi*, Radix Ginseng is used together with drugs that eliminate pathogenic factors.

Radix Ginseng is divided into various kinds according to differences in places of production and processing methods. Traditionally, *bai shen* and *shen shai shen* are used to treat cases of deficiency of both *qi* and *yin*; *hong shen* and *bie zhi shen* are often used to treat cases of *yang qi* deficiency. *Shen xu*, the fibrous roots, has a same but weaker action as that of the main root.

Radix Codonopsis Pilosulae(党参 *dang shen*)

Radix Codonopsis Pilosulae is the root of the perennial herb Codonopsis Pilosula (Franch.) Nannf. of Campanulaceae. Produced mainly in Shanxi, Shaanxi, Gansu and Sichuan provinces, it is collected in spring and summer, and dried in the sun with the stem and foreign matter removed.

Taste and Property: Sweet, and slightly warm.
Attributive Meridian: Spleen and lung meridians.
Actions and Indications:

To nourish the middle *jiao* and replenish *qi*. Indicated for spleen and stomach deficiency marked by poor appetite and loose stools , for which it is combined with Rhizoma Atractylodis Macrocephalae and Radix Astragali; For lung *qi* deficiency with cough and shortness of breath, it is often used with Fructus Schisandrae; and for blood deficiency with weak constitution, it is combined with drugs that nourish the blood to replenish *qi* and promote the generation of blood.

Dosage: 10-15 g, or 30 g at the most.

Remarks: Radix Codonopsis Pilosulae and Radix Ginseng have essentially the same actions, and so Radix Codonopsis Pilosulae is frequently used as a substitute for Radix Ginseng in ancient prescriptions. Nevertheless, the ability of the former to replenish *qi* is much weaker than the latter, and so in critical cases of collapse the latter should be applied.

Radix Astragali(黄芪 *huang qi*)

Radix Astragali is the root of the perennial herb Astragalus membranaceus Bge. var. mongholicus (Bge.) Hsiao, or A. membranaceus (Fisch.) Bge. of Leguminosae. Produced mainly in Shanxi, Gansu and Heilongjiang provinces as well as the Inner Mongolia Autonomous Region, it is collected in spring and autumn, and dried in the sun with the fibrous roots and root cap removed.

Taste and Property: Sweet, and slightly warm.
Attributive Meridian: Spleen and lung meridians.
Actions and Indications:

(1) To replenish *qi* and invigorate *yang*. Indicated for deficiency of spleen and stomach *qi* marked by sallow complexion, loss of appetite and loose stools. For such cases, it is often combined with Radix Codonopsis Pilosulae, Rhizoma Atractylodis Macrocephalae and Radix Glycyrrhizae to strengthen the spleen and replenish *qi*. For prolapse of *qi* of the middle *jiao*, it is often used with Rhizoma Cimicifugae and Radix Bupleuri, as in Decoction for Strengthening the Middle *Jiao* and Benefiting *Qi*, to replenish *qi* and invigorate *yang*.

(2) To consolidate the body surface and check perspiration. Used for patients with weak defensive *qi* marked by spontaneous sweating, or those with weak constitution who are susceptible to attack by exogenous wind. For such cases, it is often combined with Radix Ledebouriellae and Rhizoma Atractylodis Macrocephalae, as in Jade Screen Powder, to replenish *qi*, consolidate the defensive *qi* and check perspiration; or else used with Herba Ephedrae, Concha Ostreae and Fructus Tritici Levis (light).

(3) To promote diuresis and relieve edema. Indicated for edema due to spleen deficiency or edema due to wind, for which it is combined with Radix Stephaniae Tetrandrae,

Atractylodis Macrocephalae and Radix Glycyrrhizae, as in Decoction of Stephaniae Tetrandrae and Astragali, to replenish *qi*, strengthen the spleen and promote diuresis.

(4) To discharge pus and promote granulation. Indicated for abscess with insufficient *qi* and blood, or else abscess that does not heal properly after rupture with discharge of dilute pus. For unruptured abscess, it is used with Radix Angelicae Sinensis, Spina Gleditsiae and Squama Manitis; for unhealed ruptured abscess, it is combined with Radix Codonopsis Pilosulae, Angelicae Sinensis and Cortex Cinnamomi.

This drug is also indicated for cases with numbness of the limbs and hemiplegia due to *qi* deficiency and blood stagnation.

Dosage and Preparation: 10-15 g, or as much as 30 g. Used in crude form for spontaneous sweating, edema, abscess and ulcers, and baked for weakness of the spleen and stomach as well as insufficient *qi* and blood.

Remarks: Both Radix Ginseng and Radix Astragali are essential for replenishing *qi*, and they are often used simultaneously. But the former is much stronger and is indispensable for preventing collapse, while the latter is more effective for invigorating *yang*, and can consolidate the body surface's defensive *qi*, regulate water metabolism, dispel pus and promote granulation.

Rhizoma Atractylodis Macrocephalae(白术 *bai zhu*)

Rhizoma Atractylodis Macrocephalae is the rhizome of the perennial herb Atractylodis macrocephala Koidz. of Compositae. Produced mainly in Zhejiang, Hubei, Hunan and Jiangxi provinces, it is collected in the period from the Frost's Descent to the Beginning of Winter when the lower leaves turn yellow and wither and the upper leaves become fragile; with the stem, leaves and foreign matter removed, it is then dried in the sun or baked dry.

Taste and Property: Sweet and bitter, and warm.
Attributive Meridian: Spleen and stomach meridians.
Actions and Indications:

(1) To replenish *qi* and strengthen the spleen. Indicated for spleen and stomach deficiency marked by poor appetite, distention and fullness in the epigastrium and abdomen and loose stools, for which it is often combined with Radix Codonopsis Pilosulae, Radix Glycyrrhizae and Poria. For cases complicated by food stagnation, it is used with Fructus Aurantii Immaturus, as in Pill of Aurantii Immaturus and Atractylodis Macrocephalae, so as to remove stagnant food and remedy the deficiency at the same time.

(2) To eliminate dampness and promote diuresis. Indicated for spleen deficiency leading to fluid, dampness and phlegm retention, as well as edema, for which it is often combined with Ramulus Cinnamomi, Poria and Rhizoma Alismatis, as in Powder of Five Drugs Containing Poria, and Decoction of Poria, Ramulus Cinnamomi, Atractylodis Macrocephalae and Glycyrrhizae.

It also checks perspiration, and is indicated for spontaneous sweating due to deficiency of the defensive *qi*, for which it is often prescribed along with Radix Astragali. Moreover, it prevents miscarriage, and is often combined with Radix Scutellariae for threatened abortion.

Remarks: Both Rhizoma Atractylodis Macrocephalae and Rhizoma Atractylodis strengthen the spleen and eliminate dampness. The former is sweet, bitter and mild, and acts mainly to nourish the spleen and check perspiration; the latter is acrid, bitter, dry and strong, and acts mainly to dry dampness and induce perspiration. Therefore, Atractylodis Macrocephalae is often used for spleen deficiency or deficiency of the defensive *qi* with spontaneous sweating, while Rhizoma Atractylodis is usually applied for excess syndromes with dampness retained in the middle *jiao* or exterior syndromes complicated by dampness.

Rhizoma Dioscoreae(山药 *shan yao*)

Rhizoma Dioscoreae is the rhizome of the perennial trailing plant Dioscorea opposita Thunb. of Dioscoreaceae. Produced mainly in Henan, Jiangsu and Hunan provinces as well as the Guangxi Zhuang Autonomous Region, it is collected after the Frost's Descent and washed clean, the coarse epidermis is scraped off, and it is polished and cut into slices.

Taste and Property: Sweet, and mild.

Attributive Meridian: Spleen, lung and kidney meridians.

Actions and Indications:

(1) To strengthen the spleen. Indicated for spleen and stomach deficiency marked by loss of appetite, lassitude, chronic diarrhea, infantile malnutrition and leukorrhagia, for which it is often combined with Rhizoma Atractylodis Macrocephalae and Radix Codonopsis Pilosulae.

(2) To replenish *yin* and nourish the lung and kidney. Indications: (a) Chronic cough due to lung deficiency or chronic cough and dyspnea due to lung and kidney deficiency, for which it is often used with Radix Adenophorae, Radix Ophiopogonis, Fructus Schisandrae and Fructus Corni. (b) Seminal emission, hectic fever due to *yin* deficiency and frequent urination due to kidney deficiency. For such cases, it is often combined with Corni, Radix Rehmanniae Preparata and Fructus Rosae Laevigatae.

This drug is also indicated for diabetes.

Dosage: 10-30 g.

Remarks: Both Rhizoma Atractylodis Macrocephalae and Rhizoma Dioscoreae nourish and strengthen the spleen and are applied for disorders due to spleen deficiency. But the former can eliminate dampness, and is indicated for disorders due to spleen deficiency complicated by dampness; the latter is moistening and replenishes *yin*, and is indicated for cases due to deficient lung and kidney *yin*. The difference in the dry and moist properties of these two drugs merits attention.

Radix Glycyrrhizae(甘草 *gan cao*)

Radix Glycyrrhizae is the root and rhizome of the perennial herb Glycyrrhiza uralensis Fisch., G. inflata Bat., or G. glabra L. of Leguminosae. Produced mainly in Gansu and

Shanxi provinces as well as the Inner Mongolia Autonomous Region, it is collected in spring and autumn, and dried in the sun with the fibrous roots and foreign matter removed.

Taste and Property: Sweet, and mild.
Attributive Meridian: Spleen, heart and lung meridians.
Actions and Indications:

(1) To nourish the heart and spleen. Indications: (a) Sallow complexion, poor appetite and loose stools due to spleen and stomach deficiency, for which it is often combined with Radix Codonopsis Pilosulae, Rhizoma Atractylodis Macrocephalae and Poria. (b) Palpitation upon slight exertion and knotted and intermittent pulse due to deficient heart *qi*, for which it is often combined with Ramulus Cinnamomi, Radix Ophiopogonis, Codonopsis Pilosulae and Fructus Schisandrae.

(2) To moisten the lung and relieve cough. Indicated for cases with cough, in which it is often used with expectorants and antitussives. For its mild property, it can be applied for cough due to either cold or heat.

(3) To purge fire and remove toxins. Indications: (a) Carbuncles, for which it is often prescribed along with antipyretics and antiphlogistics, such as Flos Lonicerae and Fructus Forsythiae. (b) Drug and food poisoning. When no particular detoxicant is available, fresh Radix Glycyrrhizae and Semen Phaseoli Radiati, 60 g each, can be prepared into a decoction for oral administration. (c) Pharyngitis, for which it is often used with Radix Platycodi.

(4) To relieve spasm and pain. Indications: (a) Epigastric pain, abdominal pain and spasm of the gastrocnemius muscle due to deficiency of the middle *jiao*, for which it is often combined with Radix Paeoniae Alba to relieve spasm and pain. (b) To reduce the toxic and side effects of other drugs.

It can also be used together with Fructus Tritici Levis and Fructus Jujubae for hysteria, as in Decoction of Glycyrrhizae, Tritici Levis and Jujubae.

Dosage and Preparation: 2-5 g as adjuvant; about 10 g as a major ingredient; and 30-60 g as an antidote in emergent cases. Used in crude form to purge fire and eliminate toxins, and baked to nourish the heart and spleen.

Precaution: The drug is very sweet and can promote the production of dampness, and overdosage may lead to a full and stuffy feeling in the middle *jiao*. It is contraindicated for cases with excessive dampness marked by abdominal distention and edema. Prolonged use in large dosage may result in edema. It is incompatible with Radix Kansui, Radix Euphorbiae Pekinensis, Flos Genkwa and Sargassum.

Fructus Jujubae(大枣 *da zao*)

Fructus Jujubae refers to the fruit of the deciduous shrub or tree Ziziphus jujuba Mill. of Rhamnaceae. Produced mainly in Hebei, Henan, Shandong and Shaanxi provinces, it is collected in autumn when the fruit is ripe and dried in the sun.

Taste and Property: Sweet, and warm.
Attributive Meridian: Spleen and stomach meridians.
Actions and Indications:

(1) To nourish the spleen and stomach. Indicated for spleen and stomach deficiency, for which it is often combined with Radix Codonopsis Pilosulae, Rhizoma Atractylodis Macrocephalae and Poria.

(2) To moderate the action of other drugs. It is often used in prescriptions with potent and drastic actions to reduce the side effects of other ingredients. For example, in Decoction of Lepidii seu Descurainiae and Jujubae for Purging Liver Heat, Fructus Jujubae is used to moderate the drastic action of Semen Lepidii seu Descurainiae; in Decoction of Jujubae, Radix Kansui, Radix Euphorbiae Pekinensis and Flos Genkwa to promote diuresis, Fructus Jujubae is used to protect stomach *qi*. It is also used to treat hysteria.

Jujubae nourishes the blood and is often used for blood deficiency. In recent years, it has been used in a large dosage for the treatment of anaphylactoid purpura and thrombocytopenia.

Dosage: 3-10 pieces, or 10-15 g.
Precaution: As it is sweet and promotes dampness, it can give rise to a full and stuffy feeling in the middle *jiao*; it is contraindicated for cases with epigastric and abdominal distention and fullness due to excessive dampness, food stagnation, parasitic infestation and caries.

Mel(**蜂蜜** *feng mi*)

This is the liquid carbohydrate made from the nectar by honey bees Apis cerana Fabricius., or A. mellifera Linnaeus of Apidae. Produced in most parts of China, it is collected in spring and autumn. The honeycomb is cut off, kept in a cloth, the honey is obtained by squeezing or centrifuging, and then filtered.

Synonym: *Bai mi*.
Taste and Property: Sweet, and mild.
Attributive Meridian: Lung, spleen and large intestine meridians.
Actions and Indications:

(1) To nourish the middle *jiao* and relieve spasm and pain. It is indicated for spleen and stomach deficiency and epigastric and abdominal pain due to deficiency of the middle *jiao*. It is prepared into a decoction for oral administration and frequently used as an excipient in tonic pills and extracts.

(2) To moisten the lung and relieve cough. Indicated for dry cough due to lung dryness and chronic cough due to consumptive diseases, as well as dryness and pain in the throat. For such cases, it is used either alone or in combination with Radix Rehmanniae, Radix Ginseng and Poria, as in Fine Jade Extract. Expectorants are usually mixed and baked with honey to enhance their effect of moistening the lung and relieving cough.

(3) To promote bowel movements. Indicated for constipation in aged and debilitated patients due to intestinal dryness or fluid consumption.

Mel can also purge heat and eliminate toxins, and used externally for carbuncles and burns, and orally for poisoning by Radix Aconiti and Radix Aconiti Lateralis Preparata.
Dosage and Preparation: 15-30 g, taken directly with water, or prepared into pills and extract.
Remarks: Radix Glycyrrhizae, Fructus Jujubae and Mel are all very sweet and mild, and can nourish the middle *jiao*, relieve spasm and pain, moisten the dryness and eliminate toxins. *The Inner Canon of the Yellow Emperor* says, "Drugs sweet in taste can relieve urgency," indicating that they relieve spasm and pain, moderate the action of other drugs and relieve urgency (as in hysteria). All three drugs have their strong points, but Radix Glycyrrhizae is particularly effective in relieving urgency.

Drugs with a strong sweet taste are usually sticky, and overdose may affect the transporting and transforming function of the spleen and produce dampness and turbidity, resulting in distention and fullness of the epigastrium and abdomen and poor appetite. These drugs are therefore contraindicated for cases due to spleen deficiency, excessive dampness and stuffiness and fullness in the middle *jiao*.

Section 2
Tonics for *Yang* Deficiency

Cornu Cervi Pantotrichum (鹿茸 *lu rong*)

Cornu Cervi Pantotrichum is the hairy, unossified young antlers of the male Cervus nippon Temminck, or stag C. elaphus Linnaeus of Cervidae. Found in northeastern and northwestern China, Inner Mongolia and Xinjiang Uygur autonomous regions as well as the mountainous areas of southwestern China, many are domestically raised. In summer and autumn, the pilose unossified antlers are cut off, bathed in boiling water and aired dry until the stagnant blood is completely removed, then dried in the shade or by baking.

Taste and Property: Sweet and salty, and warm.
Attributive Meridian: Liver and kidney meridians.
Actions and Indications:

To reinforce kidney *yang*, replenish essence and blood, and strengthen the muscles and bones. It is indicated for cases due to insufficient kidney *yang* and deficiency of essence and blood. These include: (a) Chronic diseases marked by general lassitude and spiritlessness, lumbago and cold limbs, polyuria with clear urine, impotence, spermatorrhea and leukorrhagia with clear discharge, for which it is often used with Radix Rehmanniae Preparata, Cortex Eucommiae and Herba Cistanches. (b) Infantile maldevelopment marked by weakness of the muscles and bones, incomplete closure of the fontanel, and retarded speech and movement, for which it is often combined with Rehmanniae Preparata and Fructus Corni. (c) Chronic diseases with blood deficiency and liver and kidney deficiency, for which it is often used with Radix Ginseng, Radix Astragali, Rehmanniae Preparata and Radix Angelicae Sinensis. (d) Deficiency of the extra-meridians with incessant uterine bleeding, for which it is often prescribed along with Colla Corii Asini, Os

Sepiae, Angelicae Sinensis and Plastrum Testudinis.

It also warms and nourishes the body and discharges pus, and is indicated for unhealed ruptured abscesses and deep-rooted carbuncles.

Dosage and Preparation: 0. 6-2 g, ground into powder or prepared into pills.

Precaution: Cornu Cervi Pantotrichum has a potent warming and nourishing action. A prompt large dosage may render *yang* hyperactive and disturb the blood, resulting in dizziness, redness in the eyes, hematemesis and epistaxis. It is contraindicated for cases marked by deficient *yin* and hyperactive *yang* as well as heat in the blood system.

APPENDIX

1. **Cornu Cervi**(鹿角 *lu jiao*)

This is the ossified horn of the deer or stag. Salty and warm, it enters the liver and kidney meridians, and can warm and nourish kidney *yang*. It has similar but weaker effect as Cornu Cervi Pantotrichum. It also activates blood circulation, removes blood stasis and cures carbuncles, abscesses and ulcers. The recommended dosage is 5-10 g, applied orally or topically.

2. **Colla Cornu Cervi**(鹿角胶 *lu jiao jiao*)

This is a kind of glue extracted by decocting from the antlers. Sweet, salty and warm, it enters the liver and kidney meridians, and can nourish kidney *yang*, replenish essence and blood and check bleeding. It is indicated for cases of kidney *yang* insufficiency, essence and blood deficiency, hematemesis, hematuria and metrorrhagia of the deficiency-cold type. The recommended dosage is 5-10 g, melted in water for oral administration, or prepared into pills, powder and extract.

3. **Cornu Cervi Degelatinatum**(鹿角霜 *lu jiao shuang*)

This is the powder made from the residue in processing antler glue. It is salty and warm, enters the liver and kidney meridians, and warms and nourishes kidney *yang* and has an astringent action. It is indicated for incontinence of urine, metrorrhagia and leukorrhagia due to kidney *yang* deficiency. It can also be applied externally as a hemostatic for cases of trauma. The recommended dosage is 10-15 g.

Remarks: Cornu Cervi Pantotrichum nourishes kidney *yang* and replenishes essence and blood, and is indicated for kidney *yang* deficiency and deficiency of essence and blood. It is different from Radix Aconiti Lateralis Preparata and Cortex Cinnamomi, both of which are hot and dry and are more effective in warming and promoting "fire of the life gate."

The effects of the other three drugs derived from the antlers are basically the same—warming and nourishing kidney *yang*. But, Cornu Cervi also activates blood circulation and relieves swelling, Colla Cornu Cervi is more effective for nourishing blood and checking bleeding, and Cornu Cervi Degelatinatum possesses an astringent effect.

Herba Cistanches(肉苁蓉 *rou cong rong*)

Herba Cistanches is the squamous fleshy stem of the perennial parasitic plant Cistanche deserticola Y. C. Ma of Orobanchaceae. Produced mainly in Gansu and Qinghai provinces as well as Inner Mongolia and Xinjiang Uygur autonomous regions, it is collected in spring before the plant sprouts above the ground, the inflorescence is removed, and then it is cut into sections and dried in the sun.

Synonym: *Da yun.*
Taste and Property: Sweet and salty, and warm.
Attributive Meridian: Kidney and large intestine meridians.
Actions and Indications:

(1) To nourish the kidney and reinforce *yang*. It is indicated for disorders due to insufficient kidney *yang*, such as impotence, pain in the lumbar area and weakness in the legs as well as infertility in women. For such cases, it is often combined with Fructus Psoraleae and Radix Morindae Officinalis.

(2) To promote bowel movements. Indicated for constipation due to intestinal dryness, as seen in the aged, convalescents and puerperants with blood loss, for which it is prescribed along with Radix Angelicae Sinensis and Fructus Cannabis.

Dosage: 10-15 g, and as much as 30 g.
Remarks: Most drugs that reinforce *yang* are warm and dry, but Herba Cistanches is warm and moist, and can be used as a laxative for relieving constipation. It is particularly indicated for constipation in the aged due to *yang* deficiency, but it is contraindicated for spleen deficiency with loose stools.

Herba Epimedii(淫羊藿 *yin yang huo*)

Herba Epimedii refers to the aerial part of the perennial herb Epimedium brevicornum Maxim., and other plants of the same genus of Berberidaceae. Produced mainly in Shaanxi, Liaoning, Shanxi and Sichuan provinces, it is collected in summer and autumn and dried in the sun.

Synonym: *Xian ling pi.*
Taste and Property: Acrid and sweet, and warm.
Attributive Meridian: Liver and kidney meridians.
Actions and Indications:

(1) To nourish the kidney and reinforce *yang*. Indicated for impotence, infertility and frequent urination due to insufficient kidney *yang*, for which it is often used with Rhizoma Curculiginis, Fructus Corni and Fructus Rubi.

(2) To strengthen the muscles and bones and eliminate wind-dampness. Indicated for long-standing cases of *bi*-syndrome due to wind-dampness, cold and pain in the lumbus and knee joints, spasm of the limbs and hemiplegia, for which it is often combined with Radix Clematidis, Radix Angelicae Sinensis and Rhizoma Chuanxiong.

Dosage: 5-10 g.

Cortex Eucommiae(杜仲 *du zhong*)

Cortex Eucommiae is the bark of the deciduous tree Eucommia ulmoides Oliv. of Eucommiaceae. Produced mainly in Sichuan, Yunnan and Guizhou provinces, it is collected in the April-June period, with the coarse epidermis scraped off, it is piled up to let moisture evaporate until the inner side of the bark turns dark brown, and then dried in the sun.

Taste and Property: Sweet and slightly acrid, and warm.
Attributive Meridian: Liver and kidney meridians.
Actions and Indications:

(1) To nourish the liver and kidney and strengthen the muscles and bones. Indicated for kidney and liver insufficiency manifested as achiness and weakness of the lumbar region and knees, for which it is often combined with Radix Rehmanniae Preparata, Radix Dipsaci and Radix Achyranthis Bidentatae.

(2) To prevent miscarriage. Indicated for uterine bleeding during pregnancy, lumbago with restlessness of the fetus, or habitual abortion, for which it is often prescribed along with Dipsaci, Rhizoma Atractylodis Macrocephalae and Radix Boehmeriae.

It can also be used for dizziness due to liver deficiency.

Dosage and Preparation: 10-15 g; baked.
Remarks: Liver controls the tendons and kidney controls the bones, and the lumbus houses the kidney. Liver and kidney insufficiency thus usually leads to soreness of the lumbus and knee joints and weakness of the legs. Cortex Eucommiae can nourish the liver and kidney and strengthen the tendons and bones, and is important for the treatment of liver and kidney insufficiency that causes lumbar pain and weak legs. Its ability to prevent miscarriage is related to this, because liver and kidney sufficiency ensures the consolidation of the fetus. Its action differs from that of Fructus Amomi and Fructus Perillae since it invigorates *qi* circulation, and from that of Radix Scutellariae since it purges heat.

Radix Dipsaci(续断 *xu duan*)

Radix Dipsaci is the root of the perennial herb of Dipsacus asper Wall. of Dipsacaceae. Produced mainly in Sichuan, Hubei, Hunan and Guizhou provinces, it is collected in autumn; with the root cap and fibrous roots removed, it is baked until partially dry over a slow fire and then piled up for evaporation until its interior side turns green, then again baked dry.

Synonym: *Chuan duan*.
Taste and Property: Bitter and acrid, and slightly warm.
Attributive Meridian: Liver and kidney meridians.
Actions and Indications:

(1) To nourish the liver and kidney. Indicated for insufficiency of the liver and kidney exhibiting lumbago and soreness of knee joints or rheumatic pain, for which it is often combined with Cortex Eucommiae and Radix Achyranthis Bidentatae.

(2) To promote reunion of fractured bones. It is indicated for fracture, sprain and

trauma, for which it is often used with Rhizoma Drynariae, Pyritum and Eupolyphaga seu Steleophaga.

(3) To prevent miscarriage and stop uterine bleeding. It is indicated for uterine bleeding during pregnancy, restlessness of the fetus and metrorrhagia, for which it is often combined with Radix Rehmanniae Preparata, Colla Corii Asini and Folium Artemisiae Argyi.

Dosage and Preparation: 10-15 g, used in crude form or after baking.

Remarks: This drug is similar to Cortex Eucommiae in action but has a weaker effect, and they are often combined for lumbago and weakness of the lower limbs. As Dipsaci can promote the reunion of fractured bones, and is frequently used to treat fracture and trauma.

Rhizoma Cibotii(狗脊 *gou ji*)

Rhizoma Cibotii is the rhizome of the perennial fern of Cibotium barometz (L.) J. Sm. of Dicksoniaceae. Produced mainly in Sichuan, Zhejiang and Fujian provinces, it is collected in late autumn and early winter when the aerial part withers, then it is dried in the sun, or steamed first and dried again.

Taste and Property: Bitter and sweet, and warm.

Attributive Meridian: Liver and kidney meridians.

Actions and Indications:

To nourish the liver and kidney, strengthen the tendons and bones and eliminate wind and dampness. Indications: (a) Insufficiency of the liver and kidney marked by soreness of the lumbus and knee joints with impaired movement, as well as weakness of the lower limbs, for which it is often combined with Radix Rehmanniae Preparata, Cortex Eucommiae and Radix Dipsaci. (b) *Bi*-syndrome due to wind, cold and dampness, manifested as lumbago and arthralgia in the lower limbs, for which it is often prescribed along with Radix Angelicae Pubescentis, Herba Asari, Radix Achyranthis Bidentatae and Semen Coicis.

Dosage: 10-15 g.

Fructus Psoraleae(补骨脂 *bu gu zhi*)

Fructus Psoraleae is the ripe fruit of the annual herb Psoralea corylifolia L. of Leguminosae. Produced mainly in Henan, Sichuan and Shaanxi provinces, it is collected in autumn when the fruit is ripe.

Synonym: *Po gu zhi*.

Taste and Property: Acrid and bitter, and warm.

Attributive Meridian: Spleen and kidney meridians.

Actions and Indications:

(1) To nourish the kidney and promote *yang*, and stop diarrhea. Indications: (a) Insufficiency of kidney *yang* marked by lumbar pain, impotence, seminal emission, noctur-

nal enuresis and frequent urination, for which it is often combined with Herba Epimedii, Semen Cuscutae, Radix Dipsaci and Rhizoma Dioscoreae. (b) Diarrhea due to cold in and deficiency of the spleen and kidney, for which it is often used with Semen Myristicae, as in Pill of Two Miraculous Drugs.

(2) To promote the kidney's ability to receive *qi*, and relieve dyspnea. Indicated for kidney failure marked by shortness of breath and dyspnea aggravated upon exertion, for which it is often combined with Radix Ginseng, Semen Juglandis and Fructus Schisandrae.

Dosage: 6-15 g.

Fructus Alpiniae Oxyphyllae(益脂仁 *yi zhi ren*)

Fructus Alpiniae Oxyphyllae is the ripe fruit of the perennial plant Alpinia oxyphylla Miq. of Zingiberaceae. Produced mainly in Guangdong Province and the Guangxi Zhuang Autonomous Region, it is collected at the end of summer and the beginning of autumn when the green fruit turns red, then dried in the sun or under low temperature.

Taste and Property: Acrid, and warm.

Attributive Meridian: Spleen and kidney meridians.

Actions and Indications:

(1) To nourish the kidney, consolidate the essence and reduce urination. It is indicated for kidney deficiency marked by seminal emission, nocturnal enuresis and frequent urination, for which it is often combined with Semen Cuscutae, Fructus Rubi and Rhizoma Dioscoreae.

(2) To warm the spleen, check diarrhea and salivation. Indications: (a) Spleen *yang* deficiency marked by abdominal pain and diarrhea, for which it is often prescribed along with Rhizoma Atractylodis Macrocephalae, Rhizoma Zingiberis and Radix Glycyrrhizae Preparata. (b) Failure of the spleen to astringe body fluid, leading to profuse salivation, and also infantile salivation. For these cases, it is often used with Radix Codonopsis Pilosulae, Poria, Rhizoma Pinelliae and Pericarpium Citri Reticulatae.

Dosage and Preparation: 3-10 g, baked until the spermodern is charred black; with the spermodern removed, the seed is pounded into pieces.

Remarks: Both Fructus Alpiniae Oxyphyllae and Fructus Psoraleae warm and nourish the spleen and kidney. The former is more effective at warming the spleen and astringing fluid, and is indicated for cases of spleen deficiency marked by diarrhea, profuse salivation and nocturnal enuresis; the latter is better at warming the kidney, and is indicated for cases of kidney deficiency marked by impotence and soreness in the lumbar region and knee joints.

Cordyceps(冬虫夏草 *dong chong xia cao*)

Cordyceps refers to a compound consisting of the basal part of the fungus Cordyceps sinensis (Berk.) Sacc. of Clavicipitaceae, which grows as a parasite on the larva of Hepialus armoricanus Oberthru Hepialusaeceae. Produced mainly in Qinghai, Guizhou, Yunnan and Sichuan provinces, it is collected in early summer when the hypha grows above ground but the spores have not yet scattered, then it is dried in the sun or under low temperature.

Taste and Property: Sweet, and warm.
Attributive Meridian: Lung and kidney meridians.
Actions and Indications:

To nourish the lung and kidney, relieve dyspnea and cough. Indications: (a) Kidney *yang* deficiency marked by impotence, seminal emission and soreness in the lumbar region and knee joints. As it invigorates kidney *yang* and lung *yin*, it is applied either alone or in combination with Semen Cuscutae, Herba Cistanches and Radix Morindae Officinalis. (b) Dyspnea, cough and shortness of breath due to lung deficiency or deficiency of both the lung and the kidney, for which it is prescribed along with Radix Ginseng, Semen Juglandis and Radix Astragali. For cough with bloody sputum, night sweating and spontaneous sweating due to insufficient *qi* and *yin*, it is combined with Colla Corii Asini, Radix Ophiopogonis and Rhizoma Bletillae.
Dosage and Preparation: 5-10 g, prepared into oral decoction, pills or powder. It can also be stewed with chicken or duck and taken as food.

Gecko(蛤蚧 *ge jie*)

Gecko is the dried body of Gekko gecko of Linnaeus of Geckonidae, with the viscera removed. Produced mainly in Guangxi Zhuang Autonomous Region as well as Guangdong and Yunnan provinces, it is captured mostly in May and June. The belly is cut open, the viscera removed and the blood dried off (not washed); the whole body is flattened and straightened by putting a cross-like bamboo stay in the open belly and then dried under low temperature.

Taste and Property: Salty, and warm.
Attributive Meridian: Lung and kidney meridians.
Actions and Indications:

(1) To nourish the liver and kidney and relieve dyspnea and cough. Indicated for insufficiency of the lung and kidney marked by cough or dyspnea, or cough due to consumptive disease. For such cases, it is often combined with Radix Ginseng and Semen Juglandis.

(2) To promote kidney *yang* and replenish essence and blood. It is indicated for kidney deficiency with impotence, for which it is used alone and infused in wine, or else combined with Ginseng and Cornu Cervi Pantotrichum.
Dosage and Preparation: 3-6 g in decoction, and 1-1.5 g in powder. It can also be infused in wine.
Remarks: Since the lung dominates *qi* and the kidney receives *qi*, by nourishing the lung and kidney, Gecko promotes the *qi*-receptive function and relieves dyspnea, and is an important drug for dyspnea of the deficiency type. When used with Ginseng, it produces a

better therapeutic effect. Usually, its head, feet and scales are removed and only the hind part is used because it is thought to be more effective.

Semen Juglandis(胡桃肉 *hu tao rou*)

Semen Juglandis is the kernel from the nuts of the deciduous tree Juglans regia L. of Juglandaceae. Produced mainly in Hebei, Shanxi and Shandong provinces, it is collected in September and October when the fruit is ripe, the fleshy exocarp is removed, it is dried in the sun and then the spermodern is removed to get the kernel.

Synonym: *He tao ren.*
Taste and Property: Sweet, and warm.
Attributive Meridian: Kidney, lung and large intestine meridians.
Actions and Indications:

(1) To promote *qi* circulation and relieve dyspnea. It is indicated for dyspnea due to lung and kidney deficiency, for which it is often combined with Radix Ginseng, as in Decoction of Ginseng, Juglandis and Fructus Psoraleae.

(2) To nourish the kidney and strengthen the lumbar region. Indicated for kidney deficiency marked by lumbago and pain in the knee joints, for which it is often used with Cortex Eucommiae and Psoraleae, as in *Qing E* Pill.

It can also be used as a laxative for constipation due to internal dryness in the aged and debilitated patients.

Dosage: 10-30 g.
Remarks: Semen Juglandis has similar ability to nourish the lung and kidney, promote the *qi*-receptive function and relieve dyspnea as Gecko, but with weaker effect. It is particularly effective for nourishing the kidney and strengthening the lumbar region, and is frequently used for lumbago due to kidney deficiency. Now, it is used clinically for urinary stones.

Section 3
Tonics for Blood Deficiency

Radix Angelicae Sinensis(当归 *dang gui*)

Radix Angelicae Sinensis is the root of the perennial plant Angelica sinensis (Oliv.) Diels of Umbelliferae. Produced mainly in Gansu, Sichuan and Yunnan provinces, it is dug and collected in late autumn; with the fibrous roots and foreign matter removed and after being slightly evaporated, the roots are tied in small bundles, smoked over a gentle fire and then aired dry.

Taste and Property: Sweet and acrid, and warm.
Attributive Meridian: Liver and heart meridians.
Actions and Indications:

(1) To nourish the blood. Indicated for blood deficiency, for which it is often combined with Radix Paeoniae Alba, Radix Rehmanniae Preparata and Rhizoma Chuanxiong, as in Four Drugs Decoction.

(2) To regulate menstruation. Indicated for irregular menstruation, dysmenorrhea and amenorrhea due to either blood deficiency or blood stagnation, since it replenishes blood and activates blood flow.

(3) To activate blood circulation and relieve pain. Indicated for pain due to blood stagnation, trauma, rheumatic pain, carbuncles and abscesses, for which it is often combined with other drugs that activate blood circulation and remove blood stasis. It is also effective for pain due to blood deficiency or abdominal pain due to deficiency and cold.

(4) To promote bowel movements. Indicated for constipation due to blood deficiency in patients with protracted diseases, the aged, the debilitated or the puerperant. For such cases, it is prescribed along with Fructus Cannabis, Rehmanniae Preparata and Herba Cistanches.

Dosage and Preparation: 5-12 g, used in crude form or after baking.

Remarks: Radix Angelicae Sinensis nourishes blood and activates blood circulation, and is indicated for blood deficiency and blood stagnation, especially irregular menstruation, dysmenorrhea, amenorrhea before and after childbirth. It is an important medicine for gynecological diseases. This drug is acrid, aromatic and dispersive, and is good at relieving pain. It is combined with other drugs for blood stagnation and deficiency marked by headache, abdominal pain, lumbago and pain in the limbs. It is contraindicated for spleen deficiency for its laxative effect.

Radix Rehmanniae Preparata(熟地黄 *shu di huang*)

Radix Rehmanniae Preparata is the prepared root of the perennial herb Rehmannia glutinosa Libosch. of Scrophulariaceae. Produced mainly in Henan and Zhejiang provinces, it is collected in autumn, washed clean, baked dry, then mixed with rice wine and steamed.

Taste and Property: Sweet, and slightly warm.

Attributive Meridian: Heart, liver and kidney meridians.

Actions and Indications:

(1) To nourish the blood. Indicated for various disorders due to blood deficiency, for which it is often prescribed along with Radix Angelicae Sinensis, Radix Paeoniae Alba and Rhizoma Chuanxiong.

(2) To replenish *yin*. Indicated for liver and kidney *yin* deficiency marked by dizziness, tinnitus, lumbago, seminal emission and diabetes, for which it is often used with Rhizoma Dioscoreae and Fructus Corni; for *yin* deficiency with hyperactive *yang* marked by hectic fever, it is combined with Plastrum Testudinis, Cortex Phellodendri and Rhizoma Anemarrhenae, as in Pill to Replenish *Yin*.

It also promotes the generation of essence and marrow, and is indicated for deafness, blurred vision and premature white hair due to deficiency of essence and blood.

Dosage: 10-15 g., or as much as 30 g.
Precaution: As the drug is sticky, it may impair digestion. Therefore, it is usually prescribed along with drugs that activate *qi* circulation, such as Pericarpium Citri Reticulatae, Fructus Amomi and Radix Aucklandiae, to reduce the adverse effect. It is contraindicated for spleen deficiency with dampness marked by poor appetite and loose stools.
Remarks: After being mixed with wine and steamed, Radix Rehmanniae loses its ability to cool the blood, and Radix Rehmanniae Preparata becomes slightly warm and serves to nourish the blood and replenish *yin*. It is important for heart and liver blood as well as liver and kidney *yin* deficiency. If prescribed along with drugs that warm kidney *yang*, such as Radix Aconiti Lateralis Preparata and Cortex Cinnamomi, for insufficient kidney *yang*, it helps reduce the two drugs' dry and *yin*-consuming effects.

Both Radix Angelicae Sinensis and Radix Rehmanniae Preparata can nourish blood. Yet, the former also activates blood circulation, relieves pain, regulates menstruation and lubricates the intestines, while the latter also replenishes *yin*.

Radix Polygoni Multiflori(何首乌 *he shou wu*)

Radix Polygoni Multiflori is the tuber root of the perennial plant Polygonum multiflorum Thunb. of Polygonaceae. Produced mainly in Jiangsu, Henan and Hubei provinces, it is collected in autumn and winter, washed clean with both ends cut off, and cut half-to-half or into thick slices. If being dried in the sun or after being slightly baked, it is called raw Polygoni Multiflora; if mixed with the juice of black soybean and steamed, then dried in the sun until black, it is called Polygoni Multiflora Preparata.

Taste and Property: Sweet and bitter, and astringent and slightly warm.
Attributive Meridian: Liver and kidney meridians.
Actions and Indications:

(1) To nourish the liver and kidney and replenish essence and blood. Indications: (a) Liver blood deficiency marked by dizziness, blurred vision, palpitation and insomnia, for which it is combined with Radix Rehmanniae Preparata and Radix Angelicae Sinensis. (b) Deficiency of liver and kidney *yin* essence exhibiting soreness and weakness of the lumbar region and knee joints, seminal emission and premature white hair, for which it is often used with Rehmanniae Preparata and Fructus Corni. It can also be used for *yin* deficiency with hyperactive *yang* marked by dizziness and numbness of the limbs.

(2) To promote bowel movements. Indicated for constipation due to blood deficiency and intestinal dryness, for which it is often combined with Radix Rehmanniae, Radix Angelicae Sinensis and Fructus Cannabis.

(3) To cure skin infections. Indicated for scrofula and carbuncles, for which it is often used with Fructus Forsythiae and Radix Scrophulariae.
Dosage and Preparation: 10-15 g. Prepared to replenish essence and blood, and used in crude form to promote bowel movements and relieve carbuncles.
Precaution: Contraindicated for cases with spleen deficiency marked by loose stools, and cases with phlegm-dampness.

Radix Paeoniae Alba(白芍 *bai shao*)

Radix Paeoniae Alba is the epidermis root of the cultivated perennial plant Paeonia lactiflora Pall. of Ranunculaceae. Produced mainly in Zhejiang, Anhui and Sichuan provinces, the root of the three- or four-year-old plant is dug and collected in summer and autumn, washed clean with the rhizome and fibrous roots removed, and the rough epidermis scraped off, cooked slightly in boiling water, and finally dried in the sun.

Taste and Property: Bitter and sour, and slightly cold.
Attributive Meridian: Liver and spleen meridians.
Actions and Indications:

(1) To nourish the blood and astringe *yin*. Indications: (a) Blood deficiency, for which it is often combined with Radix Angelicae Sinensis and Radix Rehmanniae Preparata. (b) Disharmony between the *ying* (nutrient) and *wei* (defensive) systems and deficiency of the exterior marked by spontaneous sweating, for which it is often combined with Ramulus Cinnamomi; for *yin* deficiency leading to the floating up of *yang* marked by spontaneous sweating and night sweating, it is often combined with Os Draconis and Concha Ostreae.

(2) To soothe the liver, relieve spasm and pain. Indicated for liver *qi* stagnation marked by hypochondriac pain, for which it is often used with Radix Bupleuri and Radix Glycyrrhizae; for epigastric and abdominal pain, and spasm and pain in the limbs, it is often used together with Radix Glycyrrhizae, as in Decoction of Paeoniae Alba and Glycyrrhizae.

(3) To replenish *yin* and pacify the liver. Indicated for insufficient liver *yin* leading to hyperactive liver *yang* marked by headache, dizziness, tinnitus and blurred vision; for such cases it is often used with Radix Rehmanniae, Radix Achyranthis Bidentatae and Cortex Moutan Radicis.

Dosage and Preparation: 6-12 g, used in crude form or baked with wine or vinegar.
Precaution: Incompatible with Rhizoma et Radix Veratri.
Remarks: The liver is a rigid organ that needs the nourishment of *yin* and blood. Radix Paeoniae Alba enters the liver meridian to nourish liver blood and *yin*, and therefore is important for nourishing and soothing the liver. It serves as an agent to counteract stagnant liver *qi*, relieve muscular spasms and abdominal pain, and calm hyperactive liver *yang*.

Colla Corii Asini(阿胶 *e jiao*)

Colla Corii Asini is the black gelatin by decocting the hairless skin of the animal Equus asinus L. of Equidae, a domestic animal to be found in all parts of China, especially in Shandong and Zhejiang provinces.

Synonym: *Lu pi jiao.*
Taste and Property: Sweet, and mild.

Attributive Meridian: Lung, liver and kidney meridians.
Actions and Indications:

(1) To nourish the blood. Indicated for blood deficiency, for which it is often prescribed along with Radix Codonopsis Pilosulae, Radix Astragali, Radix Angelicae Sinensis and Radix Paeoniae Alba.

(2) To stop bleeding. Indicated for hematemesis, hemoptysis, hematochezia, hematuria and metrorrhagia, for which it is combined with other hemostatics and other drugs in line with specific symptoms.

(3) To replenish *yin* and relieve dryness. Indications: (a) Lung *yin* deficiency and lung dryness marked by dry cough and dry throat, for which it is often used with Radix Adenophorae, Radix Ophiopogonis and Fructus Aristolochiae. (b) Febrile diseases with damaged *yin* and hyperactive liver fire marked by spasm of the limbs. For such cases, it is often combined with Radix Paeoniae Alba, Ramulus Uncariae cum Uncis, Concha Ostreae and Carapax Trionycis. (c) *Yin* deficiency leading to hyperactive fire marked by restlessness, insomnia, thready and taut pulse, for which it is often combined with Rhizoma Coptidis and egg yolk.

Dosage and Preparation: 5-15 g, melted and taken with water, or baked with powder of Gecko or Pollen Typhae to form granules and then prepared into decoction.
Precaution: This drug is sticky and hinders digestion. It is contraindicated for patients with spleen and stomach deficiency and indigestion, as well as cases of bleeding due to blood stagnation.

Arillus Longan(桂圆肉 *gui yuan rou*)

Arillus Longan is the aril of the evergreen tree Euphoria longan (Lour.) Steud. of Sapindaceae. Produced mainly in Guangdong, Fujian and Taiwan provinces as well as the Guangxi Zhuang Autonomous Region, it is gathered in early autumn when the fruit is ripe, baked dry or dried in the sun; with the exocarp and kernel removed, the aril is taken and dried in the sun.

Synonym: *Long yan rou*.
Taste and Property: Sweet, and warm.
Attributive Meridian: Heart and spleen meridians.
Actions and Indications:

To nourish blood, calm the mind and nourish the heart and spleen. Indicated for heart and spleen deficiency and insufficient *qi* and blood marked by palpitation, insomnia and amnesia, for which it is often prescribed along with Fructus Ziziphi Spinosae and Radix Polygalae and drugs that replenish *qi* and nourish blood. It can also be taken alone and taken continuously for a long time.

Section 4
Tonics for *Yin* Deficiency

Radix Adenophorae(南沙参 *nan sha shen*)

Radix Adenophorae is the root of the perennial herb Adenophora tetraphylla (Thunb.) Fisch., or A. stricta Miq. of Campanulaceae. Produced mainly in Jiangsu, Zhejiang, Anhui, Yunnan and Sichuan provinces, it is dug and collected in summer and autumn; with the fibrous roots removed and the rough epidermis scraped off, it is washed clean and then dried.

Taste and Property: Sweet and slightly bitter, and cold.
Attributive Meridian: Lung and stomach meridians.
Actions and Indications:

(1) To replenish lung *yin*, moisten the lung and resolve phlegm. Indicated for lung *yin* insufficiency marked by cough with sputum, dry throat and hoarseness, for which it is often prescribed along with Bulbus Fritillariae and Radix Ophiopogonis.

(2) To nourish the stomach and promote fluid generation. Indicated for stomach *yin* insufficiency marked by thirst, gastric discomfort with acid regurgitation, and red and uncoated tongue, for which it is often combined with Herba Dendrobii and Radix Ophiopogonis.

Dosage: 10-15 g.
Precaution: It is incompatible with Rhizoma et Radix Veratri.

Radix Glehniae(北沙参 *bei sha shen*)

Radix Glehniae is the root of the perennial herb Glehnia littoralis Fr. Schmidt ex Miq. of Umbelliferae. Produced mainly in Shandong, Hebei, Liaoning and Jiangsu provinces, it is dug and collected in summer and autumn; with the fibrous roots removed, it is washed clean, bathed in boiling water and dried with the epidermis removed.

Taste and Property: Sweet and bitter, and slightly cold.
Attributive Meridian: Lung and stomach meridians.
Actions and Indications:

(1) To nourish lung *yin*. Indicated for lung *yin* insufficiency marked by dry cough or difficult expectoration, dry throat and hoarseness of voice, for which it is often prescribed along with Bulbus Fritillariae and Radix Ophiopogonis.

(2) To nourish the stomach and promote fluid generation. Indicated for damaged stomach *yin* marked by thirst, crimson tongue, or gastric discomfort with acid regurgitation, for which it is often combined with Ophiopogonis and Herba Dendrobii.

Dosage: 10-15 g.
Remarks: There are two kinds of *sha shen*: Radix Adenophorae and Radix Glehniae. The

drug recorded in *Shen Nong's Classic of Herbalism* refers actually to modern Radix Adenophorae. Mention of Glehniae appears in *Comments on Herbalism* written in the Qing Dynasty. Both replenish lung and stomach *yin*. Radix Adenophorae is weaker at replenishing *yin* but can moisten the lung and resolve phlegm, and Radix Glehniae is better at replenishing *yin* but has no effect in resolving phlegm.

Radix Ophiopogonis(麦门冬 *mai men dong*)

Radix Ophiopogonis is the tuber root of the perennial herb Ophiopogon japonicus (Thunb.) Ker-Gawl. of Liliaceae. Produced mainly in Sichuan, Zhejiang and Hubei provinces, it is collected in summer, dried in the sun for 3-4 days and piled up to capture moisture again aad dried in the sun.

Taste and Property: Sweet and slightly bitter, and cold.
Attributive Meridian: Heart, lung and stomach meridians.
Actions and Indications:

(1) To replenish lung *yin*. Indicated for lung *yin* insufficiency marked by dry cough and hemoptysis, for which it is often prescribed along with Bulbus Lilli, Radix Adenophorae and Radix Rehmanniae.

(2) To replenish stomach *yin* and promote fluid generation. Indicated for consumption of stomach *yin* marked by thirst and crimson tongue, for which it is often used with Herba Dendrobii and Adenophorae.

(3) To nourish heart *yin*. Indicated for heart *yin* insufficiency marked by palpitation, restlessness and insomnia, for which it is often combined with Radix Ginseng, Fructus Schisandrae and Rhizoma Polygonati Odorati.

Dosage: 5-15 g.

Radix Asparagi(天门冬 *tian men dong*)

Radix Asparagi is the tuber root of the perennial plant Asparagus cochinchinensis (Lour.) Merr. of Liliaceae. Produced mainly in Guizhou and Sichuan provinces as well as the Guangxi Zhuang Autonomous Region, it is collected in autumn and winter, washed clean; then with the basal part of the stem and fibrous roots removed, it is cooked in boiling water and its epidermis is removed when still hot, then washed again and dried.

Taste and Property: Sweet and bitter, and cold.
Attributive Meridian: Lung and stomach meridians.
Actions and Indications:

(1) To nourish lung *yin*, moisten dryness and check cough. Indicated for lung *yin* deficiency or lung dryness marked by cough with sticky sputum, difficult expectoration or blood-tinged sputum, for which it is often used with Radix Ophiopogonis, Radix Adenophorae and Bulbus Fritillariae.

(2) To replenish kidney *yin*. Indicated for kidney *yin* deficiency marked by hectic

fever, diabetes and seminal emission, for which it is often combined with Rhizoma Anemarrhenae, Cortex Phellodendri and Radix Rehmanniae Preparata.

This drug is also used for febrile diseases with damaged *yin*, thirst and constipation, and heat due to *yin* deficiency. For such cases, it is often prescribed along with Radix Rehmanniae, Radix Scrophulariae and Ophiopogonis.

Dosage: 5-15 g.

Remarks: Both Radix Ophiopogonis and Radix Asparagi are sweet, cold and moist, and act to nourish *yin* and moisten the lung. They are often used in combination for lung *yin* deficiency marked by dry cough, as in Extract of Ophiopogonis and Asparagi. But Radix Ophiopogonis nourishes the stomach and purge heart fire, and is used for insufficient stomach *yin* and deficient heart *yin*, while Asparagi is colder and replenishes kidney *yin*, and is used for kidney *yin* deficiency marked by hectic fever, diabetes and seminal emission. Both are cold and moist, and so are contraindicated for cases of spleen deficiency with dampness.

Herba Dendrobii(石斛 *shi hu*)

Herba Dendrobii is the fresh or dried stem of the perennial evergreen herb Dendrobium nobile Lindl. of Orchidaceae or other plants of the same genus. Produced mainly in Sichuan, Guizhou, Yunnan and Anhui provinces as well as the Guangxi Zhuang Autonomous Region, it can be collected any time of the year, though the quality is better if collected in autumn, baked or sunned dry.

Taste and Property: Sweet and bland, and slightly cold.

Attributive Meridian: Stomach meridian.

Actions and Indications:

To nourish stomach *yin* and promote fluid generation. Indications: (a) Febrile diseases with consumption of fluid, exhibiting low fever, dryness in the mouth and tongue, red tongue with little coating as well as thready and rapid pulse. For such cases, it is often combined with Radix Rehmanniae, Radix Scrophulariae and Radix Ophiopogonis. (b) Stomach *yin* insufficiency marked by poor appetite, gastric discomfort with acid regurgitation, retching or hiccup, and uncoated and smooth tongue, for which it is often used with Ophiopogonis, Folium Eriobotryae and Caulis Bambusae in Taeniam.

It also nourishes the kidney, improves vision and strengthens the muscles and bones, and is indicated for impaired vision or soreness and weakness in the lower back and knee joints due to deficiency of kidney *yin*.

Dosage: 5-15 g, doubled when used fresh.

Remarks: Herba Dendrobii is important for nourishing stomach *yin* and promoting fluid generation. The fresh herb is better at purging heat and promoting fluid generation, and is frequently prescribed for febrile diseases with fluid consumption, dry tongue and thirst; the dried herb is more effective for cases of thirst due to *yin* deficiency.

Rhizoma Polygonati Odorati(玉竹 *yu zhu*)

Rhizoma Polygonati Odorati is the rhizome of the perennial herb Polygonatum odoratum (Mill.) Druce of Liliaceae. Produced mainly in Hebei, Jiangsu, Liaoning and Zhejiang provinces, it is dug and collected in spring and autumn, washed clean, dried in the sun until soft, and rubbed repeatedly; it is exposed in the air until its center turns soft, then dried in the sun, or steamed, rubbed until semi-transparent, and then dried in the sun again.

Synonym: *Wei rui*.
Taste and Property: Sweet, and mild.
Attributive Meridian: Lung and stomach meridians.
Actions and Indications:

To nourish *yin*, promote fluid secretion and relieve dryness. Indicated for dryness and heat in the lung and stomach with fluid consumption marked by dry cough, dry mouth and tongue, and red tongue with little coating, for which it is often combined with Radix Ophiopogonis and Radix Adenophorae; and also for *yin* deficiency with affection of exogenous wind-heat marked by fever, cough, sore throat and thirst, for which it is often used with Herba Menthae, Semen Sojae Preparata and Radix Cynanchi Atrati.
Dosage: 10-15 g.

Rhizoma Polygonati(黄精 *huang jing*)

Rhizoma Polygonati is the rhizome of the perennial herb Polygonatum kingianum. Coll. et Hemsl., P. sibiricum Red., or P. cyrtonema Hua of Liliaceae. Produced mainly in Guizhou, Yunnan, Hunan, Zhejiang and Hebei provinces, it is collected in spring and autumn, washed clean, bathed slightly in boiling water or steamed fully and then dried.

Taste and Property: Sweet, and mild.
Attributive Meridian: Spleen, lung and kidney meridians.
Actions and Indications:

(1) To replenish *yin* and moisten the lung. Indicated for lung *yin* insufficiency and lung dryness marked by dry cough, for which it is used either alone and prepared into extract, or combined with other drugs of the same kind, such as Radix Adenophorae and Bulbus Fritillariae.

(2) To nourish the spleen. Indicated for spleen and stomach deficiency manifested as general lassitude and loss of appetite, or debility after diseases, for which it is often combined with Radix Astragali and Radix Codonopsis Pilosulae; for stomach *yin* deficiency, it is often used with Adenophorae and Radix Ophiopogonis.
Dosage: 10-30 g.
Precaution: Rhizoma Polygonati is moist and greasy, and likely causes dampness. So it is contraindicated for cases with stagnant phlegm-dampness and retained cold in the middle *jiao* accompanied by loose stools.
Remarks: Rhizoma Polygonati is sweet, moist and greasy, similar to Radix Rehmanniae

Preparata, but it is better at replenishing *yin*, moistening the lung and nourishing the spleen. Since its action is slow, it can be used as a tonic over a long period of time.

Fructus Corni（山茱萸 *shan zhu yu*）

Fructus Corni is the sarcocarp of the deciduous tree Cornus officinalis Sieb. et Zucc. of Cornaceae. Produced mainly in Zhejiang, Anhui, Shaanxi, Henan and Shanxi provinces, it is collected in late autumn and early winter when the fruit turns red, baked on a slow fire or slightly bathed in boiling water; the pips are squeezed out timely, and then dried in the sun or baked dry.

Synonym: *Shan yu rou*, *yu rou*.
Taste and Property: Sour and astringent, and slightly warm.
Attributive Meridian: Liver and kidney meridians.
Actions and Indications:

(1) To nourish the liver and kidney. Indicated for insufficiency of the liver and kidney marked by dizziness, tinnitus and lumbago, for which it is often combined with Radix Rehmanniae Preparata and Rhizoma Dioscoreae.

(2) To serve as an astringent for: (a) Spontaneous sweating and night sweating due to weak constitution, for which it is often used with Radix Astragali, Fructus Schisandrae, Os Draconis and Concha Ostreae; for profuse sweating leading to collapse, heavy doses of the drug are combined with Radix Ginseng and Radix Aconiti Lateralis Preparata to check sweating and prevent collapse. (b) Kidney deficiency marked by seminal emission, nocturnal enuresis and frequent urination, for which it is often combined with Rehmanniae Preparata, Semen Cuscutae and Fructus Rubi.

Thanks to its astringent action, Fructus Corni can also be used for dysfunction of the Chong and Ren meridians in women marked by metrorrhagia and menorrhagia.

Fructus Lycii（枸杞子 *gou qi zi*）

Fructus Lycii refers to the ripe fruit of the shrub Lycium barbarum L. of Solanaceae. Produced mainly in Ningxia Hui Autonomous Region and Gansu Province, it is gathered in summer and autumn when the fruit is ripe, aired for some time and then dried in the sun until the exocarp is dry.

Taste and Property: Sweet, and mild.
Attributive Meridian: Liver and kidney meridians.
Actions and Indications:

(1) To replenish liver and kidney *yin*. Indicated for insufficiency of the liver and kidney with seminal emission, lumbago and weakness of the knee joints, for which it is often combined with Radix Rehmanniae Preparata, Fructus Tribuli and Fructus Rubi.

(2) To nourish the liver and improve vision. Indicated for liver and kidney deficiency marked by dizziness, tinnitus and blurred vision, for which it is often used with Flos

Chrysanthemi and Rehmanniae Preparata.

Dosage: 5-10 g.

Remarks: Both Fructus Lycii and Fructus Corni nourish the liver and kidney, and especially liver *yin*. But the latter also has the astringent action, and the former also nourishes the liver and improves vision.

Herba Ecliptae(墨旱莲 *mo han lian*)

Herba Ecliptae refers to the aerial part of the annual herb Eclipta prostrata L. of Compositae. Produced mainly in Jiangsu, Jiangxi, Zhejiang and Guangdong provinces, the part above the ground is cut and collected in summer and autumn when the branches and leaves are growing luxuriantly, and then dried in the sun or shade.

Taste and Property: Sweet and sour, and cool.

Attributive Meridian: Liver and kidney meridians.

Actions and Indications:

(1) To replenish liver and kidney *yin*. Indicated for liver and kidney *yin* deficiency marked by dizziness, tinnitus, lumbago and seminal emission, for which it is often prescribed along with Fructus Ligustri Lucidi, as in *Erzhi* Pill.

(2) To cool the blood and check bleeding. Indicated for bleeding due to *yin* deficiency and blood-heat, such as hemoptysis, hematochezia, hematuria and metrorrhagia, for which it is prepared into an oral decoction or produce a juice from the fresh herb for oral administration. It can also be applied externally for trauma with bleeding.

Dosage: 10-15 g, or 30-60 g if used alone.

Fructus Ligustri Lucidi(女贞子 *nu zhen zi*)

Fructus Ligustri Lucidi is the ripe fruit of the evergreen shrub or small tree Ligustrum lucidum Ait. of Oleaceae. Produced mainly in Zhejiang, Jiangsu, Hunan, Fujian and Sichuan provinces, it is collected in winter when the fruit is ripe, steamed and then dried in the sun.

Taste and Property: Sweet and bitter, and cool.

Attributive Meridian: Liver and kidney meridians.

Actions and Indications:

To replenish liver and kidney *yin*. Indicated for liver and kidney *yin* deficiency marked by dizziness, tinnitus, blurred vision and seminal emission, for which it is often used with Herba Ecliptae, as in *Erzhi* Pill.

Dosage: 6-15 g.

Remarks: The ability of Fructus Ligustri Lucidi and Herba Ecliptae to replenish liver and kidney *yin* is not as strong as that of Radix Rehmanniae Preparata, Fructus Corni and Fructus Lycii. But they are milder, tonic and not greasy or sticky. Since they are cold, they should be used with caution for patients with spleen and stomach deficiency as well as *yang* deficiency.

Plastrum Testudinis(龟板 *gui ban*)

Plastrum Testudinis is the plastron of the fresh-water tortoise Chinemys reevesii (Gray) of Testudinidae. Produced mainly in the Yangtze River valley, the tortoise can be caught any time of the year; its plastron is boiled in water and dried in the sun.

Taste and Property: Salty, and cold.
Attributive Meridian: Liver and kidney meridians.
Actions and Indications:

(1) To replenish *yin* and pacify *yang*. Indications: (a) Kidney *yin* insufficiency leading to hyperactive *yang* in deficiency conditions marked by hectic fever and night sweating, for which it is often prescribed along with Radix Rehmanniae Preparata, Rhizoma Anemarrhenae and Cortex Phellodendri, as in Pill for Replenishing *Yin*. (b) Late stages of febrile diseases with consumption of *yin* fluid and hyperactivity of deficiency wind marked by dizziness and convulsion. For such cases, it is often combined with Concha Ostreae, Carapax Trionycis and Radix Rehmanniae.

(2) To nourish the kidney and strengthen the bones. Indicated for insufficiency of the liver and kidney marked by weakness of the lower back and limbs, weakness of the muscles and bones, and retarded and incomplete closure of the fontanel in infants, for which it is often combined with Rehmanniae Preparata, Radix Achyranthis Bidentatae and Herba Cynomorii.

(3) To strengthen the meridians and check bleeding. Indicated for *yin* deficiency and blood-heat in women marked by menorrhagia or metrorrhagia, for which it is often prescribed along with Cortex Ailanthi, Radix Paeoniae Alba and Radix Scutellariae.

Dosage and Preparation: 10-30 g, baked with sand and decocted first in preparing a decoction.

Carapax Trionycis(鳖甲 *bie jia*)

Carapax Trionycis is the shell of Trionyx sinensis Wiegmann of Trionychidae, which can be caught any time of the year, but mainly in autumn and winter. After being slaughtered, it is bathed in boiling water until the hard skin of the shell can be peeled off, the shell is then taken out, the remaining meat is removed, and the shell is dried in the sun.

Taste and Property: Salty, and cold.
Attributive Meridian: Liver meridian.
Actions and Indications:

(1) To replenish *yin* and pacify *yang*. Indications: (a) *Yin* deficiency marked by hectic fever and night sweating, in which it is often used with Radix Stellariae, Cortex Lycii Radicis and Herba Artemisiae Annuae. (b) Febrile diseases with fluid consumption and hyperactive deficiency wind marked by dizziness and convulsion, for which it is often com-

bined with Radix Rehmanniae, Concha Ostreae and Plastrum Testudinis.

(2) To soften hard masses. Indicated for abdominal masses, such as splenomegaly, for which it is often prescribed along with Radix Angelicae Sinensis, Pericarpium Citri Reticulatae Viride, Semen Persicae and Flos Carthami.

Dosage and Preparation: 10-30 g, baked with sand and decocted first in preparing a decoction.

Remarks: Both Plastrum Testudinis and Carapax Trionycis are salty and cold, replenish *yin* and pacify *yang*. But, the former is better at replenishing *yin*, and can strengthen the meridians, check bleeding, nourish the kidney and strengthen the bones; the latter is more effective in purging deficiency heat and softening hard masses.

Table 18. Action of the Tonics

	Drug	Similarities	Differences
Drugs for Tonifying *Qi*	Radix Ginseng	To replenish *qi* of the spleen and stomach	To replenish primordial *qi* potently; rescue patients from prostration; promote generation of body fluid
	Radix Codonopsis Pilosulae		Similar as Radix Ginseng action but much weaker in effect
	Radix Astragali		To elevate *yang*, consolidate superficial defensive *qi*, promote diuresis, dispel pus and promote the healing of wounds
	Rhizoma Atractylodis Macrocephalae	To tonify and strengthen the spleen	To dry dampness, promote diuresis and arrest sweating
	Rhizoma Dioscoreae		To replenish *yin*, tonify the lung and kidney
	Radix Glycyrrhizae	Very sweet, to tonify the spleen and relieve spasm and pain	To replenish heart *qi*, moisten the lung, purge fire and remove toxic materials
	Fructus Jujubae		To tonify blood
	Mel		To moisten the lung and the intestine; clear heat and toxic materials
Drugs for Tonifying *Yang*	Cornu Cervi Pantotrichum	To reinforce kidney *yang*	Potent effect in tonifying kidney *yang*, also to replenish essence and blood
	Herba Cistanches		To relieve constipation
	Herba Epimedii		Anti-rheumatic

	Drug	Similarities	Differences
Drugs for Tonifying *Yang*	Cortex Eucommiae	To tonify liver and kidney; strengthen muscles and bones	To prevent miscarriage
	Radix Dipsaci		To prevent miscarriage; promote reunion of fractured bones and muscles
	Rhizoma Cibotii		Anti-rheumatic
	Fructus Psoraleae	To warm the spleen and kidney *yang*	Mainly to warm kidney; promote function in receiving *qi* and soothe dyspnea
	Fructus Alpiniae Oxyphyllae		To warm spleen, decrease salivation, astringe essence and reduce urination
	Cordyceps	To tonify lung and kidney; relieve cough and dyspnea	To tonify kidney *yang*; replenish lung *yin*
	Gecko		Potent effect in promoting *qi*-reception and relieving dyspnea
	Semen Juglandis		To strengthen the kidney and lower back; to treat constipation
Drugs for Tonifying Blood	Radix Angelicae Sinensis	To tonify blood	To activate blood flow, regulate menses, relieve pain, and treat constipation
	Radix Rehmanniae Preparata		To replenish lung *yin* and kidney *yin*
	Radix Polygoni Multiflori		To replenish liver and kidney *yin*, tonify essence and blood; raw use for moistening intestines, removing toxic materials
	Radix Paeoniae Alba		To soothe liver, relieve spasm
	Colla Corii Asini		Important hemostatic, can replenish *yin*, moisten dryness
	Arillus Longan		Sedative

	Drug	Similarities	Differences
Drugs for Tonifying *Yin*	Radix Adenophorae	To replenish the lung *yin* and stomach *yin*; promote fluid generation	To resolve phlegm
	Radix Glehniae		Stronger than Radix Adenophorae in tonifying *yin*, no effect of resolving phlegm
	Radix Ophiopogonis		To replenish heart *yin*
	Radix Asparagis		To replenish kidney *yin*
	Herba Dendrobii		Important drug for nourishing stomach *yin* and promoting fluid generation
	Rhizoma Polygonati Odorati		Often used in *yin* deficiency cases with exterior affection
	Rhizoma Polygonati		To tonify spleen
	Fructus Corni	To tonify liver *yin* and kidney *yin*	Astringent for seminal emission, nocturnal enuresis, uterine bleeding, and spontaneous sweating
	Fructus Lycii		To nourish liver and improve vision
	Herba Ecliptae		To cool blood and stop bleeding
	Fructus Ligustri Lucidi		
	Plastrum Testudinis	To replenish *yin* and pacify *yang*	Mainly to tonify kidney *yin*, strengthen meridians, and check bleeding
	Carapax Trionycis		To clear deficient heat; also soften hard masses

Note: Other sections deal with additional tonic drugs, such as Radix Rehmanniae, Radix Scrophulariae, Radix Aconiti Lateralis Preparata, Cortex Cinnamomi, Rumulus Taxilli, Cortex Acanthopanacis, Fructus Schisandrae, Semen Nelumbinis and Semen Euryales.

CHAPTER TWENTY-ONE
ASTRINGENTS

Drugs that possess astringent action and treat excessive discharge are known as astringents (*shou se yao*).

Astringents are usually sour and styptic. They arrest perspiration, astringe the lung and intestines, arrest spontaneous emission, reduce urination, stop bleeding and check leukorrhea, and are indicated for cases with spontaneous sweating, night sweating, chronic cough, deficiency dyspnea, chronic diarrhea and dysentery, seminal emission, nocturnal enuresis, metrorrhagia and leukorrhagia. Some astringents can be applied externally to promote granulation, and are indicated for ulcerated lesions that do not heal properly.

Astringents are mainly used to relieve secondary symptoms; according to the principle of "searching for the primary cause of a disease in treatment," they should be combined with tonics to strengthen the vital energy, so that both the secondary symptoms and the primary cause are treated.

Improper use of astringents in cases when excessive pathogenic factors have not yet been completely eliminated will cause them to linger. They are therefore not indicated for such cases as cough due to attack of the lung by exogenous pathogens, profuse sweating due to excessive internal heat, diarrhea or dysentery in which the stasis of the intestines is not yet relieved, and leukorrhagia due to dampness-heat.

Fructus Schisandrae(五味子 *wu wei zi*)

Fructus Schisandrae refers to the ripe fruit of the deciduous woody vine Schisandra chinensis (Turcz.) Baill., or S. sphenanthera Rehd. et Wils. of Magnoliaceae. The former is mainly produced in Liaoning, Jilin and Heilongjiang provinces, the latter mainly in Sichuan, Hubei and Shaanxi provinces. It is collected in autumn when the fruit is ripe, then dried in the sun or steamed first and then dried.

Taste and Property: Sour, and warm.
Attributive Meridian: Lung, kidney and heart meridians.
Actions and Indications:

(1) To astringe the lung and relieve cough and dyspnea. Indicated for cough and dyspnea due to lung and kidney deficiency, for which it is often combined with Radix Rehmanniae Preparata and Fructus Corni. If combined with Herba Ephedrae, Rhizoma Zingiberis and Herba Asari, it is effective for cough and dyspnea due to retained cold-

phlegm in the lung.

(2) To replenish *qi*, promote fluid generation and arrest sweating. Indications: (a) *Qi* and *yin* injured by heat, marked by profuse sweating, lassitude, shortness of breath, thirst and feeble pulse, for which it is often used with Radix Ginseng and Radix Ophiopogonis, as in Powder for Restoring the Pulse. (b) Diabetes, for which it is often combined with Radix Astragali, Rhizoma Anemarrhenae and Radix Trichosanthis. (c) Night sweating and spontaneous sweating, for which it is prescribed along with Radix Ginseng, Ephedrae and Concha Ostreae.

(3) To astringe the intestines and check diarrhea. Indicated for deficiency cold in the spleen and stomach marked by lingering diarrhea, for which it is often combined with Fructus Psoraleae, Semen Myristicae and Fructus Evodiae, as in Pill of Four Miraculous Drugs.

(4) To arrest seminal emission and reduce urination. Indicated for kidney deficiency marked by seminal emission and nocturnal enuresis, for which it is often prescribed along with Ootheca Mantidis, Os Draconis and Semen Cuscutae.

Dosage: 2-6 g.

Remarks: Although Fructus Schisandrae has all the five tastes, as its name implies, it is mainly sour. Its astringent quality treat cough and dyspnea, arrest sweating, and relieving diarrhea, seminal emission and nocturnal enuresis. In addition, it also replenishes *qi*, promotes fluid generation and replenish kidney *qi*; its effect on cough, dyspnea, seminal emission and nocturnal enuresis deprive not only from its astringent action but also its replenishment of kidney *qi*.

Fructus Mume(乌梅 *wu mei*)

Fructus Mume is the processed unripe fruit of the deciduous tree Prunus mume (Sieb.) Sieb. et Zucc. of Rosaceae. Produced mainly in Sichuan, Zhejiang, Fujian and Hunan provinces, it is collected in May, baked dry under low temperature and covered tightly until it turns black.

Taste and Property: Sour, and mild.

Attributive Meridian: Liver, lung and large intestine meridians.

Actions and Indications:

(1) To astringe the lung and relieve cough. Indicated for lung deficiency marked by long-standing cough with little sputum, for which it is often combined with Semen Armeniacae Amarum and Colla Corii Asini.

(2) To promote fluid generation and relieve thirst. Indicated for deficiency-heat syndromes marked by polydipsia and summer-heat syndromes with fluid consumption marked by thirst, for which it is used either alone and prepared into a decoction, or else combined with Radix Trichosanthis, Radix Ophiopogonis, Radix Ginseng, Radix Astragali and Radix Puerariae, as in Jade Spring Pill.

(3) To astringe the intestines and stop diarrhea. Indicated for long-standing diarrhea and chronic dysentery, for which it is often combined with Semen Myristicae, Fructus

Chebulae, Radix Codonopsis Pilosulae and Rhizoma Atractylodis Macrocephalae.

(4) To regulate the stomach and eliminate ascarides. Indicated for abdominal pain caused by ascariasis or cold limbs and vomiting due to biliary ascariasis, for which it is often prescribed along with Rhizoma Coptidis and Pericarpium Zanthoxyli, as in Bolus of Mume.

The drug can also check bleeding and is indicated for hematochezia, hematuria and metrorrhagia.

Dosage and Preparation: 3-10 g, baked until charred to check bleeding, and used crude for other purposes.

Galla Chinensis(五倍子 *wu bei zi*)

Galla Chinensis is the gall produced by Melaphis chinensis (Bell) Baker, which grows as a parasite on the leaves of the deciduous shrub or tree Rhus chinensis Mill. of Anacardiaceae, or other plants of the same genus. Produced mainly in Sichuan, Guizhou, Shaanxi, Hubei and Fujian provinces, it is collected in September and October, cooked in boiling water for 3-5 minutes to kill the young insects inside the gall, and then dried in the sun.

Taste and Property: Sour and astringent, and cold.

Attributive Meridian: Lung, kidney and large intestine meridians.

Actions and Indications:

(1) To astringe the lung and relieve cough. Indicated for long-standing cough due to lung deficiency and expectoration of blood-tinged sputum due to injury to the lung caused by deficiency fire, for which it is often prescribed along with Fructus Schisandrae and Radix Ophiopogonis.

(2) To arrest sweating. Indicated for night sweating, for which it is used singly and ground into powder that is made into paste to be applied externally on the umbilicus, or else prepared into an oral decoction with other drugs.

(3) To astringe the intestines and relieve diarrhea. Indicated for long-standing diarrhea and dysentery, for which it is used either alone or in combination with Schisandrae and Fructus Chebulae. It can also be applied for rectal prolapse caused by chronic diarrhea, for which it is prepared into a decoction with Alumen for steaming and washing the rectum.

(4) To astringe seminal emission. Indicated for kidney deficiency marked by seminal emission and nocturnal enuresis, for which it is often prescribed along with Schisandrae, Os Draconis and Concha Ostreae.

(5) To stop bleeding. Indicated for hemoptysis, epistaxis, hematochezia and metrorrhagia. It can also be ground into powder for external use to treat bleeding due to trauma.

It is also used externally for carbuncles, ulcerative gingivitis and aphthae.

Dosage and Preparation: 1. 5-6 g, prepared into pills or powder for oral administration. Moderate amount for external application, as decoction for local steaming and washing, or as topical application.

Fructus Tritici Levis(浮小麦 *fu xiao mai*)

Fructus Tritici Levis refers to the unripe, dried and light caryopsis of the annual plant Triticum aestivum L. of Gramineae, which is produced in all parts of China. It is obtained by washing a large amount of wheat, the floated are collected and then dried in the sun.

Taste and Property: Sweet, and cool.
Attributive Meridian: Heart meridian.
Actions and Indications: To arrest sweating. Indicated for cases of spontaneous and night sweating due to weak constitution, for which it is used alone and prepared into an oral decoction, or combined with Concha Ostreae, Radix Ephedrae and Radix Astragali, as in Powder of Concha Ostreae. For night sweating, it is used along with Cortex Lycii Radicis.
Dosage: 10-15 g, and 30-60 g if used alone.

Radix Oryzae Glutinosae(糯稻根 *nuo dao gen*)

Radix Oryzae Glutinosae is the root and rhizome of the annual plant Oryza sativa L. of Gramineae, which grows in all parts of China. It is collected in autumn, washed clean and dried in the sun.

Taste and Property: Sweet, and mild.
Attributive Meridian: Heart and lung meridians.
Actions and Indications:

To arrest sweating. Indicated for spontaneous and night sweating due to weak constitution, for which it is used singly and prepared into an oral administration or else combined with Fructus Tritici Levis (light) and Concha Ostreae Usta.
Dosage: 15-30 g.
Remarks: Fructus Tritici Levis (light), Radix Oryzae Glutinosae and Radix Ephedrae are common antihydrotics for spontaneous and night sweating. Each can be combined with Os Draconis and Concha Ostreae to enhance the antihydrotic effect, or else with drugs that replenish *qi*, and nourish *yang* and *yin* in line with the specific symptoms.

Cortex Ailanthi(椿白皮 *chun bai pi*)

Cortex Ailanthi is the bark of the root or stem of the deciduous tree Ailanthus altissima (Mill.) Swingle of Simaroubaceae. Produced in most parts of China, it can be obtained at any time of the year. The bark is peeled off, the rough outer epidermis is scraped off, and then it is dried in the sun.

Synonym: *Chu gen pi*, *chun gen pi*.
Taste and Property: Bitter and astringent, and cold.
Attributive Meridian: Large intestine and liver meridians.

Actions and Indications:

(1) To purge heat, eliminate dampness, astringe the intestines and relieve leukorrhagia. Indications: (a) Diarrhea due to dampness-heat, chronic diarrhea and dysentery, for which it is used either alone or in combination with other related drugs. It is also effective for hematochezia. (b) Leukorrhagia with red and white discharge due to dampness-heat, for which it is often used with Cortex Phellodendri.

(2) To stop bleeding. Indicated for menorrhagia and metrorrhagia due to heat in the blood. For such cases, it is often combined with Phellodendri and Plastrum Testudinis.

Dosage: 10-15 g.

Remarks: Cortex Ailanthi not only astringes the intestines but also purges heat and eliminate dampness, and is commonly used to treat diarrhea, dysentery and leukorrhagia caused by dampness-heat.

Pericarpium Granati(石榴皮 *shi liu pi*)

Pericarpium Granati is the pericarp of the deciduous shrub or tree Punica granatum L. of Punicaceae. Produced in most parts of China, it is collected in autumn when the fruit is ripe, the pericarp is peeled off and dried in the sun.

Taste and Property: Sour and astringent, and warm.

Attributive Meridian: Stomach and large intestine meridians.

Actions and Indications:

(1) To astringe the intestines and relieve diarrhea. Indicated for chronic diarrhea and dysentery, and rectal prolapse, for which it can be used alone and prepared into decoction or powder for oral administration, or used in combination with Semen Myristicae and Fructus Chebulae.

(2) To kill parasites. Indicated for teniasis, ascariasis and oxyuriasis, for which it is often prescribed along with Fructus Mume, or applied alone.

Dosage: 3-10 g.

Fructus Chebulae(诃子 *he zi*)

Fructus Chebulae is the ripe fruit of the deciduous tree Terminalia chebula Retz., or T. chebula Retz. var. tomentella Kurt. of Combretaceae. Originally produced in India, Malaysia and Burma, it is now cultivated in Yunnan and Guangdong provinces as well as the Guangxi Zhuang Autonomous Region of China. It is collected in July and August and dried in the sun.

Synonym: *He li le.*

Taste and Property: Bitter, sour and astringent, and warm.

Attributive Meridian: Lung and large intestine meridians.

Actions and Indications:

(1) To astringe the intestines and relieve diarrhea. Indicated for chronic diarrhea and

dysentery. For cases due to heat, it is combined with Rhizoma Coptidis; and for cases due to cold, with Rhizoma Zingiberis.

(2) To astringe the lung and relieve cough and sore throat. Indicated for lung deficiency marked by protracted cough, hoarse voice and sore throat, for which it is often combined with Radix Platycodi and Radix Glycyrrhizae. For cases due to lung fire, it is often prescribed along with Pericarpium Trichosanthis, Bulbus Fritillariae Cirrhosae and Radix Scrophulariae.

Dosage and Preparation: 3-10 g, wrapped with wet coverings and roasted to astringe the intestines, and used in crude form to astringe the lung.

Remarks: Fructus Chebulae not only astringes the lung but also suppresses the abnormal ascent of *qi* and fire, thus relieving sore throat and hoarse voice. It is essential for aphonia.

Semen Myristicae(肉豆蔻 *rou dou kou*)

Semen Myristicae is the ripe seed of Myristica fragrans Houtt. of Myristicaceae. Produced mainly in Malaysia and Indonesia, it is also cultivated in China's Guangdong Province. The seeds are collected in April-June and November-December periods; the ripe fruit is picked from the tree and the seed is taken out and soaked in lime water for one day, then baked dry over a slow fire.

Synonym: *Rou guo.*

Taste and Property: Acrid, and warm.

Attributive Meridian: Spleen, stomach and large intestine meridians.

Actions and Indications:

(1) To astringe the intestines and relieve diarrhea. Indicated for chronic diarrhea due to spleen deficiency, for which it is often combined with Radix Codonopsis Pilosulae, Rhizoma Atractylodis Macrocephalae and Rhizoma Zingiberis. For morning diarrhea due to deficiency-cold in the spleen and kidney, it is often combined with Fructus Psoraleae, Fructus Schisandrae and Fructus Evodiae, as in Pill of Four Miraculous Drugs.

(2) To warm the middle *jiao* and activate *qi* circulation. Indicated for spleen and stomach deficiency and cold with retarded *qi* circulation, marked by epigastric and abdominal distention and pain, poor appetite and vomiting; here it is often used with Radix Aucklandiae, Rhizoma Pinelliae and Zingiberis.

Dosage and Preparation: 3-10 g in decoction and 1. 5-3 g in powder. Wrapped in dough and roasted to get rid of oil.

Remarks: Semen Myristicae and Semen Amomi Rotundus are two different drugs. The former, which is warm and dry, can astringe the intestines, relieve diarrhea, warm the middle *jiao* and activate *qi* circulation, and is indicated for chronic diarrhea due to deficiency and cold. The latter, aromatic and capable to eliminate dampness, pacify the stomach and check vomiting, is indicated for vomiting due to dampness retained in the middle *jiao*.

Semen Myristicae, when used crude, often causes nausea and vomiting; this side effect can be reduced by wrapping it in dough and then roasted.

Halloysitum Rubrum(赤石脂 *chi shi zhi*)

Halloysitum Rubrum is a mineral mainly composed of hydrated aluminum silicate $Al_4(Si_4O_{10})(OH)_8 \cdot 4H_2O$. Produced mainly in Fujian, Shandong and Henan provinces, it can be mined any time of the year, with foreign matter removed.

Taste and Property: Sweet and astringent, and warm.
Attributive Meridian: Large intestine meridian.
Actions and Indications:

(1) To astringe the intestines and relieve diarrhea. Indicated for long-standing diarrhea and dysentery due to deficiency and cold, as well as such cases accompanied by incontinence of stools and rectal prolapse, for which it is often used with Rhizoma Zingiberis Preparata and Fructus Oryzae Sativae, as in *Taohua* Decoction, or else with Radix Codonopsis Pilosulae, Rhizoma Atractylodis Macrocephalae, Radix Aconiti Lateralis Preparata and Radix Glycyrrhizae.

(2) To check bleeding and relieve leukorrhagia. Indicated for metrorrhagia and leukorrhagia with red and white discharge. For such cases, it is often prescribed along with Os Sepiae and Cacumen Biotae. It can also be used for hematochezia, and used externally for bleeding due to trauma.

Dosage and Preparation: 10-20 g, wrapped in a piece of cloth and decocted, or prepared into pills and powder. Moderate amount for external use.

Remarks: Halloysitum Rubrum, with strong astringent effect on the intestines, is indicated for chronic diarrhea and dysentery without symptoms of stagnation, and is especially important for incontinence of stools and severe diarrhea. It serves as an astringent and antidiarrhea agent for symptomatic treatment, and is often combined with Radix Ginseng, Rhizoma Zingiberis and Atractylodis Macrocephalae for causative treatment. In addition, it is especially effective for bleeding in the lower part of the body, as in metrorrhagia and hematochezia. Now, it is frequently applied for hematemesis or hematochezia due to peptic ulcers.

Semen Nelumbinis(莲子 *lian zi*)

Semen Nelumbinis is the ripe seed of the perennial aquatic plant Nelumbo nucifera Gaertn. of Nymphaeaceae. Produced mainly in Jiangsu, Zhejiang, Hunan and Fujian provinces as well as other areas in southern China where there are many lakes and ponds, it is usually collected in autumn when the fruit is ripe, and dried in the sun with the exopleura removed.

Taste and Property: Sweet and astringent, and mild.
Attributive Meridian: Spleen, kidney and heart meridians.
Actions and Indications:

(1) To nourish the spleen and relieve diarrhea. Indicated for spleen deficiency marked

by chronic diarrhea or dysentery and poor appetite, for which it is often combined with Rhizoma Atractylodis Macrocephalae, Radix Codonopsis Pilosulae, Rhizoma Dioscoreae and Poria. It can also be used for leukorrhagia due to spleen deficiency.

(2) To nourish the kidney and arrest kidney essence. Indicated for seminal emission due to kidney deficiency. For such cases, it is often used with Os Draconis and Fructus Alpiniae Oxyphyllae.

It also nourishes the heart and calms the mind, and is used for palpitation and insomnia.

Dosage and Preparation: 10-15 g, crushed with the plumule removed.

Semen Euryales(芡实 *qian shi*)

Semen Euryales is the ripe seed of the annual aquatic plant Euryale ferox Salisb. of Nymphaeaceae. Produced mainly in Jiangsu, Hunan, Hubei and Shandong provinces, it is collected in late autumn and early winter when the petioles and leaves have withered; the exocarp is broken and the seed is removed, then the exopleura is peeled off and dried in the sun.

Synonym: *Ji tou mi.*

Taste and Property: Sweet and astringent, and mild.

Attributive Meridian: Spleen and kidney meridians.

Actions and Indications:

(1) To nourish the kidney and astringe kidney essence. Indicated for seminal emission due to kidney deficiency, for which it is often combined with Fructus Rosae Laevigatae, as in Pill Containing Two Drugs.

(2) To nourish the spleen and check diarrhea. Indicated for diarrhea due to spleen deficiency, for which it is often used with Radix Codonopsis Pilosulae, Rhizoma Atractylodis Macrocephalae, Rhizoma Dioscoreae and Semen Dolichoris Album.

(3) To astringe vaginal discharge and arrest leukorrhea. Indicated for leukorrhagia due to spleen deficiency marked by thin vaginal discharge, for which it is often prescribed along with Dioscoreae, Codonopsis Pilosulae, Atractylodis Macrocephalae and Os Sepiae; and also for leukorrhagia due to dampness-heat marked by thick yellow discharge, for which it is often combined with Cortex Phellodendri, Cortex Ailanthi and Semen Plantaginis.

Dosage: 10-15 g.

Remarks: Semen Nelumbinis and Semen Euryales have similar actions in nourishing the spleen and relieving diarrhea, nourishing the kidney and arresting seminal emission. But the former is better at nourishing the spleen, the latter at arresting kidney essence.

Fructus Rosae Laevigatae(金樱子 *jin ying zi*)

Fructus Rosae Laevigatae is the ripe fruit of the evergreen climbing shrub Rosa laevigata Michx. of Rosaceae. Produced mainly in Guangdong, Hunan, Zhejiang and Jiangxi provinces, it is collected between October and November when the fruit is ripe, and dried in the sun with the thorns removed.

Taste and Property: Sour and astringent, and mild.
Attributive Meridian: Kidney and large intestine meridians.
Actions and Indications:

(1) To arrest seminal emission and reduce urination. Indicated for kidney deficiency marked by seminal emission, nocturnal enuresis and frequent urination, for which it is often used with Semen Euryales, or sometimes with Rhizoma Dioscoreae, Ootheca Mantidis and Radix Linderae.

(2) To astringe the intestines and relieve diarrhea. Indicated for chronic diarrhea and dysentery, for which it is often prescribed along with Rhizoma Atractylodis Macrocephalae, Radix Codonopsis Pilosulae, Poria and Euryales.

This drug can also relieve leukorrhagia and metrorrhagia.

Dosage and Preparation: 6-12 g, as a decoction or else for oral administration.

Ootheca Mantidis(桑螵蛸 *sang piao xiao*)

Ootheca Mantidis is the egg case of the insect Tenodera sinensis Saussure, Statilia maculata (Thunberg), or Hierodula patellifera (Serville) of Mantidae. Produced in most parts of China, it is collected from late autumn to spring, steamed and dried in the sun or by baking with foreign matter removed.

Taste and Property: Sweet and salty, and mild.
Attributive Meridian: Kidney meridian.
Actions and Indications:

To nourish the kidney, promote *yang*, arrest seminal emission and reduce urination. Indicated for kidney *yang* deficiency marked by impotence, premature ejaculation, seminal emission, frequent urination and nocturnal enuresis, for which it is often combined with other drugs that nourish the kidney, such as Radix Rehmanniae Preparata, Fructus Psoraleae and Semen Cuscutae. When combined with Os Draconis and Concha Ostreae, its ability to arrest seminal emission and reduce urination will be enhanced.

Dosage: 5-10 g.
Precaution: It is contraindicated for patients with *yin* deficiency and hyperactive fire, as well as heat in the urinary bladder.

Os Sepiae(乌贼骨 *wu zei gu*)

Os Sepiae is the internal shell of the cuttlefish Sepiella maindronide Rochebrune, or Sepia esculenta Hoyle of Sepiadae. Produced mainly in the coastal areas of Liaoning, Jiangsu and Zhejiang provinces, the cuttlefish is caught from April to August; its internal shell is washed clean, dried in the sun and exposed to dew day and night in order to eliminate its fishy smell.

Synonym: *Hai piao xiao.*
Taste and Property: Salty and astringent, and slight warm.
Attributive Meridian: Liver, stomach and kidney meridians.
Actions and Indications:

(1) To stop bleeding. Indicated for bleeding from the lung and stomach, hematuria and metrorrhagia, for which it is used either alone or in combination with other hemostatics. For bleeding due to trauma, it is processed into powder for external use.

(2) To relieve leukorrhagia. Indicated for leukorrhagia due to spleen and kidney deficiency, for which it is often combined with Radix Codonopsis Pilosulae, Rhizoma Atractylodis Macrocephalae and Cornu Cervi Degelatinatum.

(3) To cure stomach hyperacidity. Indicated for epigastric pain with acid regurgitation, for which it is often prescribed along with Bulbus Fritillariae, as in Powder of Os Sepiae and Fritillariae. For cases accompanied by hematemesis and hematochezia, it is often used with Rhizoma Bletillae, as in Powder of Os Sepiae and Bletillae.

(4) To arrest seminal emission. It is indicated for seminal emission due to kidney deficiency, for which it is often combined with Fructus Corni, Semen Cuscutae and Fructus Tribuli.

(5) To cure lesions. Indicated for weeping eczema and unhealed sores, for which it is often combined with Rhizoma Coptidis, Cortex Phellodendri, Indigo Naturalis and Gypsum Fibrosum Usta.

Dosage and Preparation: 3-10 g in decoction, and 1. 5-3 g in powder. Moderate amount for external application.
Precaution: Overdosage and prolonged administration may result in constipation; this can be avoided by adding laxatives.

Table 19. Actions of Astringents

Drug	Similarities	Differences
Fructus Schisandrae	To astringe the lung and relieve cough	To arrest perspiration, relieve diarrhea and emission, reduce urination; replenish *qi* and fluids; tonify kidney
Fructus Mume		To promote production of fluids, relieve diarrhea, treat ascariasis
Galla Chinensis		To check sweating, relieve diarrhea and emission, reduce urination

Drug	Similarities	Differences
Fructus Tritici Levis	To arrest perspiration	
Radix Oryzae Glutinosae		
Cortex Ailanthi	To astringe the lung and relieve diarrhea	To eliminate dampness-heat; relieve leukorrhagia; hemostatic
Pericarpium Granati		Anthelmintic
Fructus Chebulae		To astringe the lung, relieve cough and sorethroat
Semen Myristicae		To warm middle *jiao* and activate the circulation of *qi*
Halloysitum Rubrum		Potent action in asorrhging the intestine; check bleeding and leukorrhagia
Semen Nelumbinis	To relieve seminal emission and reduce urination	To tonify the spleen, relieve diarrhea; nourish heart
Semen Euryales		To tonify the spleen, relieve diarrhea and leukorrhagia
Fructus Rosae Laevigatae		To astringe lung, relieve diarrhea, leukorrhagia and metrorrhagia
Ootheca Mantidis		To tonify kidney *yang*
Os Sepiae		To check bleeding, relieve leukorrhagia, counteract gastric hyperacidity; promote granulation

Note: Other sections deal with additional drugs that have an astringent action, including Os Draconis, Concha Ostreae, Radix Ephedrae and Fructus Corni.

ANNEX
A GLOSSARY OF THE EFFICACY OF CHINESE DRUGS

(Arranged in the order wind, cold, summer-heat, dampness, phlegm, dryness, fire, *qi*, blood, *yin* and *yang*)

Pathogenic Wind

To dispel wind (祛风 *qu feng*): To eliminate pathogenic wind from the body surface, channels, muscles and joints by using drugs that dispel wind. Most of these drugs are acrid and warm, can eliminate pathogenic wind and relieve pain, spasm and itching, and indicated for headache caused by pathogenic wind, pain in *bi*-syndrome, tetanus and pruritus. Examples: Herba Schizonepetae, Radix Ledebouriellae, Rhizoma seu Radix Notopterygii, Radix Angelicae Dahuricae and Rhizoma Chuanxiong.

To eliminate wind-dampness (祛风湿 *qu feng shi*): To eliminate pathogenic wind and dampness from the surface and the meridians. Drugs that eliminate wind-dampness purge wind, relieve pain, remove obstruction in the meridians, ease the tendons and strengthen the muscles and bones. They are indicated for *bi*-syndrome due to wind-dampness marked by lumbago, weakness of the lower limbs and hemiplegia. Examples: Radix Ledebouriellae, Rhizoma seu Radix Notopterygii, Radix Angelicae Pubescentis, Radix Clematidis, Radix Gentianae Macrophyllae, Fructus Chaenomelis, Ramulus Taxilli and Agkistrodon seu Bungarus.

To eliminate wind-phlegm (祛风痰 *qu feng tan*): To resolve phlegm, eliminate wind and relieve spasm. Most are acrid and warm, and are indicated for wind-phlegm syndrome marked by vertigo, epilepsy, deviation of the mouth and eyes and hemiplegia due to wind-stroke. Example: Rhizoma Arisaematis.

To dispel wind-cold (散风寒 *san feng han*): To dispel exogenous pathogenic wind and cold. Drugs that dispel wind-cold are acrid and warm, can relieve exterior syndrome by dispelling wind-cold from the surface, and are indicated for exterior syndrome due to wind-cold, headache due to wind-cold and pain in the limbs. Examples: Herba Ephedrae, Ramulus Cinnamomi, Folium Perillae, Herba Schizonepetae, Radix Ledebouriellae and Rhizoma Zingiberis Recens.

To dispel wind-heat (散风热 *san feng re*): To dispel exogenous pathogenic wind-heat.

Drugs that dispel wind-heat are acrid and cool, can relieve exterior syndrome by dispelling wind-heat from the surface and purge heat, and are indicated for exterior syndrome due to wind-heat, headache due to wind-heat and sore throat. Examples: Herba Menthae, Fructus Arctii, Periostracum Cicadae, Folium Mori and Flos Chrysanthemi.

To subdue wind (息风 *xi feng*): To suppress liver wind; this is also known as "calming the liver and subduing wind." Drugs that subdue wind relieve spasms and convulsions, and are indicated for febrile diseases with arousal of liver wind, apoplexy, epilepsy and deviation of the mouth and eyes. Examples: Cornu Saigae Tataricae, Ramulus Uncariae cum Uncis, Rhizoma Gastrodiae, Scorpio and Bombyx Batryticatus.

Remarks: Pathogenic wind is either exogenous or endogenous. Exogenous wind should be dispelled, and endogenous wind subdued. The two aspects should be distinguished.

Pathogenic Cold

To warm the interior (温里 *wen li*): To warm the interior and dispel interior cold. Drugs that warm the interior are acrid, hot (or warm) and dry. With a strong ability to eliminate cold, they are indicated for various kinds of interior cold syndromes by dispelling cold and relieving pain, warming the middle *jiao*, warming *yang* and restoring *yang*.

To dispel cold and relieve pain (散寒止痛 *san han zhi tong*): To relieve pain by warming and dispelling pathogenic cold. Cold is characterized by contraction and stagnation, and pain occurs when the *qi* passage is obstructed by cold. Drugs that dispel cold and relieve pain are acrid and hot, and are indicated for cold-pain in the epigastrium and abdomen, and *bi*-syndrome due to cold and dampness. Examples: Radix Aconiti Lateralis Preparata, Radix Aconiti, Cortex Cinnamomi, Rhizoma Zingiberis, Herba Asari, Fructus Evodiae and Pericarpium Zanthoxyli.

To warm the middle jiao (温中 *wen zhong*): Drugs that warm the middle *jiao* are acrid and hot or warm, and can eliminate pathogenic cold from the spleen and stomach and restore their normal functions so as to relieve pain, vomiting and diarrhea and strengthen the spleen and stomach. They are indicated for pain in the epigastrium and abdomen, vomiting and diarrhea due to attack of the middle *jiao* by cold, cold-pain in the epigastrium and abdomen, as well as vomiting and diarrhea due to disturbance of *yang-qi*. Examples: Rhizoma Zingiberis, Cortex Cinnamomi, Rhizoma Alpiniae Officinarum, Fructus Evodiae, and Pericarpium Zanthoxyli.

To warm the lung and resolve phlegm(温肺化饮 *wen fei hua yin*): To resolve phlegm by warming and dispersing cold from the lung. Drugs that warm the lung and resolve phlegm are acrid and hot or warm, are indicated for cough and dyspnea with copious dilute sputum due to retention of cold and phlegm in the lung. Examples: Rhizoma Zingiberis and Herba Asari.

Pathogenic Summer-Heat

To purge summer-heat(清暑热 *qing shu re*): Summer-heat is a *yang* factor that can be eliminated with cold drugs. Most of the drugs that purge summer-heat are sweet and cold. They are indicated for stroke of summer-heat manifested as fever, polydipsia, sweating, reddish urine, red tongue with yellow coating, and bounding and rapid pulse. Examples: Gypsum Fibrosum, Herba Artemisiae Annuae, Flos Lonicerae and Talcum.

To eliminate summer-heat and disperse dampness (祛暑化湿 *qu shu hua shi*): Drugs that eliminate summer-heat and disperse dampness are acrid, aromatic and warm. They are indicated for attack by summer-heat and dampness marked by chills, fever, vomiting and diarrhea. Examples: Herba Elsholtziae and Herba Agastaches.

Remarks: Drugs that purge summer-heat are cold, and are indicated for summer-heat syndrome. In addition, drugs that eliminate summer-heat and disperse dampness are acrid, warm and aromatic, and are particularly used to disperse dampness, are indicated for summer-heat-dampness syndrome. But, among the drugs that purge summer-heat, Herba Artemisiae Annuae is bitter, cold and aromatic, and Talcum can facilitate elimination of dampness, and so they can also be used in summer-heat-dampness syndrome.

Pathogenic Dampness

To disperse dampness(化湿 *hua shi*): To eliminate dampness in the upper *jiao*. Dampness is characterized by viscidity and stagnation, which obstruct the *qi* passages. There will be no retention of dampness if *qi* circulates normally. Most drugs that disperse dampness are acrid, aromatic and warm, and eliminate dampness by activating *qi* circulation. They are indicated for syndromes in which dampness blocks the middle *jiao*, dampness-heat syndrome and summer-heat-dampness syndrome. Examples: Herba Agastaches, Herba Eupatorii, Fructus Amomi Rotundus, Rhizoma Atractylodis and Cortex Magnoliae Officinalis.

To dry dampness and strengthen the spleen(燥湿健脾 *zao shi jian pi*): To eliminate dampness by promoting the spleen's ability to transport and transform. The spleen prefers dryness and is intolerable to dampness. Dampness blocking the middle *jiao* leads to impaired splenic functions and further gives rise to dampness. Drugs that dry dampness and strengthen the spleen are bitter and warm, and can eliminate dampness in the middle *jiao*. They are indicated for dampness blocking the middle *jiao*, dampness-heat syndrome, phlegm-fluid syndrome and edema. Examples: Rhizoma Atractylodis and Rhizoma

Atractylodis Macrocephalae.

Remarks: Treatment for dampness includes drying dampness and strengthening the spleen as well as drying dampness and resolving phlegm. The former lays stress on strengthening the spleen and the latter on resolving phlegm.

To purge heat and dry dampness(清热燥湿 *qing re zao shi*): Drugs that purge heat and dry dampness are bitter and cold. They are indicated for syndromes due to dampness-heat, such as diarrhea, dysentery and jaundice due to dampness-heat and wet sores. Examples: Rhizoma Coptidis, Radix Scutellariae, Cortex Phellodendri, Radix Gentianae and Radix Sophorae Flavescentis.

Remarks: The above two terms are both meant to eliminate dampness. But drugs that dry dampness and strengthen the spleen are bitter and warm, and are indicated for cold-dampness syndromes; drugs that purge heat and dry dampness are bitter and cold, and are indicated for dampness-heat syndromes.

To promote diuresis and eliminate dampness(利水渗湿 *li shui shen shi*): This is often abbreviated as *li shi*. Drugs that promote diuresis and eliminate dampness are sweet, bland and slightly cold, or bitter and cold. They are indicated for disorders due to retained water and dampness, such as dysuria, edema, stranguria and jaundice. Examples: Poria, Rhizoma Alismatis, Semen Plantaginis, Talcum and Caulis Akebiae.

To purge heat and eliminate dampness(清热利湿 *qing re li shi*): Drugs that promote diuresis and eliminate dampness also purge heat, and so their efficacy is also described as *qing li shi re* (eliminating dampness-heat). Most drugs that eliminate dampness-heat are bitter and cold, and are indicated for dampness-heat syndromes, such as stranguria due to heat, wet sores and jaundice. Examples: Fructus Gardeniae, Caulis Akebiae, Semen Plantaginis, Spora Lygodii and Folium Pyrrosiae.

Remarks: The main difference between *qing re zao shi* (purging heat and drying dampness) and *qing re li shi* (purging heat and eliminating dampness) is that the former eliminates dampness by drying, and the latter by promoting diuresis.

To relieve stranguria(通淋 *tong lin*): To remove obstructions in the water passage and relieve impaired urination. Drugs that relieve stranguria are bitter or sweet and cold. They not only promote diuresis but also purge dampness-heat from the lower *jiao*. Moreover, some remove stones in the urinary tract, thus relieving dribbling and painful urination due to accumulated dampness-heat in the urinary ladder or urinary stones. They are indicated for stranguria due to heat and stones, and stranguria complicated by hematuria. Examples: Semen Plantaginis, Caulis Akebiae, Talcum, Herba Lysimachiae, Folium Pyrrosiae and Spora Lygodii.

To promote diuresis and eliminate dampness with bland-tasted drugs(淡渗利湿 *dan shen li shi*): To eliminate dampness by diuretics that are sweet, bland and cold (or mild). They are indicated for dysuria, edema and phlegm retention. Examples: Poria, Polyporus Umbellatus, Rhizoma Alismatis, Semen Coicis and Talcum.

To eliminate dampness and relieve jaundice (利湿退黄 *li shi tui huang*): To eliminate dampness-heat and relieve jaundice. Most drugs for this purpose are bitter and cold, and can promote diuresis and purge dampness-heat from the liver and gallbladder. They are indicated for jaundice due to dampness-heat. Examples: Herba Artemisiae Scopariae, Fructus Gardeniae, Radix Gentianae Macrophyllae, Herba Lysimachiae and Rhizoma Polygoni Cuspidati.

To promote diuresis and relieve edema (利水消肿 *li shui xiao zhong*): To relieve edema by promoting diuresis; this is one of the effects of the drugs that promote diuresis and eliminate dampness. They are indicated for edema and ascites. Examples: Poria, Polyporus Umbellatus, and Rhizoma Alismatis. Because the lung functions as the upper organ of water metabolism, drugs that relieve exterior syndrome by dispersing the lung, such as Herba Ephedrae and Herba Elsholtziae, can also promote diuresis and relieve edema.

To eliminate fluid by purgation(逐水 *zhu shui*): Drastic purgatives eliminate accumulated fluid and dampness by means of their strong cathartic action, and some also possess diuretic action. They are indicated for edema and ascites. Examples: Radix Kansui, Flos Genkwa, Radix Euphorbiae Pekinensis and Semen Pharbitidis.

Remarks: Both diuretics and purgatives eliminate accumulated fluid and dampness and relieve edema, but the former are mild and the latter drastic.

Phlegm

To eliminate phlegm (祛痰 *qu tan*): Drugs that eliminate phlegm can expel phlegm to relieve cough. They are indicated for productive cough and lung abscess. Examples: Radix Platycodi and Radix Polygalae.

To dry dampness and resolve phlegm (燥湿化痰 *zao shi hua tan*): Among drugs that resolve phlegm, those that are warm and dry and used to treat dampness-phlegm syndrome are called drugs for drying dampness and resolving phlegm. They are acrid and warm, and are indicated for syndromes of dampness-phlegm marked by cough with copious white sputum, stuffiness in the chest and greasy tongue coating. Examples: Rhizoma Pinelliae and Rhizoma Arisaematis.

To purge heat and resolve phlegm(清热化痰 *qing re hua tan*): Among drugs that resolve phlegm, those that are cold and purge heat are called drugs for purging heat and resolving phlegm, also referred to as "purging heat phlegm" (清化热痰 *qing hua re tan*). They are sweet or bitter and cold, and are indicated for heat-phlegm syndrome marked by cough with yellow sticky sputum, and for febrile diseases and apoplexy with phlegm-heat blocking the heart marked by unconsciousness and delirium. Examples: Fructus Trichosanthis, Bulbus Fritillariae, Concretio Silicea Bambusae, Caulis Bambusae in Taeniam and Succus Bambusae.

To resolve phlegm and soften hard masses (化痰软坚 *hua tan ruan jian*): To resolve accumulated phlegm and soften hard masses. Most of them are sea products, which are salty and cold, and are indicated for goiter and scrofula. Examples: Thallus Eckloniae and Sargassum.

To weigh down phlegm (坠痰 *zhui tan*): To remove phlegm with heavy drugs which have the action of sinking. They are indicated for excess syndrome due to phlegm manifested as epilepsy, manic-depressive psychosis and dyspneic cough. Example: Lapis Chloriti.

Pathogenic Dryness

To moisten dryness (润燥 *run zao*): Most of the drugs that moisten dryness are sweet, moist and cold. They moisten the lung to relieve cough, moisten the stomach to promote fluid generation and moisten the intestines to relax the bowels.

To moisten the lung to relieve cough (润肺止咳 *run fei zhi ke*): Most of these drugs are sweet and cold. They are indicated for cough due to dryness in the lung and *yin* deficiency marked by dry cough and dry mouth and tongue. Examples: Mel, Radix Glycyrrhizae, Colla Corii Asini, Radix Glehniae, Radix Asparagi and Rhizoma Polygonati Odorati. Moreover, some of the drugs that purge heat and resolve phlegm, such as Fructus Trichosanthis and Succus Bambusae, also moisten the lung.

To promote fluid generation (生津 *sheng jin*): Most drugs that promote fluid generation are sweet and cold, and are indicated for thirst, dryness in the throat and diabetes. According to their different properties, these drugs can be classified into those that purge heat and those that nourish *yin*. The former are indicated for fluid consumption due to excessive heat, thirst and polydipsia. Examples: Gypsum Fibrosum, Rhizoma Anemarrhenae, Rhizoma Phragmitis and Radix Trichosanthis. The latter nourish lung and stomach *yin*, and are indicated for damage to lung and stomach *yin* and insufficient body fluid. Examples: Herba Dendrobii, Radix Ophiopogonis, Radix Adenophorae, Radix Rehmanniae and Radix Scrophulariae. Moreover, sour drugs such as Fructus Mume and Fructus Schisandrae also promote fluid generation.

To moisten the intestines to relax the bowels (润肠通便 *run chang tong bian*): Also called "purgation by moistening" (润下 *run xia*) or "moistening dryness and lubricating the intestines"（润燥滑肠 *run zao hua chang*）. Most are seeds that are sweet, moistening and rich in oil. They can relax the bowels without causing drastic purgation, and are indicated for constipation in the aged and debilitated, and also constipation due to dryness in intestines and fluid consumption. Examples: Fructus Cannabis, Semen Pruni, Semen Trichosanthis, Semen Armeniacae Amarum, Semen Persicae, Semen Biotae, Semen Cassiae, Mel, Radix Angelicae Sinensis and Herba Cistanches.

Pathogenic Fire

To purge heat and eliminate fire（清热泻火 *qing re xie huo*）: Cold drugs purge heat and bitter ones purge and suppress hyperactive fire. This is abbreviated as "purging fire"（泻火 *xie huo*）, "suppressing fire"（降火 *jiang huo*）, or "purging fire"（清火 *qing huo*）. These drugs are indicated for excessive pathogenic heat in febrile diseases and excessive endogenous heat, to purge fire in the lung, heart, stomach, liver and kidney, respectively.

To purge lung fire（清肺火 *qing fei huo*）: Drugs that purge lung fire are indicated for cough with expectoration of yellow sputum and shortness of breath due to heat in the lung. Examples: Radix Scutellariae, Talcum, Rhizoma Anemarrhenae and Rhizoma Phragmitis.

To eliminate heart fire（清心火 *qing xin huo*）: Drugs that purge heart fire are indicated for excessive heat in the Heart Meridian marked by high fever, coma, delirium, restlessness, insomnia and aphthae, as well as hematemesis and epistaxis due to excessive heat in the blood. Examples: Rhizoma Coptidis, Radix Scutellariae, Radix et Rhizoma Rhei, Fructus Gardeniae and Fructus Forsythiae.

To eliminate stomach fire（清胃火 *qing wei huo*）: Drugs that purge stomach fire are indicated for various syndromes due to stomach heat. For instance, Gypsum Fibrosum and Rhizoma Anemarrhenae can be used for the treatment of the Yangming Meridian syndrome of the excess and heat types in febrile diseases, and headache and toothache caused by stomach fire; Rhizoma Coptidis can be used for vomiting and fullness in the epigastrium due to stomach fire.

To purge liver fire（清肝火 *qing gan huo*）: Drugs that purge liver fire are indicated for hyperactive liver fire marked by headache, hypochondriac pain, red eyes and infantile convulsion. Examples: Radix Gentianae, Fructus Gardeniae, Spica Prunellae, Cortex Moutan Radicis and Radix et Rhizoma Rhei.

To eliminate kidney fire（清肾火 *qing shen huo*）: Also called "purging ministerial fire"（清相火 *qing xiang huo*）. Drugs for this purpose are indicated for hectic fever, night sweating and seminal emission due to insufficient kidney *yin* and hyperactive ministerial fire (kidney fire). Examples: Rhizoma Anemarrhenae and Cortex Phellodendri.

To purge heat and cool the blood (清热凉血 *qing re liang xue*): To purge pathogenic heat from the *xue* (blood) system. Drugs that purge heat and cool the blood are sweet or bitter and cold, and are indicated for epidemic febrile diseases with attack of the *ying* (nutrient) and *xue* systems by pathogenic factors, marked by fever, eruptions, coma, delirium and dark red tongue, as well as for hematemesis and epistaxis due to excessive heat in the blood. Examples: Cornu Rhinocerotis, Radix Rehmanniae, Radix Scrophulariae, Cortex Moutan Radicis, Radix Paeoniae Rubra, Fructus Gardeniae, Radix Arnebiae seu Lithospermi and Indigo Naturalis.

To purge heat and toxicins (清热解毒 *qing re jie du*): Most of the drugs that purge heat and toxicins are bitter and cold though some are sweet and cold. They are indicated for various diseases caused by heat and toxicins, such as epidemic febrile diseases due to excessive toxic heat marked by persistent fever, skin infections, sore throat, diarrhea and dysentery due to toxic heat and poisonous snakebites. Examples: Radix et Rhizoma Rhei, Rhizoma Coptidis, Flos Lonicerae, Fructus Forsythiae, Herba Taraxaci, Folium Isatidis, Radix Pulsatillae and Herba Lobeliae Chinensis.

To purge deficiency heat (清虚热 *qing xu re*): Also called "eliminating deficiency heat" (退虚热 *tui xu re*). Deficiency heat syndrome includes fever due to deficiency of *yin*, *yang*, *qi* and blood. Most drugs that purge deficiency heat are sweet and cold, though some are bitter and cold. They are indicated for hectic fever, night sweating and flushed face due to *yin* deficiency leading to hyperactive *yang*, the late stages of febrile diseases with *yin*-fluid consumption marked by fever at night but defervescence in the morning, and infantile malnutrition accompanied by fever. Examples: Radix Rehmanniae, Rhizoma Anemarrhenae, Herba Artemisiae Annuae, Cortex Lycii Radicis, Radix Cynanchi Atrati, Radix Stellariae and Radix Gentianae Macrophyllae.

To conduct fire downward (引火下行 *yin huo xia xing*): To conduct rising heat and fire downward. For instance, Radix Achyranthis Bidentatae conducts fire downward and is used for headache and vertigo due to hyperactive liver *yang*, swelling and pain of the gums due to an upward attack of stomach fire, and hematemesis and epistaxis due to excessive heat in the blood. Powder of Fructus Evodiae mixed with vinegar and applied externally onto the center of the soles can treat aphthae by conducting the fire downward.

Remarks: Other terms that relate to the elimination of heat include *qing re zao shi*, *qing re hua tan*, *qing re li shi* and *qing xue re*. They are discussed in other sections.

Qi

To regulate qi (理气 *li qi*): To regulate *qi* circulation. Most drugs that regulate *qi* are acrid, warm and aromatic, and can activate *qi*, break stagnant *qi* and suppress the adverse ascent of *qi*. They are indicated for syndromes due to *qi* stagnation and the adverse ascent of *qi*.

To activate qi (行气 *xing qi*): To promote *qi* circulation and remove obstruction in *qi* passages; also called "facilitating *qi* (利气 *li qi*). Most drugs that activate *qi* are sweet, warm and aromatic, and can strengthen the spleen and stomach, and promote transportation and transformation, improve digestion, and relieve distention, fullness and pain. They are indicated for *qi* stagnation syndromes exhibiting distensive pain in the epigastrium, abdomen and hypochondria, and poor appetite, by easing the middle *jiao qi*, dispersing liver *qi*, or breaking stagnant *qi*.

To activate qi *and ease middle* jiao (行气宽中 *xing qi kuan zhong*): Splenic and stomach *qi* stagnation often results in distention and fullness in the epigastrium and abdomen. Drugs that activate stagnant spleen and stomach *qi* are acrid, warm and aromatic, and can remove stagnant *qi* and strengthen the spleen and stomach, thus relieving the distention and fullness in the epigastrium and abdomen. Some also disperse lung *qi* and relieve stuffiness in the chest, also referred to as "activate *qi* and ease the chest" (行气宽胸 *xing qi kuan xiong*). Examples: Folium Perillae, Exocarpium Citri Reticulatae, Radix Aucklandiae, and Fructus Aurantii.

To disperse stagnant liver qi (疏肝解郁 *shu gan jie yu*): To relieve stagnation by dispersing liver *qi*. Such drugs are acrid, warm and aromatic (very few are bitter and cold). They are indicated for liver *qi* stagnation marked by hypochondriac distensive pain, distention and pain or lumps in the breasts, hernial pain and irregular menstruation. Examples: Radix Bupleuri, Rhizoma Cyperi, Pericarpium Citri Reticulatae Viride, Fructus Toosendan, Radix Curcumae, and Rhizoma Chuanxiong.

To break stagnant qi (破气 *po qi*): Drugs with powerful effect in activating *qi* are called "drugs for breaking stagnant *qi*." They are particularly effective for removing food stasis and *qi* stagnation. Examples: Cortex Magnoliae Officinalis, Fructus Aurantii Immaturus, and Pericarpium Citri Reticulatae Viride.

To suppress the adverse ascent of qi (降气 *jiang qi*): Also known as "lowering *qi*" (下气 *xia qi*), including suppressing the adverse ascent of the stomach and lung *qi*. Drugs that suppress stomach *qi* are indicated for vomiting, belching and hiccup due to the adverse ascent of stmach *qi*, and drugs that suppress lung *qi* are indicated for cough and dyspnea due to the adverse ascent of lung *qi*. Examples: Flos Inulae, Lignum Aquilariae Resinatum, Haematitum, Folium Eriobotryae, Cortex Magnoliae Officinalis, Rhizoma Pinelliae, and Rhizoma Cynanchi Stauntonii. Most suppress both stomach *qi* and lung *qi*, but some only suppress either one.

To purge the lung and relieve dyspnea (泻肺定喘 *xie fei ding chuan*): To purge lung fire or fluid to relieve dyspnea. Drugs that purge the lung and relieving dyspnea are indicated for cough, dyspnea and edema caused by heat or fluid accumulated in the lung. Examples: Cortex Mori Radicis, and Semen Lepidii seu Descurainiae.

To promote the kidney's ability to receive qi *and relieve dyspnea* (纳气定喘 *na qi ding chuan*): Also called "warming the kidney and promoting its ability to receive *qi*" (温肾纳气 *wen shen na qi*). "The lung is the administrator of *qi* and the kidney is the root of *qi*," as the ancient medical literature says. Liver *yang* insufficiency impairs the kidney's ability to receive *qi*, resulting in shortness of breath and dyspnea which are aggravated on exertion. Drugs that promote this function warm and nourish kidney *yang* and restore kidney function. They are indicated for dyspnea due to kidney deficiency. Examples: Gecko, Semen Juglandis, and Fructus Psoraleae.

To replenish qi (补气 *bu qi*): To strengthen the antipathogenic *qi*, also called "benefiting *qi*" (益气 *yi qi*). Most drugs that replenish *qi* are sweet and warm, and can nourish spleen, lung and heart *qi*. They are indicated for weak spleen *qi*, marked by general lassitude, poor appetite and loose stools; weak lung *qi*, marked by shortness of breath, dyspnea, feeble voice and spontaneous sweating; and weak heart *qi*, marked by palpitation, shortness of breath, knotted and intermittent pulse and collapse. Examples: Radix Ginseng, Radix Codonopsis Pilosulae, Radix Astragali, Rhizoma Atractylodis Macrocephalae, Rhizoma Dioscoreae, and Radix Glycyrrhizae.

To strongly replenish primordial qi (大补元气 *da bu yuan qi*): Drugs for this purpose have fairly potent effect in strengthening resistance. They are indicated for cases with primordial *qi* deficiency, especially prostration of primordial *qi*. Example: Radix Ginseng.

To replenish qi *and consolidate the exterior* (补气固表 *bu qi gu biao*): To consolidate the *wei* (defensive) system and surface of the body by replenishing *qi*. Weakness of defensive *qi* in the surface often leads to spontaneous sweating. Drugs that replenish *qi* and consolidate the exterior are indicated for exterior syndrome of the deficiency type with spontaneous sweating. Example: Radix Astragali.

To replenish and promote granulation (补气托疮 *bu qi tuo chuang*): To promote pus discharge and healing of lesions by replenishing the antipathogenic *qi*. Drugs that replenish *qi* to promote granulation are indicated for diffused and unruptured sores or ruptured and unhealed sores with discharge of thin pus due to antipathogenic *qi* deficiency. Examples: Radix Astragali, and Cortex Cinnamomi.

To strengthen the spleen (健脾 *jian pi*): To strengthen the spleen and promote its transporting function. There are various causative factors for impaired transporting function, such as dampness accumulated in the spleen, stagnant *qi* circulation and weakness of the spleen. All drugs that dry dampness, activate *qi* and nourish the spleen also strengthen the spleen. They are indicated for cases with impaired transporting function of the spleen marked by poor appetite, diarrhea, edema and abdominal distention. They can strengthen the spleen either by drying dampness (Rhizoma Atractylodis and Rhizoma Atractylodis Macrocephalae), activating *qi* (Pericarpium Citri Reticulatae and Fructus Amomi), or replenishing *qi* (Radix Codonopsis Pilosulae, and Radix Astragali).

Remarks: Nourishing the spleen and strengthening the spleen are correlated but different. Not all the drugs that nourish the spleen can be used to strengthen it, such as Radix Glycyrrhizae and Fructus Jujubae, and vice versa.

Blood

To check bleeding (止血 *zhi xue*): Drugs that check bleeding are indicated for internal and traumatic hemorrhage, either by cooling the blood, by astringing, by removing blood stasis, or by warming the meridians.

To stop bleeding by cooling the blood (凉血止血 *liang xue zhi xue*): Drugs for this purpose are cold, and can purge heat from the blood system. They are indicated for bleeding due to excessive heat in the blood. Examples: Herba seu Radix Cirsii Japonici, Herba Cephalanoploris, Radix Sanguisorbae, Radix Boehmeriae, Rhizoma Imperatae, and Radix et Rhizoma Rhei.

Remarks: The main difference between drugs that check bleeding by cooling the blood and those that purge heat and cool the blood is that the former are more effective at checking bleeding, and the latter at purging heat.

To stop bleeding by astringing (收敛止血 *shou lian zhi xue*): Among drugs for stopping bleeding, those have also the astringent effect are known as drugs for stopping bleeding by astringing. Most are astringent. They are indicated for cases of bleeding without the presence of blood stasis. Examples: Vagina Trichycarpi Carbonisatus, and Rhizoma Bletillae.

To remove blood stasis and stop bleeding (化瘀止血 *hua yu zhi xue*): Among drugs that stop bleeding, those that also remove blood stasis are known as drugs for removing blood stasis and stopping bleeding. They have the advantage of stopping bleeding without causing blood stasis. They are especially advisable for blood stagnation accompanied by extravasation and persistent bleeding.

To warm the meridians and stop bleeding (温经止血 *wen jing zhi xue*): *Among drugs that stop bleeding, those that also eliminate cold are known as drugs for warming the meridians and stopping bleeding. They are mainly indicated for bleeding due to deficiency cold. Examples: Rhizoma Zingiberis Preparata, and Folium Artemisiae Argyi.*

To activate blood circulation and remove blood stasis (活血祛瘀 *huo xue qu yu*): Also known as *huo xue hua yu* and *huo xue xing yu*. Drugs that activate blood circulation and remove blood stasis are indicated for retarded blood circulation and blood stasis, manifested as pain in the chest, hypochondrium, epigastrium and abdomen, abdominal mass, dysmenorrhea, postpartum abdominal pain, *bi*-syndrome, carbuncles and abscess. Examples: Radix et Rhizoma Rhei, Radix Salviae Miltiorrhizae, Flos Carthami, Semen Persicae, Radix Angelicae Sinensis, and Rhizoma Chuanxiong.

To activate qi *and blood circulation* (活血行气 *huo xue xing qi*): Also known as *xing qi huo xue*. Drugs that activate *qi* and blood circulation are conventionally called "*qi*-activating agents among drugs for blood disorders," and have an analgesic effect in addition to their ability to activate blood circulation and remove blood stasis. They are indicated for pain due to *qi* and blood stagnation. Examples: Rhizoma Chuanxiong, Olibanum, Myrrha, Rhizoma Corydalis, Radix Curcumae, and Rhizoma Zedoariae.

To break and remove blood stasis (破血逐瘀 *po xue zhu yu*): Activating blood circulation and removing blood stagnation are also called *po xue* or *po yu*. Drugs that break and remove blood stasis are indicated for blood stasis syndrome in patients whose antipathogenic *qi* is not yet deficient. Examples: Rhizoma Sparganii, Rhizoma Zedoariae, Hirudo, and Eupolyphaga seu Steleophaga.

To restore menstruation (通经 *tong jing*): Drugs that restore menstruation activate blood circulation and remove blood stasis. They are indicated for amenorrhea due to obstruction by blood stasis. Examples: Herba Leonuri, Flos Carthami, and Radix Achyranthis Bidentatae.

To nourish the blood (补血 *bu xue*): Also called *yang xue*(养血). Drugs that nourish the blood are sweet and warm or mild. They are indicated for blood deficiency marked by sallow complexion, pale lips and nails, dizziness, blurred vision, palpitation, insomnia and irregular menstruation. Examples: Radix Angelicae Sinensis, Radix Rehmanniae Preparata, Radix Polygoni Multiflori, Radix Paeoniae Alba, Colla Corii Asini, and Fructus Lycii.

To replenish qi *and promote blood regeneration* (补气生血 *bu qi sheng xue*): Since *qi* promote blood regeneration and is known as the "commander of blood," drugs that replenish *qi* are also indicated for blood deficiency. Examples: Radix Ginseng, Radix Codonopsis Pilosulae, and Radix Astragali.

Yin

To replenish yin (补阴 *bu yin*): Also known as "nourishing *yin*" (养阴 *yang yin* or 滋阴 *zi yin*). Most drugs that replenish *yin* are sweet and cold, and are indicated for various kinds of *yin* deficiency syndrome. Replenishing *yin* involves replenishing lung, heart, stomach, liver and kidney yin.

To replenish lung yin (补肺阴 *bu fei yin*): Also known as "nourishing lung *yin*" (养肺阴 *yang fei yin*). Drugs that replenish lung *yin* are sweet and cold. They are indicated for lung *yin* deficiency marked by cough with little sputum or difficult expectoration, or blood-tinged sputum, dry throat and hoarse voice. Examples: Radix Adenophorae, Radix Glehniae, Radix Ophiopogonis, and Rhizoma Polygonati Odorati.

To replenish stomach yin (补胃阴 *bu wei yin*): Also called "nourishing stomach *yin*" (养胃阴 *yang wei yin*). Drugs that replenish stomach *yin* are sweet and cold. They are indicated for stomach *yin* insufficiency marked by thirst, polydipsia, epigastric pain, retching, and dry and red or uncoated tongue. Examples: Herba Dendrobii, Radix Ophiopogonis, and Rhizoma Polygonati Odorati.

To replenish heart yin (补心阴 *bu xin yin*): Also called "nourishing heart *yin*" (养心阴 *yang xin yin*). Drugs that replenish heart *yin* are sweet and cold. They are indicated for heart *yin* deficiency marked by palpitation, restlessness and insomnia. Examples: Radix Ophiopogonis, and Rhizoma Polygonati Odorati.

To replenish liver yin (补肝阴 *bu gan yin*): Also called "nourishing liver *yin*" (养肝阴 *yang gan yin*). Drugs that replenish liver *yin* are cold or slightly warm. They are indicated for liver *yin* deficiency marked by hypochondriac pain, dizziness and blurred vision. Examples: Fructus Lycii, Fructus Corni, and Radix Paeoniae Alba.

To replenish kidney yin (补肾阴 *bu shen yin*): Also called "nourishing kidney *yin*" (滋肾阴 *zi shen yin*). Drugs that replenish kidney *yin* are sweet, salty, cold or slightly warm. They are indicated for kidney *yin* insufficiency marked by lumbago, seminal emission, blurred vision and tinnitus, or for *yin* deficiency leading to hyperactive *yang* marked by hectic fever. Examples: Radix Rehmanniae, Radix Rehmanniae Preparata, Plastrum Testudinis, and Fructus Ligustri Lucidi.

To nourish yin *and suppress fire* (滋阴降火 *zi yin jiang huo*): To nourish *yin* fluid and suppress deficiency fire. Most drugs that nourish *yin* and suppress fire are sweet and cold, though a few are bitter and cold. They are indicated for *yin* deficiency leading to hyperactive fire marked by hectic fever, seminal emission and night sweating. Examples: Radix Rehmanniae, Radix Scrophulariae, and Rhizoma Anemarrhenae.

Yang

To pacify yang (潜阳 *qian yang*): To pacify liver *yang*, an abbreviation for easing the liver and pacifying *yang*. Most drugs that pacify *yang* are minerals and animal shells (especially those of mollusks). They are indicated for dizziness and headache caused by hyperactive liver *yang*. Examples: Os Draconis, Magnetitum, Haematitum, Concha Haliotidis, and Concha Margaritifera Usta. Plastrum Testudinis and Carapax Trionycis nourish *yin* in order to pacify *yang* and are used when liver and kidney *yin* deficiency leads to hyperactive *yang*.

To lift yang (升阳 sheng *yang*): To lift the *yang qi* of the middle *jiao*, also called "lifting *yang* and collapsed *qi*" (升阳举陷 *sheng yang ju xian*) or "lifting middle *jiao qi*" (升举中气 *sheng ju zhong qi*). Drugs that lift *yang* are indicated for collapse of middle *jiao qi* marked by rectal prolapse, hysteroptosis or gastroptosis. Examples: Radix Bupleuri, Rhizoma Cimicifugae, and Radix Astragali.

Remarks: Pacifying yang and lifting *yang* are contrary to each other. The former lowers the upward disturbance of hyperactive liver *yang*, while the latter lifts the collapsed *yang qi* of the middle *jiao*.

To activate yang (通阳 *tong yang*): To warm and activate *yang qi*. Pathogenic cold and phlegm and fluid retention may obstruct the circulation of *yang qi* and affect the *qi* passages. Drugs that activate *yang qi* are acrid and warm, and can eliminate pathogenic cold, disperse phlegm and fluid, and promote *qi* circulation. They are indicated for cases with retained phlegm and fluid in the lung and stomach, dysuria, and stuffiness and pain in the chest. Examples: Ramulus Cinnamomi, and Bulbus Allii Macrostemi.

To warm yang (温阳 *wen yang*): To dispel pathogenic cold and support *yang qi*, also called "supporting *yang*" (助阳 *zhu yang*). Drugs that warm *yang* are acrid and hot, and are indicated for *yang* deficiency syndrome. They include drugs that warm heart, spleen and kidney *yang*. To warm heart *yang* (温心阳 *wen xin yang*): Drugs that warm heart *yang* are acrid and hot. They are indicated for weak heart *yang* marked by palpitation, shortness of breath, chest pain, pallor, cyanosis of the lips, cold limbs and aversion to cold. Example: Radix Aconiti Lateralis Preparata.

To warm spleen yang (温脾阳 *wen pi yang*): Drugs that warm spleen *yang* are acrid and hot. They are indicated for weak spleen *yang* marked by abdominal pain, diarrhea, cold limbs and feeble pulse. Examples: Rhizoma Zingiberis, and Radix Aconiti Lateralis Preparata.

To warm kidney yang (温肾阳 *wen shen yang*): Also known as "nourishing kidney fire" (补肾火 *bu shen huo*) or "strengthening fire of the gate of life" (补命门火 *bu ming men huo*). Drugs that warm kidney *yang* are acrid and hot. They are indicated for weak kidney *yang* marked by coldness and pain in the lower back and knees, frequent urination or dysuria, and edema. Examples: Radix Aconiti Lateralis Preparata, and Cortex Cinnamomi.

To nourish kidney yang (补肾阳 *bu shen yang*): Drugs that nourish kidney *yang* are sweet, salty or pungent, and warm, and can nourish kidney *yang*, replenish the kidney essence and blood, and strengthen the lumbar region and knees. They are indicated for kidney *yang* deficiency marked by impotence and infertility. Examples: Cornu Cervi Pantotrichum, Herba Cistanches, Radix Morindae Officinalis, Cortex Eucommiae, and Herba Epimedii.

To strengthen yang (壮阳 *zhuang yang*): To strengthen the sexual function. Drugs that strengthen *yang* can nourish kidney *yang* and promote sexuality. They are indicated for impotence resulting from kidney *yang* insufficiency. Examples: Cornu Cervi Pantotrichum, Herba Cistanches, Semen Morindae Officinalis, and Herba Epimedii.

To restore yang *and prevent collapse* (回阳救逆 *hui yang jiu ni*): Also called *hui yang*. Drugs that restore *yang* and prevent collapse are acrid and hot. They are indicated for *yang* depletion with profuse sweating, cold limbs and feeble pulse. Examples: Radix Aconiti Lateralis Preparata, and Rhizoma Zingiberis.

To conduct fire back to its origin (引火归原 *yin huo gui yuan*): If the fire of the life gate is weak, *yang qi* will float up (known as floating *yang* or floating fire). Drugs that warm kidney *yang* can conduct deficiency fire back to the kidney. For instance, Cortex Cinnamomi and Radix Aconiti Lateralis Preparata can do so by warming kidney *yang*, and are indicated for cases with heat in the upper portion of the body and cold in the lower due to excessive *yin* leading to floating *yang*, manifested as a feverish sensation in the face, flushed cheeks, sore throat, coldness in the lower limbs, thready and weak pulse.

Others

To purge and remove intestinal stasis (泻下攻积 *xie xia gong ji*): Most drugs that purge and remove intestinal stasis are bitter and cold. They are indicated for constipation due to accumulated heat. Examples: Radix et Rhizoma Rhei, Natrii Sulfas, Aloe, and Folium Sennae; these are known as cold purgatives. Others, such as Fructus Crotonis, can effectively remove cold stasis and are known as warm purgatives.

To promote digestion (消食 *xiao shi*): Drugs that promote digestion can remove food stasis and improve appetite. They are indicated for food stasis and dyspepsia due to weakness of the spleen and stomach. Examples: Fructus Crataegi, Endothelium Corneum Gigeriae Galli, Massa Fermentata Medicinalis, Fructus Oryzae Germinatus, Fructus Hordei Germinatus, Semen Raphani, Semen Arecae, Fructus Aurantii Immaturus, and Semen Pharbitidis.

To expel parasites (驱虫 *qu chong*): To expel and destroy such intestinal parasites as roundworm, hookworm, pinworm, tapeworm and fasciolopsis. Drugs for this purpose are known as anthelmintics. Examples: Fructus Quisqualis, Cortex Meliae, Semen Arecae,

Semen Cucurbitae, Omphalia, and Gemma Agrimoniae.

To kill parasites (杀虫 *sha chong*): This has three aspects: (1) To expel and kill intestinal parasites, as do anthelmintics. (2) To kill parasites in the skin, such as ringworm and mite. Drugs for this purpose are indicated for scabies and tinea infection. Examples: Sulfur, Realgar, Calomels, Fructus Cnidii, and Radix Sophorae Flavescentis. (3) To kill trichomonad. These drugs are indicated for trichomonas vaginitis. Examples: Fructus Cnidii, Gemma Agrimoniae, and Radix Sophorae Flavescentis.

To pacify roundworms (安蛔 *an hui*): "Worms are often pacified by sour drugs." Irritated roundworms can be pacified by Fructus Mume, which is sour, thus relieving the acute abdominal pain. This is often used in biliary ascariasis.

To astringe (收涩 *shou se*): Astringents are mostly sour, and can arrest excessive flow of body fluid and *qi* and check abnormal seminal emission. They are used to treat syndromes due to overconsumption and loss of fluid, *qi* and essence. They check sweating, astringe lung *qi* to stop cough, astringe the large intestine to stop diarrhea, astringe essence to relieve seminal emission, relieve leukorrhagia and check exudation of sores.

To check sweating (止汗 *zhi han*): Drugs that check sweating are known as antihydrotics. They are indicated for spontaneous and night sweating due to weak constitution. Examples: Os Draconis, Concha Ostreae, Fructus Schisandrae, Fructus Tritici Levis (light), and Radix Oryzae Glutinosae.

To astringe lung qi *to stop cough* (敛肺止咳 *lian fei zhi ke*): Such drugs are usually sour and astringent. They are indicated for protracted cough due to lung deficiency. Examples: Fructus Schisandrae, Fructus Mume, and Fructus Chebulae.

To astringe the large intestine to stop diarrhea (涩肠止泻 *se chang zhi xie*): Such drugs are mostly sour and astringent. They are indicated for protracted diarrhea and dysentery or patients with involuntary fecal discharge. Examples: Fructus Schisandrae, Fructus Mume, Fructus Chebulae, Halloysitum Rubrum, Semen Myristicae, and Pericarpium Granati.

To astringe essence and reduce urination (涩精缩尿 *se jing suo niao*): These drugs check abnormal seminal emission, nocturnal enuresis and incontinent urine due to kidney deficiency. Most are sour and astringent. Examples: Fructus Rosae Laevigatae, Semen Euryales, Os Draconis, and Concha Ostreae.

To astringe sores (敛疮 *lian chuang*): Drugs that astringe sores promote the granulation and healing of skin lesions. They are indicated for ruptured and unhealed sores. Examples: Os Draconis, and Os Sepiae.

To relieve spasm and pain (缓急 *huan ji*): Sweet drugs relieve acute pain and spasms, and also moderate the potency of other drugs. They are indicated for epigastric and abdominal pain due to deficiency of the middle *jiao* and spasmodic pain of the calf. Examples: Radix Glycyrrhizae, Fructus Jujubae, and Mel.

To soften the liver (柔肝 *rou gan*): The liver is a *zang* organ characterized by hardness, and should be well nourished by *yin* and blood. When liver *yin* and blood are well nourished, the liver *qi* is softened or harmonized. Drugs that soften the liver (*qi*) are indicated for cases of long-standing liver *qi* stagnation, damage to *yin* and blood, and undernourishment of the liver marked by hypochondriac distensive pain, dryness in the mouth, and red tongue with little coating. Examples: Radix Paeoniae Alba, and Fructus Lycii.

To open orifice (开窍 *kai qiao*): Drugs that open orifice are acrid, warm and aromatic, characterized by their motive and dispersive actions, and can restore consciousness. They are indicated for loss of consciousness seen in febrile diseases, and apoplexy. Examples: Moschus, Borneolum Syntheticum, Calculus Bovis, and Rhizoma Acori Graminei.

To remove nasal obstruction (通窍 *tong qiao*): Most drugs for this purpose are acrid and warm, and can remove nasal obstruction. They are indicated for chronic sinusitis and nasosinusitis. Examples: Herba Asari, Radix Angelicae Dahuricae, Flos Magnoliae, Fructus Xanthii. Herba Asari ground into powder for nasal insufflation induces sneezing, and is also used for this purpose.

BOOK TWO

SCIENCE OF TRADITIONAL CHINESE PRESCRIPTION

Written by: Li Fei, Sun Meizhen, Hui Jiyuan, Zhang Haoliang, Zuo Yanfu, Liu Xuehua and Chao Yinci

Translated by: Li Yanwen, Huang Yuezhong and Chen Xianqing

Edited by: Ou Ming

CONTENTS

INTRODUCTION

Science of Traditional Chinese Prescription deals with the theory and method of forming prescriptions and their clinical application. It is an important part of the theoretical system of traditional Chinese medicine, as well a basic course in the study of traditional Chinese medicine.

A prescription, which consists of necessary drugs in appropriate amounts, is made up in accordance with syndrome differentiation and on the basis of principles unique to traditional Chinese medicine. The application of such prescriptions can be traced back to primitive society, when our ancestors began to know how to use natural drugs to treat and protect themselves against diseases. At the outset, only one herb was used in a dose. But through long years of clinical practice, they gradually came to understand that mutually compatible drugs could be used together with better results, and various prescriptions were then formed and used more effectively.

Recorded in *Prescriptions for Fifty-Two Kinds of Diseases* (unearthed from the No. 3 Han Dynasty Tomb at Mawangdui, Changsha, Hunan Province in 1973) are nameless rough prescriptions composed of a few herbs. It is the extant oldest dispensatory in China. *The Inner Canon of the Yellow Emperor*, written in the Spring and Autumn Period as well as the Warring States Period (770-221 B. C.), summarized the theories and principles for syndrome differentiation, treatment, and the composition and compatibility of ingredients in a prescription. *Treatise on Cold Diseases and Miscellaneous Disorders*, written by Zhang Zhongjing in the Eastern Han Dynasty (A. D. 25-220), is considered the classical dispensatory, which creatively brings together syndrome differentiation, treatment, prescription and drugs used in treating a disease, laying the foundation for the formation and development of the science of traditional Chinese prescription.

This science underwent rapid development up to the Jin and Tang dynasties, when books dealing herbal prescriptions appeared one after another. Among them were *Handbook of Prescriptions for Emergencies*, written by Ge Hong in the Jin Dynasty, in which proved recipes and inexpensive prescriptions popular among the people were collected; *Essentially Treasured Prescriptions for Emergencies* and *Supplement to Essentially Treasured Prescriptions* by Sun Simiao, and *Clandestine Essentials from the Imperial Library* by Wang Tao in the Tang Dynasty. These books collected valuable prescriptions not only from successive dynasties but also from abroad; they made it possible for the prescriptions of many well-known physicians in the Han and Tang dynasties to be handed down. Today they are still valuable reference materials for the study of medical prescriptions before the Tang Dynasty.

Well-known prescription books appeared in the Song Dynasty, including *Imperial Benevolent Prescriptions of the Taiping Period* and *Imperial Medical Encyclopedia*. In the former, 16,834 prescriptions were recorded; in the latter, about 20,000. Both books incorporated valuable prescriptions used before the Song Dynasty. Also popular was *Benevolent Prescriptions from the Pharmaceutical Bureau of the Taiping Period*, a pharmacopoeia of herbal medicines first compiled in China under the auspices of the imperial court with slightly fewer than 800 prescriptions. But the prescriptions recorded were collected from all over the country; they were tested and verified by the then Bureau of Imperial Physicians, thus serving as the basis for the preparation of ready-made herbal medicines. Besides, there were Qian Yi's *Medical Elucidation of Pediatrics*, Chen Yan's *Treatise on the Tripartite Pathogenesis of Diseases*, and Yan Yonghe's *Prescriptions of Life Saving*. All the recipes recorded in these three books were practical and effective, and are still widely used today.

The four eminent physicians in the Jin and Yuan dynasties and the school of epidemic febrile diseases in the Ming and Qing dynasties all made great contributions to the progress of the science of traditional Chinese prescription. The chapter "Prescriptions" in *Concise Exposition on Cold Diseases*, written by Cheng Wuji in the Jin Dynasty, is the first monograph dealing with the compatibility of herbal drugs in a prescription, which analyzes and studies the principles developed by Zhang Zhongjing in forming a prescription in line with the principles recorded in *The Inner Canon of the Yellow Emperor*. *Study on Prescriptions*, written by Wu Kun in the Ming Dynasty, expounds in depth the various aspects of composing a prescription, such as its nomenclature, composition, effects, indications, explanation, modifications, and contraindications, and has become a valuable reference book for studying the theory of prescription. Recording 61,739 prescriptions, *Prescriptions of Universal Benevolence*, compiled by Zhu Su in the Ming Dynasty, is a collection of valuable prescriptions popular before the Ming Dynasty. There are also quite a few medical works describing effective prescriptions from the perspective of treatment, the origin or the effect, and they include Zhang Jingyue's *A New Book of Eight Principles for Herbal Prescription*, Xu Dachun's *Classification of Prescriptions of Treatise on Cold Diseases*, Wang Ang's *Variorum of Prescriptions* and Zhang Bingcheng's *A Concise Book of Established Prescriptions*, all of which are still important literature for the study of the science of traditional Chinese prescription. In addition, Wang Ang's *Verses of Classified Common Recipes*, in which the names of the ingredient drugs, the effects and the indications of prescriptions are written into a poem with seven characters to a line, is concise and comprehensive. It has therefore been widely transmitted from generation to generation.

Since 1949, the science of traditional Chinese prescription has witnessed new development. Not only have many new effective prescriptions been produced, but the therapeutic mechanism of ancient prescriptions has been studied in depth. Moreover, a series of textbooks and monographs have been compiled and published, laying down a sound foundation for further development in this field.

In studying the science of traditional Chinese prescription, it is important to memorize a certain number of commonly used prescriptions. It is more important, however, to acquire sufficient understanding of the principles governing the composition of the prescriptions as well as other related theories before trying to recite them. Only in this way can one use the right prescription for the right disease.

CHAPTER ONE

PRESCRIPTION AND THERAPEUTIC PRINCIPLES

Prescription is one of the four important aspects (theory, therapeutic principle, prescription and drugs) of traditional Chinese medicine. It is established on the basis of the differentiation of syndromes. In order to learn the theory and method for composing a prescription, it is important, first of all, to understand the relation between the prescription and therapeutic principles.

In the formation and development of traditional Chinese medicine, therapeutic principles were generalized on the basis of an accumulation of clinical experience gained in long years of medical practice. So, prescriptions appeared before the summarization of therapeutic principles. When the latter were crystalized into basic theory, it, in turn, served as guiding principles for the composition and application of prescriptions. Take the treatment of common cold, for example. If the disease is determined as the exterior heat syndrome caused by an attack of wind-heat through a comprehensive analysis of the data obtained from the application of the four diagnostic methods and a differentiation of syndromes, it would be treated by expelling the pathogenic factors from the surface with acrid and cool drugs. Proceeding from this principle, the physician selects the appropriately established prescription and modifies it according to the particular case. This indicates that the prescription is the expression of the therapeutic principles in clinical practice and the principles serve as the theoretical basis for the prescription of drugs. In clinical practice, eight therapeutic methods are commonly used:

1. **Diaphoretic therapy** (*han fa*): This is a method to expel pathogenic factors from the superficial portion of the body by inducing perspiration, which is used for cases at the onset of the exterior syndrome caused by an attack of exogenous pathogens, as well as for measles with inadequate eruption, edema in the upper part of the body, the initial stage of skin infections, or cases in which the pathogenic factor should be dispelled from the interior to the exterior. However, as the conditions for each individual case are different, the diaphoretic prescription may be composed of acrid drugs with a warm nature or acrid drugs with a cold nature. Furthermore, the diaphoretic method can also be combined with other methods, such as the heat-purging; purgative, warming, and tonic ones.

2. **Emetic therapy** (*tu fa*): This uses emetics or physical stimulation to induce vomiting in order to eliminate retained phlegm, undigested food or toxin from the throat, esophagus or stomach. However, this therapy is liable to damage stomach *qi*. It is chiefly used for cases in which pathogenic factors are predominant, or acute and serious cases. Besides, it should be used with great care for senile and debilitated persons and pregnant

women.

3. **Purgative therapy** (*xia fa*): This method is for releasing dry stool, eliminating excessive endogenous heat, undigested food, accumulated cold and fluid through the application of purgatives. It is indicated for cases of interior-excess syndrome, including the retention of dry stool, phlegm, food and fluid due to pathogenic factors in the stomach and intestine. Since the severity and nature of the diseases, the associated etiological factors and the body resistance of the patients vary, the prescriptions may be composed of cold-natured, warm-natured, lubricant or potent purgatives. It can also be combined with tonic and other therapies.

4. **Regulative therapy** (*he fa*): This means to regulate the functions of the internal organs to eliminate pathogenic factors. It is indicated for Shaoyang diseases in which the pathogenic factors stay between the exterior and the interior. As stated in *Concise Exposition on Cold Diseases*, for exogenous pathogen in the exterior, the diaphoretic therapy should be used, while for exogenous pathogen in the interior, the purgative therapy should be used. But, for a case in which the pathogen is neither in the interior nor in the exterior but between them, neither the diaphoretic nor the emetic and purgative method is applicable; here the regulative therapy is recommended. This is also indicated for cases of disharmony between the internal organs and cases of imbalance between *qi* and blood, cases of mixed cold and heat syndromes, or cases of mixed deficiency and excess syndromes. In clinical practice, the prescriptions for regulative therapy vary for different diseases, such as regulative prescriptions for regulating Shaoyang, those for regulating the liver and spleen, and those for regulating the gastrointestines.

5. **Warming therapy** (*wen fa*): This therapy expels cold, restores *yang-qi*, activates the meridians and promotes blood circulation. It is indicated for interior-cold syndrome. In terms of etiology, this syndrome may be caused by a direct attack of cold, damage of *yang-qi* due to erroneous treatment, or endogenous cold due to deficient *yang-qi*. In terms of location, the interior-cold syndrome may be in the viscera or the meridians. So, the warming therapy may be modified for different cases: to expel cold by warming the middle *jiao*, recuperate depleted *yang*, rescue the patient from collapse, or expel cold by warming the meridians. In addition, an interior-cold syndrome is often complicated by *yang-qi* deficiency, thus warming therapy is often used together with tonic therapy.

6. **Heat-purging therapy** (*qing fa*): This means purging heat with cold or cool drugs. It is applicable to interior-heat syndrome. Clinically, the interior-heat syndrome is divided into different types: heat residing in *qifen*, in *yingfen*, in *xuefen* and in the viscera, and excessive heat that produces toxins. Accordingly, the heat-purging therapy is modified to achieve different results, such as purging heat from *qifen*, purging heat from *yingfen* and cooling the blood, purging heat from both *qifen* and *xuefen*, purging heat and toxins, purging summer-heat, and purging heat from the viscera. It is used for a wide range of diseases, particularly seasonal febrile diseases. In the later stage of a seasonal febrile disease, if *yin* is damaged by excessive heat, or becomes deficient after prolonged illness and produces hectic fever, the heat-purging therapy is used together with the *yin*-invigorating therapy.

7. **Resolving therapy** (*xiao fa*): This therapy removes *qi* stagnation, blood stasis,

phlegm retention, dampness retention, undigested food, and parasitic infestation. In a broad sense, elimination of phlegm and dampness, regulation of *qi*, regulation of blood circulation and removal of parasites are all covered by this therapy. In a narrow sense, however, it refers to relieving dyspepsia and abdominal mass due to *qi* and blood stagnation. Clinically, this therapy is often used together with the tonic or the purgative therapy.

8. **Tonic therapy** (*bu fa*): This is to invigorate *qi*, blood, *yin* and *yang* with tonic drugs so as to correct the dysfunction of the viscera or *qi*, blood, *yin* and *yang*. It is indicated for various types of deficiency syndromes when no apparent pathogenic factors exist. When the resistance is weakened and incapable of eliminating the pathogens, this therapy can be used either individually or in combination with other therapeutic methods to strengthen the antipathogenic *qi* and expel the pathogens. It is used variously to invigorate *qi*, blood, *yin* or *yang*, and to strengthen the heart, liver, spleen, lung and kidney. Moreover, it is divided into drastic and mild types. Besides, based on the theory of mutual promotion between the five elements, indirect tonic therapies were invented, such as invigorating the spleen (earth) to strengthen the lung (metal), and strengthening the kidney (water) to nourish the liver (wood).

Except for emetic therapy, the other seven methods are frequently used in clinical practice. In complicated cases, two or more are often used together to achieve the desired results. Nevertheless, all the eight therapeutic methods should be used flexibly in accordance with the specific conditions of individual cases.

CHAPTER TWO
THE CLASSIFICATION OF PRESCRIPTIONS

There are many ways to classify the prescriptions of traditional Chinese medicine; the major ones include the "seven prescriptions" theory, the "ten prescriptions" theory, the theories to classify prescriptions according to syndromes, *zang-fu* organs, therapeutic principles, etiology, and therapeutic effects.

The "seven prescriptions" (*qi fang*) theory originates in *The Inner Canon of the Yellow Emperor*. It is a method of classifying prescriptions according to the severity, location and cause of diseases, the odd or even number of drugs included in the prescriptions, the virulence of pathogens and the physical conditions of the patients. Based on this theory, the prescriptions are grouped under seven categories, namely, large, small, mild, potent, odd-numbered, even-numbered and compound. The "large" prescriptions refer to those which are composed of a large number of drugs in large quantities and which are used to treat diseases due to virulent pathogens. The "small" prescriptions refer to those composed of a small number of drugs in small quantities and applied for diseases due to less virulent pathogens. The "mild" prescriptions are those composed of drugs with mild action and a light flavor and which are indicated for chronic and debilitating diseases and for prolonged application. The "potent" prescriptions are those composed of drugs with potent action and a strong flavor and applied to treat acute and serious diseases. The "odd-numbered" prescriptions refer to those composed of a single drug or drugs in odd numbers, while the "even-numbered" prescriptions are those composed of two drugs or drugs in even numbers. The "compound" prescriptions refer to those composed of two or more different prescriptions and applied for diseases with complications.

The "ten prescriptions" (*shi ji*) theory, first appeared in *A Supplement to Collection on Herbalism* by Chen Zangqi of the Tang Dynasty, is to classify prescriptions based on their actions. *Daguan Herbalism* quoted from *A Supplement to Collection on Herbalism* said that the Chinese medicinal herbs had ten actions, i. e. , releasing, obstruction removing, tonic, purgative, mild, potent, astringent, lubricant, drying and moistening. These actions of Chinese herbal drugs were used to classify prescriptions in *Discussion on Canon of Medicine* by Zhao Ji in the Song Dynasty and *Preface to Concise Exposition on Cold Diseases* by Cheng Wuji in the Jin Dynasty. However, the "ten prescriptions" theory could not generalize all commonly used prescriptions, and so cold, hot, lifting and lowering prescriptions were added later, forming the theory of "fourteen prescriptions." In the Ming Dynasty, Xu Sihe, in his *Complete Medical Works*, added to the original ten fourteen more categories, i. e. , regulating, harmonizing, relieving, promoting, cold, warm, summer-heat, fire, appeasing, capturing, calming, alleviating, bland and clear, forming the theory of "twenty-four prescriptions."

The classification of prescriptions according to syndromes was first proposed in the *Prescriptions for Fifty-two Kinds of Diseases*. Other representative works in this field include *Clandestine Essentials from the Imperial Library* written in the Tang Dynasty, *Imperial Benevolent Prescriptions of the Taiping Period* written in the Song Dynasty, *Prescriptions of Universal Benevolence* and *Study on Prescriptions* appeared in the Ming Dynasty, and *Lantai's Collection of Typical Prescriptions* written in the Qing Dynasty.

The classification of prescriptions according to different *zang-fu* organs was embodied in many medical books, including *Essentially Treasured Prescriptions for Emergencies* written in the Tang Dynasty and *Treatise on the Tripartite Pathogenesis of Diseases* written in the Song Dynasty.

The most representative work to classify prescriptions on the basis of therapeutic principles is *A Complete Collection of Jingyue's Treatises* compiled in the Ming Dynasty. In the book, Zhang Jingyue summarized all prescriptions into eight groups, namely, consolidating, harmonizing, assaulting, dissipating, cooling, heating, astringent and corresponding ones. It also stated that the consolidating prescriptions are used to remedy the deficiency, the harmonizing prescriptions are used to adjust the imbalance, the assaulting prescriptions expel the excessive pathogenic factors, the dissipating ones relieve the exterior syndrome, the cooling ones eliminate fire and heat, the heating ones expel cold, the astringent ones keep essence and body fluid, and the corresponding ones relieve syndromes accordingly. However, as the eight groups could not cover and summarize all prescriptions, the book also separately listed prescriptions for women, for children, for eruptive diseases and for surgical diseases. Although Cheng Zhongling mentioned in *Insights into Medicine* that the prescriptions can be summarized in line with the eight therapeutic principles (diaphoretic, harmonizing, purgative, digestive, emetic, heat-purging, warming and invigorating), what he did was just to give some examples.

Based on the different actions of the prescriptions, Wang Ang of the Qing Dynasty classified in his work *Variorum of Prescriptions* all prescriptions into 22 categories, i. e., invigorating, diaphoretic, emetic, internal pathogen eliminating, interior reinforcing, reconciling, *qi* regulating, blood regulating, wind expelling, cold expelling, summer-heat eliminating, dampness removing, moistening, pathogenic fire purging, phlegm eliminating, food retention removing, astringing, parasiticide, vision improving, skin infection treatment, as well as prescriptions for gynopathy and for emergencies. This principle for prescription classification is concise and easily applicable in clinical practice. It has been modeled by Wu Yiluo in his *Practical Conventional Prescriptions* and Zhang Bingcheng in his *Prescriptions in Verse*.

For the convenience of study and application, this book classifies the prescriptions into sixteen categories in line with their different actions; some of the prescriptions are further classified into subgroups.

CHAPTER THREE
COMPOSITION OF A PRESCRIPTION

In terms of development, a prescription was, at the beginning, composed of only one drug and later composed of two or more. Some prescriptions gradually became established ones for special diseases, and later they were further modified and improved in clinical practice according to differentiation of syndromes.

Different drugs possess different properties; each has its own special effects and deficiencies. There is a saying in traditional Chinese medicine, "An individual drug possesses its own special effect, while a prescription exerts a miraculous cure by putting different drugs together." So, a prescription is composed of drugs carefully selected in line with their compatibility. The purposes of composing a prescription are: 1) to enhance the therapeutic effects of individual drugs by promoting their synergism, or to enable the drugs to produce a new therapeutic result by changing their original properties; 2) to select drugs according to the differentiation of syndromes to cure complicated cases in an overall way; and 3) to inhibit the adverse effects of some potent drugs or to counteract the toxicity of poisonous ones. Therefore, drugs selected for a prescription should not only supplement but also suppress one another. Only in this way can the advantages of a prescription be brought into play.

1. The Principle for Composing a Prescription

A prescription should be made in line with the correct diagnosis based on the differentiation of syndromes and the drugs to be included in the prescription must be selected in accordance with the principle governing the composition of prescriptions. The principle for the composition of prescriptions was first recorded in *The Inner Canon of the Yellow Emperor* and further developed and improved through clinical practice in the succeeding ages. The principle stipulates that a prescription should include four different kinds of drugs, referred to as the chief (*jun* 君), adjuvant (*chen* 臣), assistant (*zuo* 佐) and guide (*shi* 使), according to the different roles they play in the prescription.

Chief drug (*jun yao*): Being essential in a prescription, it aims at dealing with the cause and the chief symptoms of a disease, and plays the principal curative role.

Adjuvant drug (*chen yao*): It helps strengthen the curative action of the chief drug.

Assistant drug (*zuo yao*): It refers to: 1) the ingredient for treating the accompanying disease (diseases) or syndrome (syndromes); 2) the ingredient to counter the potent effects or toxicity of the chief and adjuvant drugs; and 3) the ingredient to counteract the action of the chief ingredient but play a supporting role in the treatment.

Guide drug (*shi yao*): It refers to: 1) the ingredient leading the effects of other drugs to the diseased part; and 2) the ingredient to balance the action of other drugs in the prescription.

In a prescription, the four kinds of drugs are determined in accordance with the action of the drugs selected. As for the composition, whether they should all be included or how many ingredients should be used depend on the condition of the disease, the therapeutic needs and the action of drugs selected. Generally speaking, the chief drug is indispensable. In a simple prescription, it is not necessary to have them all included. In some prescriptions, the chief drug or the adjuvant drug itself possesses the action of the assistant or the guide drug, and therefore it is not necessary to include other drugs as the assistant and guide ingredients.

Basic Questions says, "A prescription composed of one chief drug and two adjuvant drugs is called a mild prescription; one composed of one chief drug and three adjuvant drugs and five assistant drugs is called a moderate prescription; and one composed of one chief drug, three adjuvant drugs and nine assistant drugs is called a strong prescription." But in clinical application, this is not necessarily the case. In general, fewer drugs are used as chief ingredients than as adjuvant and assistant ones. No matter what drug is used as the chief ingredient, its dosage should be larger than all each ingredients.

To show the application of the principle for composing a prescription, let's take Decoction of Ephedrae for example.

The Decoction of Ephedrae, which originates in *Treatise on Cold Diseases*, is used to relieve exterior syndromes by means of diaphoresis, and facilitating the flow of lung *qi* to relieve asthma. It is indicated for exterior-excess syndromes due to exposure to cold, with such symptoms as chills, fever, headache, general achiness, anhidrosis, asthma, thin and white tongue coating and superficial tense pulse. The composition of Decoction of Ephedrae is as following:

Chief drug—Herba Ephedrae: tastes acrid and is warm in nature; used to treat exterior syndromes by means of diaphoresis, and relieving the inhibited flow of lung *qi* and asthma.

Adjuvant—Ramulus Cinnamomi: tastes acrid and sweet, and is warm in nature; helps Herba Ephedrae induce sweating to expel pathogenic factors from the exterior, warms the meridians and regulates *yingfen* and *weifen* to relieve pain.

Assistant—Semen Armeniacae Amarum: tastes bitter and is warm in nature; suppresses the adversely upward flow of lung *qi* to help Herba Ephedrae in relieving asthma, dispel wind-cold to help Herba Ephedrae and Ramulus Cinnamomi in expelling pathogenic factors in the exterior.

Guide—Radix Glycyrrhizae Preparata: tastes sweet and is warm in nature; coordinates the actions of the chief, adjuvant and assistant drugs.

2. Modification of an Established Prescription

In writing out a prescription, apart from following the above-mentioned principle, some other factors, such as the state of the disease, the constitution, age and sex of the patient and the climatic and geographical conditions, should also be considered and modifications should be made accordingly. In other words, it is necessary to follow the principle but not adhere to the originally established prescription mechanically. In general, prescriptions are modified in three ways:

(1) Modification of the Number of Drugs

By increasing or decreasing the number of drugs in an established prescription, a new one is formed and the compatibility of the drugs is changed, leading to changes in therapeutic effects. For instance, Decoction of Ephedrae, composed of Herba Ephedrae, Ramulus Cinnamomi, Semen Armeniacae Amarum and Radix Glycyrrhizae Preparata, is developed to treat exterior-excess syndrome caused by exposure to cold; its chief action is to induce perspiration and expel the pathogen from the exterior. But for cases due to exposure to wind-cold characterized by dysfunction of lung *qi*, with the symptoms of stuffy nose, hoarse voice, productive cough, full sensation in the chest and even shortness of breath, white tongue coating and superficial pulse, it should be treated by means of releasing the inhibited lung *qi* and expelling cold. The prescription recommended for this case is the Three Crude Drugs Decoction, which is a modification of the Decoction of Ephedrae through the removal of Ramulus Cinnamomi. For a case due to exposure to wind-cold with accompanying *qi* stagnation and phlegm retention, which produces the same symptoms as the previous case in addition to asthma, difficult expectoration, and more serious full sensation in the chest, it should be treated by not only releasing the inhibited lung *qi* and expelling cold, but also by regulating the flow of *qi* and resolving phlegm. In this case, another prescription modified on the basis of the Decoction of Ephedrae, called *Huagai* Powder, is recommended. It is composed of all the ingredients of the Decoction of Ephedrae except the removal of Ramulus Cinnamomi and the addition of Fructus Perillae, Pericarpium Citri Reticulatae, Poria Rubra and Cortex Mori Radicis Preparata.

The modification of an established prescription by means of increasing or decreasing the number of drugs may or may not change the action of the original prescription. The two modified prescriptions mentioned above—the Three Crude Drugs Decoction and the *Huagai* Powder—are both based on the Decoction of Ephedrae, with some ingredients removed or added. Yet, they are still prescriptions for relieving the exterior syndrome with acrid and warm drugs. There is no change in nature. Then, let us make a comparison between the Decoction of Ephedrae and the Decoction of Ephedrae, Armeniacae Amarum, Glycyrrhizae and Gypsum Fibrosum. In the former, Herba Ephedrae is the chief ingredient with Ramulus Cinnamomi serving as the adjuvant ingredient, and its action is to induce perspiration and expel the pathogen from the exterior; while in the latter, Herba Ephedrae is the chief drug with Gypsum Fibrosum as the adjuvant, and its action is to purge heat from the lung and relieve asthma. The former is a prescription for expelling the pathogenic factors from the exterior with acrid and warm drugs, while the latter is a prescription for expelling pathogenic factors from the exterior with acrid and cool drugs. The two are different in nature and produce different actions. In this case, the modification made to the established prescription brings about a change in nature.

(2) Modification of the Quantity of the Ingredients

This means to alter the compatibility between the ingredients of an established prescription by changing their quantities, thus changing its action and indications. Table 1 and Table 2 are a comparison between two prescriptions, which have the same ingredients but in different quantities.

Table 1. Comparison of Decoction for Treating *Yang* Exhaustion and Decoction of Dredging Meridians for Cold Extremities

Prescription	Ingredient			Action	Indication
	Radix Aconiti Lateralis	Rhizoma Zingiberis	Radix Glycyrrhizae Preparata		
Decoction for Treating *Yang* Exhaustion	1 piece	1.5 *liang*	2 *liang*	recuperating the depleted *yang* and rescuing the patient from danger	cold limbs due to dominant *yin* and deficient *yang*, chilliness with the body huddling up, watery diarrhea with indigested food, deep and fine pulse
Decoction of Dredging Meridians for Cold Extremities	1 piece (larger)	3 *liang*	2 *liang*	recuperating the depleted *yang* and activating pulse beat	cold limbs due to dominant *yin* repelling *yang*, no chilliness, flushed complexion, watery diarrhea with indigested food, fading pulse

Table 2. Comparison of Decoction for Mild Purgation and Decoction of Three Drugs Containing Magnoliae Officinalis

Prescription	Ingredient			Action	Indication
	Chief	Adjuvant	Assistant & Guide		
Decoction for Mild Purgation	Radix et Rhizoma Rhei 4 *liang*	Fructus Aurantii Immaturus 3 pieces	Cortex Magnoliae Officinalis 2 *liang*	clearing away heat by increasing bowel movement with purgatives	excess syndrome of Yangming hollow-organ (heat-accumulation): hectic fever, delirium, constipation, abdominal pain and tenderness

Prescription	Ingredient			Action	Indication
	Chief	Adjuvant	Assistant & Guide		
Three Drugs Decoction Containing Magnoliae Officinalis	Cortex Magnoliae Officinalis 8 *liang*	Fructus Aurantii Immaturus 5 pieces	Radix et Rhizoma Rhei 4 *liang*	increasing bowel movement by activating *qi*	*qi*-stagnation syndrome with constipation: progressive abdominal distention and pain, constipation

* One *liang* equals approximately 30 grams.

In Table 1, although the ingredients of the two prescriptions are the same (Radix Aconiti Lateralis as the chief ingredient, Rhizoma Zingiberis as the adjuvant, and Radix Glycyrrhizae Preparata as the assistant and guide), the quantity of Rhizoma Zingiberis in the Decoction of Dredging Meridians for Cold Extremities is doubled so that its action is different.

In Table 2, the components of both prescriptions are the same but their dosages are different. Cortex Magnoliae Officinalis is used in an exceedingly large dose and acts as the chief ingredients in the Three Drugs Decoction, so that an action different from that of Decoction for Mild Purgation is obtained.

(3) Modification of the Form of the Prescription

By preparing the ingredients of a prescription into different forms, the same prescription may produce different effects, and it may be used to treat different diseases. For example, Bolus for Regulating the Middle *Jiao* is a kind of honeyed bolus used to treat deficiency cold in the spleen and stomach, composed of equal amounts of Rhizoma Zingiberis, Radix Gingseng, Rhizoma Atractylodis Macrocephalae and Radix Glycyrrhizae Preparata. If these ingredients are prepared as a decoction, it may be more potent and produce a quicker result, suitable for an acute or a serious case.

The three kinds of modification of an established prescription can be made independently or simultaneously. The former two are usually applied together clinically. This shows that in writing out a prescription, not only the established principle should be followed, modifications should also be made flexibly for individual cases so as to reduce the harmful effects of the drugs and achieve the desired results. Provided we have a good command of the theory and method of prescription composition, we will know how to select right drugs to compose a prescription in clinical practice.

CHAPTER FOUR

FORMS OF PREPARATION

Chinese medicinal prescriptions are composed of various drugs in line with their compatibility. In order to achieve the best therapeutic results, it is necessary to prepare the prescriptions into different forms according to the condition of patients and the specific characteristics of the drugs. Here, only the more commonly used forms are described.

Decoction (*tang ji*): The processed pieces of drugs are soaked and then boiled with water for a period of time. The liquid obtained is known as decoction, e.g., Decoction of Ephedrae and Decoction of Ramulus Cinnamomi. Usually, decoction is for oral administration, yet it can be applied externally for steaming and washing. Its advantages are easy absorption, fast action and flexibility in adjusting the number or amount of the ingredient drugs. It is one of the forms most widely used in clinical practice.

Powder (*san ji*): The drugs are ground into fine or coarse powder before application. It may be taken directly with boiled water, such as Powder of Ten Drugs' Ashes, or be boiled with water to get the liquid for oral use, such as Powder of Lonicerae and Forsythiae. Some powders are only for external use, such as Powder for Promoting Tissue Regeneration. Furthermore, some are used for eye application and throat insufflation, such as Eyedrop with Eight Ingredients and Powder of Borneolum Syntheticum and Borax. The powder form has the advantages of simplicity in processing, convenience for use, economy of medicinal materials and longer preservation.

Pill (*wan ji*): This form is made by grinding the drugs into fine powder and then mixing with excipients, such as honey, water, or rice paste, flour paste, wine, vinegar and medicinal liquid. Some condensed pills are made of the extract of drugs mixed with other medicinal powder or excipients. The advantages of the pills are slow absorption, longstanding action, small dosage, and convenience for use and storage. It is often used for chronic and debilitating diseases, such as Pill of Six Drugs Containing Rehmanniae Preparata, and Pill for *Yin*-Replenishing. Some are also used for emergency treatment, such as Bolus of Calculus Bovis for Resurrection and Pill of Storax, which contain fragrant drugs that cannot be boiled with water. There are four kinds of commonly used pills, i.e., honeyed pill, watered pill, pasted pill and condensed pill.

Extract (*gao ji*): It is prepared by boiling the drugs repeatedly three times and discarding the dregs. The solution is further condensed before sugar or honey is added to form a semi-liquid preparation. Generally, it serves as an oral tonic suitable for longstanding and debilitating illnesses. Examples are Extract of Ginseng and Astragali, and Extract of Eriobotryae.

Ointment (*ruan gao*): It is a sort of drug preparation with a fatty base, which can be readily applied to the skin and mucous membranes. The ointment is semi-solid at room temperature and is softened when it is applied to the surface of the body, where the effective elements of drugs are gradually absorbed. It is for external application and mainly used to cure skin infections. One example is Three-Yellow Ointment.

Plaster (*ying gao*): It is prepared by boiling the selected drugs with vegetable oil, discarding the dregs and adding yellow lead and white wax. The mixture is spread on a piece of paper or cloth and cooled. It becomes solid at room temperature and melts at 36-37℃. The plaster is prepared for contusions and strains, rheumatism and skin infections. Example: Dog Skin Plaster.

Dan (*dan ji*): It is a general term for some preparations made of refined or precious drugs. *Dan* for oral use may be prepared as fine powder or pellets, but the term is used instead of "powder" or "pill" because the ingredient drugs are rather precious or have been refined. An example is the Bolus of Precious Drugs. *Dan* for external use is usually composed of refined mineral powders. Examples: *Hongsheng Dan* and *Baijiang Dan*.

Liquor (*jiu ji*): It is an alcoholic solution prepared by soaking or simmering the drugs in white or yellow wine for a certain period of time. The liquor may be taken orally or applied externally, and it is used as tonics, or for rheumatism, contusions and strains. Two examples are the Tonic Wine of Ten Drugs and Wine of Os Tigris and Chaenomelis.

Medicated tea (*cha ji*): The drugs are pulverized and mixed with sticker to form granules or cakes, which serve as drinks by adding boiling water. This preparation is often used for common cold or indigestion. Example: *Wushi* Tea.

Distillate (*yao lu*): A preparation obtained by distilling fresh drugs containing volatile substances. It tastes bland and usually serves as drinks in summer time. Examples: Distillate of Flos Lonicerae, and Distillate of Artemisiae Annuae.

Troche (*ding ji*): The drugs are pulverized and mixed with honey or excipients to form small tablets or cakes. The troche is ground into powder or prepared with water as juice for oral or topical use. Example: *Zijin* Troche.

Paper strip (*tiao ji*): The medicinal powder is adhered on a small tough paper strip which is inserted into deep ulcers or fistulas to promote tissue regeneration and healing of the lesion. Example: Medicinal Strip for Obliterating Fistula.

Thread (*xian ji*): A cotton or silk thread is boiled with medicinal solution and then dried. It is used for ligation of fistula and piles to promote the healing of fistula and the shrinkage and fall of fistula.

Wool (*jiu ji*): It is a woolly preparation usually made of dry moxa leaves and is used as a material to be burnt in moxibustion therapy.

Syrup (*tang jiang ji*): The drugs are boiled with water to form a decoction. After the dregs are removed, the decoction is further condensed before it is added with sugar to form a medicated syrup. This kind of preparation is particularly suitable for children.

Tablet (*pian ji*): The medicinal powder or extract is mixed with certain excipients and pressed into small pellets containing the same dosage. For drugs with bitter taste and bad smell, the tablets may be sugar-coated and for those which effective elements are easily destroyed by gastric acid, it may be covered with some kind of coating that can be absorbed by the human body. Nowadays, the tablet form is widely used. Examples: Tablet of Mori and Chrysanthemi for Common Cold, and Tablet of Lonicerae and Forsythiae for Detoxification.

Instant granule (*chong ji*): The appropriate drugs are prepared into extract, mixed with sugar, starch or paste, and dried to form granules, which can be taken instantly when dissolved in hot water. It should be stored in sealed containers or plastic packages to prevent dampness. This preparation, fast-acting and convenient, is also widely used. Examples: Instant Granule of Mori and Chrysanthemi for Common Cold, and Instant Granule of Isatidis.

Injection (*zhen ji*): The drugs are extracted, refined and prepared as sterilized solution for subcutaneous, intramuscular and intravenous injection. This preparation is fast-acting and can directly enter the human body without going through the digestive system. Many injections made of herbal medicines are available now, such as Injectio Bupleuri, and Injectio Salviae Miltiorrhizae Co.

In addition, there are also the forms of sponge, oil, aerosol, suppository, frost, capsule as well as miscellaneous forms for external use. All of them are available on the market.

CHAPTER FIVE

THE USAGE OF PRESCRIPTION

The usage of a prescription includes two aspects: the method of decoction and the method of administration, both of which exert some influence upon the therapeutic effect.

1. Method of Decoction

Boiling the medicinal herbs to produce a decoction is the most commonly used method in clinical practice. Physicians of past ages paid great attention to the method of decocting medicines. Xu Dachun, a famous physician in the Qing Dynasty, pointed out in *The Origin and Development of Chinese Medicine*, "The therapeutic effect of a prescription depends entirely on the method of decocting, which should be known to all."

The utensil for decocting medicines: Earthenware is usually used, because it will not cause chemical changes to the medicines. Tin and iron utensils are not recommended, since boiling medicines in metallic utensils may cause sediment, reduce the solubility of medicines, and even induce incompatible chemical reaction that produces undesirable side effects.

Water for decocting medicines: In ancient times, flowing water, spring water, rice-washing water, wine, etc., were used. Nowadays, clean water, such as running water, well water and distilled water, are recommended. The amount of water is adjusted according to the amount of the drugs. Generally, the water level should be approximately two centimeters over the drugs.

Fire for decocting medicines: In general, strong fire is used at first until the water boils, then followed by slow fire for a certain duration.

Procedures of decocting medicines: After the drugs are put in the container, water is added to a level above the drugs. When the water boils, the fire should be reduced to avoid overflowing and charring of the drugs. The cover of the container should not be lifted frequently to avoid escape of the odor and the volatile elements. Generally, a strong fire is required for diaphoretics and heat-purging fragrant drugs for a short period of time, and a slow fire is needed for tonics for a longer period of time. For poisonous medicines, such as Radix Aconiti, Radix Aconiti Lateralis Preparata and Radix Euphorbiae Fischerianae, the boiling should be long enough to reduce their toxicity. In preparing a decoction, some drugs need special treatment. They are described below.

(1) Drugs to be decocted first: Shells and minerals, such as Plastrum Testudinis,

Carapax Trionycis, Concha Haliotidis, Concha Ostreae, Haematitum, Os Draconis, Magnetitum, Gypsum Fibrosum, should be decocted for 10-20 minutes before other drugs are added. Drugs with plenty of mud and sand, such as Terra Flava Usta and Radix Oryzae Glutinosae, and those of light weight and large volume, such as Rhizoma Phragmitis and Spica Prunellae, should also be decocted first and the supernatant fluid is then used to decoct other drugs.

(2) Drugs to be decocted later: Fragrant drugs with volatile elements, such as Herba Menthae, Fructus Amomi and Fructus Amomi Rotundus, should be added for just two or three minutes when the other drugs are already well decocted.

(3) Drugs to be wrapped for boiling: Halloysitum Rubrum Talcum, Semen Plantaginis, Flos Inulae and any other drugs that are directly irritant to the throat and digestive tract should be wrapped with a piece of gauze before they are decocted together with other drugs.

(4) Drugs to be simmered or decocted alone: Some valuable drugs are simmered or decocted alone so as to prevent their effective elements from being absorbed by other drugs. For example, Radix Ginseng should be sliced and put in a covered container and simmered for two or three hours. Cornu Saigae Tataricae and Cornu Rhinocerotis should be sliced and decocted alone for two hours to get the solution for drinking, or ground with water or into powder for oral administration.

(5) Drugs to be melted by heat: Some glutinous and sticky drugs, such as Colla Corii Asini, Colla Cornu Cervi and Saccharum Granorum, are easily melted and stuck to the bottom of the pot when decocted. Therefore, they should be melted separately or in the hot decoction prepared just before administration.

(6) Drugs to be taken with the prepared decoction: Some powder, pellets, pills, fresh juice and some fragrant or precious drugs should be taken with the decoction. They include Calculus Bovis, Moschus, Pulvis Lignum Aquilariae Resinatum, Pulvis, Cinnamomi, Pulvis Notoginseng, fresh lotus root juice, and fresh radish juice.

2. Method of Administration

Generally, drugs should be taken before meal. But, those irritant to the stomach should be taken after meal. Tonics are to be taken when the stomach is empty and antimalarial drugs taken three to four hours before the attack, while sedatives are to be taken before bedtime. Pills, powder and medicated wine for chronic diseases should be taken at regular intervals. In addition, some decoctions may be taken as daily drinks when necessary.

In order to achieve the desired therapeutic results, drugs are usually administered two or three times a day. As for decoction, it should be boiled twice as two doses, and one or two doses may be taken a day according to the condition of the patient and the severity of the disease.

The decoction is usually taken when it is still warm. After a decoction for relieving the exterior syndrome is taken, the patient should be covered with a quilt to induce perspiration and avoid exposure to wind. The decoction for purging heat used in treating heat syndrome should be taken cool and that for warming the interior to treat the cold syndrome should be taken hot. The decoction of a hot nature for cold syndrome accompanied by false heat syndrome should be taken cold, while the decoction of a cold nature for heat syndrome accompanied by false cold syndrome should be taken hot. If the patient vomits after taking the decoction, add some ginger juice to the decoction or rub the tongue with fresh ginger piece or chew some dried orange peel before taking the decoction, or take the decoction cool in small and divided doses. For comatose patients, nasal feeding is advisable.

The decoction containing potent or poisonous drugs should be taken in a small dose at first and the dosage should be increased gradually. The administration should be suspended when the desired result is obtained to avoid intoxication. In addition, the method of administration may be altered in line with the condition of the patient and the nature of drugs during the course of treatment.

CHAPTER SIX

PRESCRIPTIONS FOR RELIEVING EXTERIOR SYNDROME

Prescriptions for relieving the exterior syndrome (*jie biao ji*) are mainly composed of drugs that can induce perspiration, expel the pathogens from the exterior, and let out skin eruptions. The use of such prescriptions falls into the category of diaphoretic therapy.

Exterior syndrome is due to the affection of the body surface by the six exogenous pathogenic factors. It has such symptoms as chills, fever, headache, general achiness, and superficial pulse; it is classified into the cold type and the heat type. The former is named exterior-cold syndrome and should be treated by expelling the pathogenic factors from the exterior with acrid and warm drugs. The latter is called exterior-heat syndrome and should be treated by expelling the pathogenic factors from the exterior with acrid and cold drugs. A case complicated by a deficiency of *qi*, blood, *yin* or *yang* should be treated by expelling the pathogens from the exterior in combination with the tonic therapy. Therefore, prescriptions for relieving the exterior syndrome are divided into three kinds: prescriptions for expelling the pathogens from the exterior with acrid and warm drugs, prescriptions for expelling the pathogens from the exterior with acrid and cold drugs, and prescriptions with both drugs expelling the pathogens from the exterior and drugs strengthening the antipathogenic *qi*.

Prescriptions for relieving the exterior syndrome with acrid and warm drugs (*xin wen jie biao ji*) are suitable for exterior syndrome due to wind-cold, which exhibits chills, fever, rigidity of the nape with headache, aching of the limbs, absence of thirst, sweating or no sweating, thin and white tongue coating, superficial and tense pulse, or superficial and slow pulse. Major acrid and warm drugs for expelling pathogens from the exterior include Herba Ephedrae, Ramulus Cinnamomi, Herba Schizonepetae, Radix Ledebouriellae and Folium Perillae. They are often used as the chief drugs to make up a prescription with drugs for relieving cough and asthma, purging heat, preserving *yin* and regulating the *yingfen*, warming the lung and reducing phlegm, in order to relieve the exterior syndrome. Representative prescriptions of this kind are Decoction of Ephedrae, Decoction of Ramulus Cinnamomi, Decoction of Nine Ingredients Containing Notopterygii and Small Blue Dragon Decoction.

Prescriptions for relieving the exterior syndrome with acrid and cool drugs (*xin liang jie biao ji*) are fit for exterior syndrome due to wind-heat, which exhibits fever, slight chills, headache, thirst, sore throat or cough, thin and white tongue coating or yellowish tongue coating, and superficial and rapid pulse. For this kind of exterior syndrome, prescriptions are usually composed of acrid and cool drugs, such as Herba Menthae, Fructus

Arctii, Folium Mori, Flos Chrysanthemi, Radix Puerariae and Rhizoma Cimicifugae, in combination with drugs for reducing phlegm and relieving cough, purging heat, and promoting the production of body fluid. The representative prescriptions are Decoction of Mori and Chrysanthemi, Powder of Lonicerae and Forsythiae, and Decoction of Ephedrae, Armeniacae Amarum, Glycyrrhizae and Gypsum Fibrosum.

Prescriptions for relieving exterior syndrome and strengthening antipathogenic *qi* (*fu zheng jie biao ji*) are suitable for cases of general debility complicated by the attack of exogenous pathogenic factors. To treat such cases, it is necessary to expel the pathogens from the exterior and strengthen the antipathogenic *qi* at the same time. Therefore, drugs for expelling the pathogens are usually used in combination with drugs for supplementing *qi* and restoring *yang* or drugs for nourishing *yin* and blood. Representative prescriptions of this kind are Anti-phlogistic Powder and Modified Decoction of Polygonati Odorati.

Ingredient drugs in this kind of prescriptions are mostly acrid in taste and volatile in nature, so they should not be boiled for a long time, lest their actions be weakened. After taking the decoction, the patient should avoid exposure to wind and cold, put on more clothes or keep warm in bed, so as to induce perspiration. However, the perspiration should be moderate, neither too much nor too little. Too little sweating cannot expel the pathogenic factors, but too much is likely to cause a loss of *qi* and body fluid. In severe cases, too much sweating may lead to exhaustion of *yin* or *yang*.

Clinically, such prescriptions should only be applied in the treatment of exterior syndromes caused by exogenous pathogens. If an interior syndrome appears while the exterior syndrome has not been cured, it is imperative to relieve the exterior syndrome first and treat the interior one later, or prescribe drugs that can cure both the exterior and interior syndromes simultaneously.

It should be noticed that prescriptions for relieving exterior syndrome cannot be used for cases in which the pathogens have already entered the interior, or the skin eruptions have not been let out, or lesions have been ulcerated, and for deficiency syndrome with edema, or too much loss of water due to vomiting and diarrhea.

Decoction of Ephedrae

麻黄汤 *ma huang tang*

(from *Treatise on Cold Diseases*)

Herba Ephedrae	9 g
Ramulus Cinnamomi	6 g
Semen Armeniacae Amarum	9 g
Radix Glycyrrhizae Preparata	3 g

Administration: Decocted for oral use. Be sure to keep warm with more clothes or bedding after taking the decoction to induce slight perspiration.

Action: Inducing perspiration to expel pathogenic factors from the exterior, and releasing the inhibited lung *qi* to relieve asthma.

Indications: Exterior-excess syndrome caused by exogenous wind-cold, with such symptoms as chills, fever, headache, general achiness, asthma, no sweating, thin and whitish tongue coating, and superficial and tense pulse.

Explanation: When wind-cold affects the body surface, a struggle erupts between the exogenous wind-cold and the antipathogenic *qi*, resulting in chills, fever, headache and general achiness. The lung is in charge of *qi* circulation and connected with the skin and hair. When the pores are blocked and the lung *qi* cannot circulate properly, asthma appears with the absence of sweating. Therefore, it is necessary to induce sweating to expel the pathogenic wind-cold from the exterior and release the inhibited lung *qi*. In the prescription, Herba Ephedrae, after which the prescription is named, is the chief ingredient with the ability to induce sweating, expel the wind-cold, and release the inhibited lung *qi* to relieve asthma. Ramulus Cinnamomi serves as the adjuvant ingredient; it induces sweating, expels the pathogenic factors from the muscles and skin, disperses cold by warming the meridians, and helps strengthen the action of Herba Ephedrae. Semen Armeniacae Amarum, as the assistant ingredient, releases stagnant lung *qi* and relieves cough and asthma. And Radix Glycyrrhizae Preparata, as the guide ingredient, is capable of balancing the effects of the other drugs, supplementing *qi* and regulating the middle *jiao*.

Clinically, symptoms and signs such as chills, fever, absence of sweating, asthma, superficial and tense pulse are the key manifestations calling for the application of this prescription, which, however, may be modified for different cases. For a case with severe dyspneic cough due to exposure to wind-cold, Ramulus Cinnamomi can be removed in order to lessen the effect of inducing sweating; for a case complicated by the attack of pathogenic dampness and manifested as arthralgia, Rhizoma Atractylodis and Rhizoma Atractylodis Macrocephalae can be added to expel cold and dampness.

This prescription is not recommended for exterior-deficiency syndromes caused by wind-cold, exterior syndrome caused by wind-heat and patients debilitated by prolonged illness.

Appendant Prescriptions

(1) Three Crude Drugs Decoction

三拗汤 *san ao tang*

(from *Benevolent Prescriptions from the Pharmaceutical Bureau of the Taiping Period*)

This prescription is composed of Herba Ephedrae, Semen Armeniacae Amarum and Radix Glycyrrhizae in equal amounts. The drugs are ground into coarse powder, 15 g for each dose. Decoct the powder in water with five pieces of Rhizoma Zingiberis Recens for oral use. Be sure to keep warm to induce slight perspiration. It acts to expel cold from the exterior, release the inhibited lung *qi* and relieve cough; it is indicated for exterior syndrome caused by wind-cold with such symptoms as stuffy nose, hoarse voice, disinclination to talk, productive cough, a full sensation in the chest, and shortness of breath.

(2) *Huagai* Powder

华盖散 *hua gai san*
(from *Benevolent Prescriptions from the Pharmaceutical Bureau of the Taiping Period*)

The prescription is composed of Herba Ephedrae, Cortex Mori Radicis (prepared with honey), Fructus Perillae (fried), Semen Armeniacae Amarum (fried), Poria Rubra, and Pericarpium Citri Reticulatae, 30 g each; and Radix Glycyrrhizae Preparata, 15 g. Grind the drugs into coarse powder, take 9 g for each dose and decoct with water. Take the warm decoction after meal. It acts to release the inhibited lung *qi*, expel the pathogenic factors from the exterior, remove phlegm and relieve cough. It is indicated for exterior syndrome caused by wind-cold, exhibiting chills, fever, cough, dyspnea, difficult expectoration, a full sensation in the chest, and superficial and tense pulse.

The above two prescriptions are both modifications of the Decoction of Ephedrae. With Ramulus Cinnamomi removed, both have a milder diaphoretic effect but stronger antitussive and antidyspneic effects, and the ability to expel wind-cold from the lung. Consequently, they are both indicated for cases characterized by dyspneic cough. Compared with the Three Crude Drugs Decoction, the *Huagai* Powder has more ingredients, such as Cortex Mori Radicis, Fructus Perillae, Pericarpium Citri Reticulatae and Poria Rubra. It is thus more effective in regulating *qi*, eliminating phlegm, relieving the inhibited circulation of lung *qi* and dyspnea.

Decoction of Ramulus Cinnamomi
桂枝汤 *gui zhi tang*
(from *Treatise on Cold Diseases*)

Ramulus Cinnamomi	9 g
Radix Paeoniae Lactiflorae	9 g
Radix Glycyrrhizae Preparata	6 g
Rhizoma Zingiberis Recens	9 g
Fructus Jujubae	5 pieces (big)

Administration: Decoct with water for oral administration. Take a small amount of hot thin porridge or hot water after taking the decoction to help enforce its effects, and induce mild perspiration with more clothes or bedding.

Action: Inducing sweating, expelling pathogens from the muscles and skin, and regulating the *ying* and *wei* systems.

Indications: Exterior-deficiency syndrome caused by wind-cold with such symptoms as fever, headache, sweating, aversion to wind, thin and white tongue coating, and superficial slow pulse.

Explanation: Wind-cold affecting the body usually rests in the superficial part and gives rise to chills and fever without sweating. If fever with sweating appears but the aversion to wind does not ebb, it is due to weakened resistance caused by a disharmony between the *ying* and *wei* systems. The case should be treated by expelling the pathogens from the exterior, inducing sweating and harmonizing *ying* and *wei* systems. In this prescription, Ramulus Cinnamomi, after which the prescription is named, is the chief ingredient, and it acts to expel the pathogenic factors from the exterior, induce sweating, warm the meridians and relieve pain; Paeoniae Lactiflorae serves as the adjuvant to nourish *yin* and regulate the *ying* system, helping Ramulus Cinnamomi eliminate the pathogenic factors from the exterior but not damaging *yin*. Ramulus Cinnamomi and Paeoniae Lactiflorae used together can strengthen each other's action, producing better results in harmonizing the *ying* and *wei* systems. Zingiberis Recens is acrid and warm, and can help Ramulus Cinnamomi expel cold from the exterior; Jujubae is sweet and mild, and not only can nourish *qi* and regulate the middle *jiao*, but can also invigorate the spleen and promote the secretion of body fluid. These two in combination serve as the assistant ingredients to strengthen the actions of Ramulus Cinnamomi and Paeoniae Alba to regulate the *ying* and *wei* systems. Glycyrrhizae Preparata, serving as the guide ingredient, can balance the effects of the other ingredients.

"Taking a small amount of hot thin porridge after medication" means using the essence of food to increase the potency of the drugs and benefit stomach *qi* at the same time. "Drinking hot water and putting on more clothes" means inducing perspiration by keeping warm. Moderate sweating is suitable while too much sweating will consume *qi* and damage fluid.

This prescription can be applied for cases of convalescence, puerperium, debility resulting in disharmony between the *ying* and *wei* systems with the symptoms of fever, spontaneous sweating, and slight aversion to wind and cold. For a case accompanied by dyspneic cough, Semen Armeniacae Amarum and Cortex Magnoliae Officinalis are added to relieve dyspnea; for a case with disharmony between *yin* and *yang* leading to nocturnal emission, vertigo, night and spontaneous sweating, Os Draconis and Concha Ostreae are added to suppress excessive *yang* and restore the astringent function of the body.

This prescription should not be used for exterior-excess syndrome without sweating, or exterior-cold and interior-heat syndromes with irritability but without sweating, or the early stage of a seasonal febrile disease with the symptoms of fever, thirst, sore throat and rapid pulse.

Decoction of Nine Ingredients Containing Notopterygii

九味羌活汤 *jiu wei qiang huo tang*

(from *Zhang Yuansu's Prescriptions*, recorded in *It's Hard to Know This*)

Rhizoma seu Radix Notopterygii	9 g
Radix Ledebouriellae	9 g
Rhizoma Atractylodis	9 g
Herba Asari	3 g
Rhizoma Chuanxiong	6 g

Radix Angelicae Dahuricae	6 g
Radix Rehmanniae	3 g
Radix Scutellariae	3 g
Radix Glycyrrhizae	3 g

Administration: Boil the drugs with water for oral use.

Action: Inducing perspiration, eliminating dampness and purging interior heat.

Indications: Exterior syndrome caused by exogenous wind, cold and dampness with such symptoms as chills, fever, absence of sweating, headache, general achiness, slight thirst, bitter taste in the mouth, white tongue coating, and superficial pulse.

Explanation: This prescription is used to treat exterior syndrome caused by wind, cold and dampness with heat accumulation in the interior. When wind, cold and dampness attack the body surface, a conflict between the pathogens and antipathogenic *qi* erupts, leading to chills, fever, headache, absence of sweating; when cold and dampness affect the muscles and meridians, poor circulation of blood and *qi* occurs, resulting in general achiness; bitter taste and slight thirst indicate heat accumulated in the interior. The treatment should focus on expelling wind, cold and dampness from the exterior and purging interior heat at the same time.

Notopterygii, the chief drug in the prescription, is acrid, warm and fragrant, and is effective in eliminating wind, cold and dampness. Ledebouriellae and Atractylodis, serving as the adjuvant ingredients, induce sweating and eliminate dampness, and are used to help Notopterygii expel the pathogens from the exterior. Asari, Chuanxiong and Angelicae Dahuricae are used as assistant ingredients to expel wind and cold, and promote the circulation of *qi* and blood so that the headache and general achiness can be relieved. Rehmanniae and Scutellariae are also used as assistant ingredients to purge interior heat and counteract the dry property of acrid and warm drugs to prevent the body fluid from being damaged. Serving as the guide ingredient, Glycyrrhizae balances the effects of these drugs.

This prescription is frequently used to treat common cold in all seasons caused by wind, cold and dampness, and is suitable for exterior-excess syndrome characterized by the absence of sweating and complicated by the existence of interior heat. It can be modified according to the symptoms and signs of individual cases clinically. For a mild case in which general achiness caused by dampness is not serious, remove Atractylodis and Asari to lessen the prescription's dry-warm property; for a serious general achiness, double the amount of Notopterygii to promote *qi* and blood circulation so that the achiness can be relieved; for a case characterized by a full sensation in the chest due to accumulated dampness, remove Rehmanniae and add Fructus Aurantii and Cortex Magnoliae Officinalis to promote *qi* circulation and eliminate dampness; and for a case with symptoms of absence of interior heat, such as bitter taste and slight thirst, remove Rehmanniae and Scutellariae.

Small Blue Dragon Decoction

小青龙汤 *xiao qing long tang*

(from *Treatise on Cold Diseases*)

Herba Ephedrae	9 g
Radix Paeoniae Lactiflorae	9 g
Herba Asari	3 g
Rhizoma Zingiberis	3 g
Radix Glycyrrhizae Preparata	6 g
Ramulus Cinnamomi	9 g
Rhizoma Pinelliae Preparata	9 g
Fructus Schisandrae	6 g

Administration: Boil the drugs with water for oral use.

Action: Expelling the pathogens from the exterior and relieving phlegm retention, cough and dyspnea.

Indications: Phlegm-fluid retention syndrome caused by wind-cold, characterized by chills, fever, absence of sweating, dyspneic cough with copious thin sputum, or edema over the head and the limbs, smooth white tongue coating, and superficial pulse.

Explanation: This prescription is frequently used to treat dyspneic cough caused by wind-cold and phlegm-fluid retention. When wind-cold affects the surface, such manifestations as chills, fever without sweating, and superficial pulse eventually appear; attack by cold leads to phlegm retention in the interior and affects the lung, which causes the adverse rising of lung *qi*, dyspneic cough ensues; because phlegm retention is of a cold nature, the sputum appears thin and frothy. In this case, phlegm retention cannot be relieved only by expelling the pathogenic factors from the exterior. Conversely, the pathogenic factors cannot be expelled only by relieving phlegm retention. So, the syndrome should be treated simultaneously by inducing perspiration to expel the pathogens from the surface and relieving phlegm retention with warm-natured drugs. In this prescription, Ephedrae and Cinnamomi are used together to induce perspiration, expel the pathogens from the exterior, relieve the inhibited lung *qi* and dyspnea; Cinnamomi is associated with Paeoniae Lactiflorae to regulate the *ying* and *wei* systems and prevent oversweating induced by Ephedrae and Cinnamomi and prevent possible damage to the antipathogenic *qi*; Zingiberis, Asari and Pinelliae Preparata act to warm the lung and relieve phlegm retention. Of them, Asari can also help Ephedrae and Cinnamomi expel the pathogens from the exterior. In order to prevent the warm-natured and diaphoretic drugs from damaging *qi* and body fluid, Schisandrae is used to restrain the lung *qi*, producing the results of relieving cough and dyspnea and preventing the lung *qi* from dissipating. Glycyrrhizae Preparata is used to balance the effects of all the other ingredients. In a word, this prescription is composed of two kinds of drugs: drugs for inducing perspiration to expel the pathogens from the exterior, and drugs for warming the lung to relieve phlegm retention. Of these two kinds, the former are the major ingredients and the latter are the auxiliary ones. Clinically, this prescription can be given no matter whether there is sweating or not. In a case when the exogenous cold has been expelled but cough and dyspnea still remain, remove Cinnamomi so as to weaken the action of inducing sweating and expelling the pathogens; Ephedrae is stir-fried with honey to increase the effect of relieving the inhibited lung *qi* and dyspnea. The modified prescription is indicated for productive cough with thin and clear sputum, pale tongue with white and smooth coating. For a case accompanied by interior heat, Gypsum Fibrosum should be added to purge interior heat and relieve irritability.

Powder of Elsholtziae

香薷散 *xiang ru san*

(from *Benevolent Prescriptions from the Pharmaceutical Bureau of the Taiping Period*)

Herba Elsholtziae	30 g
Semen Dolichoris Album (fried)	15 g
Cortex Magnoliae Officinalis (prepared with ginger)	15 g

Administration: Grind the drugs into coarse powder, take 9 g of the powder and boil it with water, drink the cooled decoction with a little amount of wine. It may also be prepared by boiling the drugs directly with water to produce a decoction, with the dosage reduced proportionally to the original formula.

Action: Removing summer-heat from the exterior, eliminating dampness and regulating the middle *jiao*.

Indications: Attack by cold of the surface and by dampness of the interior in summer time, exhibiting chills, fever without sweating, headache, lassitude, oppressed feeling in the chest, nausea, or abdominal pain, vomiting, or diarrhea, greasy white tongue coating and superficial pulse.

Explanation: Enjoying the cool outdoors at a summer night makes one liable to be affected by exogenous cold, in which case the pores are blocked and therefore chills, fever without sweating, headache, superficial pulse occur; excessive intake of cold and raw food may lead to damage of the interior by dampness, causing dysfunction of the spleen and stomach, thus giving rise to the oppressed feeling in the chest, nausea, lassitude, or even abdominal pain, vomiting and diarrhea; a greasy white tongue coating signifies the existence of cold and dampness. The treatment should expel cold from the exterior and eliminate dampness from the interior (spleen and stomach). Elsholtziae, which is acrid, warm and fragrant, is used as the chief ingredient in the prescription. It acts to expel pathogenic cold from the exterior, disperse summer-heat and dampness; Magnoliae Officinalis, which serves as the adjuvant drug, is bitter and warm, and acts to promote *qi* and ease the middle *jiao* to relieve dampness retention; Dolichoris Album, which serves as the assistant and guide, is effective in strengthening the spleen, regulating the middle *jiao*, removing dampness by means of diuresis and eliminating summer-heat. These three drugs used together not only can expel pathogenic cold from the exterior but also relieve dampness retention and regulate the middle *jiao*. For a case with stuffy and running nose, add Bulbus Allii Fistulosi and Semen Sojae Preparatum to increase the effect of expelling pathogenic cold from the exterior.

Appendant Prescription

Modified Decoction of Elsholtziae

新加香薷饮 *xin jia xiang ru yin*

(from *Essentials of Seasonal Febrile Diseases*)

This prescription is composed of 6 g of Herba Elsholtziae, 9 g of Flos Lonicerae, 9 g of Flos Dolichoris, 6 g of Cortex Magnoliae Officinalis, and 9 g of Fructus Forsythiae. These drugs are boiled with water for oral administration. It acts to eliminate summer-heat, relieve the exterior syndrome, purge heat and eliminate dampness, and is indicated for affection by summer-heat and dampness in summer, which exhibits fever, headache, chills without sweating, thirst, flushed face, oppressed feeling in the chest, vexation, thin greasy tongue coating, and superficial and rapid pulse.

Because summer-heat is a *yang* pathogenic factor, Flos Dolichoris, Flos Lonicerae and Fructus Forsythiae are therefore added to purge summer-heat.

Decoction of Mori and Chrysanthemi

桑菊饮 *sang ju yin*

(from *Essentials of Seasonal Febrile Diseases*)

Folium Mori	7.5 g
Flos Chrysanthemi	3 g
Semen Armeniacae Amarum	6 g
Fructus Forsythiae	5 g
Herba Menthae	2.5 g
Radix Platycodi	6 g
Radix Glycyrrhizae	2.5 g
Rhizoma Phragmitis	6 g

Administration: Decoct the drugs with water for oral use; or prepare them into pills or tablets, four to eight pieces each time, twice a day.

Action: Expelling wind-heat, releasing the inhibited lung *qi* and relieving cough.

Indications: The onset stage of a wind-warm disease appears as mild cases of exterior-heat syndrome, marked by cough, mild fever, slight thirst, red tongue tip and thin yellow tongue coating, and superficial and rapid pulse.

Explanation: Wind-warm disease is a kind of seasonal febrile disorders occurring in winter and spring, usually caused by wind-heat, as its name suggests. The case is usually mild with the pathogens affecting the body surface, so mild fever appears; wind-heat is likely to damage body fluid, but when it is not serious, thirst is slight; wind-heat invades the body through mouth and nose, leading to obstruction of the lung *qi*, giving rise to cough as the major symptom. Treatment aims to expel wind-heat from the exterior and release the inhibited lung *qi*. Mori and Chrysanthemi, which are sweet, cool and light, are used as the chief ingredients to disperse wind-heat from the upper *jiao*; Menthae, which is acrid and cool, and serves as the adjuvant drug, aids Mori and Chrysanthemi to enhance their effects of expelling pathogens from the exterior. Armeniacae Amarum and Platycodi, which act to release the inhibited lung *qi*, ease the throat, relieve cough and eliminate sputum; Forsythiae, which is bitter and cold, purges heat; and Phragmitis, which is sweet and cold, purges heat and promotes the production of body fluid to quench thirst—all are used as assistant ingredients. Glycyrrhizae serves as the guide ingredient to balance the effects of the other drugs and help ease the throat as well.

This is a mild prescription used to relieve exterior syndrome with acrid and cool drugs, and is indicated for the initial stage of wind-warm disease characterized by cough. If the case is severe and complicated by heat in *qifen*, exhibiting high fever and noisy breathing like dyspnea, Gypsum Fibrosum and Rhizoma Anemarrhenae are added to increase the heat-eliminating effect. For frequent cough and dominant heat in the chest, Radix Scutellariae is added to purge lung heat and relieve cough. For severe thirst, Radix Trichosanthis is added to purge heat and promote the production of fluid. For cough and thick sputum, Pericarpium Trichosanthis and Bulbus Fritillariae Thunbergii are added to eliminate heat and sputum.

Powder of Lonicerae and Forsythiae
银翘散 *yin qiao san*
(from *Essentials of Seasonal Febrile Diseases*)

Fructus Forsythiae	30 g
Flos Lonicerae	30 g
Radix Platycodi	18 g
Herba Menthae	18 g
Herba Lophatheri	12 g
Radix Glycyrrhizae (crude)	15 g
Schizonepetae	12 g
Semen Sojae Preparatum	15 g
Fructus Arctii	18 g

Administration: Grind the drugs into coarse powder, boil 18 g of the powder and 15 g of Rhizoma Phragmitis with water for oral use, or directly prepare the drugs into decoction, with the dosage of the ingredients reduced proportionally.

Action: Expelling the pathogenic factors from the exterior, purging heat and removing toxins.

Indications: The onset stage of seasonal febrile diseases appearing as wind-heat exterior syndrome, exhibiting fever, mild chills, no or little sweating, headache, thirst, cough, sore throat, red tip of the tongue with thin and white coating or thin and yellow coating, and superficial and rapid pulse.

Explanation: At the onset of seasonal febrile diseases, the pathogens only affect *weifen*, where they conflict with the antipathogenic *qi*, giving rise to fever, mild chills and headache. When wind-heat affects the throat, lung *qi* is inhibited and cough and sore throat occur. When wind-heat damages body fluid, thirst appears. The therapeutic principle at this stage should be to expel the pathogens from the exterior, purge heat and toxins. In this prescription, the chief ingredients are Lonicerae and Forsythiae, which are effective for purging heat and toxins, releasing stagnant lung *qi* and expelling pathogens at the surface; Menthae, Schizonepetae and Sojae are adjuvant ingredients, helping to expel the pathogens from the exterior. Schizonepetae, which is warm and, when combined with acrid and cool drugs, can enhance the prescription's action to expel the pathogens from the exterior. Used together, Platycodi, Arctii and Glycyrrhizae can release inhibited lung *qi*, dissipate phlegm and cure sore throat; Lophatheri and Phragmitis, serving as the assistant drugs, purge heat and promote the production of fluid. Glycyrrhizae is the guide drug to balance the effects of the other drugs.

This is a mild prescription for relieving exterior syndrome with acrid and cool drugs. It is chiefly composed of two kinds of drugs: drugs for purging heat and toxins, and drugs for expelling wind from the surface, in combination with drugs for relieving sore throat and promoting fluid secretion. It is indicated for the initial stage of wind-heat syndrome in which heat prevails, exhibiting fever, thirst, sore throat, red tip of the tongue, and superficial rapid pulse. Modifications can be made in line with the specific conditions of individual cases. For a case accompanied by an oppressed feeling in the chest, Herba Agastaches and Radix Curcumae are added to eliminate dampness; for a case with severe thirst, Radix Trichosanthis is added to purge heat and promote fluid secretion; for a case with epistaxis, Schizonepetae and Sojae Preparatum are removed, and Rhizoma Imperatae and burned Cacumen Biotae are added to cool the blood and stop bleeding.

Here is a comparison between Powder of Lonicerae and Forsythiae and Decoction of Mori and Chrysanthemi. Both share some drugs, such as Fructus Forsythiae, Herba Menthae, Radix Platycodi, Radix Glycyrrhizae and Rhizoma Phragmitis. But in the former, there are some other drugs, such as Flos Lonicerae, Herba Lophatheri, Herba Schizonepetae, Semen Sojae Preparatum and Fructus Arctii, to expel wind from the exterior and purge heat and toxins; in the latter, there is Folium Mori, Flos Chrysanthemi and Semen Armeniacae Amarum, to expel wind-heat, release the inhibited lung *qi* and relieve cough.

Decoction of Ephedrae, Armeniacae Amarum, Glycyrrhizae and Gypsum Fibrosum

麻黄杏仁甘草石膏汤 *ma huang xing ren gan cao shi gao tang*

(from *Treatise on Cold Diseases*)

Herba Ephedrae	6 g
Semen Armeniacae Amarum	9 g
Radix Glycyrrhizae Preparata	6 g
Gypsum Fibrosum (broken into pieces and decocted first)	18 g

Administration: Decoct with water for oral administration.

Action: Releasing stagnant lung *qi*, purging lung heat and relieving dyspnea.

Indications: Lung excess-heat syndrome with dyspnea caused by attack of wind, exhibiting such symptoms as fever, thirst, sweating or no sweating, cough, dyspnea, thin and white or yellow tongue coating, and smooth and rapid pulse.

Explanation: The syndrome that can be treated with the prescription is due to superficial pathogens entering the interior and then turning into heat, leading to predominant heat in the lung. Excessive lung heat causes an adversely upward flow of *qi* and is liable to damage body fluid, giving rise to fever with sweating, cough, dyspnea or even flaring of the alae nasi, and smooth and rapid pulse. Treatment aims to release stagnant lung *qi*, purge lung heat and relieving dyspnea. In this prescription, Ephedrae expels pathogenic factors from the exterior, releases stagnant lung *qi* and relieves dyspnea. Thanks to its warm nature, however, it is used together with Gypsum Fibrosum to purge stagnant heat. The two drugs, opposite in nature yet complementary to each other, serve as the chief drugs. Armeniacae Amarum, which is used as the assistant drug, is combined with Ephedrae to relieve cough and dyspnea, while Glycyrrhizae, capable of balancing the effects of the other ingredients, is used as the guide.

This is a major prescription for purging lung heat and releasing stagnant lung *qi*. The clinical evidence calling for its application includes fever, dyspneic cough, and smooth and rapid pulse. It is applicable no matter whether sweating is present or not. For a case with high fever, severe cough and dyspnea, the dosage of Gypsum Fibrosum is increased and Folium Isatidis, Radix Scutellariae and Fructus Forsythiae are added to purge lung heat; for a case with yellow and thick sputum, Fructus Trichosanthis and Bulbus Fritillariae Thunbergii are added to purge heat and resolve sputum.

This prescription and Decoction of Ephedrae are both applicable to dyspnea of the excess syndrome. The former is composed of acrid and cool drugs, in combination with Ephedrae and Gypsum Fibrosum to purge lung heat; it is indicated for dyspnea of the excess type due to lung heat. The latter is composed of acrid and warm drugs, and combined with Ephedrae and Ramulus Cinnamomi to expel cold from the surface; it is indicated for dyspnea of the excess type due to wind-cold.

Antiphlogistic Powder

败毒散 *bai du san*

(from *Medical Elucidation of Pediatrics*)

Radix Bupleuri	30 g
Radix Peucedani	30 g
Rhizoma Chuanxiong	30 g
Fructus Aurantii	30 g
Rhizoma et Radix Notopterygii	30 g
Radix Angelicae Pubescentis	30 g

Poria	30 g
Radix Platycodi (fried)	30 g
Radix Ginseng	30 g
Radix Glycyrrhizae	15 g

Administration: Grind the drugs into coarse powder. Take 6 g of the powder and decoct it with a small amount of Rhizoma Zingiberis Recens and Herba Menthae; or prepare the drugs directly into a decoction with the dosages reduced proportionally.

Action: Eliminating wind and dampness, benefiting *qi* and relieving exterior syndrome.

Indications: Deficiency of antipathogenic *qi* with exposure to wind, cold and dampness, exhibiting chills, fever, absence of sweating, stiff neck, headache, general achiness, oppressed feeling in the chest, stuffy nose, productive cough, greasy and white tongue coating, and superficial pulse that feels weak on heavy pressure.

Explanation: Due to weak constitution, the antipathogenic *qi* is too weak to eliminate the pathogens from the body when the body is affected by wind, cold and dampness, and chills, fever without perspiration, stiff neck and general achiness occur. When wind-cold invades the lung, the lung *qi* is obstructed, causing stuffy nose, hoarseness and productive cough; and *qi* flow blocked by stagnant phlegm results in an oppressed feeling in the chest. In accordance with the principle of expelling pathogens from the surface in an exterior syndrome and restoring *qi* when there is *qi* deficiency, treatment seeks to eliminate wind and dampness, benefit *qi* and relieve the exterior syndrome. In the prescription, Notopterygii and Angelicae Pubescentis serve as the chief drugs to eliminate cold and dampness; Chuanxiong and Bupleuri are used as the adjuvant ingredients—the former acts to promote blood circulation, eliminate wind and relieve pain, and the latter to relieve the exterior syndrome and fever. Aurantii, Platycodi, Peucedani and Poria, all of which are used as assistant drugs to release the lung *qi*, relieve cough and eliminate sputum. Ginseng is also used as an assistant ingredient to help strengthen the antipathogenic *qi*, expel the pathogens from the body by inducing perspiration; Glycyrrhizae, serving as the guide, balances the effects of the other ingredients.

Originally, this prescription was for children. Because of the insufficient antipathogenic *qi* in children, a small amount of Ginseng is used. Later, it is used to treat all cases with the above symptoms, especially the aged, parturient, convalescent, and debilitated patients suffering from exposure to wind, cold and dampness. In cases of pyogenic skin infection caused by excessive virulent heat with local redness, swelling and pain, remove Ginseng and add Flos Lonicerae and Fructus Forsythiae to purge the virulent heat and relieve pyogenic infection. For a serious case of exterior syndrome due to wind-cold, remove Ginseng and add Herba Schizonepetae and Radix Ledebouriellae to strengthen the effect of expelling cold. This prescription is chiefly composed of acrid, fragrant, warm and dry drugs. So, it should not be used for cases not caused by wind, cold and dampness despite the presence of chills, fever and anhidrosis.

Appendant Prescription

Antiphlogistic Powder with Schizonepetae and Ledebouriellae
荆防败毒散 *jing fang bai du san*
(from *Wonderful Prescriptions for Keeping Health*)

This prescription is composed of 5 g of Rhizoma seu Radix Notopterygii, 5 g of Radix Angelicae Pubescentis, 5 g of Radix Bupleuri, 5 g of Radix Peucedani, 5 g of Fructus Aurantii, 5 g of Poria, 5 g of Herba Schizonepetae, 5 g of Radix Ledebouriellae, 5 g of Radix Platycodi, 5 g of Rhizoma Chuanxiong, and 2 g of Radix Glycyrrhizae. To be decocted with water for oral administration, it acts to expel pathogens from the exterior by inducing sweating and relieving pyogenic infection and pain. It is indicated for exterior syndrome caused by wind, cold and dampness, exhibiting chills, fever, stiff neck, headache, general achiness, absence of thirst and sweating, stuffy nose and hoarseness, productive cough, thin and white tongue coating, and superficial pulse. It is also indicated for the initial stage of pyogenic skin infection with local redness, heat, swelling and pain, which is associated with the exterior syndrome.

Decoction of Ephedrae, Aconiti Lateralis and Asari
麻黄附子细辛汤 *ma huang fu zi xi xin tang*
(from *Treatise on Cold Diseases*)

Herba Ephedrae	6 g
Radix Aconiti Lateralis Preparata	3 g
Herba Asari	3 g

Administration: Decoct with water for oral administration.

Action: Restoring *yang* to expel superficial pathogens.

Indications: Exterior syndrome caused by exogenous pathogens with *yang* deficiency, exhibiting severe chills, slight fever, and deep pulse.

Explanation: In cases of an attack by wind and cold, the pathogens stay in the surface of the body, causing exterior syndrome with chills and fever. But, since there is also deficiency of *yang qi*, chills is severe while fever is slight, and the pulse is not superficial but deep. Although the exterior syndrome should be treated by inducing sweating, the *yang qi* deficiency makes it impossible to expel the pathogens from the exterior, and so the proper treatment is to strengthen *yang qi* to expel the pathogens from the exterior. In this case, the pathogens are eliminated and the *yang qi* restored at the same time. In the prescription, Ephedrae and Aconiti Lateralis are used as the chief ingredients—the former is used to expel cold from the exterior, and the latter to warm the meridians and restore *yang*. Asari, which serves as the adjuvant ingredient and is acrid and warm, expels the pathogens and restores *yang qi*, thus helping strengthen the actions of Ephedrae and Aconiti Lateralis.

Modified Decoction of Polygonati Odorati
加减葳蕤汤 *jia jian wei rui tang*
(from *The Revised Popular Treatise on Cold Diseases*)

Rhizoma Polygonati Odorati	9 g
Bulbus Allii Fistulosi	6 g
Radix Platycodi	5 g
Radix Cynanchi Atrati	3 g
Semen Sojae Preparatum	9 g
Herba Menthae	3 g
Radix Glycyrrhizae Preparata	2 g
Fructus Jujubae	2 pieces

Administration: Decoct with water for oral use.

Action: Nourishing *yin* and relieving exterior syndrome.

Indications: *Yin* deficiency associated with exterior syndrome, exhibiting headache, fever, slight aversion to wind and cold, no or little sweating, cough, dry throat, thirst, vexation, red tongue, and rapid pulse.

Explanation: *Yin* deficiency usually produces internal heat. When a *yin*-deficient constitution is attacked by wind, the above-mentioned symptoms appear. *Yin* deficiency always results in insufficient production of body fluid (including sweat). Therefore, it is improper simply to induce sweating, for the body fluid may be consumed and *yin* damaged. Instead, a combined remedy to nourish *yin* and expel the pathogens should be chosen. In this prescription, Polygonati Odorati, a tonic that is not greasy, is used as the chief ingredient to nourish *yin* and moisten dryness and replenish the source of sweat; Allii Fistulosi, Sojae Preparatum and Menthae serve as the adjuvant ingredients to relieve the exterior syndrome and release the inhibited lung *qi*; Platycodi, which eliminates phlegm and eases the throat, and Cynanchi Atrati, which purges heat and relieves vexation, are used as the assistant ingredients; and Glycyrrhizae and Jujubae, which are sweet and capable of promoting fluid production, can help Polygonati Odorati nourish *yin* and moisten dryness, and also serve as the guide to regulate the effects of the other drugs. The combination of all these drugs can induce sweating but not damage *yin*, and nourish *yin* but not cause retention of pathogens. For severe exterior syndrome, Radix Ledebouriellae and Radix Puerariae are added to expel exogenous pathogens; for a case complicated by cough, difficult expectoration and dry throat, Fructus Arctii and Pericarpium Trichosanthis are added to ease the throat and eliminate phlegm; for cases with severe thirst and vexation, Herba Lophatheri and Radix Trichosanthis are added to purge heat and promote fluid production.

Summary

Included in this chapter are eleven principal and four appendant prescriptions, all of which are classified into three categories:

(1) Prescriptions composed of acrid and warm drugs to relieve exterior syndrome:

Prescriptions falling into this category include Decoction of Ephedrae, Decoction of Cinnamomi, Decoction of Nine Ingredients Containing Notopterygii, and Small Blue Dragon Decoction. They all act to expel cold from the exterior and are indicated for exterior syndrome due to exposure to wind and cold. Decoction of Ephedrae, for its combined use of Herba Ephedrae and Ramulus Cinnamomi, is much more potent in inducing sweating, and is indicated for exterior-excess syndromes due to exposure to wind and cold; Decoction of Ramulus Cinnamomi is less potent in this respect, but can satisfactorily expel pathogens from the muscles and regulate the *ying* and *wei* systems, and is indicated for exterior-deficiency syndrome due to exposure to wind and cold; Decoction of Nine Ingredients Containing Notopterygii not only greatly induces sweating, but also eliminates dampness and endogenous heat, and is often used for cases of common cold with wind, cold and dampness in the exterior. Small Blue Dragon Decoction relieves exterior syndrome and fluid retention, and is indicated for diseases due to wind-cold associated with fluid retention; Powder of Elsholtziae seu Moslae eliminates summer-heat and exogenous pathogens, dispels dampness and regulates the middle *jiao*, and is commonly used for disorders due to cold in summer complicated by interior dampness.

(2) Prescriptions composed of acrid and cool drugs for relieving exterior syndrome:

Both Decoction of Mori and Chrysanthemi and Powder of Lonicerae and Forsythiae relieve exterior syndrome due to exposure to wind-heat. Of the two, the former is effective for releasing the inhibited lung *qi* and cough, and is indicated for mild exterior-heat syndrome with cough as the chief symptom. The latter is effective for purging heat and toxins and expelling wind from the exterior, and is indicated for serious cases of exterior-heat syndrome with fever and thirst as the predominant symptoms. Another prescription, Decoction of Ephedrae, Armeniacae Amarum, Glycyrrhizae and Gypsum Fibrosum, releases inhibited lung *qi*, purging lung heat and relieves dyspnea, and is indicated for excessive lung heat manifested as dyspneic cough.

(3) Prescriptions for relieving exterior syndrome by supporting antipathogenic *qi*:

Antiphlogistic Powder, Decoction of Ephedrae, Aconiti Lateralis and Asari, and Modified Decoction of Polygonati Odorati are all effective for exterior syndrome due to exogenous pathogens and complicated by antipathogenic *qi* deficiency. Of the three, the first eliminates wind and dampness, benefits *qi* and relieves exterior syndrome, and is indicated for cases accompanied by antipathogenic *qi* deficiency and caused by wind, cold and dampness; the second is a typical one for restoring *yang* and expelling superficial pathogens, and is indicated for cases with *yang* deficiency and exterior-cold syndrome; and the third is effective for nourishing *yin* and expelling superficial pathogens, and is indicated for constitutional weakness due to *yin* deficiency complicated by exterior syndrome due to exposure to wind-heat.

CHAPTER SEVEN

PRESCRIPTIONS FOR PURGATION

Prescriptions for purgation (*xie xia ji*) are mainly composed of purgative drugs and act to eliminate heat, relax the bowels and relieve food stagnation and fluid retention. They are applied for interior-excess syndrome, and their use falls into the category of purgation therapy.

Because the interior-excess syndrome has different etiology, it can be divided into different types clinically, such as that marked by dry stool, by food stagnation, and by fluid retention. In terms of nature, it can be divided the heat type and the cold type. Furthermore, prescriptions for purgation are subdivided into five kinds: purgation by cold drugs, by warm drugs and by lubricant drugs, purgation by relieving fluid retention, and purgation combined with invigoration.

Prescriptions for purgation with cold drugs (*han xia ji*) are indicated for excess syndrome associated with interior heat and food stagnation, which exhibits constipation, abdominal distention or pain, hectic fever, yellow tongue coating and forceful pulse. Such prescriptions are chiefly composed of cold purgatives, such as Radix et Rhizoma Rhei and Natrii Sulfas, in combination with drugs that activate *qi*, purge heat and promote blood circulation. The examples are Decoction for Potent Purgation and Decoction of Rhei and Moutan Radicis.

Prescriptions for purgation with warm drugs (*wen xia ji*) are indicated for excess syndrome associated with interior cold and food stagnation, which exhibits constipation, abdominal pain that can be relieved by warmth, cold limbs, and deep and tense pulse. Purgatives and drugs for warming the interior are usually used together to form such prescriptions. Decoction of Rhei and Aconiti Lateralis Preparata is one example.

Prescriptions for purgation with lubricant drugs (*run xia ji*) are indicated for constipation due to fluid consumption by accumulated heat in the stomach and intestines. Such prescriptions are usually composed of lubricant drugs, such as Fructus Cannabis and Semen Pruni, in combination with cold purgatives, such as Rhei, and drugs that nourish *yin* and blood, such as Radix Rehmanniae and Radix Paeoniae Alba. One example is Bolus of Cannabis.

Prescriptions for purgation by relieving fluid retention (*zhu shui ji*) are indicated for excess syndrome with retained fluid in the interior. Drugs for relieving fluid retention, such as Radix Euphorbiae Pekinensis, Radix Kansui, Flos Genkwa and Semen Pharbitidis, are usually used together with drugs that nourish the stomach and the spleen, such as Fructus Jujubae. One example is Decoction of Jujubae.

Prescriptions for purgation with invigoration (*gong bu jian shi ji*) are indicated for interior-excess syndrome marked by deficient antipathogenic *qi* and constipation. Purgatives, such as Rhei and Natrii Sulfas, are usually used together with drugs that invigorate *qi* and enrich blood, or drugs that nourish *yin* and promote fluid production, such as Radix Ginseng, Radix Angelicae Sinensis, Radix Rehmanniae, Radix Scrophulariae and Radix Ophiopogonis. Three examples are Yellow Dragon Decoction, Decoction for Warming the Spleen, and Decoction for Fluid Increasing and Purgation.

Attention should be given to the individual clinical case. If exterior syndrome is not thoroughly relieved when interior-excess syndrome appears, it is advisable to relieve the exterior syndrome first and then cure the interior-excess syndrome, or else treat both at the same time. For exterior syndrome in aged people with delicate constitution, or when fluid consumption follows prolonged illness, and if there is *qi* and blood deficiency, purgation therapy should not be used alone. In this case, purgation should be used with invigoration. For pregnant women, purgative prescriptions should be used with caution. Moreover, three kinds of purgative prescriptions, namely, that with cold drugs, that with warm drugs and that for relieving fluid retention, are liable to damage stomach *qi*. Special attention should therefore be given to their dosage. In order to avoid damaging stomach *qi*, greasy food and other food that is not easy to digest should be avoided when purgative prescriptions are administered.

Decoction for Potent Purgation

大承气汤 *da cheng qi tang*

(from *Treatise on Cold Diseases*)

Radix et Rhizoma Rhei	12 g
Cortex Magnoliae Officinalis (prepared with ginger)	24 g
Fructus Aurantii Immaturus	15 g
Natrii Sulfas	9 g

Administration: Boil Aurantii Immaturus and Magnoliae Officinalis first and then together with Rhei. Discard the dregs, add Natrii Sulfas and then let it boil gently for a moment. Divide the decoction into two doses and take it warm.

Action: Potent purgation for eliminating accumulated heat.

Indications: Excess syndrome of the Yangming *fu* organ exhibiting constipation, abdominal flatulence, pain and tenderness, or even hectic fever, delirium, profuse sweating of the limbs, prickled tongue with dry and yellow coating, or fissured tongue with dry and black coating, and deep and forceful pulse. The prescription is also indicated for fecal impaction due to heat with watery diarrhea, or cold limbs due to excessive interior heat.

Explanation: This is a typical prescription for purgation with cold drugs. Excess syndrome of Yangming *fu* organ is an instance of excess syndrome due to interior heat, caused by the attack of the Yangming *fu* organ by heat, leading to dry stool in the intestines. The therapeutic principle for this syndrome should be to expel heat to loosen the bowels with potent purgatives. In the prescription, Rhei serves as the chief drug; it is cold and bitter, and acts to purge heat in order to relax the bowels and relieve food stagnation; Natrii Sulfas, serving as the adjuvant, is salty and cold, softens the dry feces, and strengthen the action of Rhei in purging heat to relax the bowels when used together with Rhei. When there is stagnant food in the stomach and intestines and the visceral *qi* is blocked, Magnoliae Officinalis and Aurantii Immaturus are used as the assistant and the guide to activate *qi* circulation, relieve distention and flatulence, helping Natrii Sulfas and Rhei to purge heat and relax the bowels. Clinical evidence calling for the application of this prescription is epigastric upset, fullness over the chest and abdomen, dry stool, and abdominal pain and tenderness with constipation or watery diarrhea. Besides, tongue coating and pulse condition should also be considered.

Appendant Prescription

(1) Decoction for Mild Purgation
小承气汤 *xiao cheng qi tang*
(from *Treatise on Cold Diseases*)

This prescription is composed of 12 g of Radix et Rhizoma Rhei (prepared with wine), 6 g of Cortex Magnoliae Officinalis (prepared with ginger), and 9 g of Fructus Aurantii Immaturus (fried). The drugs are decocted with water and the decoction is taken in two separate doses. It has a mild purgative action for accumulated heat, and is indicated for mild cases of excess syndrome of the Yangming *fu* organ exhibiting constipation, fullness of the chest and abdomen, hectic fever, rough and yellow tongue coating, and smooth and rapid pulse.

(2) Decoction for Purgation and Regulation of Stomach *Qi*
调胃承气汤 *tiao wei cheng qi tang*
(from *Treatise on Cold Diseases*)

It is composed of 12 g of Radix et Rhizoma Rhei (prepared with wine), 6 g of Radix Glycyrrhizae Preparata, and 12 g of Natrii Sulfas. Decoct Rhei and Glycyrrhizae first and then add Natrii Sulfas, let it boil on a gentle fire for a moment. Take the warm decoction all at once. It has a demulcent purgative action for accumulated heat, and is indicated for slow cases of excess syndrome of Yangming *fu* organ with the symptoms of constipation, vexation, thirst, fever, or fullness of the abdomen, yellow tongue coating, and smooth and rapid pulse, as well as for eruptive diseases with hemorrhage, toothache and sore throat due to the accumulation of heat in the stomach and intestines.

The above three prescriptions are all indicated for excess syndrome of the Yangming *fu* organ. Decoction for Potent Purgation has a strong purgative action, and is indicated for serious cases of heat accumulation in the Yangming *fu* organ exhibiting all the major symptoms mentioned above. Decoction for Mild Purgation has a mild action and is indicated for mild cases of heat accumulation in the Yangming *fu* organ with all main symptoms except dry stool. Decoction for Purgation and Regulation of Stomach *Qi* has a more demulcent purgative action, and is indicated for cases of heat accumulation in the Yangming *fu* organ exhibiting dry stool, abdominal pain and tenderness.

Decoction of Rhei and Moutan Radicis
大黄牡丹汤 *da huang mu dan tang*
(from *Synopsis of the Golden Cabinet*)

Radix et Rhizoma Rhei	12 g
Cortex Moutan Radicis	9 g
Semen Persicae	12 g
Semen Benincasae	30 g
Natrii Sulfas	9 g

Administration: First decoct all the drugs except Natrii Sulfas, discard the dregs and add Natrii Sulfas and let the decoction boil again. Take the decoction all at once.

Action: Purging heat, removing blood stasis, relieving swelling and resolving masses.

Indications: The early stage of acute appendicitis, exhibiting pain and tenderness in the right lower abdomen, even local mass formation, or preference for bending the right lower limb, aggravation of abdominal pain by extending the right leg, or intermittent fever, spontaneous sweating, chills, and thin and greasy yellow tongue coating.

Explanation: At the onset of acute appendicitis, dampness-heat accumulates in the intestinal tract and the circulation of *qi* and blood is blocked, giving rise to abscess. Because of the accumulation of heat and blood stasis, local abdominal pain and tenderness or even a local mass occur. The treatment aims at purging heat, removing blood stasis and eliminating the masses. In this prescription, Rhei, which serves as the chief drug, purges heat, relaxes the bowels, activates blood circulation and removes blood stasis; Moutan Radicis, as the adjuvant, purges heat, cools the blood, and also activates blood circulation and removes blood stasis; Natrii Sulfas dissipates the masses, and is used together with Rhei to strengthen the effect of purging heat and relaxing the bowels; Persicae activates blood circulation, removes blood stasis and relaxes the bowels; Benincasae purges dampness-heat, promotes pus discharge and removes masses. These three all serve as both the assistant and the guide. As a whole, this prescription consists of three kinds of drugs: bitter and cold purgatives, drugs that activate blood circulation and remove blood stasis, and drugs that purge dampness-heat. It thus has the special effects of purging dampness-heat, removing blood stasis by purgation as well as relieving pain and swelling.

In order to get a better result, some other drugs that purge heat and toxins, activate blood circulation and remove blood stasis, such as Flos Lonicerae, Herba Taraxaci, Herba Hedyotis Diffusae, Herba Patriniae, Radix Aucklandiae and Fructus Aurantii Immaturus, can also be included.

Decoction of Rhei and Aconiti Lateralis Preparata
大黄附子汤 *da huang fu zi tang*
(from *Synopsis of the Golden Cabinet*)

Radix et Rhizoma Rhei	9 g
Radix Aconiti Lateralis Preparata	9 g
Herba Asari	6 g

Administration: Decoct with water for oral administration.

Action: Relaxing the bowels to purge accumulated pathogen, warming the interior to expel cold.

Indications: Excess syndrome due to accumulation of cold marked by abdominal pain, constipation, cold limbs, fever, greasy white tongue coating, and taut and tense pulse.

Explanation: Unscrupulous intake of food and drink complicated by cold, in which the cold enters the interior through the meridians, leading to failure of transportation of nutrients, blockage of visceral *qi* and accumulation of pathogenic cold. Abdominal pain and constipation thus result. Splenic *yang* is blocked and fails to reach the limbs, causing cold limbs and fever. Greasy and white tongue coating, and taut and tense pulse are also manifestations of excess-cold syndrome. For this syndrome, the therapeutic principle is to relax the bowels to purge the accumulated pathogen, and warm the interior to eliminate cold. In the prescription, Rhei, bitter and cold, and acting to relax the bowels and purge accumulated cold, is used together with acrid and hot Aconiti Lateralis Preparata, which warms the interior to eliminate cold and is capable of checking the cold nature of Rhei. They are both used as the chief ingredients. Asari helps expel cold and relieve pain, and strengthens the effect of Aconiti Lateralis Preparata, serving as the assistant. All three drugs are used together to relax the bowels and eliminate cold, and so are suitable for the excess syndrome due to accumulated cold.

Both this prescription and Decoction of Ephedrae, Aconiti Lateralis and Asari include Aconiti Lateralis Preparata and Asari, which are used to warm the interior to expel cold. But the former, in which Aconiti Lateralis Preparata, Asari and Rhei are used together, is for purgation with warm drugs and is indicated for excess syndrome due to accumulated cold; while the latter, in which Aconiti Lateralis Preparata, Asari and Ephedrae are combined, is for relieving exterior syndrome by enforcing *yang qi*, and is indicated for exterior-cold syndrome complicated by *yang* deficiency.

Bolus of Cannabis
麻子仁丸 *ma zi ren wan*
(from *Treatise on Cold Diseases*)

Fructus Cannabis	500 g
Radix Paeoniae Lactiflorae	250 g
Fructus Aurantii Immaturus	250 g

Radix et Rhizoma Rhei	500 g
Cortex Magnoliae Officinalis (prepared with ginger)	100 g
Semen Armeniacae Amarum	250 g

Administration: Grind the drugs into fine powder and prepare it with honey into boluses. Take 9 g with warm water each time, twice a day. They may also be prepared into decoction, with their dosages reduced proportionally.

Action: Lubricating the intestine to induce bowel movements.

Indications: Cases with dryness-heat in the stomach and intestines and fluid deficiency, manifested as constipation and frequent micturition.

Explanation: Dryness-heat in the stomach and intestines and fluid deficiency may cause constipation. The spleen has the function of transporting the nutrients from the stomach. If it is affected by dryness-heat and fails to distribute fluid to the whole body, the fluid gathers in the urinary bladder, leading to frequent micturition. Dryness-heat may also consume fluid, causing dryness of the intestines and resulting in constipation. The therapeutic principle is to lubricate the intestines and promote bowel movements to relieve constipation, which is combined with purging heat and dispersing stagnation. In the prescription, Cannabis serves as the chief drug and acts to lubricate the intestines and promote bowel movements; Armeniacae Amarum, which lowers the adversely rising lung *qi* and lubricates the bowels, and Paeoniae Lactiflorae, which nourishes *yin* and regulates the interior, are used together with Cannabis to lubricate the bowels to relieve constipation. They both serve as the adjuvant. Rhei, which purges heat and relaxes the bowels, and Aurantii Immaturus and Magnoliae Officinalis, which activate *qi*, disperse stagnation and strengthen the purgative effect, are used as the assistant and guide. This is a typical recipe for purgation composed of lubricant drugs; it is lubricant but not greasy, and possesses a moderate purgative effect.

This prescription is the most suitable for constipation with dryness-heat in the gastrointestinal tract and fluid deficiency. It is also indicated for constipation due to intestinal dryness in the aged and the parturient. But, it should be used with caution for pregnant patients.

Decoction of Jujubae
十枣汤 *shi zao tang*
(from *Treatise on Cold Diseases*)

Flos Genkwa
Radix Kansui
Radix Euphorbiae Pekinensis
(in equal amount)

Administration: Grind the drugs into fine powder and take 0.5-1 g of the powder (increasing the dosage progressively) once a day in early morning on an empty stomach with a decoction prepared with 10 pieces of Fructus Jujubae. Take some gruel after purgation.

Action: Relieving fluid retention.

Indications: Fluid-retention syndrome in the thorax (*xuan yin*) marked by cough, shortness of breath, pain over the chest and hypochondriac region, headache, dizziness, and taut and deep pulse; and also edema and ascites of the excess syndrome.

Explanation: Fluid retained in the chest and hypochondriac region and obstruction of *qi* circulation causes pain in these regions. It affects the lung, leading to obstruction of lung *qi* and giving rise to cough and shortness of breath. It also displaces lucid *yang* upward, causing headache and dizziness. Deep pulse indicates an internal disorder and taut pulse implies fluid retention and pain. So in the case of fluid retained in the interior associated with pain over the chest and hypochondriac region, deep and taut pulse appears. If fluid is retained in the abdomen and *qi* circulation is obstructed, edema with ascites occurs. The treatment is to relieve fluid retention with potent purgatives. In this prescription, the combination of Kansui, Euphorbiae Pekinensis and Genkwa is very effective in relieving fluid retention and edema. This decoction invigorates the spleen and nourishes the stomach, and counteracts the toxicity and inhibits the potent effects of the other drugs, thus relieving retention but not damaging the antipathogenic *qi*.

This is a prescription for relieving fluid retention with potent purgatives. If incessant diarrhea occurs after taking the powder or decoction, take some gruel. For patients with weak constitution, apply this and a tonic prescription alternately—the purgative one first and then the tonic one, or vice versa. Remember that this prescription is contraindicated for pregnant women.

Appendant Prescription

Pill for Treating Phlegm Syndrome

控涎丹 *kong xian dan*

(from *Treatise on the Tripartite Pathogenesis of Diseases*)

This is composed of equal amounts of Radix Kansui, Radix Euphorbiae Pekinensis and Semen Sinapis Albae. Grind the drugs into fine powder and prepare the powder with water into pills of mung-bean size. Take 1-3 g each time in early morning on an empty stomach with thin ginger decoction or date decoction. It acts to eliminate phlegm and relieve retained fluid, and is indicated for cases with phlegm-fluid retention in the chest marked by sudden intolerable wandering pain in the chest, the back, the neck and the waist, or severe headache, fatigue and somnolence, tastelessness, thick sputum, a wheezing sound in the throat in night, and salivation.

In this prescription, Sinapis Albae is acrid and warm, and has the effects of activating *qi* circulation and eliminating phlegm; it is especially effective for phlegm-fluid retention in the chest and hypochondrium. When it is used together with Kansui and Euphorbiae Pekinensis, Sinapis Albae is especially effective for relieving retained phlegm.

Yellow Dragon Decoction
黄龙汤 *huang long tang*
(from *Six Books on Cold Diseases*)

Radix et Rhizoma Rhei	12 g
Natrii Sulfas	9 g
Fructus Aurantii Immaturus	6 g
Cortex Magnoliae Officinalis	12 g
Radix Glycyrrhizae	3 g
Radix Ginseng	6 g
Radix Angelicae Sinensis	4 g

Administration: Add 3 g of Radix Platycodi, 3 pieces of Rhizoma Zingiberis Recens and 2 pieces of Fructus Jujubae to the prescription, and decoct with water for oral administration.

Action: Purging heat, promoting bowel movements, invigorating *qi* and nourishing the blood.

Indications: Interior-excess syndrome due to accumulation of heat with deficiency of *qi* and blood, marked by watery diarrhea or constipation, abdominal distention, pain and tenderness, fever, thirst, delirium, listlessness, shortness of breath, dry yellow or dry black tongue coating, and feeble pulse.

Explanation: Watery diarrhea or constipation associated with abdominal distention, pain and tenderness, fever, delirium, and dry yellow or dry black tongue coating are the manifestations of excess syndrome due to accumulated heat in the *zang* organs. Listlessness, shortness of breath and feeble pulse indicate deficient antipathogenic *qi* and blood. This should be treated by purgation combined with reinforcement. In the prescription, Rhei, Natrii Sulfas, Aurantii Immaturus, Magnoliae Officinalis make up the Decoction for Potent Purgation, which can purge heat, induce bowel movements to eliminate the accumulated heat promptly, while at the same time preserving the antipathogenic *qi*. Ginseng and Angelicae Sinensis invigorate *qi* and nourish the blood, and so help the antipathogenic *qi* purge the accumulated heat. Platycodi is added to release the inhibited lung *qi* and loosen the bowels. Zingiberis Recens, Jujubae and Glycyrrhizae are used to support stomach *qi* and regulate the actions of the other drugs. Therefore, this prescription is both for purgation and also for supporting the antipathogenic *qi*.

Decoction for Warming the Spleen
温脾汤 *wen pi tang*
(from *Essentially Treasured Prescriptions for Emergencies*)

Radix et Rhizoma Rhei	12 g
Radix Aconiti Lateralis Preparata	9 g
Rhizoma Zingiberis	6 g

Radix Ginseng	6 g
Radix Glycyrrhizae	6 g

Administration: Decoct the drugs with water for oral administration (put in Radix et Rhizoma Rhei later than other drugs).

Action: Warming and recuperating spleen *yang*, and relieving masses.

Indications: Cases with spleen *yang* deficiency, manifested as constipation due to accumulation of cold, or diarrhea with mucous and bloody stools, abdominal pain, cold limbs, and deep and taut pulse.

Explanation: Deficiency of spleen *yang* leads to generation of endogenous cold which, plus preference for cold and raw food, causes accumulation of cold in the intestines. Hence, constipation, abdominal coldness and pain occur. Deficient *yang* fails to reach the limbs, which thus become cold. If cold accumulates in the body for a long time, it may lead to spleen *qi* deficiency, manifested as diarrhea with mucous and bloody stools. If treated only by warming and recuperating spleen *yang*, it is hard to eliminate the accumulated cold; if treated only by purgation, spleen *yang* will be damaged and the accumulated cold not necessarily purged. Hence, both principles of warming spleen *yang* and purging accumulated cold should be applied. In this prescription, Rhei is a purgative for eliminating accumulated pathogens, while Aconiti Lateralis Preparata warms the interior and helps *yang* eliminate cold, and both serve as the chief ingredients; Zingiberis warms the middle-*jiao*, Ginseng and Glycyrrhizae invigorate the spleen to benefit *qi*, and so the three are used as the assistant together with Aconiti Lateralis Preparata, which strengthens the action of warming spleen *yang*. Glycyrrhizae regulates the effects of the drugs, serving as the guide. This is a prescription for purgation with warm drugs, suitable for cases of *yang* deficiency in the middle *jiao* accompanied by accumulated cold.

The dosage of Rhei in this prescription is rather large. To treat a case with more serious deficiency cold in the spleen and stomach complicated by protracted dysentery and diarrhea, it should be reduced. For a case of deficient *yang* and excessive cold with accompanying severe abdominal pain, Cortex Cinnamomi may be added to strengthen the effects of warming the interior and relieving pain.

Decoction for Fluid Increase and Purgation

增液承气汤 *zeng ye cheng qi tang*

(from *Essentials of Seasonal Febrile Diseases*)

Radix Scrophulariae	30 g
Radix Ophiopogonis	24 g
Radix Rehmanniae	24 g
Radix et Rhizoma Rhei	9 g
Natrii Sulfas	5 g

Administration: Boil the drugs with water and then mix the decoction with Natrii Sulfas for oral use.

Action: Nourishing *yin*, increasing fluid, purging heat and relaxing the bowels.

Indications: Seasonal febrile diseases with accumulated heat and *yin* deficiency marked by constipation.

Explanation: In cases of seasonal febrile disease, heat accumulates in the gastrointestinal tract and consumes fluid, leading to constipation. This should be treated by nourishing *yin* and promoting fluid production with drugs that are sweet and cold, and by softening the indurative masses and inducing bowel movements with salty and bitter drugs. When *yin*-fluid is produced and dry stool is purged, the accumulated heat is relieved. In this prescription, Scrophulariae, Rehmanniae and Ophiopogonis (the ingredients of Fluid-Increasing Decoction) nourish *yin*, increase fluid secretion, moisten the intestines and promote bowel movements. Rhei and Natrii Sulfas purge heat, moisten the intestines and soften the dry feces. This is in fact a prescription for purgation associated with reinforcement.

Essentials of Seasonal Febrile Diseases points out that for febrile diseases of the Yangming accompanied by constipation due to the consumption of fluid, Fluid-Increasing Decoction is recommended to increase fluid production. If dry stool still remains, this indicates serious dryness, and thus Decoction for Fluid Increasing and Purgation should be used.

This prescription is mainly used for constipation due to accumulated heat and deficient *yin*. It is also suitable for long-standing cases of hemorrhoids with constipation due to accumulated heat and deficient *yin*.

Summary

This chapter has presented eight principal and three appendant prescriptions, all of which are classified into five types according to their actions:

(1) Prescriptions for purgation with cold drugs:

The typical examples of this type are Decoction for Potent Purgation and Decoction of Rhei and Moutan Radicis. The former mainly aims at eliminating heat by potent purgation and is indicated for excess syndrome of the Yangming *fu* organ due to interior heat, with such typical symptoms as epigastric upset, full sensation in the chest and abdomen, dry stool, and abdominal pain and tenderness with constipation or watery diarrhea. The latter mainly aims at purging heat, removing blood stasis, relieving swelling and dispersing stagnation, and is indicated for the early stage of acute appendicitis.

(2) Prescriptions for purgation with warm drugs:

Decoction of Rhei and Aconiti Lateralis Preparata is an example, and it purges accumulated cold, warms the interior and relieves pain, and is indicated for abdominal pain and constipation due to accumulated cold.

(3) Prescriptions for purgation with lubricant drugs:

Bolus of Cannabis falls into this category. It moistens the intestines to promote bowel movements and is also effective for purging heat and dispersing stagnation, suitable for constipation due to dryness-heat in the gastrointestinal tract and insufficient fluid.

(4) Prescriptions for purgation by relieving fluid retention:

Decoction of Jujubae is an example. It has potent effect and is indicated for fluid retention syndrome in the thorax, edema and flatulence of the excess type.

(5) Prescriptions for both purgation and invigoration:

Yellow Dragon Decoction, Decoction for Warming the Spleen and Decoction for Fluid Increasing and Purgation belong to this category. The first invigorates *qi* and nourishes the blood, and is indicated for excess syndrome with accumulated heat in the interior and *qi* and blood deficiency. The second is effective to purge the accumulated heat and warm spleen *yang*, and is indicated for constipation with accumulated cold due to spleen *yang* deficiency, or prolonged diarrhea with mucous and bloody stools. The third purges heat, promotes bowel movements, and also nourishes *yin* and increases fluid secretion, and so it is indicated for seasonal febrile diseases with heat accumulation and *yin* deficiency marked by constipation.

CHAPTER EIGHT
PRESCRIPTIONS OF RECONCILIATORY ACTION

Prescriptions of reconciliatory action (*he jie ji*) are indicated for Shaoyang diseases, disharmony between the liver and spleen and between the stomach and intestines. They fall into the regulative therapy.

Originally, such prescriptions were invented especially for Shaoyang diseases with heat retention in the gallbladder. Since the gallbladder is closely related to and paired with the liver, they influence each other when either is diseased, and even affects the spleen and stomach, leading to disharmony between the liver and spleen, and between the stomach and intestines. There are consequently three sub-categories of prescriptions.

(1) Prescriptions for regulating Shaoyang (he jie shao yang ji):

Such prescriptions are indicated for Shaoyang syndrome, a febrile disease caused by exogenous pathogens and marked by alternating episodes of chills and fever, chest and hypochondriac upset, vexation, vomiting, poor appetite, bitter taste, dry throat and dizziness. Radix Bupleuri, Herba Artemisiae Annuae and Radix Scutellariae are the commonly used drugs and they are usually combined with drugs that suppress the adversely rising *qi* and relieve vomiting. The examples are Decoction of Bupleuri for Regulating Shaoyang, Decoction of Bupleuri for Regulating Shaoyang and Yangming, and Decoction of Artemisiae Annuae and Scutellariae for Purging Dampness-Heat from Gallbladder.

(2) Prescriptions for reconciling the disharmony between the liver and spleen (*tiao he gan pi ji*):

They are indicated for cases with stagnant liver *qi* and disharmony between the liver and spleen, exhibiting such symptoms as fullness in the chest and hypochondrium, pain in the hypochondrium, abdominal pain and diarrhea. Drugs that disperse stagnant liver *qi* and regulate the spleen, such as Radix Bupleuri, Radix Paeoniae Alba, Rhizoma Atractylodis Macrocephalae and Poria are usually used in the prescriptions. *Xiaoyao* Powder and Powder for Treating Diarrhea with Abdominal Pain are two examples.

(3) Prescriptions for harmonizing the stomach and intestines (*tiao he chang wei ji*):

They are indicated for cases with gastrointestinal dysfunction and coexistence of cold and heat syndromes, marked by epigastric fullness, nausea, vomiting, abdominal pain or diarrhea with increased borborygmus. Rhizoma Pinelliae Preparata and Rhizoma Zingiberis are usually used together with Radix Scutellariae and Rhizoma Coptidis. One example is the Decoction of Pinelliae for Purging Stomach Fire.

However, this kind of prescriptions is not suitable when pathogens are still in the exterior and have not entered Shaoyang, or when they have entered the interior but heat in

Yangming is predominant. Moreover, it is also inappropriate for chills and fever caused by overstrain, improper diet, and *qi* and blood deficiency.

Decoction of Bupleuri for Regulating Shaoyang
小柴胡汤 *xiao chai hu tang*
(from *Treatise on Cold Diseases*)

Radix Bupleuri	12 g
Radix Scutellariae	9 g
Radix Ginseng	9 g
Radix Glycyrrhizae Preparata	6 g
Rhizoma Zingiberis Recens	9 g
Fructus Jujubae	4 pieces
Rhizoma Pinelliae Preparata	9 g

Administration: Decoct with water for oral administration.

Action: Eliminating pathogens from Shaoyang.

Indications: Shaoyang syndrome marked by alternating episodes of chills and fever, fullness in the chest and hypochondrium, poor appetite, restlessness, vomiting, bitter taste, dry throat, dizziness, thin white tongue coating, and taut pulse.

Explanation: This is a major prescription for eliminating pathogens from Shaoyang. Shaoyang, according to differential diagnosis based on the theory of six meridians, is located between the exterior (Taiyang) and the interior (Yangming). When exogenous pathogens attack Shaoyang, a conflict occurs between the pathogens and the antipathogenic *qi*, giving rise to alternating episodes of chills and fever. Moreover, the Shaoyang Meridian passes through the chest and hypochondrium; when pathogens are present in Shaoyang, the meridian *qi* is blocked and a full sensation over the chest and hypochondrium occurs. When gallbladder heat affects the stomach, stomach *qi* fails to descend, causing poor appetite and vomiting. Other symptoms, such as bitter taste, dry throat, dizziness and restlessness, are also caused by gallbladder heat affecting the upper part of the body. In this prescription, Bupleuri is used as the chief ingredient to expel the pathogens from the semi-exterior; Scutellariae is used as the adjuvant to disperse accumulated heat from the semi-interior; the two act together to eliminate the pathogens from Shaoyang. Pinelliae Preparata and Zingiberis Recens are used together to regulate the stomach and suppressing the adversely rising *qi*; Ginseng, Glycyrrhizae Preparata and Jujubae, serving as the assistant, invigorate and support the antipathogenic *qi*, and prevent the pathogens from entering the interior; Glycyrrhizae Preparata is used as the guide, coordinating the effects of all other drugs.

This is a representative prescription for Shaoyang syndrome. The clinical evidence calling for the use of this prescription is alternating episodes of chills and fever, fullness over the chest and hypochondrium, bitter taste, dry throat, white tongue coating, and taut pulse. For malaria with such chief symptoms and signs as alternating episodes of chills and fever (chills more severe than fever), vomiting, pain in the hypochondrium, white tongue coating and the absence of thirst, Radix Dichroae and Fructus Tsaoko are added. This prescription is also applicable for female patients with alternating episodes of chills and fever, bitter taste, dry throat and dizziness, resulting from exposure to wind during menstruation or after giving childbirth.

Decoction of Bupleuri for Regulating Shaoyang and Yangming
大柴胡汤 *da chai hu tang*
(from *Synopsis of the Golden Cabinet*)

Radix Bupleuri	12 g
Radix Scutellariae	9 g
Radix Paeoniae Lactiflorae	9 g
Rhizoma Pinelliae Preparata	9 g
Fructus Aurantii Immaturus	9 g
Radix et Rhizoma Rhei	9 g
Fructus Jujubae	4 pieces
Rhizoma Zingiberis Recens	12 g

Administration: Boil with water for oral administration.

Action: Eliminating pathogens from Shaoyang and purging accumulated heat from the interior.

Indications: Coexistence of Shaoyang and Yangming diseases, marked by alternating episodes of chills and fever, fullness over the chest and hypochondrium, incessant vomiting, restlessness, distention or pain in the epigastric region, constipation or diarrhea of the heat type, yellow tongue coating, and forceful and taut pulse.

Explanation: This is a chief prescription for coexisted Shaoyang and Yangming diseases. When pathogens are not eliminated from Shaoyang, there may be alternating episodes of chills and fever, and fullness over the chest and hypochondrium. Gallbladder heat in Shaoyang may lead to incessant vomiting and restlessness when it affects Yangming. Distention or pain over the epigastric region, constipation or diarrhea of the heat type are all due to pathogens that affect Yangming along with heat accumulated in the interior. The treatment should concentrated on regulation while aided by purgation. In the prescription, Bupleuri is the chief drug, and it is used together with Scutellariae to eliminate pathogens from Shaoyang and purge heat. Rhei and Aurantii Immaturus, which serve as the adjuvant ingredients, are used to purge heat accumulated in Yangming. Paeoniae Lactiflorae, helping Rhei and Aurantii Immaturus relieve abdominal pain, and Zingiberis Recens, helping Pinelliae Preparata suppress the adverse flow of stomach *qi* and relieve vomiting, are used as the assistant. Jujubae, serving as the guide, invigorates the spleen, regulates stomach *qi* and balance the effects of the other drugs.

Alternative episodes of chills and fever, distention and pain over the chest and hypochondrium or in the epigastric region, constipation, and yellow tongue coating are evidence calling for the application of this prescription. For severe fullness in the chest and pain over the hypochondrium, Radix Curcumae and Pericarpium Citri Reticulatae Viride are added; for dominant gallbladder heat and the formation of stones, Herba Lysimachiae and Spora Lygodii are added to promote bile secretion and remove stones.

Decoction of Artemisiae Annuae and Scutellariae for Eliminating Dampness-Heat from the Gallbladder

蒿芩清胆汤 *hao qin qing dan tang*

(from *The Revised Popular Treatise on Cold Diseases*)

Herba Artemisiae Annuae	6 g
Caulis Bambusae in Taeniam	9 g
Rhizoma Pinelliae Preparata	5 g
Poria Rubra	9 g
Radix Scutellariae	9 g
Fructus Aurantii	5 g
Pericarpium Citri Reticulatae	5 g
Mixed powder of Talcum, Radix Glycyrrhizae and Indigo Naturalis (wrapped in a piece of gauze)	6 g

Administration: Boil with water for oral administration.

Action: Clearing gallbladder heat, eliminating dampness, regulating stomach function and eliminating phlegm.

Indications: Cases of dampness-heat in the gallbladder meridian and phlegm retained in the middle *jiao*, exhibiting alternating episodes of chills and fever (with fever being predominant), bitter taste, chest depression, vomiting of bilious fluid or yellowish mucous sputum, or even hiccup, distention and pain in the chest and hypochondrium, red tongue with greasy white or greasy yellow coating, and smooth, taut and rapid pulse.

Explanation: This prescription is commonly used to treat Shaoyang diseases accompanied by high fever and phlegm retention in the middle *jiao*. When the pathogen is in Shaoyang, excessive heat will be witnessed in the gallbladder meridian, leading to alternating episodes of chills and fever (with fever being predominant). When gallbladder heat attacks the stomach, phlegm and dampness are retained in the interior and stomach *qi* rises adversely, leading to vomiting of bilious fluid or yellowish mucous sputum, and hiccup. Chest depression, distention and pain in the chest and hypochondrium all result from the stagnant heat and retained phlegm, which disturb *qi* circulation. In the prescription, Artemisiae Annuae is fragrant and acts to eliminate accumulated heat from Shaoyang; Scutellariae is bitter and cold, and eliminates accumulated fire from the gallbladder. Both are used as chief ingredients. Caulis Bambusae in Taeniam, Pinelliae Preparata, Citri Reticulatae, and Aurantii combined together are used to purge gallbladder heat, regulate stomach *qi*, eliminate phlegm and suppress the adversely rising *qi*; they all serve as the adjuvant ingredients. Poria Rubra and the mixed powder of Talcum, Glycyrrhizae and Indigo Naturalis, serving as the assistant and guide, purge dampness-heat and guide heat downward. All the drugs combined have special effects of purging accumulated heat from

Shaoyang, relieving retained phlegm, and regulating gallbladder and stomach *qi*. Evidence calling for the application of this prescription is alternating episodes of chills and fever with fever being predominant, bitter taste, chest upset, vomiting of bilious fluid or yellowish mucous sputum. For severe vomiting, Rhizoma Coptidis and Fructus Evodiae are added to strengthen the effects of purging heat and dampness and suppressing the adversely rising stomach *qi*.

Xiaoyao Powder

逍遥散 *xiao yao san*

(from *Benevolent Prescriptions from the Pharmaceutical Bureau of the Taiping Period*)

Radix Glycyrrhizae Preparata	15 g
Radix Angelicae Sinensis	30 g
Poria	30 g
Radix Paeoniae Alba	30 g
Rhizoma Atractylodis Macrocephalae	30 g
Radix Bupleuri	30 g

Administration: Grind the drugs into fine powder and take 6-9 g of the powder with the decoction of burnt Rhizoma Zingiberis Recens and Herba Menthae. The drugs can also be prepared into pills, 6-9 g per dose; or prepared into decoction, with their dosage reduced proportionally.

Action: Dispersing stagnant liver *qi*, invigorating the spleen and nourishing the blood.

Indications: Blood deficiency syndrome with stagnant liver *qi* marked by pain in the hypochondrium, headache, dizziness, dry mouth and throat, poor appetite, listlessness, or alternating episodes of chills and fever, or irregular menstruation, distention of the breast, light red tongue, and taut and feeble pulse.

Explanation: The prescription is a common recipe for blood deficiency syndrome with stagnation of liver *qi*, and disharmony between the liver and the spleen. In cases of blood deficiency with stagnation of liver *qi*, the stagnant *qi* fails to nourish the liver, leading to hypochondriac pain, headache, dizziness, dry mouth and throat, and distensive pain of the breast. If the diseased liver affects the spleen, the spleen will not function properly in transporting and converting nutrient substances, causing poor appetite and listlessness. Such cases should be treated by dispersing stagnant liver *qi*, accompanied by nourishing the blood and invigorating the spleen. In the prescription, Bupleuri serves as the chief ingredient and acts to disperse stagnant liver *qi*. Angelicae Sinensis and Paeoniae Alba, as adjuvant, nourish the blood and invigorate the liver. Poria, Atractylodis Macrocephalae and Glycyrrhizae Preparata, which can invigorate the spleen and regulate the middle *jiao*, serve as the assistant drugs to help disperse stagnant liver *qi*. Burnt Zingiberis Recens is used as the guide, helping Poria and Atractylodis Macrocephalae regulate the middle *jiao*. Menthae is capable of helping Bupleuri to relieve stagnant liver *qi*.

Clinically, hypochondriac pain, poor appetite, listlessness, and taut and feeble pulse are the evidence calling for the application of the prescription. Since stagnant liver *qi*, spleen deficiency, and deficiency of the nutrient and blood are liable to cause irregular menstruation, the prescription is also frequently used to regulate it.

Appendant Prescription

Modified *Xiaoyao* Powder
加味逍遥散 *jia wei xiao yao san*
(from *Summary of Internal Medicine*)

This prescription is also called *Xiaoyao* Powder with Moutan Radicis and Gardeniae (*dan zhi xiao yao san* 丹栀逍遥散), which is composed by adding to the *Xiaoyao* Powder 3 g of Cortex Moutan Radicis and 3 g of Fructus Gardeniae. To be decocted for oral administration, it disperses stagnant liver *qi*, purges heat, nourishes the blood and regulates menstruation, and is indicated for blood deficiency syndrome with stagnant liver *qi* and heat production, manifested as irregular menstruation, distensive pain in the lower abdomen, irritability, headache and dry eyes.

Powder for Diarrhea with Abdominal Pain
痛泻要方 *tong xie yao fang*
(from *Complete Collection of Jingyue's Treatises*)

Rhizoma Atractylodis Macrocephalae (fried)	90 g
Radix Paeoniae Alba (fried)	60 g
Pericarpium Citri Reticulatae (fried)	45 g
Radix Ledebouriellae	60 g

Administration: The drugs may be prepared as pills or powder for oral administration, or as a decoction, with the dosage of the ingredients reduced proportionally.

Action: Regulating the function of the liver and spleen, relieving diarrhea and pain.

Indications: Diarrhea with abdominal pain due to dysfunction of the liver and spleen, accompanied by increased borborygmus, thin white tongue coating, and taut and slow pulse.

Explanation: This prescription is especially indicated for diarrhea with abdominal pain due to excess of the liver and deficiency of the spleen, leading to a disorder of the ascending-descending function. It should be treated by regulating the function of the liver and spleen. In the prescription, Atractylodis Macrocephalae invigorates the spleen and removes dampness, and Paeoniae Alba calms the liver and relieves diarrhea; both are used as the chief ingredients. Citri Reticulatae regulates the flow of *qi* and benefits the middle *jiao*, helping Atractylodis Macrocephalae invigorate the spleen, and Ledebouriellae, acrid and diaphoretic, eliminates dampness from the spleen and disperses stagnant liver *qi*. Both are used as the assistant drugs. The four drugs are used together to coordinate liver and spleen function, promote the normal circulation of *qi* and restore spleen function, thus relieving all the above symptoms.

The clinical evidence calling for the application of the prescription is diarrhea with abdominal pain that is relieved after diarrhea, and taut and slow pulse. In a chronic case of diarrhea, Rhizoma Cimicifugae (fried) is added to raise lucid *yang* so as to enhance the anti-diarrheic effect.

Decoction of Pinelliae for Purging Stomach Fire
半夏泻心汤 *ban xia xie xin tang*
(from *Treatise on Cold Diseases*)

Rhizoma Pinelliae Preparata	9 g
Radix Scutellariae	9 g
Rhizoma Zingiberis	9 g
Radix Ginseng	9 g
Radix Glycyrrhizae Preparata	6 g
Rhizoma Coptidis	3 g
Fructus Jujubae	4 pieces

Administration: Boil with water for oral administration.

Action: Keeping stomach *qi* downward and relieving epigastric fullness.

Indications: Epigastric fullness without pain, vomiting or retching, diarrhea, increased borborygmus, thin and greasy yellow tongue coating, and taut and rapid pulse.

Explanation: This was originally designed for epigastric fullness resulting from the misuse of purgation therapy for Shaoyang syndrome. When Shaoyang is affected, it should be treated with regulation therapy. The misuse of purgation therapy damages the middle *jiao qi* and thus pathogenic heat in Shaoyang moves inward. Cold associated with epigastric heat and stagnant *qi* thus occurs, leading to fullness in the epigastric region without pain. Splenic *qi* is also damaged, affecting the ascending-descending function and leading to vomiting and diarrhea. Cold and heat syndromes should therefore be relieved simultaneously, and the ascending-descending function should be restored. In the prescription, Scutellariae and Coptidis are bitter and cold, and are used as the chief ingredients to eliminate heat. Pinelliae Preparata is capable of regulating stomach *qi*, relieving epigastric fullness, suppressing the rising *qi* and relieving vomiting, while Zingiberis is warm, capable of eliminating cold and helping Pinelliae Preparata relieve fullness; both of them are used as the adjuvant. Ginseng, serving as the assistant, replenishes middle *jiao qi*. Glycyrrhizae Preparata and Jujubae invigorate spleen and stomach *qi*; both serve as the guide. As a whole, the prescription consists of acrid and bitter, warm and cold drugs that suppress the adverse upward flow of *qi*, relieve fullness and perform both the invigorative and purgative actions at the same time. It is especially effective for cases of painless epigastric fullness.

Moreover, the prescription can eliminate dampness-heat and harmonize the stomach and intestines. It is also applicable for retention of dampness-heat in the middle *jiao*, stomach and intestinal dysfunction, and simultaneous occurrence of cold and heat in both deficiency and excess syndromes. However, it should not be used for painless epigastric fullness due to phlegm and heat.

Summary

Selected in this chapter are six principal and one appendant prescriptions, all of which are classified into three sub-categories:

(1) Prescriptions for eliminating pathogens from Shaoyang:

Decoction of Bupleuri for Regulating Shaoyang, Decoction of Bupleuri for Regulating Shaoyang and Yangming, and Decoction of Artemisiae Annuae and Scutellariae for Clearing Away Dampness-Heat from Gallbladder eliminate pathogens from Shaoyang. The first one is the chief representative, and also has the effect of strengthening the antipathogenic *qi*; it is indicated for Shaoyang syndrome of exogenous febrile disease. The second, in addition to eliminating pathogens from Shaoyang, also purges accumulated heat from Yangming and is indicated for diseases involving both the Yangming and Shaoyang meridians simultaneously. The third purges heat from the gallbladder, eliminates dampness, regulates stomach *qi* and removes phlegm, and is indicated for dampness-heat in the gallbladder meridian and retained phlegm.

(2) Prescriptions for regulating the stomach and intestines:

Xiaoyao Powder and Powder for Diarrhea with Abdominal Pain are typical ones. The former disperses stagnant liver *qi*, nourishes the blood and invigorates the spleen, and is indicated for blood deficiency syndrome with stagnant liver *qi* and disharmony between the liver and the spleen, exhibiting hypochondriac pain, headache, dizziness, irregular menstruation, and distention of the breast. The latter has the principal effect of harmonizing the liver and the spleen, relieving diarrhea and pain, and is indicated for diarrhea with abdominal pain caused by liver excess and spleen deficiency.

(3) Prescriptions for regulating the stomach and intestines:

Decoction of Pinelliae for Purging Stomach Fire is an example. It regulates the flow of stomach *qi* and suppresses the adverse upward flow of *qi*, and is indicated for epigastric fullness caused by simultaneous occurrence of cold and heat and deficiency and excess in the stomach and intestines.

CHAPTER NINE
PRESCRIPTIONS FOR ELIMINATING HEAT

Prescriptions composed of drugs for purging heat, purging fire, cooling the blood and removing toxins and indicated for interior-heat syndrome, are called prescriptions for purging heat.

Interior-heat syndrome may be caused by exogenous or endogenous factors. The former refers to external pathogens that invade the body and turn into heat or fire; the latter refers to visceral excess or emotional disorders. Prescriptions introduced in this chapter are appropriate for treating interior-heat syndrome free from external affection as well as internal stagnation. Unrelieved exterior syndrome should be treated with prescriptions for relieving exterior syndrome; for excess syndrome that has already developed from interior heat, purgative prescriptions should be used; and for exterior syndrome that has not been relived while excess syndrome is developed, prescriptions for expelling pathogens from both the exterior and interior simultaneously are recommended.

Since the interior-heat syndrome has different manifestations in different cases, prescriptions for purging heat can be classified into six sub-categories.

(1) Prescriptions for purging heat from *qifen* (*qing qi fen re ji*):

They are indicated for the syndrome in which heat is at *qifen*, marked by high fever, thirst, profuse sweating, yellow tongue coating, bouncing or smooth and rapid pulse, or marked by continuous fever after illness, and restlessness. Drugs that purge heat and purge fire, such as Gypsum Fibrosum, Rhizoma Anemarrhenae, Herba Lophatheri and Fructus Gardeniae, are combined with drugs that benefit *qi* and promote fluid production. Two examples are White Tiger Decoction and Decoction of Lophatheri and Gypsum Fibrosum.

(2) Prescriptions for purging heat from *yingfen* and cooling the blood (*qing re liang xue ji*):

Such prescriptions are indicated for the syndrome in which pathogenic heat has entered *yingfen* or *xuefen*, exhibiting thirst or absence of thirst, coma, delirium, hemorrhage, skin rashes, crimson tongue and rapid pulse. Drugs that purge heat from *yingfen* and cooling the blood, such as Cornu Rhinocerotis and Radix Rehmanniae, are combined with drugs that purge heat and toxins and drugs that cool the blood and remove blood stasis. The examples are Decoction for Clearing Away Heat in the *Yingfen* and Decoction of Cornu Rhinocerotis and Rehmanniae.

(3) Prescriptions for purging heat and toxins (*qing re jie du ji*):

They are indicated for such serious cases as pestilence, acute febrile disease caused by virulent heat, or else pyogenic infection, which are usually marked by irritability, mania, hemorrhage, skin rashes, or redness and swelling of the head and face, or erosion of buccal mucosa and sore throat. Drugs that purge heat and toxins, such as Rhizoma Coptidis, Radix Scutellariae, Cortex Phellodendri and Fructus Gardeniae, are usually combined with drugs that purge heat or acrid and cool drugs of dispersive effect. Decoction of Coptidis for Detoxification and Decoction for General Antiphlogistic are two examples.

(4) Prescriptions for purging heat from *zang-fu* organs (*qing zang fu re ji*):

Such prescriptions are indicated for heat-syndromes caused by heat affecting the *zang-fu* organs. The symptoms vary with the location of the heat, and the prescriptions vary accordingly. The prototypes are Powder for Promoting Diuresis, Decoction of Gentianae for Purging Liver Fire, Powder for Clearing Away Stomach Heat, Powder for Expelling Lung Heat, Decoction of Puerariae, Scutellariae and Coptidis, and Decoction of Pulsatillae.

(5) Prescriptions for purging summer-heat (*qing re qu shu ji*):

These are indicated for diseases due to exposure to summer-heat, which is usually characterized by fever, restlessness, profuse sweating, thirst, or vomiting and diarrhea, or fatigue and feeble pulse. Drugs that purge summer-heat, such as Exocarpium Citrulli, Folium Nelumbinis, Petiolus Nelumbinis and Gypsum Fibrosum, are combined with drugs that expel pathogens from the exterior, promote diuresis, benefit *qi* and nourishing *yin*. Examples: Six-to-One Powder and Decoction for Clearing Away Summer-Heat and Benefiting *Qi*.

(6) Prescriptions for purging deficiency heat (*qing xu re ji*):

These are indicated for the late stage of febrile diseases with persistent heat and damaged *yin* fluid, exhibiting fever in the evening, and red tongue with little coating; they are also indicated for deficiency-heat syndrome due to deficient liver and kidney *yin* marked by prolonged fever. They are mainly composed of drugs that nourish *yin*, such as Carapax Trionycis, Herba Artemisiae Annuae, Radix Rehmanniae Rhizoma Anemarrhenae and Cortex Lycii Radicis. The examples are Decoction of Artemisiae Annuae and Carapax Trionycis, and Powder for Relieving Deficiency-Heat Syndrome.

In clinical application, some points warrant attention: (1) Prescriptions for purging heat are suitable only for interior-heat syndrome without any manifestations of exterior syndrome and without any internal stagnation. For cases with heat in the surface, the heat should first be expelled; for excess syndrome that has already developed from interior heat, the treatment should be purging the heat; for persistent exterior heat and dominant interior heat, treatment aims at expelling exterior heat and interior heat simultaneously. (2) The different heat-clearing prescriptions should be used accordingly on the basis of correct differentiation of the nature of the individual interior-heat syndrome (e.g., deficiency type or excess type), the location of the disease (e.g., at *qifen*, *yingfen* or *xuefen*), and in which *zang* or *fu* organ the heat is dominant. (3) It is important to differentiate whether the heat syndrome is true or false. If the case appears to be a heat syndrome but has the nature of a cold syndrome, it is not appropriate to use the heat-eliminating prescriptions. (4) Since heat is a *yang* pathogenic factor, it is liable to damage *yin*. So for cases in which *yin* is damaged by dominant internal heat, it is not appropriate to merely use bitter and cold drugs; other relevant drugs should be added accordingly. (5) For cases with dominant internal heat and vomiting immediately after taking the heat-eliminating prescriptions, add some ginger juice, or take the decoction when it is hot. (6) Prescriptions presented in this chapter are mainly composed of cold or cool drugs, which are liable to damage *yang qi* and the stomach. Hence, they should be used with caution and not in large dosage or for a long time.

White Tiger Decoction

白虎汤 *bai hu tang*

(from *Treatise on Cold Diseases*)

Rhizoma Anemarrhenae	18 g
Gypsum Fibrosum	30 g
Radix Glycyrrhizae Preparata	6 g
Fructus Oryzae Sativae	9 g

Administration: Boil the ingredients with water until the Oryzae Sativae is dissolved. Discard the dregs and take the decoction warm.

Action: Purging heat and promoting fluid production.

Indications: Exogenous febrile diseases with dominant heat in the Yangming Meridian, or seasonal febrile diseases with heat at *qifen*, marked by fever, flushed face, serious thirst, sweating, aversion to heat, and bouncing, large and forceful pulse.

Explanation: This prescription is indicated for excess-heat syndrome with the pathogens of exogenous febrile diseases transforming themselves into heat and entering the Yangming Meridian, or with the pathogens of seasonal febrile diseases entering *qifen*. Because of the domination of internal heat, fever and flushed face appear; heat makes the fluid escape outward, and thus profuse sweating and aversion to heat occur; intense heat consumes fluid, leading to serious thirst; when heat is excessive at *qifen* in the Yangming Meridian, a conflict between the pathogens and the antipathogenic *qi* occurs, leading to bouncing, large and forceful pulse. In the prescription, Gypsum Fibrosum, which is sweet, acrid and cold, purges heat and relieves vexation, and is used as the chief ingredient. Anemarrhenae, serving as the adjuvant, not only can help Gypsum Fibrosum purge excessive internal heat, but also nourish the damaged *yin*. Glycyrrhizae and Oryzae Sativae nourish the stomach and promote fluid production, and also prevent the extremely cold drugs from damaging the stomach. The four drugs used together produce a desirable effect.

This is a major prescription for excess-heat syndrome with heat at *qifen*. Clinical manifestations calling for its application are high fever, profuse sweating, serious thirst, and bouncing, large and forceful pulse.

The prescription is contraindicated for cases with (1) unrelieved exterior syndrome; fever but no sweating; (2) fever but no thirst; (3) excessive sweating but pale complexion; and (4) pulse bouncing and large but forceless upon heavy pressure.

Appendant Prescriptions

(1) White Tiger Decoction with Ginseng
白虎加人参汤 *bai hu jia ren shen tang*
(from *Treatise on Cold Diseases*)

Add 10 g of Radix Ginseng to the White Tiger Decoction and boil with water for oral administration. It acts to purge heat, benefit *qi* and promote fluid production. It is indicated for cases with typical manifestations suited to the application of White Tiger Decoction in addition to incessant serious thirst, profuse sweating, and large but forceless pulse, all of which are due to *qi* and fluid consumption.

(2) White Tiger Decoction with Ramulus Cinnamomi
白虎加桂枝汤 *bai hu jia gui zhi tang*
(from *Synopsis of the Golden Cabinet*)

Add 9 g of Ramulus Cinnamomi to White Tiger Decoction and boil with water for oral administration. It acts to purge heat, promote *qi* circulation and relieve pain, and is indicated for wind-dampness-heat *bi*-syndrome (*feng shi re bi*), exhibiting fever, vexation, swelling and pain of the joints, thirst; white tongue coating, and taut and rapid pulse.

(3) White Tiger Decoction with Atractylodis
白虎加苍术汤 *bai hu jia cang zhu tang*
(from *A Classified Book on Treating Cold Diseases*)

Add 9 g of Rhizoma Atractylodis to White Tiger Decoction and boil with water for oral administration. It acts to purge heat and dampness, and is indicated for dampness-warm diseases, marked by fever, chest upset, profuse sweating, and red tongue with white greasy coating.

The above three prescriptions are all based on White Tiger Decoction. The first aims at purging heat, benefiting *qi* and promoting fluid production. Ginseng is added to treat *qi* and fluid consumption due to dominant heat. This prescription is also suitable for summer-heat disease marked by profuse sweating and *qi* and fluid consumption. The second aims at purging heat, promoting *qi* circulation and relieving pain; it is indicated for heat-type *bi*-syndrome exhibiting prolonged fever, swelling and pain of the joints. The third, capable of purging heat and drying dampness, is applicable to dampness-warm disease with more heat than dampness.

Decoction of Lophatheri and Gypsum Fibrosum
竹叶石膏汤 *zhu ye shi gao tang*
(from *Treatise on Cold Diseases*)

Herba Lophatheri	12 g
Gypsum Fibrosum	30 g
Rhizoma Pinelliae Preparata	9 g
Radix Ophiopogonis	18 g
Radix Ginseng	6 g
Radix Glycyrrhizae Preparata	6 g
Fructus Oryzae Sativae	9 g

Administration: Boil the drugs except Oryzae Sativae with water and remove the dregs. Add Oryzae Sativae to the decoction and decoct again until the Oryzae Sativae is thoroughly cooked. Take the decoction warm with the Oryzae Sativae removed.

Action: Purging heat, promoting fluid production, benefiting *qi* and regulating the stomach.

Indications: The late stage of febrile diseases when fever has not subsided entirely and *qi* and fluid consumption has not yet been remedied, exhibiting fever, sweating, chest upset, nausea, dry mouth with a desire to drink, red tongue with little coating, and feeble and rapid pulse.

Explanation: When heat is not entirely eliminated in the late stage of a febrile disease, fever, sweating and chest upset appear; the stomach *qi* fails to descend, causing the adverse rising of *qi* and resulting in nausea; the consumption of *qi* and fluid in the late stage of a febrile disease causes dry mouth with the desire to drink, red tongue with little coating, and feeble and rapid pulse. In the prescription, Lophatheri and Gypsum Fibrosum are used as the chief ingredients to purge heat and relieve chest upset. Ginseng and Ophiopogonis, as the adjuvant, benefit *qi* and nourish *yin*. Pinelliae Preparata is used as the assistant to regulate stomach *qi* in order to relieve nausea. Glycyrrhizae and Oryzae Sativae are used as the guide to regulate the middle *jiao qi* and nourish stomach *qi*. The combination of all the drugs exerts the ideal effects of purging heat and invigorating the body.

This prescription is a modification of the White Tiger Decoction, with Rhizoma Anemarrhenae removed and Ginseng, Ophiopogonis, Lophatheri and Pinelliae Preparata added. Both this prescription and the White Tiger Decoction purge heat and promote fluid production, and are applicable to the syndrome with heat at *qifen*. Yet, this one also acts to benefit *qi*, nourish *yin* and regulate the stomach *qi*, and is indicated for febrile diseases in the late stage when *qi* and *yin* are consumed but fever stil! remains. The White Tiger Decoction is more effective in purging heat, and indicated for cases with high fever and extreme thirst, profuse sweating, as well as large and bouncing pulse.

Decoction for Eliminating Heat in the *Yingfen*

清营汤 *qing ying tang*

(from *Essentials of Seasonal Febrile Diseases*)

Cornu Rhinocerotis	2 g
Radix Rehmanniae	15 g
Radix Scrophulariae	9 g
Radix Ophiopogonis	9 g
Gemma Bambusae	3 g
Radix Salviae Miltiorrhizae	6 g
Rhizoma Coptidis	5 g
Flos Lonicerae	9 g
Fructus Forsythiae	6 g

Administration: Decoct the drugs except Cornu Rhinocerotis with water and remove the dregs. Grind Cornu Rhinocerotis into fine powder or grind it in a mortar to get juice, which is then mixed with the decoction for oral administration.

Action: Purging heat and toxins from *yingfen*, nourishing *yin* to release heat.

Indications: Heat syndrome involving *yingfen*, exhibiting fever which is higher at night, occasional delirium, restlessness, insomnia, thirst or no thirst, skin rashes, dry crimson tongue, and thready and rapid pulse.

Explanation: This is appropriate for the initial stage of heat syndrome involving *yingfen*. Heat attacking *yingfen* causes fever that is higher at night. *Ying qi* circulates to the heart, and if it is affected by heat, the heart is also disturbed, leading to restlessness, insomnia and occasional delirium. Heat in *yingfen* makes the blood extravasate, resulting in skin eruptions. In this prescription, Cornu Rhinocerotis is the chief ingredient, serving to purge heat from *yingfen*. Rehmanniae, Ophiopogonis and Scrophulariae are the adjuvant, used to nourish *yin* and purge heat. In the initial stage of heat syndrome involving *yingfen*, it is possible to eliminate the heat, and so Coptidis, Lophatheri, Lonicerae and Forsythiae are used as the assistant ingredients to eliminate heat and toxins. Salviae Miltiorrhizae is capable of cooling the blood and promoting blood circulation, and thus used to remove blood stasis. The combination of all the drugs not only purges heat from *yingfen*, but also nourishes *yin* and promotes blood circulation.

Although this prescription is meant to eliminate heat from *yingfen*, it can also be used to purge heat from *qifen*, as well as for heat syndrome involving *yingfen* in its initial stage with heat still in *qifen*.

Cornu Rhinocerotis can be replaced by Cornu Bubali; the dosage is 30-60 g.

Decoction of Cornu Rhinocerotis and Rehmanniae

犀角地黄汤 *xi jiao di huang tang*

(from *Essentially Treasured Prescriptions for Emergencies*)

Cornu Rhinocerotis	3 g
Radix Rehmanniae	30 g
Radix Paeoniae Lactiflorae	12 g
Cortex Moutan Radicis	9 g

Administration: Decoct the drugs except Cornu Rhinocerotis with water and remove the dregs. Grind Cornu Rhinocerotis in a mortar to get its juice and mix the juice with the decoction for oral administration.

Action: Purging heat and toxins, cooling the blood and removing blood stasis.

Indications: Heat syndrome involving *xuefen*, exhibiting coma, delirium, dim purplish rashes or hematemesis, epistaxis, hematochezia, hematuria, crimson tongue with rough and prickly coating, and thready and rapid pulse.

Explanation: In heat syndrome involving *xuefen*, the heart is disturbed by blood-heat, resulting in coma and delirium. When blood-heat affects the upper part of the body, hematemesis and epistaxis appear; when it affects the lower part of the body, hematochezia and hematuria occur; when it affects the surface to a serious extent, dim purplish rashes appear. In the prescription, Cornu Rhinocerotis clears heat from pericardium, cools the blood and removes toxins, while Rehmanniae cools the blood, nourishes *yin* and purges heat; both are used as the chief. Paeoniae Lactiflorae regulates *yingfen* and purges heat, and Moutan Radicis cools the blood and removes blood stasis; these are used as the assistant.

Clinically, for cases with hematemesis or epistaxis, Rhizoma Imperatae and Caulis Bambusae in Taeniam are added; for cases with hematochezia, Radix Sanguisorbae and Flos Sophorae are added; and for cases with hematuria, Herba Cephalanoploris and Rhizoma Imperatae are added. This prescription is suitable only for heat syndrome involving *xuefen* with hemorrhage, not for bleeding with *yang* deficiency and deficiency of the spleen and stomach.

Compare this decoction with Decoction for Eliminating Heat in the *Yingfen*. The former aims at purging heat and toxins, cooling the blood and removing blood stasis, and is indicated for heat syndrome involving *xuefen*. The latter is composed of drugs that purge heat from *yingfeng* and cool the blood and drugs that purge heat from *qifen*, so that the *yingfen* heat can be released through *qifen*.

Decoction of Coptidis for Detoxification

黄连解毒汤 *huang lian jie du tang*

(from *Clandestine Essentials from the Imperial Library*)

Rhizoma Coptidis	9 g
Radix Scutellariae	6 g
Cortex Phellodendri	6 g
Fructus Gardeniae	9 g

Administration: Decoct the drugs with water for oral administration.

Action: Purging fire and eliminating toxins.

Indications: Excess-heat syndrome with hyperactive heat in the triple *jiao*, exhibiting high fever, irritability, dry mouth and throat, delirium, insomnia, or various bleeding and skin rashes, or skin infection, red tongue with yellow coating, and rapid and strong pulse.

Explanation: This is a frequently used prescription for hyperactive heat in the triple *jiao*. Because of the hyperactivity, fever and irritability occur; disturbance of the mind by heat gives rise to insomnia and delirium; when heat attacks the blood, making it flow upwards, hematemesis and epistaxis appear; skin rashes occur when heat injures the collaterals; when heat affects the muscles, blood and *qi* become sluggish and skin infection results. In the prescription, Coptidis purges heart fire, and is combined with Scutellariae to purge heat from the middle and upper *jiao*; Phellodendri purges fire from the lower *jiao*; and Gardeniae purges heat from the triple *jiao*. The four drugs combined not only purge fire but also eliminate toxins, resulting in the relief of all symptoms.

Clinically, for bleeding and skin rashes, drugs that cool the blood and remove blood stasis, such as Radix Rehmanniae, Radix Scrophulariae and Cortex Moutan Radicis, are added to strengthen the effects; for dysentery due to dampness-heat, or jaundice due to accumulated heat, both of which are the result of excessive heat, a modified form of this prescription can be applied; for skin infection, the drugs can be ground into fine powder for topical application.

Besides, this prescription is composed of bitter and cold drugs, suitable only for cases when heat is dominant but body fluid has not been damaged. It is not suitable for cases in which *yin*-fluid is damaged by heat and the tongue is crimson and uncoated.

Appendant Prescription

Decoction for Purging Stomach Fire
泻心汤 *xie xin tang*
(from *Synopsis of the Golden Cabinet*)

The prescription is composed of 6 g of Radix et Rhizoma Rhei, 3 g of Rhizoma Coptidis, and 3 g of Radix Scutellariae. The drugs are decocted with water for oral administration. It purges fire, removes toxins, relaxes bowel movements and stops bleeding, and is indicated for heat syndrome with hyperactive heart and stomach fire, which extravasates the blood and leads to hematemesis, epistaxis and hemafecia; or heat syndrome with red, swollen and painful eyes and aphthae due to accumulated heat that disturbs the upper part of the body; or carbuncles caused by dominant heat.

Decoction for General Antiphlogistic
普济消毒饮 *pu ji xiao du yin*
(from *Prescriptions of Universal Benevolence*)

Radix Scutellariae (fried with wine)	15 g
Rhizoma Coptidis (fried with wine)	15 g
Pericarpium Citri Reticulatae	6 g
Radix Glycyrrhizae	6 g

Radix Scrophulariae	6 g
Radix Bupleuri	6 g
Radix Platycodi	6 g
Fructus Forsythiae	3 g
Radix Isatidis	3 g
Lasiosphaera seu Calvatis	3 g
Fructus Arctii	3 g
Herba Menthae	3 g
Bombyx Batryticatus	2 g
Rhizoma Cimicifugae	2 g

Administration: Decoct the drugs with water for oral administration; or grind them into fine powder for oral use by dividing the powder into several doses.

Action: Purging heat and toxins, eliminating pathogenic wind from the body.

Indications: Epidemic diseases with swollen head (*da tou wen*), exhibiting chills, fever, redness, swelling and pain of the head, throat ailments, dry mouth, red tongue with yellow coating, and rapid and forceful pulse.

Explanation: Epidemic diseases with swollen head are caused by virulent wind-heat, which accumulates in the upper *jiao* and affects the head, leading to the redness, swelling and pain. When wind-heat affects the surface, chills and fever occur; when it affects the lung and stomach, throat ailments and dry mouth result. In this case, the therapeutic principle should be purging heat and toxins, and expelling wind from the body. In the prescription, Scutellariae and Coptidis serve as the chief ingredients in a large dose to purge heat from the upper *jiao*. Arctii, Forsythiae, Menthae and Bombyx Batryticatus, as the adjuvant, expel wind-heat from the head. Scrophulariae, Lasiosphaera seu Calvatis, Isatidis, Platycodi and Glycyrrhizae purge heat and toxins and relieve throat ailments, and Citri Reticulatae regulates *qi* circulation—all serve as the assistant ingredients. Cimicifugae and Bupleuri are used as the guide to expel wind-heat and lead the effects of the other drugs to go to the head.

This prescription is particularly effective for epidemic heat syndrome characterized by swollen head. It is also recommended for mumps, acute tonsillitis, and skin infections in the head and face.

Powder for Promoting Diuresis

导赤散 *dao chi san*

(from *Medical Elucidation of Pediatrics*)

Radix Rehmanniae
Radix Glycyrrhizae
Caulis Akebiae
(in equal amount)

Administration: Grind the drugs into coarse powder. Take 9 g of the powder each time and decoct it in water with a moderate amount of Herba Lophatheri and take the warm decoction after meals.

Action: Purging heart fire and promoting diuresis.

Indications: Heat attacking the heart meridian, exhibiting a feverish sensation in the chest, flushed cheeks, thirst with an inclination for cold drinks, aphthae; or oliguria, dysuria, red tongue, and rapid pulse.

Explanation: When pathogenic heat attacks the heart meridian, it causes heart fire. Flaming of heart fire leads to the feverish sensation; when heart fire affects the upper part of the body, it leads to flushed checks, thirst and aphthae; when it attacks the small intestines, it leads to oliguria and dysuria. In the prescription, Rehmanniae is used as the chief ingredient for purging heat, cooling the blood and nourishing *yin*. Akebiae and Lophatheri, as the adjuvant, purge heart fire by promoting diuresis, and relieve restlessness. Glycyrrhizae is used as both the assistant and guide to purge heat, eliminate fire and treat stranguria.

This is a common prescription for purging heart fire and promoting diuresis. Clinical evidence calling for its application includes aphthae or oliguria and dysuria, and red tongue and rapid pulse. For a marked feverish sensation in the chest, Rhizoma Coptidis and Fructus Gardeniae are added; for stranguria complicated by hematuria, Herba Cephalanoploris and Herba Ecliptae are added.

Decoction of Gentianae for Purging Liver Fire

龙胆泻肝汤 *long dan xie gan tang*

(from *Variorum of Prescriptions*)

Herba Gentianae (fried with wine)	6 g
Radix Scutellariae (fried)	9 g
Fructus Gardeniae (fried with wine)	9 g
Rhizoma Alismatis	12 g
Caulis Akebiae	9 g
Semen Plantaginis	9 g
Radix Angelicae Sinensis (soaked in wine)	3 g
Radix Rehmanniae (fried with wine)	6 g
Radix Bupleuri	6 g
Radix Glycyrrhizae	6 g

Administration: Decoct the drugs with water for oral administration; or prepare them into pills and take 6-9 g each time, twice a day.

Action: Purging excess fire from the liver, and purging dampness-heat from the lower *jiao*.

Indications: Cases due to upward attack of excess-fire from the liver and gallbladder, exhibiting headache, congestion of the conjunctiva, deafness, hypochondriac pain and bitter taste; or downward affection of dampness-heat from the liver meridian, exhibiting stranguria with turbid urine, pruritus vulvae, leukorrhagia, red tongue with yellow greasy coating, and taut and rapid pulse.

Explanation: The liver and gallbladder form the interior-exterior pair and are connected with each other by the network of meridians. The liver meridian starts from the foot, goes through the genitalia and hypochondrium and then up to the head, connecting the ears and eyes by its branches. When excess-fire is flaming up along the liver meridian, headache, congestion of the conjunctiva and deafness occur. When retained fire leads to *qi* stagnation, hypochondriac pain occurs. When dampness-heat affects the genitals, stranguria, pruritus vulvae and leukorrhagia with stinking yellow discharge occur. In the prescription, Gentianae is used as the chief ingredient to purge excess-fire from the liver and gallbladder and eliminate dampness-heat from the liver meridian. Scutellariae and Gardeniae, as the adjuvant, help Gentianae strengthen the effects of purging excess-fire and dampness-heat. Alismatis, Akebiae and Plantaginis purge dampness-heat by promoting diuresis, while Angelicae Sinensis and Rehmanniae nourish *yin* and blood, purge fire and promote diuresis without damaging *yin* and blood—all are used as the assistant ingredients. Bupleuri disperses the stagnant liver *qi*, and Glycyrrhizae regulates the effects of the other drugs, and both serve as the guide. The combination of these drugs produces the desirable effects of both purgation and invigoration, so that the liver fire can be purged and dampness-heat eliminated.

Powder for Eliminating Stomach Heat
清胃散 *qing wei san*
(from *Secret Records of the Cabinet of Orchids*)

Radix Rehmanniae	12 g
Radix Angelicae Sinensis	6 g
Cortex Moutan Radicis	9 g
Rhizoma Coptidis	5 g
Rhizoma Cimicifugae	6 g

Administration: Decoct the drugs with water twice, and take the cool decoction in separate doses.

Action: Purging stomach heat and cooling the blood.

Indications: Cases with heat accumulated in the stomach, exhibiting toothache radiating to the head, feverish cheeks, dental preference for cold and aversion to heat, bleeding; or bleeding from the gum, swollen and painful lips, tongue or cheeks, or halitosis, dry mouth, red tongue with yellow coating, and smooth, large and rapid pulse.

Explanation: The prescription is for disorders caused by the accumulation of heat in the stomach and the flare-up of stomach fire. The gum is the place where the Yangming Meridian passes; when hyperactive stomach fire moves upward along the meridian, it leads to swollen and painful gum and cheeks. The stomach is an organ full of *qi* and blood;

when there is heat in the stomach, there is also heat in *xuefen*, leading to bleeding, ulceration and swelling of the gums. Other manifestations, such as halitosis and dry mouth and tongue, are also caused by an accumulation of heat in the stomach. In the prescription, Coptidis is bitter and cold, and purges fire, and it is used as the chief. Rehmanniae and Moutan Radicis cool the blood and purging heat, and serve as the adjuvant. Angelicae Sinensis is used as the assistant to nourish the blood in order to relieve swelling and pain. Cimicifugae is used as the guide to purge fire and lead the effects of the other drugs to Yangming. All the drugs used together produce the ideal effects of purging stomach fire and cooling the blood. For cases with constipation, Radix et Rhizoma Rhei is added to lead the heat downward.

Appendant Prescription

Jade Maid Decoction
玉女煎 *yu nu jian*
(from *Complete Collection of Jingyue's Treatises*)

This prescription is composed of 15-30 g of Gypsum Fibrosum, 9-15 g of Radix Rehmanniae Preparata, 6 g of Radix Ophiopogonis, 4.5 g of Rhizoma Anemarrhenae, and 4.5 g of Radix Achyranthis Bidentatae. The drugs are decocted with water for oral administration. It purges stomach fire and nourish *yin*, and is indicated for cases of stomach heat syndrome along with *yin* deficiency, marked by headache, toothache, bleeding of the gum, feverishness accompanied with restlessness, thirst, red tongue with dry yellow coating, and thready and rapid pulse.

Both this prescription and Powder for Eliminating Stomach Heat cure toothache. The former aims at purging stomach heat and nourishing *yin*, and is suitable for excessive stomach fire and deficient kidney *yin*, while the latter aims at purging stomach fire and cooling the blood, and is indicated for accumulation of heat in the stomach.

Decoction of Phragmitis
苇茎汤 *wei jing tang*
(from *Essentially Treasured Prescriptions for Emergencies*)

Rhizoma Phragmitis	30 g
Semen Coicis	30 g
Semen Benincasae	24 g
Semen Persicae	10 g

Administration: Decoct the drugs with water for oral administration.

Action: Purging lung heat, eliminating phlegm, removing blood stasis and discharging pus.

Indications: Lung abscess (*fei yong*), exhibiting cough with discharge of foul purulent sputum, dull pain in the chest aggravated by cough, red tongue with yellow greasy coating, and smooth and rapid pulse.

Explanation: Lung abscess is caused by the accumulation of phlegm-heat and blood stasis in the lung. When the lung is affected by heat, lung *qi* becomes sluggish, blood stagnates and heat accumulates, leading to cough with expectoration of foul and purulent sputum. Blood stasis and heat accumulated in the lung produce a dull pain in the chest. In the prescription, Phragmitis, serving as the chief and principal drug for lung abscess, purges lung heat. Benincasae, as the adjuvant, eliminates phlegm-heat and discharges pus. Coicis purges heat and promotes diuresis, and Persicae promotes blood circulation and removes blood stasis—both serve as the assistant and guide. These drugs combined can produce the ideal effects of purging lung heat, removing phlegm, blood stasis and pus, thereby relieving lung abscess.

This is appropriate for lung abscess whether or not pus has formed. If pus has not yet formed, Herba Taraxaci, Herba Houttuyniae, Flos Lonicerae, Fructus Forsythiae and Rhizoma Fagopyri Cymosi are added to purge heat and toxins; if formed, Radix Platycodi, Bulbus Fritillariae Thunbergii, Herba Patriniae and Radix Glycyrrhizae are added to remove phlegm and pus, helping to relieve the abscess.

Powder for Expelling Lung Heat

泻白散 *xie bai san*

(from *Medical Elucidation of Pediatrics*)

Cortex Lycii Radicis	30 g
Cortex Mori Radicis	30 g
Radix Glycyrrhizae Preparata	3 g
Oryzae Sativae	9 g

Administration: Decoct the drugs with water until Oryzae Sativae is dissolved. Discard the dregs and take the decoction before meals.

Action: Purging lung heat, relieving cough and dyspnea.

Indications: Cases with cough due to lung heat, exhibiting dyspnea, feverish skin which gets more serious in the afternoon, red tongue with yellow coating, and thready and rapid pulse.

Explanation: This is specially suitable for cases of cough and dyspnea caused by heat and fire retained in the lung. The lung controls *qi* circulation, and the lung *qi* should be kept pure and descendent. When pathogenic fire is retained in the lung, lung *qi* fails to descend, which leads to cough. The lung is connected with the skin and hair, and so retained lung fire gradually damages *yin*, leading to feverish skin which becomes more serious in the afternoon. In the prescription, Mori Radicis is used as the chief to purge lung heat and relieve cough and dyspnea. Lycii Radicis, as the adjuvant, is used to purge lung fire and relieve deficiency-heat syndrome. Glycyrrhizae and Oryzae Sativae serve as the assistant and guide to nourish the stomach, regulate the middle *jiao* and replenish lung *qi*. This prescription aims at relieving the primary and secondary symptoms at the same time by means of purging and nourishing at the same time.

For cases of predominant lung heat, Rhizoma Anemarrhenae and Radix Scutellariae are added; for thirst, Radix Adenophorae, Radix Ophiopogonis and Radix Trichosanthis are added.

Decoction of Puerariae, Scutellariae and Coptidis
葛根黄芩黄连汤 *ge gen huang qin huang lian tang*
(from *Treatise on Cold Diseases*)

Radix Puerariae	15 g
Radix Glycyrrhizae Preparata	6 g
Radix Scutellariae	9 g
Rhizoma Coptidis	9 g

Administration: Decoct Puerariae with water first until the decoction boils for several minutes, then add other drugs to boil with the decoction. Discard the dregs and take the decoction warm in two separate doses.

Action: Purging heat and relieving diarrhea.

Indications: Diarrhea at the onset, accompanied by fever, diarrhea with foul discharge, feverishness in the chest, dry mouth, thirst, dyspnea with sweating, yellow tongue coating, and rapid pulse.

Explanation: The prescription is frequently used to treat diarrhea at its onset. When internal heat is predominant, fever, thirst and feverishness in the chest appear. When the large intestine is affected by heat, diarrhea with foul discharge occurs. When heat fumigates the lung and affects the surface, dyspnea with sweating results. In the prescription, Puerariae is used in a large dosage as the chief to purge heat and relieve diarrhea, and also make lucid *yang* go upward. Scutellariae and Coptidis are used as the adjuvant to purge heat from the intestines and relieve diarrhea. Glycyrrhizae is sweet and mild, capable of coordinating the effects of the other drugs and used as both the assistant and guide. Since Puerariae is acrid and cool, and able to expel pathogens from the surface, this prescription is also indicated for cases of diarrhea complicated by unrelieved exterior-syndrome.

The clinical evidence calling for the application of this prescription is fever, diarrhea with foul discharge, a burning sensation in the anus, yellow tongue coating and rapid pulse. For cases with abdominal pain, Radix Aucklandiae and Radix Paeoniae Alba are added to promote *qi* circulation, regulate blood circulation and relieve pain.

Decoction of Pulsatillae
白头翁汤 *bai tou weng tang*
(from *Treatise on Cold Diseases*)

Radix Pulsatillae	15 g
Cortex Phellodendri	12 g
Rhizoma Coptidis	6 g
Cortex Fraxini	12 g

Administration: Decoct the drugs with water for oral administration.

Action: Purging heat and toxins, cooling the blood and relieving dysentery.

Indications: Cases of dysentery, characterized by abdominal pain, tenesmus, a burning sensation in the anus, bloody purulent stool, thirst with an inclination to drink, red tongue with yellow coating, and taut and rapid pulse.

Explanation: Dysentery that can be cured with this prescription is due to dampness-heat retained in the intestines. Here the intestines are damaged, leading to bloody purulent discharge. When heat and toxins accumulate, *qi* circulation is blocked and abdominal pain and tenesmus occur. When the large intestine is affected by pathogenic heat, a burning sensation in the anus results. In the prescription, Pulsatillae is used as the chief to purge heat, cool the blood and relieve dysentery. Coptidis, Phellodendri and Fraxini are used to help strengthen the removal of toxins and relief of dysentery.

Six-to-One Powder

六一散 *liu yi san*

(from *Expounding Prescriptions*)

Talcum	180 g
Radix Glycyrrhizae	30 g

Administration: Grind the drugs into fine powder, wrap 9 g of the powder with a piece of gauze and decoct in water, or mix the powder with honey and warm water for oral administration, twice a day.

Action: Purging summer-heat and promoting diuresis to eliminate dampness.

Indications: Summer-heat-dampness syndrome, exhibiting fever, restlessness and thirst, dysuria or diarrhea; or dampness-heat in the urinary bladder, exhibiting oliguria, dysuria, or stranguria due to urinary stones.

Explanation: In disorders caused by summer-heat and dampness, summer-heat is attributed to *yang* and is related to the heart. When it attacks the body, fever and restlessness occur; when it consumes body fluid, thirst results; when it affects the urinary bladder, dysuria happens; when it is retained in the stomach and intestines, vomiting and diarrhea occur. If dampness-heat is retained in the urinary tract for a long time, stranguria due to urinary stones is the result. In the prescription, Talcum, sweet, cold, heavy and lubricant, serves as the chief ingredient. It not only purges summer-heat but also promotes diuresis and relieves stranguria. Glycyrrhizae purges heat and regulates the middle *jiao*, and produces an ideal effect in promoting fluid production when used together with Talcum; it is used as the assistant and guide.

This is a basic prescription for summer-heat-dampness syndrome and is used clinically with other prescriptions. For a case that is caused only by summer-heat, or if there is no difficulty in micturition, this prescription is not recommended.

Appendant Prescriptions

(1) Powder for Eliminating Summer-Heat and Dampness
益元散 *yi yuan san*
(from *Expounding Prescriptions*)

This is composed of Talcum, Radix Glycyrrhizae and Cinnabaris. Grind the drugs into fine powder and mix the powder in decoction of Medulla Junci for oral administration. It purges heart fire and summer-heat and tranquilizes the mind, and is indicated for summer-heat-dampness syndrome with the symptoms of restlessness, insomnia and dreaminess.

(2) Green Jade Powder
碧玉散 *bi yu san*
(from *Expounding Prescriptions*)

This is composed of Talcum, Radix Glycyrrhizae and Indigo Naturalis. It purges summer-heat, and is indicated for summer-heat-dampness syndrome with red eyes and sore throat or aphthae.

(3) Cock-Waking Powder
鸡苏散 *ji su san*
(from *Expounding Prescriptions*)

This prescription is composed of Talcum, Radix Glycyrrhizae and Herba Menthae. It acts to disperse wind and purge summer-heat, and is indicated for summer-heat-dampness syndrome accompanied by mild chills and headache.

Decoction for Eliminating Summer-Heat and Benefiting *Qi*
清暑益气汤 *qing shu yi qi tang*
(from *Compendium of Seasonal Febrile Diseases*)

Radix Panacis Quinquefolii	5 g
Herba Dendrobii	15 g
Radix Ophiopogonis	9 g
Rhizoma Coptidis	3 g
Herba Lophatheri	6 g
Petiolus Nelumbinis	15 g
Rhizoma Anemarrhenae	6 g

Radix Glycyrrhizae	3 g
Fructus Oryzae Sativae	15 g
Exocarpium Citrulli	30 g

Administration: Decoct the drugs with water for oral administration.

Action: Purging summer-heat, benefiting *qi*, nourishing *yin* and promoting fluid production.

Indications: Summer-heat syndrome with consumption of both *qi* and fluid, exhibiting fever, profuse sweating, restlessness, thirst, scanty reddish urine, lassitude, shortness of breath, listlessness, and feeble and rapid pulse.

Explanation: In summer-heat syndrome with consumption of *qi* and fluid, summer-heat is predominant, resulting in fever and restlessness. When heat steams inside the body, the fluid escapes outward, causing profuse sweating. Summer-heat is attributed to *yang* and liable to damage *qi* and fluid, hence thirst with a desire to drink, fatigue, shortness of breath and listlessness occur. In the prescription, Panacis Quinquefolii benefits *qi* and promotes fluid production, and Citrulli purges summer-heat—both are used as the chief. Nelumbinis helps Citrulli purge summer-heat, while Dendrobii and Ophiopogonis help Panacis Quinquefolii nourish *yin* and purge heat—all three are used as the adjuvant. Coptidis, Anemarrhenae and Lophatheri purge heat and relieve restlessness, while Oryzae Sativae and Glycyrrhizae benefit the stomach and regulate the middle *jiao*—all are used as the assistant and guide.

This prescription is particularly designed for summer-heat syndrome marked by the consumption of both *qi* and fluid. The clinical evidence calling for its administration are fever, profuse sweating, restlessness, thirst, fatigue, shortness of breath, and feeble and rapid pulse. This prescription is also recommended for long-standing cases of summer fever in children due to insufficient *qi* and fluid. But for summer-heat-dampness diseases, Dendrobii and Ophiopogonis, which nourish *yin*, should be removed.

Decoction of Artemisiae Annuae and Carapax Trionycis

清蒿鳖甲汤 *qing hao bie jia tang*

(from *Essentials of Seasonal Febrile Diseases*)

Herba Artemisiae Annuae	6 g
Carapax Trionycis	15 g
Radix Rehmanniae	12 g
Rhizoma Anemarrhenae	6 g
Cortex Moutan Radicis	9 g

Administration: Decoct the drugs in water for oral administration.

Action: Nourishing *yin* and releasing heat.

Indications: The late stage of seasonal febrile diseases marked by consumption of *yin* fluid and retention of heat in *yingfen*, exhibiting evening fever which subsides in the morning, no sweating when fever subsides, red tongue with little coating, and thready and rapid pulse.

Explanation: In the late stage of febrile diseases when pathogenic heat still resides deeply in *yingfen*, there is evening fever that subsides in the morning, and no sweating when the fever subsides. The other manifestations are indications of consumption of *yin*-fluid. For such cases, it is not proper to only use bitter and cold drugs to purge heat, nor is it proper to only use drugs that nourish *yin*. The best way is to nourish *yin* and simultaneously release the heat deep in *yingfen*. In the prescription, Artemisiae Annuae is fragrant, and able to release deep heat, while Carapax Trionycis nourishes *yin*, and both of them are used as the chief. Rehmanniae and Anemarrhenae help Carapax Trionycis nourish *yin* and relieve fever, and Moutan Radicis, acrid and cold, helps Artemisiae Annuae release deep heat — all three are used as the assistant and guide.

Clinically, this prescription is also indicated for long-standing low fever of unknown reasons but attributable to *yin* deficiency. For such cases, Radix Cynanchi Atrati and Cortex Lycii Radicis can be added when necessary.

Powder for Relieving Deficiency-Heat Syndrome
清骨散 *qing gu san*
(from *Standard for Diagnosis and Treatment*)

Radix Stellariae	5 g
Rhizoma Picrorhizae	3 g
Radix Gentianae Macrophyllae	3 g
Carapax Trionycis (fried with vinegar)	3 g
Cortex Lycii Radicis	3 g
Herba Artemisiae Annuae	3 g
Rhizoma Anemarrhenae	3 g
Radix Glycyrrhizae	2 g

Administration: Decoct with water for oral administration.

Action: Purging deficiency heat.

Indications: Consumptive diseases, such as hectic fever due to *yin* deficiency, exhibiting flushed cheeks, red lips, feverishness in the palms and soles, restlessness, thirst, red tongue with little coating, and thready and rapid pulse.

Explanation: This prescription is appropriate for consumptive diseases caused by consumption of liver and kidney *yin* and the irritation of deficiency fire. The kidney controls the bones and stores essence, while the liver stores blood; they have the same origin. Deficient *yin* results in internal heat, thus leading to hectic fever and feverishness in the palms and soles. When deficiency fire attacks the upper part of the body, restlessness, dry mouth, flushed cheeks and red lips occur. The other manifestations, such as red tongue with little coating and thready and rapid pulse, are also indications of deficient *yin* and hyperactive fire. In the prescription, Stellariae is used as the chief to relieve hectic fever due to *yin* deficiency. Picrorhizae, Anemarrhenae and Lycii Radicis purge internal heat, while Artemisiae Annuae and Gentianae Macrophyllae release deficiency heat—all are used as the adjuvant. Carapax Trionycis, used as the assistant, nourishes *yin* and suppresses *yang*. Glycyrrhizae coordinates the effects of the other drugs, and is used as the guide.

This prescription is effective for liver and kidney *yin* deficiency, and for hectic fever due to *yin* deficiency. Clinical evidence calling for its application is hectic fever, red tongue with little coating, and thready and rapid pulse. For cases associated with shortness of breath and inclination to talk, which are indications of *qi* and *yin* deficiency, Radix Astragali is added to benefit *qi* and relieve hectic fever; for cases with loose stool due to spleen deficiency, bitter and cold drugs, such as Picrorhizae, Gentianae Macrophyllae and Anemarrhenae are removed, and Semen Dolichoris and Rhizoma dioscoreae are added to invigorate the spleen and benefit *yin*.

Summary

Included in this chapter are sixteen principal and eight appendant prescriptions. According to their different actions, they are classified into six categories.

(1) Prescriptions for purging heat from *qifen*:

The examples are White Tiger Decoction and Decoction of Lophatheri and Gypsum Fibrosum. The former purges heat and promotes fluid production, and is indicated for hyperactive heat in *qifen*, which exhibits high fever, sweating, restlessness, thirst, and bounding and large pulse. The latter purges heat, benefits *qi*, nourishes *yin* and regulates stomach *qi*; it is indicated for consumption of both *qi* and *yin* with heat persisting after a febrile disease, exhibiting fever, profuse sweating, chest upset and nausea.

(2) Prescriptions for purging heat from *yingfen* and cooling the blood:

Decoction for Eliminating Heat in the *Yingfen* and Decoction of Cornu Rhinocerotis and Rehmanniae are two examples. The former purges heat from *yingfen* and nourishes *yin*, and is indicated for cases of pathogenic warm-heat beginning to enter *yingfen*, exhibiting fever that is higher at night, occasional delirium, skin rashes, and dry and crimson tongue. The latter purges heat and toxins, cools the blood and removes blood stasis, and is indicated for cases of heat entering *xuefen* and extravasation of blood, exhibiting coma, delirium, dark purple rashes, hematemesis and epistaxis.

(3) Prescriptions for purging heat and toxins:

Decoction of Coptidis for Detoxification and Decoction for General Antiphlogistic are two examples. The former is composed of bitter and cold drugs for purging fire, and is indicated for cases of hyperactive fire in the triple *jiao*, in which heat is predominant while *yin*-fluid has not yet been damaged. The latter eliminates pathogenic wind, and is indicated for epidemic heat syndrome marked by swollen head due to wind-heat in the upper *jiao*.

(4) Prescriptions for purging heat from the viscera:

Prescriptions of this category are specially designed for heat syndromes involving various *zang-fu* organs. Powder for Promoting Diuresis purges heart fire and promotes diuresis, releasing heat from the heart meridian and dampness-heat from the small intestine through urination; it is indicated for aphthae due to a flare-up of heart fire, and for oliguria with reddish urine or stranguria caused by heart fire attacking the small intestine. Decoction of Gentianae for Purging Liver Fire aims at purging excess fire and eliminating dampness-heat from the liver and gallbladder, and is indicated for headache, bitter taste, red, swollen and painful eyes, deafness caused by excess liver and gallbladder fire affecting the upper part of the body, or stranguria with turbid urine, leukorrhagia, pruritus vulvae caused by a downward attack of dampness-heat from the liver and gallbladder. Powder for Eliminating Stomach Heat purges stomach heat and cools the blood, and is indicated for toothache or bleeding in the gums due to stomach fire. Both Decoction of Phragmitis and Powder for Expelling Lung Heat purge lung heat. The former removes blood stasis and discharges pus, and is indicated for lung abscess with expectoration of blood and pus; the latter relieves cough and dyspnea, and is indicated for cough and dyspnea due to lung heat. Decoction of Puerariae, Scutellariae and Coptidis purges heat and relieves diarrhea, and is indicated for diarrhea at its onset, exhibiting fever and a feverish sensation in the chest. Decoction of Pulsatillae purges heat, eliminates toxins, cools blood and relieves dysentery, and is indicated for dysentery with bloody stool due to heat that affects *xuefen*.

(5) Prescriptions for purging summer-heat:

Both Six-to-One Powder and Decoction for Eliminating Summer-Heat and Benefiting *Qi* purge summer-heat. The former purges summer-heat and promotes diuresis, and is mainly indicated for summer-heat-dampness syndrome. The latter purges summer-heat and also nourishes *yin* and promotes fluid production, and is indicated for the consumption of both *qi* and fluid due to attack by summer-heat, exhibiting fever, sweating, thirst, restlessness and fatigue.

(6) Prescriptions for purging deficiency heat:

Decoction of Artemisiae Annuae and Carapax Trionycis and Powder for Relieving Deficiency-Heat Syndrome are two examples. They nourish *yin* and relieve fever. The former nourishes *yin* and releases pathogenic heat, and is indicated for the late stage of febrile diseases with heat residing in *yingfen*, night fever which subsides in the morning, and absence of sweating when the fever subsides, and also for long-standing fever due to *yin* deficiency. The latter purges deficiency heat and relieves hectic fever, and is indicated for consumptive diseases, such as hectic fever due to liver and kidney *yin* deficiency, and the irritation of deficiency fire in the body.

CHAPTER TEN
PRESCRIPTIONS FOR WARMING THE INTERIOR

Mainly composed of drugs for warming the interior and eliminating cold, prescriptions for warming the interior (*wen li ji*) warm the interior and support *yang*, eliminate cold and promote blood circulation, and are used for interior-cold syndromes. Their use constitutes the warming therapy.

Diseases caused by cold can be divided into exterior-cold and interior-cold syndromes. The former should be treated with prescriptions for relieving exterior-syndrome, composed of acrid and warm drugs; this has been discussed in a separate chapter. The present chapter deals with the therapeutic principle and prescriptions for interior-cold syndrome.

Interior-cold syndrome may be caused by endogenous cold in cases of *yang* deficiency; exposure to exogenous cold, with the cold affecting the three *yin* meridians and the *zang-fu* organs; or overdose of cold drugs results in damage to *yang qi*. Prescriptions for warming the interior are recommended for interior-cold syndrome of any origin, according to the principle that "cold-syndrome should be treated with warm-natured drugs." But since different cases vary in seriousness and in location, such prescriptions can be grouped under the following three categories:

Prescriptions for warming the middle *jiao* and eliminating cold (*wen zhong qu han ji*) are indicated for deficiency cold in the middle *jiao*. The stomach and spleen lie in the middle *jiao* and are responsible for digestion and fluid transportation. If the spleen and stomach are attacked by cold when suffering from *yang-qi* deficiency, their functions are weakened, affecting the ability of the visceral *qi* to ascend and descend and giving rise to such manifestations as distensive stomach pain, fatigue, cold limbs, eructation, nausea, vomiting, or abdominal pain with diarrhea, tastelessness, absence of thirst, smooth and white tongue coating, and deep and thready, or deep and slow pulse. For such cases, Rhizoma Zingiberis, Fructus Evodiae, Pericarpium Zanthoxyli and Rhizoma Zingiberis Recens are usually combined with drugs that invigorate *qi* and the spleen. The examples are Bolus for Regulating the Middle *Jiao*, Decoction of Evodiae and Decoction for Mildly Warming the Middle *Jiao*.

Prescriptions for recuperating the depleted *yang* and rescuing the patient from danger (*hui yang jiu ni ji*) are indicated for kidney *yang* deficiency, excessive *yin*-cold, or exhaustion of *yang*, exhibiting cold limbs, chills, vomiting, abdominal pain, diarrhea with undigested food, listlessness, and deep and faint pulse. Such prescriptions are usually composed of acrid and hot drugs, such as Radix Aconiti Lateralis Preparata, Rhizoma Zingiberis and Cortex Cinnamomi, along with drugs that invigorates *qi*. Two examples are Decoction for Treating *Yang* Exhaustion, and Decoction of Ginseng and Aconiti Lateralis Preparata.

Prescriptions for warming the meridians to expel cold (*wen jing san han ji*) are indicated for syndromes due to blood deficiency accompanied by damage of the meridians by exogenous cold and poor blood circulation. Such prescriptions are mainly composed of Ramulus Cinnamomi, Herba Asari, etc. , along with drugs that invigorate *qi* and nourish the blood. An example is Decoction of Angelicae Sinensis for Warming Cold Limbs.

Prescriptions for warming the interior are mostly composed of acrid and hot drugs. In clinical application, on the one hand, it is necessary to distinguish the nature of the syndromes; for heat syndrome with false-cold symptoms, they are not recommended. On the other, the dosage should be moderate for patients with apparent *yin* and blood deficiency, so as to avoid further damage to *yin*.

Bolus for Regulating the Middle *Jiao*
理中丸 *li zhong wan*
(from *Treatise on Cold Diseases*)

Radix Ginseng	9 g
Rhizoma Zingiberis	9 g
Radix Glycyrrhizae Preparata	9 g
Rhizoma Atractylodis Macrocephalae	9 g

Administration: Grind the drugs into fine powder and prepare the powder into honeyed bolus, take 9 g of the bolus with warm water each time, twice a day; or prepare the drugs as a decoction, with the dosages of the ingredients reduced proportionally.

Action: Warming the meridians to expel cold, invigorating *qi* and strengthening the spleen.

Indications: Deficiency cold in the middle *jiao*, manifested as diarrhea, absence of thirst, vomiting, abdominal pain, poor appetite, white tongue coating, and thready pulse; and bleeding due to spleen *yang* deficiency, intermittent infantile convulsion, salivation after illness, and chest *bi*-syndrome.

Explanation: The spleen transports and transforms nutrients, while the stomach receives food and sends digested food downward. When *yang* deficiency in the spleen and stomach leads to spleen and stomach dysfunction, vomiting, diarrhea, abdominal pain and poor appetite occur. The case should be treated by warming the meridians to expel cold, invigorating *qi* to strengthen the spleen, helping restore the normal function of the spleen and stomach. In the prescription, Zingiberis serves as the chief to warm the spleen and stomach to expel cold. Ginseng, as the adjuvant, invigorates primordial *qi* and help transport and transform nutrients. Atractylodis Macrocephalae and Glycyrrhizae are used as the assistant and the guide to strengthen the spleen and eliminate dampness, benefit *qi* and regulate the middle *jiao*. In this way, the cold in the middle *jiao* is eliminated by acrid and hot drugs, and the normal function of the middle *jiao* is restored by sweet and warm drugs, once the lucid *yang* has ascended and the turbid *yin* descended.

Various kinds of bleeding, accompanied by pallor, fatigue, shortness of breath, thready, or feeble, large and forceless pulse are due to spleen and stomach deficiency resulting in the failure of the spleen to control the blood to circulate within the vessels. Better results will be obtained if Zingiberis is baked and Radix Astragali and Colla Corii Asini are added.

Intermittent infantile convulsion always results from congenital deficiency and improper postnatal nursing, overdose of cold drugs in the course of a disease, or improper nursing after a serious disease—all of which may lead to damage of spleen and stomach *yang*. Such cases manifest emaciation, cold limbs, vomiting, diarrhea, lassitude, poor appetite, pale tongue with white coating, thready and slow, or deep, thready and slow pulse, simply due to deficiency cold in the middle *jiao*. They can also be treated with this prescription.

It can additionally be used for salivation due to deficiency cold in the spleen with failure to control body fluid, and for chest *bi*-syndrome due to deficient *yang* in the upper *jiao* and excessive *yin*-cold.

In a word, this prescription is suitable for a variety of diseases due to deficiency cold in the middle *jiao*, according to the principle of "treating different diseases with the same therapy." Although the prescription is named Bolus for Regulating the Middle *Jiao*, the drugs are usually prepared into an oral decoction. Ginseng Decoction, recorded in *Synopsis of the Golden Cabinet*, has the same ingredients, and is used to treat chest *bi*-syndrome.

Appendant Prescriptions

(1) Pill of Aconiti Lateralis for Regulating the Middle *Jiao*

附子理中丸 *fu zi li zhong wan*

(from *Yan's Treatise on Prescriptions for Children's Diseases*)

This is composed of 30 g of Radix Ginseng, 30 g of Rhizoma Atractylodis Macrocephalae, 30 g of Rhizoma Zingiberis Preparata, 30 g of Radix Glycyrrhizae Preparata and 30 g of Radix Aconiti Lateralis Preparata. Grind the drugs into fine powder and prepare the powder into honeyed bolus, each weighing 3 g. Take one each time with warm water before meals. It acts to warm *yang*, eliminate cold, invigorate the spleen and kidney. It is indicated for deficiency cold in the spleen and kidney, exhibiting cold stomach pain, chronic diarrhea and cholera morbus.

This prescription is more effective than Bolus for Regulating the Middle *Jiao* in warming *yang* to expel cold because of the additional drug Aconiti Lateralis. Thus, it is more effective for syndromes due to deficiency cold in the spleen and kidney.

(2) Pill of Aconiti Lateralis and Cinnamomi for Regulating the Middle *Jiao*

附桂理中丸 *fu gui li zhong wan*

(from *Treatise on the Tripartite Pathogenesis of Diseases*)

This is composed of the ingredients of Bolus for Regulating the Middle *Jiao* in addition to Radix Aconiti Lateralis Preparata and Cortex Cinnamomi. It is better at warming the interior to expel cold than are the above two prescriptions, and thus is indicated for more serious cases of *yang* deficiency in the spleen and kidney.

(3) Decoction of Coptidis for Regulating the Middle *Jiao*
连理汤 *lian li tang*
(from *Symptoms and Etiology*, *Pulse Condition and Treatment*)

This is composed of the ingredients of Bolus for Regulating the Middle *Jiao* in addition to Rhizoma Coptidis, and is indicated for deficiency cold in the spleen and stomach with acid eructation.

Decoction of Evodiae
吴茱萸汤 *wu zhu yu tang*
(from *Treatise on Cold Diseases*)

Fructus Evodiae	5 g
Radix Ginseng	9 g
Fructus Jujubae	4 pieces
Rhizoma Zingiberis Recens	18 g

Administration: Decoct the drugs with water for oral administration.

Action: Warming the middle *jiao*, invigorating primordial *qi*, suppressing adversely rising *qi* to relieve vomiting.

Indications: (1) Deficiency cold in the stomach exhibiting nausea and fullness in the chest, or stomachache and acid regurgitation; (2) Jueyin headache with retching and salivation; and (3) Shaoyin diseases with vomiting, diarrhea, cold limbs and restlessness.

Explanation: This is a common prescription for warming the middle *jiao* and suppressing adversely rising *qi*, indicated for vomiting due to deficiency cold in the stomach and adversely rising turbid *yin* at Yangming, Shaoyin or Jueyin. In the prescription, Evodiae is acrid, bitter and hot, and warms the stomach to expel cold, relieves stagnant liver *qi* and suppresses adversely rising *qi*; it is therefore used as the chief. Ginseng invigorates primordial *qi* and nourishes the stomach, and serves as the adjuvant. Zingiberis Recens warms the stomach to expel cold, while Jujubae benefits *qi* and invigorates the spleen. These two help the chief and adjuvant ingredients warm the stomach and invigorate *qi*. Moreover, their combination regulates the *yingfen* and *weifen*, and both serve as the assistant and guide. Vomiting of clear fluid, pale tongue with smooth and white coating, and thready and slow pulse or thready and taut pulse are clinical evidence calling for its application.

Decoction for Mildly Warming the Middle *Jiao*
小建中汤 *xiao jian zhong tang*
(from *Treatise on Cold Diseases*)

Radix Paeoniae Lactiflorae (fried with wine)	18 g
Ramulus Cinnamomi	9 g
Radix Glycyrrhizae Preparata	6 g
Rhizoma Zingiberis Recens	9 g
Fructus Jujubae	4 pieces
Saccharum Granorum	30 g

Administration: Decoct the drugs (except Saccharum Granorum) with water twice, then remove the dregs, add Saccharum Granorum and let it melt over a slow fire. Take the decoction warm in two or three separate doses.

Action: Warming the middle *jiao*, invigorating *qi*, regulating the interior and relieving abdominal pain.

Indications: Consumptive diseases due to insufficient *qi* and blood, exhibiting intermittent abdominal pain relieved by warmth and pressure, pale tongue with white coating, thready, taut and slow pulse; or palpitation, restlessness, pallor; or soreness and feverishness in the limbs, dry mouth, etc.

Explanation: Consumptive diseases with abdominal pain relieved by warmth and pressure are caused by consumption of *qi* and blood and deficiency cold in the middle *jiao*. The spleen is the source of nutrients for physical development. When there is deficiency cold in the spleen, insufficient *qi* and blood and imbalance between *ying qi* and *wei qi* appear, leading to sore and feverish limbs, and dry mouth. The heart is the mother organ of the spleen. When spleen deficiency affects the heart, palpitation, restlessness and lusterless complexion result. It is therefore necessary to treat the case mainly by invigorating the spleen and warming the middle *jiao*, along with nourishing *yin* and regulating the interior to relieve pain. In the prescription, Saccharum Granorum, sweet and warm, and serving as the chief, benefits spleen *qi* to nourish spleen *yin* and warms the middle *jiao*. Cinnamomi warms *yang qi*, and Paeoniae Lactiflorae benefits *yin*-blood, and both are used as the adjuvant. Glycyrrhizae is sweet and warm; and helps Saccharum Granorum and Cinnamomi benefit *qi* and warm the middle *jiao*. It is combined with Paeoniae Lactiflorae to relieve pain, serving as the assistant. Zingiberis Recens warms the stomach and Jujubae invigorates the spleen; both are also used as the assistant and combined to regulate *yingfen* and *weifen*. The combination of these ingredients not only activates *yang* but also nourishes *yin*, and so are effective for warming the middle *jiao*, invigorating *qi*, regulating the interior and relieving abdominal pain.

Decoction for Mildly Warming the Middle *Jiao* is composed of the same ingredients as Decoction of Cinnamomi except that the former doubles the dosage of Paeoniae Lactiflorae and is added with Saccharum Granorum. In the latter, Cinnamomi is used as the chief and belongs to the category of prescriptions that expel superficial pathogens with acrid and warm drugs, while the former uses Saccharum Granorum as the chief, and is a prescription that warms the middle *jiao* and invigorates *qi*.

This prescription is also indicated for deficiency-heat syndrome after illness or delivery due to the imbalance between *yin* and *yang*, marked by fatigue, pale complexion and shortness of breath.

Appendant Prescription

Decoction of Astragali for Strengthening the Middle *Jiao*
黄芪建中汤 *huang qi jian zhong tang*
(from *Synopsis of the Golden Cabinet*)

It is composed of the same ingredients as Decoction for Mildly Warming the Middle *Jiao*, added with 5 g of Radix Astragali, and has the same method of administration. It acts to warm the middle *jiao*, invigorate *qi*, regulate the interior and relieve abdominal pain, and is indicated for consumptive diseases due to insufficient *qi* and blood with abdominal pain.

In accordance with the principles that "deficiency syndrome should be treated with tonic therapy" and "general debility should be invigorated with warm drugs," Astragali is used to benefit *qi* and invigorate the middle *jiao*, helping replenish both *yin* and *yang*. It is applicable for more serious cases, especially those with deficient *qi*, spontaneous perspiration and intermittent fever.

Decoction for Treating *Yang* Exhaustion
四逆汤 *si ni tang*
(from *Treatise on Cold Diseases*)

Radix Aconiti Lateralis	5-10 g
Rhizoma Zingiberis	6-9 g
Radix Glycyrrhizae Preparata	6 g

Administration: Decoct Aconiti Lateralis with a moderate amount of water for an hour, then add the other two drugs and decoct them together, and take the decoction when it is warm; or prepare the drugs into an intramuscular or intravenous injection, 2-4 ml each time.

Action: Recuperating the depleted *yang* and rescuing the patient from danger.

Indications: Shaoyin diseases showing extremely cold limbs, chills, vomiting with no thirst, diarrhea with abdominal pain, listlessness, sleepiness, smooth and white tongue coating, and weak and thready pulse; and Taiyang diseases erroneously treated by inducing sweating, leading to *yang* exhaustion.

Explanation: When pathogenic cold affects Shaoyin, kidney *yang* becomes deficient and, *yin* and *yang* separate from each other; this leads to extremely cold limbs, chills, and sleepiness as external manifestations, and vomiting with no thirst, diarrhea with abdominal pain, smooth and white tongue coating, and weak and thready pulse as internal ones. This is a critical case of overabundant *yin* and deficient *yang*, and it is imperative to use large dosages of acrid and hot drugs. In this prescription, Aconiti Lateralis is therefore used as the chief to help heart *yang* promote blood circulation, to invigorate kidney *yang* to benefit the life-gate fire, and to warm *yang* to eliminate pathogenic cold. Zingiberis, used as the adjuvant, warms spleen *yang* and eliminates internal cold, and helps Aconiti Lateralis strengthen the effect of warming *yang* in order to eliminate cold. Glycyrrhizae is used as the assistant; it benefits *qi*, invigorates the spleen, removes toxins and moderate the potent effects of the other two drugs. If vomiting appears upon taking the warm decoction, take it cold.

Appendant Prescription

Decoction of Ginseng for Treating *Yang* Exhaustion
四逆加人参汤 *si ni jia ren shen tang*
(from *Treatise on Cold Diseases*)

It is composed of the same ingredients as Decoction for Treating *Yang* Exhaustion, added with 3 g of Radix Ginseng (to be decocted separately). The method of administration is the same as that for Decoction for Treating *Yang* Exhaustion. It acts to recuperate the depleted *yang* and benefit *qi* in order to rescue the patient from danger, and is indicated for cases with extremely cold limbs, chills, diarrhea with abdominal pain, and weak and thready pulse; or else those with diarrhea relieved but the other symptoms still present.

In this prescription, Ginseng is added to benefit *qi*, recuperate the depleted *yang* and promote fluid production; It is especially effective for cases with exhaustion of *qi* and consumption of fluid.

Decoction of Ginseng and Aconiti Lateralis
参附汤 *shen fu tang*
(from *Annotations on Effective Prescriptions for Women*)

Radix Ginseng	30 g
Radix Aconiti Lateralis Preparata	15 g

Administration: Decoct with water for oral administration.

Action: Benefiting *qi*, recuperating depleted *yang* and rescuing the patient from danger.

Indications: Cases of exhaustion of primordial *qi* and depletion of *yang*, exhibiting extremely cold limbs, sweating, vertigo, shortness of breath, pale complexion, and deep and weak pulse.

Explanation: This is a well-known prescription, based on the principle of warming and invigorating *yang* and benefiting *qi* to recuperate *yang*. Here, Ginseng, sweet and warm, invigorates the primordial *qi* of the spleen and lung, benefits *qi* and recuperates the depleted *yang*; Aconiti Lateralis Preparata, acrid and hot, warms and invigorates kidney *yang*. They reinforce each other to invigorate the heart and lung in the upper part of the body, the spleen and stomach in the middle and the kidney in the lower, as well as to recuperate the depleted *yang*. Clinically, it is also effective for sudden onset of metrorrhagia, traumatic hemorrhage and collapse due to massive hemorrhage. Once *yang qi* is restored, this decoction should be discontinued, in order to avoid an over-intake of pure *yang* drugs which, on the contrary, may lead to the consumption of *yin* and blood. The quantity of the drugs should be modified according to the individual case. In some, a proper amount of Os Draconis and Concha Ostreae may be added to strengthen the effect of recuperating the depleted *yang*.

Decoction of Angelicae Sinensis for Warming Cold Limbs
当归四逆汤 *dang gui si ni tang*
(from *Treatise on Cold Diseases*)

Radix Angelicae Sinensis	9 g
Ramulus Cinnamomi	9 g
Radix Paeoniae Lactiflorae	9 g
Herba Asari	3 g
Radix Glycyrrhizae Preparata	6 g
Caulis Akebiae	6 g
Fructus Jujubae	12 pieces

Administration: Decoct with water for oral administration.

Action: Warming the meridians to expel cold, nourishing the blood to promote blood circulation.

Indications: Attack by cold in cases of blood deficiency and poor blood circulation, exhibiting extremely cold limbs, pale tongue with white coating, and deep and thready pulse; as well as pain in the waist, thigh, leg and foot due to invasion of cold in the meridians.

Explanation: A frequently used prescription for nourishing blood and promoting blood circulation, it is indicated for attack by cold in cases of blood deficiency. Here the blood fails to circulate smoothly and to warm and nourish the four limbs, leading to cold hands and feet, as well as deep and thready pulse. The therapeutic principle is to warm the meridians to expel cold, and nourish the blood to promote circulation. Therefore, Angelicae Sinensis is used to enrich the blood and regulate blood circulation; it is combined with Paeoniae Lactiflorae to strengthen the effect of relieving blood deficiency. Cinnamomi is used to warm the meridians to expel cold; it is combined with Asari to expel both internal and external cold. Glycyrrhizae and Jujubae benefit *qi* and invigorate the spleen, not only helping Angelicae Sinensis and Paeoniae Lactiflorae enrich the blood, but also helping Cinnamomi and Asari activate *yang*. Akebiae is used to regulate blood circulation in order to relieve all the above-mentioned symptoms.

Decoction for Warming *Yang*
阳和汤 *yang he tang*
(from *Treatise on Diagnosis and Treatment of External and Surgical Diseases*)

Radix Rehmanniae Preparata	30 g
Cortex Cinnamomi	3 g
Herba Ephedrae	2 g
Colla Cornu Cervi	9 g
Semen Sinapis Albae	6 g
Rhizoma Zingiberis (burnt)	2 g
Radix Glycyrrhizae	3 g

Administration: Decoct with water for oral administration.

Action: Warming *yang* and enriching the blood to expel cold and promote blood circulation.

Indications: *Yin*-type carbuncles, manifested as local and poorly demarcated swelling without any change of color and temperature, mild achiness, pale tongue with whitish coating, absence of thirst, and deep and thready pulse, or slow and thready pulse.

Explanation: This is frequently used for *yin*-type carbuncles, which are usually caused by deficiency cold at *yingfen* and *xuefen*, leading to cold and phlegm retention in the muscles, tendons, bones and meridians. The treatment seeks to warm *yang* and enrich the blood to expel cold and promote blood circulation. In the prescription, a larger dosage of Rehmanniae Preparata is used to nourish *yingfen* and *xuefen*. Colla Cornu Cervi nourishes the blood, invigorates *yang*, warms and strengthens the tendons and bones. Zingiberis (burnt) and Cinnamomi are used to warm the meridians to promote blood circulation. Ephedrae and Sinapis Albae activate *yang*, expel cold and relieve phlegm retention, and at the same time make Rehmanniae Preparata and Colla Cornu Cervi not so greasy. Glycyrrhizae is used to remove toxins and regulate the effects of other drugs.

This prescription should not be used for cases of carbuncles with pain and change of color and temperature, or with *yin* deficiency and fever, or with rupture of the lesion.

Summary

Presented in this chapter are seven principal and five appendant prescriptions, all indicated for interior-cold syndromes. In line with the location and degree of affection as well as severity of *yang* deficiency, they are classified into three sub-categories.

(1) Prescriptions for warming the middle *jiao* and eliminating cold:

This kind is indicated for deficiency cold in the middle *jiao*. Of these, Bolus for Regulating the Middle *Jiao* is a typical example for cases of deficiency cold in the middle *jiao* and diarrhea with abdominal pain; it warms the middle *jiao* to expel cold, benefit *qi* and invigorate the spleen. Decoction of Evodiae warms the middle *jiao*, restores *qi*, suppresses adversely rising *qi* to relieve vomiting, and is indicated for deficiency-cold syndromes in

Yangming, Jueyin and Shaoyin meridians, and mainly for cases with vomiting due to the rise of *yin*-cold. Decoction for Mildly Warming the Middle *Jiao* warms the middle *jiao*, invigorates *qi*, regulates the interior and relieves abdominal pain; it is effective for abdominal pain of the deficiency-cold type.

(2) Prescriptions for recuperating depleted *yang* and rescuing the patient from danger:

Prescriptions of this kind are indicated for critical cases of *yang* exhaustion caused by deficient *yang qi* and overabundant *yin*-cold, marked by cold limbs. One example is Decoction for Treating *Yang* Exhaustion, which is indicated for critical cases due to overabundant *yin* and deficient *yang*, showing the symptoms of cold extremities, vomiting, diarrhea, and weak and thready pulse, as well as the signs of the *yang* depletion. Decoction of Ginseng and Aconiti Lateralis is a well-known prescription for benefiting *qi* and recuperating *yang*, and is indicated for sudden collapse, consumption of primordial *qi*, or *yang* depletion due to massive hemorrhage.

(3) Prescriptions for warming the meridians to expel cold:

Such prescriptions are indicated for blood deficiency with cold in the meridians. Decoction of Angelicae Sinensis for Warming Cold Limbs is a representative for warming *yang*, nourishing the blood and expelling cold to promote blood circulation; it is indicated for attack by cold in cases of blood deficiency, marked by fading pulse, cold hands and feet. Decoction for Warming *Yang* is effective for warming *yang* and enriching the blood to expel cold and promote blood circulation, as indicated for *yin*-type carbuncles.

CHAPTER ELEVEN

PRESCRIPTIONS WITH TONIC EFFECT

Prescriptions with tonic effect (*bu yi ji*) are composed chiefly of tonics, which act to invigorate *qi*, blood, *yin* and *yang*, and is indicated for various kinds of deficiency syndromes. They are instances of invigorating therapy.

Since the etiology, location and the *zang-fu* organs affected in deficiency syndromes are different, the clinical manifestations and the principles of treatment of individual cases vary. In general, deficiency syndromes are classified into deficiency of *qi*, blood, both *qi* and blood, *yin* and *yang*, and the prescriptions are also grouped accordingly.

Prescriptions for invigorating *qi* (*bu qi ji*) are indicated for disorders involving deficiency of spleen and lung *qi*, exhibiting fatigue, shortness of breath, disinclination to speak, low voice, pale complexion, poor appetite, loose stools, dyspnea upon exertion, pale tongue with white coating, weak pulse, or even deficiency fever, spontaneous sweating, rectal prolapse, hysteroptosis, etc. The common *qi* tonics are Radix Ginseng, Radix Astragali, Rhizoma Atractylodis Macrocephalae and Radix Glycyrrhizae, which are combined with drugs that eliminate dampness, raise *yang* and nourish *yin* to form prescriptions for invigorating *qi*. The examples are Four Mild Drugs Decoction, Powder of Ginseng, Poria and Atractylodis Macrocephalae, Decoction for Strengthening the Middle *Jiao* and Benefiting *Qi*, and Powder for Restoring the Pulse.

Prescriptions for invigorating blood (*bu xue ji*) are indicated for disorders involving blood deficiency, exhibiting dizziness, sallow complexion, pale lips and nails, palpitations, insomnia, amnesia, irregular menstruation with scanty light-colored flow, pale tongue, and thready and rapid or unsmooth pulse. The common hematic tonics are Radix Angelicae Sinensis, Radix Paeoniae Alba, and Colla Corii Asini, which are combined with drugs that activate and regulate *qi*, activate the blood and tranquilize the mind to form the blood-invigorating prescriptions. The examples are Four Drugs Decoction, Decoction of Angelicae Sinensis for Enriching Blood and Decoction for Invigorating Spleen and Nourishing Heart.

Prescriptions for invigorating both *qi* and blood (*qi xue shuang bu ji*) are indicated for disorders with deficient *qi* and blood, exhibiting pale complexion, dizziness, palpitation, shortness of breath, fatigue, pale tongue, and feeble and thready pulse. They are usually composed of drugs that invigorate *qi*, such as Radix Ginseng, Radix Astragali and Radix Glycyrrhizae, and such hematic tonics as Radix Angelicae Sinensis, Radix Paeoniae Alba and Colla Corii Asini. The examples are Decoction of Eight Precious Ingredients and Decoction of Glycyrrhizae Preparata.

Prescriptions for invigorating *yin* (*bu yin ji*) are indicated for disorders with *yin* deficiency, exhibiting emaciation, dizziness, tinnitus, hectic fever, flushed cheeks, night sweating, insomnia, lumbago, nocturnal emission, dry cough, dryness of mouth and throat, red tongue with little coating, and thready and rapid pulse. The common drugs for nourishing *yin* are Radix Adenophorae, Radix Ophiopogonis, Plastrum Testudinis and Rhizoma Anemarrhenae, which are combined with drugs that purge heat, regulate *qi*, eliminate dampness and moisten the lung as well as expectorants and antitussives for such prescriptions. The examples are Pill of Six Drugs Containing Rehmanniae Preparata, *Yiguan* Decoction, Pill for *Yin* Replenishing, Decoction of Adenophorae and Ophiopogonis, and Decoction of Lilli for Strengthening Lung.

Prescriptions for invigorating *yang* (*bu yang ji*) are indicated for disorders with kidney *yang* deficiency, exhibiting pale complexion, soreness and weakness of the lumbus and knees, cold limbs, cold pain in the lower abdomen, difficult or frequent urination, impotence, praecox ejaculation, pale tongue with white coating, and deep, thready and weak pulse. Drugs commonly used for warming and invigorating kidney *yang* are Radix Aconiti Lateralis Preparata, Cortex Cinnamomi, Rhizoma Curculiginis, Herba Epimedii, and Radix Morindae Officinalis, which are combined with drugs that replenish kidney *yin*. An example is Pill for Invigorating Kidney *Qi*.

However, prescriptions with different tonic effects should not be considered independently. Since *qi* and blood generate each other, and *yin* and *yang* are interdependent, prescriptions for invigorating *qi* and for invigorating the blood are often used simultaneously, so are those for invigorating *yin* and *yang*.

Moreover, according to the theory of mutual promotion between the five elements, the principle to invigorating the mother organ in treating the disease of the son organ should be adopted, for instance, invigorating the kidney (water) to remedy the deficiency of liver (wood), invigorating the life-gate fire for the deficiency of the spleen (earth), invigorating the spleen (earth) for the deficiency of the lung (metal), and so on. Generally speaking, invigorating the kidney and spleen is the key of the tonic therapy, since the kidney is the prenatal basis in which true *yin* and true *yang* dwell, and the spleen is the postnatal basis that serves as the source of *qi* and blood production.

In applying tonic prescriptions, precautions should be taken in the following aspects: (1) It is necessary to determine whether the deficiency is true or false and its severity. Generally speaking, potent prescriptions are indicated for acute cases exhibiting *qi* and blood consumption to prevent collapse, and the mild ones are indicated for chronic cases to restore health gradually. (2) Tonic prescriptions are contraindicated for cases with hyperactive pathogens when the healthy energy is not yet impaired, so as to avoid the retention of the pathogens. (3) For cases of excess syndrome inappropriate for tonic therapy, spleen and stomach function should first be regulated before tonic prescriptions are given. (4) In order to fully elicit their curative effects, the ingredients of tonic prescriptions should be decocted over a slow fire for a longer period.

Four Mild Drugs Decoction

四君子汤 *si jun zi tang*

(from *Benevolent Prescriptions from the Pharmaceutical Bureau of the Taiping Period*)

Radix Ginseng	9 g
Poria	9 g
Rhizoma Atractylodis Macrocephalae	9 g
Radix Glycyrrhizae Preparata	6 g

Administration: Decoct with water for oral administration.

Action: Benefiting *qi* and strengthening the spleen.

Indications: Spleen and stomach *qi* deficiency, exhibiting pale complexion, low voice, fatigue, poor appetite, loose stools, pale tongue, and feeble and weak pulse.

Explanation: This prescription is indicated for disorders caused by spleen *qi* deficiency and disfunctional spleen and stomach. The spleen and stomach are the postnatal base and source of *qi* and blood production. Splenic deficiency may lead to insufficient *qi* and blood, manifested as pale complexion, fatigue and low voice. Spleen and stomach dysfunction may cause poor appetite and loose stools. A pale tongue with white coating and a feeble and weak pulse also signify spleen deficiency and weak *qi*. Hence, benefiting *qi* and strengthening the spleen constitute the proper treatment for such disorders. In the prescription, Ginseng serves as the chief drug and it, sweet and warm, benefits *qi*, invigorates the spleen and nourishes the stomach; Atractylodis Macrocephalae, as the adjuvant, is bitter and warm and acts to invigorate the spleen and dry dampness; Poria, sweet and bland, is the assistant and used to eliminate dampness and invigorate the spleen. The combination of Atractylodis Macrocephalae and Poria enhances the effects of invigorating the spleen and eliminating dampness. Glycyrrhizae Preparata serves as the guide; it is sweet and warm and used for benefiting *qi* and regulating the middle *jiao*. These four drugs, when used together, strengthen spleen and stomach *qi*, restore the functions of the spleen and stomach and promote *qi* and blood production.

This is a basic prescription for invigorating *qi*, and many prescriptions for invigorating *qi* and strengthening the spleen are derived from it.

Appendant Prescriptions

(1) Decoction of Six Mild Drugs

六君子汤 *liu jun zi tang*

(from *Effective Prescriptions for Gynecological Diseases*)

The prescription is composed of the ingredients of the Four Mild Drugs Decoction, to be added with 6 g of Pericarpium Citri Reticulatae and 6 g of Rhizoma Pinelliae. It invigorates the spleen and *qi*, regulates the stomach and dissolves sputum, and is indicated for cases with spleen and stomach *qi* deficiency complicated by phlegm-dampness, exhibiting fullness in the chest and epigastrium, poor appetite, nausea, vomiting, loose stools or cough with profuse thin and clear expectoration.

(2) Decoction of Six Mild Drugs with Cyperi and Amomi
香砂六君子汤 *xiang sha liu jun zi tang*
(from *Variorum of Prescriptions*)

The prescription is composed of the ingredients of the Six Mild Drugs Decoction, to be added with 6 g of Rhizoma Cyperi (substituted by 6 g of Radix Aucklandiae now) and 6 g of Fructus Amomi. It acts to invigorate the spleen, regulate the stomach and *qi* and relieve pain, and is indicated for cases with spleen and stomach *qi* deficiency, stagnant *qi* and retained dampness in the middle *jiao*, exhibiting abdominal fullness or pain, poor appetite, belching, vomiting and diarrhea.

Powder of Ginseng, Poria and Atractylodis Macrocephalae
参苓白术散 *shen ling bai zhu san*
(from *Benevolent Prescriptions from the Pharmaceutical Bureau of the Taiping Period*)

Semen Nelumbinis	500 g
Semen Coicis	500 g
Fructus Amomi	500 g
Radix Platycodi	500 g
Semen Dolichoris Album	750 g
Poria	1,000 g
Radix Ginseng	1,000 g
Rhizoma Atractylodis Macrocephalae	1,000 g
Radix Glycyrrhizae	1,000 g
Rhizoma Dioscoreae	1,000 g

Administration: Grind these drugs into fine powder, take 6 g of the powder each time with decoction of Fructus Jujubae. The dosage for children should be reduced correspondingly. The drugs can also be prepared into a decoction, with the dosages of the ingredients reduced proportionally.

Action: Benefiting *qi*, invigorating the spleen, regulating the stomach and eliminating dampness.

Indications: Spleen and stomach *qi* deficiency complicated by dampness, exhibiting weakness of limbs, emaciation, indigestion, vomiting or diarrhea, fullness in the epigastrium and chest, sallow complexion, white and greasy tongue coating, and feeble and slow pulse.

Explanation: The prescription is indicated for cases of spleen deficiency complicated by dampness. The spleen is the organ responsible for digestion and the activity of the limbs, and its dysfunction may lead to indigestion and weak limbs. Hypofunction of the spleen and stomach may cause abnormal ascent and descent of *qi* and failure to separate lucid and turbid substances, vomiting or diarrhea results. Fullness in the epigastrium and chest is an indication of functional disturbance of *qi*, and white and greasy tongue coating indicates dampness. In turn, a sallow complexion, emaciation, pale tongue all denote *qi* and blood insufficiency resulting from spleen dysfunction . Hence, the treatment for such disorders should be benefiting *qi*, invigorating the spleen, regulating the stomach and eliminating dampness. This prescription is based on the Four Mild Drugs Decoction. In it, Ginseng and Atractylodis Macrocephalae serve as the chief for invigorating *qi* and spleen; Dioscoreae and Semen Nelumbinis enhance the tonic effect of Ginseng; Dolichoris Album, Coicis and Poria assist Atractylodis Macrocephalae in invigorating the spleen, eliminating dampness and relieving diarrhea; Amomi and Platycodi help regulate the stomach, activate the spleen, regulate *qi* activities and ease the chest; Glycyrrhizae serves to harmonize the actions of all the drugs. These ingredients together cure general debility, eliminate dampness, regulate *qi* activities and restore spleen and stomach function, relieving all the above symptoms.

Decoction for Invigorating the Middle *Jiao* and Benefiting *Qi*
补中益气汤 *bu zhong yi qi tang*
(from *Comments on the Spleen and Stomach*)

Radix Astragali	10 g
Radix Glycyrrhizae Preparata	5 g
Radix Ginseng	3 g
Exocarpium Citri Reticulatae	3 g
Radix Angelicae Sinensis	2 g
Rhizoma Cimicifugae	3 g
Radix Bupleuri	3 g
Rhizoma Atractylodis Macrocephalae	3 g

Administration: Decoct with water for oral administration, or prepare as pills and take 6-9 g each time, twice or three times daily.

Action: Benefiting *qi*, reinforcing *yang qi*, regulating and invigorating the spleen and stomach.

Indications: (1) Spleen and stomach *qi* deficiency, exhibiting fever, spontaneous sweating, thirst with desire for hot drinks, disinclination to speak, lassitude, pale tongue with thin and white coating, and feeble pulse. (2) Sinking and deficiency of *qi*, manifested as rectal prolapse, hysteroptosis, long-standing diarrhea, and chronic malaria.

Explanation: This prescription is indicated for disorders due to deficiency of spleen and stomach *qi* and collapse of middle *jiao qi*. The spleen and stomach are the source of *ying*, *wei*, *qi* and blood, and their impairment may lead to fever resulting from *qi* and blood deficiency. *Qi* deficiency, which weakens the surface resistance, may induce spontaneous sweating, and failure to distribute fluid upward may elicit thirst with desire for hot drinks. Spleen *qi* deficiency may cause such symptoms as disinclination to speak, shortness of breath upon exertion, intolerance to strain, and fatigue. A pale tongue with thin and white coating, and feeble pulse also indicate *qi* deficiency. When the middle *jiao qi* sinks, it causes failure in controlling the organs and fluid. Hence, rectal prolapse, long-standing diarrhea, chronic dysentery and uterine prolapse occur. Therefore, the principle of treatment should be benefiting *qi*, reinforcing *yang qi*, regulating and invigorating the spleen and stomach. In the prescription, Astragali serves as the chief for invigorating the middle *jiao*, benefiting *qi*, reinforcing *yang qi* and strengthening surface resistance; Ginseng, Atractylodis Macrocephalae and Glycyrrhizae Preparata enhance the effects of Astragali; Citri Reticulatae and Angelicae Sinensis serve as the assistant, the former for regulating *qi* and stomach, the latter for tonic; and Cimicifugae and Bupleuri help restore the collapsed middle *jiao qi*. Combined use of these drugs strengthens the spleen and stomach, invigorates middle *jiao qi*, remedies *qi* deficiency, makes fever subside, raises the collapsed *qi*, and cures rectal and uterine prolapse.

Appendant Prescription

Decoction for Rescuing Collapse
升陷汤 *sheng xian tang*
(from *Discourse on Medical Problems Interpreted by Combining Chinese and Western Medicine*)

The prescription is composed of 18 g of Radix Astragali, 9 g of Rhizoma Anemarrhenae, 5 g of Radix Bupleuri, 5 g of Radix Platycodi and 3 g of Rhizoma Cimicifugae. The method of administration is to boil the drugs with water for oral administration. Acting to benefit *qi* and lift the collapsed *qi*, it is indicated for collapse of pectoral *qi*, manifested as shortness of breath, dyspnea, and deep and slow feeble pulse, or arrhythmia. This prescription is based on Decoction for Strengthening the Middle *Jiao* and Benefiting *Qi*. The lung controls *qi* activities, and lung *qi* collapse may lead to shortness of breath and dyspnea. The blood vessels of the whole body converge in the lung, and lung *qi* deficiency may impede blood flow, leading to deep, slow and feeble pulse. Astragali is the chief drug, which effectively invigorates lung *qi*; Platycodi regulates *qi* activities and eases the chest; Cimicifugae and Bupleuri raise the collapsed *qi*; Anemarrhenae, which is cold, serves to counteract the warmth of Astragali.

Powder (Decoction) for Restoring the Pulse
生脉散(生脉饮) *sheng mai san* (*sheng mai yin*)
(from *Differentiation of Endogenous and Exogenous Diseases*)

Radix Ginseng	6 g
Radix Ophiopogonis	6 g
Fructus Schisandrae	3 g

Administration: Decoct with water for oral administration.

Action: Benefiting *qi*, promoting fluid production, astringing *yin* fluid and stopping excessive perspiration.

Indications: Impairment of both *qi* and *yin*, exhibiting lassitude, shortness of breath, disinclination to speak, excessive perspiration, dry throat, thirst, and feeble pulse; also for long-standing cough due to lung deficiency, manifested as dry cough, shortness of breath, spontaneous sweating, dry mouth and tongue, and feeble pulse.

Explanation: This prescription is indicated for disorders due to impairment of both *qi* and *yin*. *Qi* and *yin* deficiency leads to shortness of breath, lassitude and thirst. The lung controls *qi* activities and the function of the skin, and lung *qi* deficiency weakens the surface resistance, leading to profuse perspiration which further consumes body fluid, and in turn causing dry throat and thirst. A feeble pulse may occur as a result of *qi* and *yin* deficiency. Hence, the therapeutic principle is to benefit *qi*, promote fluid production, astringe *yin*, and stop perspiration. In the prescription, Ginseng, sweet and warm, serves as the chief drug for benefiting *qi* and invigorating the lung; Ophiopogonis, sweet and cold, acts as the adjuvant to nourish *yin*, purge heat and increase fluid production; Schisandrae, sour and astringent, serves as the assistant to stop sweating and promote fluid production. The three drugs used together normalize *qi* activities and increase body fluid, so that the pulse is restored when *qi* is sufficient.

The prescription is a common remedy for impairment of both *qi* and *yin*. It is particularly suitable for cases of summer-heat syndrome with hyperhidrosis, *qi* and *yin* consumption, spiritlessness, and severe thirst. Its effect on long-standing cases of cough due to lung deficiency may be considered a causative treatment for restoring *qi* and *yin*, moistening the lung and promoting fluid production.

Four Drugs Decoction

四物汤 *si wu tang*

(from *Benevolent Prescriptions from the Pharmaceutical Bureau of the Taiping Period*)

Radix Angelicae Sinensis (soaked in wine and fried)	9 g
Rhizoma Chuanxiong	9 g
Radix Paeoniae Alba	9 g
Radix Rehmanniae Preparata	9 g

Administration: Decoct with water for oral administration.

Action: Enriching and regulating the blood.

Indications: Disorders involving deficiency and stagnation of *ying*-blood, such as irregular menstruation, amenorrhea, dysmenorrhea and blood-deficiency syndrome, exhibiting dizziness, tinnitus, lusterless lips and nails, pale tongue, and thready or thready and unsmooth pulse.

Explanation: This is indicated for disorders due to deficiency and stagnation of *ying*-

blood. Deficient blood, leading to insufficient liver blood and impaired Chong and Ren meridians, may induce oligomenorrhea, irregular menstruation, or even amenorrhea. *Ying*-blood deficiency, leading to impeded blood flow, may produce dysmenorrhea, dizziness, tinnitus, lusterless lips and nails, pale tongue, and thready or thready and unsmooth pulse. The therapeutic principle is to enrich and regulate the blood. In the prescription, Rehmanniae Preparata and Angelicae Sinensis serve as the chief ingredients to nourish *yin* and blood, and enrich and nourish the liver, respectively; Paeoniae Alba serves as the adjuvant, nourishing the blood, softening the liver and regulating *ying*; Chuanxiong acts as the assistant to regulate the blood and promote *qi* and blood circulation. The four drugs used together produce a tonic effect that can be easily absorbed. The prescription is used as a hematic tonic and a hemagogue.

This prescription is derived from Decoction of Colla Corii Asini and Artemisiae Argyi in *Synopsis of the Golden Cabinet*. It is a basic recipe for enriching the blood and regulating menstruation. It is effective for various kinds of blood-deficiency syndromes, irregular menstruation, as well as disorders during pregnancy and after childbirth.

Appendant Prescription

Decoction of Four Drugs with Persicae and Carthami
桃红四物汤 *tao hong si wu tang*
(from *Golden Mirror of Orthodox Medical Lineage*)

The prescription is composed of the same ingredients of Four Drugs Decoction, to be added with 6 g of Semen Persicae and 4 g of Flos Carthami. It nourishes the blood and activates blood circulation, and is indicated for cases of preceded menstrual cycle, menorrhagia with purplish and viscous discharge or discharge containing blood clots, and distensive abdominal pain.

Persicae and Carthami are added to remove blood stasis and activate blood circulation, so as to restore normal menstruation and relieve abdominal pain. However, overdose of the prescription should be avoided. Otherwise, metrorrhagia may occur.

Decoction of Angelicae Sinensis for Enriching the Blood
当归补血汤 *dang gui bu xue tang*
(from *Differentiation of Endogenous and Exogenous Diseases*)

Radix Astragali	30 g
Radix Angelicae Sinensis	6 g

Administration: Decoct with water for oral administration.

Action: Invigorating *qi* and promoting blood generation.

Indications: Damage to the internal organs by overstrain and *qi* and blood deficiency, exhibiting feverishness, flushed face, severe thirst, and bounding pulse that is feeble upon pressure; blood-deficiency syndrome during the menstrual period or puerperium of women with fever and headache; unhealed pyogenic skin infections after rupture.

Explanation: Damage to the internal organs by overstrain and primordial *qi* deficiency which leads to *yin*-blood deficiency and outward appearance of *yang* and cause feverishness, flushed face, severe thirst, and bounding pulse that is feeble upon pressure; all are indications of deficiency-heat syndrome. The recommended treatment is to invigorate *qi* and promote blood generation, so that *yin* and *yang* can be kept in balance and the deficiency fever subside spontaneously. Since the blood is generated from *qi*, Astragali is applied in large dosage to effectively invigorate spleen and lung *qi* to promote blood generation; Angelicae Sinensis is added to nourish the blood and regulate *ying*. *Yin* and *yang* thus grow, *qi* and blood become abundant, and the symptoms are relieved.

In cases of blood deficiency during menstruation and puerperium, fever is made to subside by benefiting *qi* and nourishing the blood; and in cases of unhealed pyogenic skin infections after rupture, granulation and healing are promoted by invigorating *qi* and nourishing the blood.

Decoction for Invigorating the Spleen and Nourishing the Heart
归脾汤 *gui pi tang*
(from *Prescriptions for Life Saving*)

Rhizoma Atractylodis Macrocephalae	30 g
Lignum Pini Poriaferum	30 g
Radix Astragali	30 g
Arillus Longan	30 g
Semen Ziziphi Spinosae (fried)	30 g
Radix Ginseng	15 g
Radix Aucklandiae	15 g
Radix Glycyrrhizae Preparata	8 g

(In the prescription recorded in *Effective Prescriptions for Gynecological Diseases*, 3 g of Radix Angelicae Sinensis and 3 g of Radix Polygalae are added)

Administration: Grind all the drugs into coarse powder, take 15 g of the powder each time and decoct it with 5 pieces of Zingiberis Recens and 3-5 pieces of Fructus Jujubae for oral administration; or prepared the powder into pills, take 9 g each time with warm water.

Action: Benefiting *qi*, enriching the blood, invigorating the spleen and nourishing the heart.

Indications: Disorders involving heart and spleen deficiency, exhibiting palpitation, amnesia, insomnia, poor appetite, fatigue, sallow complexion, pale tongue with thin whitish coating, and thready and slow pulse; also for cases of hemafecia, metrorrhagia or metrostaxis, preceded menstrual cycle, and hypermenorrhea with light-colored discharge due to spleen failure to control blood.

Explanation: This prescription is indicated for cases of heart and spleen damage by anxiety and overstrain that leads to damage and hypofunction of the heart and spleen and *qi* and blood insufficiency. The heart houses the mind and regulates blood circulation, while the spleen governs thinking, controls blood, and acts along with the stomach as the source of *qi* and blood production. Hence, spleen hypofunction leads to *qi* and blood deficiency and failure to nourish the heart, thus giving rise to palpitation, amnesia, insomnia, fatigue, poor appetite and sallow complexion. Weak spleen *qi* leads to failure of control over the blood, exhibiting hemafecia, metrorrhagia or metrostaxis. Treatment aims at benefiting *qi*, enriching the blood, invigorating the spleen and nourishing the heart. In the prescription, Ginseng, Astragali, Atractylodis Macrocephalae and Glycyrrhizae benefit *qi* and invigorate the spleen, so that the spleen function to control and produce blood can be restored; Angelicae Sinensis, Longan, Lignum Pini Poriaferum, Ziziphi Spinosae and Polygalae serve as hematic tonics and heart-nourishing agents, so that the mind can be tranquilized when the heart is nourished; Aucklandiae regulates *qi* and reinforces the spleen in order to promote the absorption of tonics; and Jujubae and Zingiberis regulate spleen and stomach function and help the production of *qi* and blood. All the drugs together generate *qi* and blood, invigorate the heart and spleen and relieve the above symptoms.

Eight Precious Ingredients Decoction

八珍汤 *ba zhen tang*

(from *Classification and Treatment of Traumatic Diseases*)

Radix Angelicae Sinensis	6 g
Rhizoma Chuanxiong	6 g
Radix Paeoniae Alba	6 g
Radix Rehmanniae Preparata	6 g
Radix Ginseng	6 g
Rhizoma Atractylodis Macrocephalae	6 g
Poria	6 g
Radix Glycyrrhizae Preparata	3 g

Administration: Prepared as an oral decoction by adding 2 pieces of Rhizoma Zingiberis Recens and 3 pieces of Fructus Jujubae.

Action: Invigorating and replenishing *qi* and blood.

Indications: Disorders of *qi* and blood deficiency, exhibiting pale or sallow complexion, dizziness, fatigue, shortness of breath, disinclination to speak, palpitation, poor appetite, pale tongue with thin whitish coating, and thready and weak or feeble and large pulse.

Explanation: Deficient *qi* and blood resulting from various diseases or bleeding disorders may lead to the above symptoms, and the treatment seeks to invigorate *qi* and blood. In the prescription, Ginseng and Rehmanniae Preparata serve as the chief for benefiting *qi* and invigorating the blood; Atractylodis Macrocephalae and Poria, as the adjuvant, enhance the ability of Ginseng to invigorate the spleen and benefit *qi*; Angelicae Sinensis and Paeoniae Alba help Rehmanniae Preparata nourish the blood and regulate *ying*; Chuanxiong activates *qi* and promotes blood circulation; and Glycyrrhizae Preparata invigorates the middle *jiao qi*, both serve as the assistant; and Zingiberis and Jujubae are applied to regulate the spleen and stomach and serve as the guide.

This prescription includes the ingredients of Four Mild Drugs Decoction and Four Drugs Decoction in addition to Zingiberis Recens and Jujubae. It is frequently used for debility after illness, various chronic diseases, disorders during pregnancy and puerperium, irregular menstruation, metrorrhagia, and intractable pyogenic skin infections, with *qi* and blood deficiency as the primary syndrome.

Appendant Prescriptions

(1) Decoction of Ten Powerful Tonic Drugs

十全大补汤 *shi quan da bu tang*

(from *Benevolent Prescriptions from the Pharmaceutical Bureau of the Taiping Period*)

The prescription is composed of 6 g of Radix Ginseng; 3 g of Cortex Cinnamomi; 6 g of Rhizoma Chuanxiong; 6 g of Radix Rehmanniae Preparata; 6 g of Poria; 6 g of Rhizoma Atractylodis Macrocephalae; 5 g of Radix Glycyrrhizae Preparata; 6 g of Radix Astragali; 6 g of Radix Angelicae Sinensis; and 6 g of Radix Paeoniae Alba. All these drugs are prepared into decoction, pills (6-9 g per dose), or spirit (10-15 ml, twice daily). It warms and invigorates *qi* and blood, and is indicated for cases of *qi* and blood deficiency exhibiting cough due to visceral impairment, poor appetite, emission, weak lumbus and knees, intractable pyogenic skin infections, metrorrhagia, etc.

(2) Decoction of Ginseng for Nourishing *Qi* and *Ying*

人参养荣汤 *ren shen yang rong tang*

(from *Benevolent Prescriptions from the Pharmaceutical Bureau of the Taiping Period*)

The prescription is composed of 30 g of Radix Angelicae Sinensis; 30 g of Pericarpium Citri Reticulatae; 30 g of Radix Ginseng; 30 g of Lignum Cinnamomi; 30 g of Radix Astragali; 30 g of Rhizoma Atractylodis Macrocephalae; 22 g of Radix Rehmanniae Preparata; 22 g of Fructus Schisandrae; and 15 g of Radix Polygalae. The drugs are ground into granules and mixed, 3 pieces of Rhizoma Zingiberis Recens and 2 pieces of Fructus Jujubae are added and decocted with 12 g of the mixture for oral administration each time; or prepare the mixture into pills with honey, take 6-9 g each time; or directly prepare the drugs into an oral decoction, with their dosages reduced proportionally. It benefits *qi*, enriches the blood, nourishes the heart and calms the mind, and is indicated for visceral impairment by overstrain, exhibiting shortness of breath, dyspnea upon exertion, palpitation, dry throat and tongue, etc.

Although the above three prescriptions are all indicated for cases of deficiency of both *qi* and blood, their effects are somewhat different. Eight Precious Ingredients Decoction has only a mild tonic effect on *qi* and blood; Decoction of Ten Powerful Drugs produces a warming and tonic effect; and Decoction of Ginseng for Nourishing *Qi* and *Ying* not only has a tonic effect on *qi* and blood but also a heart-nourishing and tranquilizing action.

Decoction of Glycyrrhizae Preparata
(Decoction for Restoring the Pulse and Nourishing *Yin*)
炙甘草汤(复脉汤) *zhi gan cao tang* (*fu mai tang*)
(from *Treatise on Cold Diseases*)

Radix Glycyrrhizae Preparata	12 g
Rhizoma Zingiberis Recens	9 g
Radix Ginseng	6 g
Radix Rehmanniae	30 g
Ramulus Cinnamomi	9 g
Colla Corii Asini	6 g
Radix Ophiopogonis	10 g
Fructus Cannabis	10 g
Fructus Jujubae	5-10 pieces

Administration: Decoct all drugs except Colla Corii Asini with water, add 10 ml of wine to the decoction, divide Colla Corii Asini into two halves and mix it with the decoction for oral administration.

Action: Benefiting *qi*, nourishing the blood and *yin*, and restoring pulse beating.

Indications: (1) *Qi* and blood deficiency, manifested as slow and irregular pulse, palpitation, emaciation, shortness of breath, pale, and dry and uncoated tongue. (2) Cough due to visceral impairment associated with bloody sputum, shortness of breath, emaciation, insomnia, spontaneous or night sweating, dry throat and tongue, dyschesia, and feeble and rapid pulse.

Explanation: *Qi* and blood deficiency may lead to *qi* stagnation in the vessels and cause failure in nourishing heart blood, exhibiting slow and irregular pulse and palpitation. Consumption of *qi* and blood may lead to undernourishment, manifested as emaciation and shortness of breath. Deficient *qi* and blood in the heart gives rise to pale, dry and uncoated tongue, while cough due to visceral impairment, bloody sputum, fatigue and shortness of breath indicate insufficient *qi* and *yin* that fail to nourish the lung. Hence, the therapeutic principle should be benefiting *qi*, nourishing *yin*, enriching the blood and restoring the pulse. In the prescription, Glycyrrhizae Preparata, sweet and warm, serves as the chief for benefiting *qi* and nourishing the heart; Ginseng and Jujubae benefit *qi*, invigorate the spleen, and nourish the heart; and Rehmanniae, Colla Corii Asini, Ophiopogonis and Cannabis nourish *yin*, enrich the blood and nourish heart *yin*—all act as the adjuvant. Ramulus Cinnamomi, Zingiberis Recens and wine, acrid, warm and dispersive, serve as the assistant to activate *yang qi* and dredge the vessels. In summary, all these drugs act to benefit heart *qi*, replenish heart blood, nourish heart *yin* and invigorate heart *yang* to restore the pulse.

This is a common prescription for cases of slow and irregular pulse and palpitation due to *qi* and blood deficiency, and it is also indicated for cases of cough due to visceral impairment. For cases of obvious impairment of lung *yin* and dryness in the lung, Zingiberis Recens, Ramulus Cinnamomi and wine are reduced or removed to prevent consumption of *yin*-fluid.

Appendant Prescription

Modified Decoction for Restoring the Pulse and Nourishing *Yin*
加减复脉汤 *jia jian fu mai tang*
(from *Essentials of Seasonal Febrile Diseases*)

The prescription is composed of 18 g of Radix Glycyrrhizae Preparata; 18 g of Radix Rehmanniae (dried); 18 g of Radix Paeoniae Alba; 15 g of Radix Ophiopogonis; 9 g of Colla Corii Asini; and 9 g of Fructus Cannabis. They are prepared as an oral decoction. It nourishes blood and *yin*, promotes fluid generation and moistens dryness, and is indicated for the late stage of seasonal febrile diseases with heat retention and *yin*-blood deficiency, exhibiting a hot sensation in the soles and palms, dry mouth and tongue, and feeble and large pulse.

This prescription is derived from Zhang Zhongjing's *Decoction for Restoring the Pulse*. At the late stage of seasonal febrile diseases when *yin*-fluid is consumed by heat, such drugs for warming *yang* and benefiting *qi* as Ramulus Cinnamomi, Zingiberis Recens, Ginseng and Jujubae are omitted, and Paeoniae Alba is added to nourish the blood and *yin* and promote fluid production.

Pill of Six Drugs Containing Rehmanniae Preparata
(originally named Pill of Rehmanniae)
六味地黄丸(地黄丸) *liu wei di huang wan* (*di huang wan*)
(from *Medical Elucidation of Pediatrics*)

Radix Rehmanniae Preparata	24 g
Fructus Corni	12 g
Rhizoma Dioscoreae	12 g
Rhizoma Alismatis	9 g
Cortex Moutan Radicis	9 g
Poria	9 g

Administration: Grind all the drugs into granules and prepare into pills with honey, and take 6-9 g each time, twice or three times daily; or directly prepare them into an oral decoction.

Action: Nourishing *yin* and invigorating the kidney.

Indications: Cases of kidney *yin* insufficiency and upward attack of deficiency fire, exhibiting soreness and weakness in the lumbus and knees, dizziness, tinnitus, deafness, night sweating, nocturnal emission, diabetes, hectic fever, a hot sensation in the soles and palms, dry throat and tongue, loose teeth, heel pain, dripping urination, red tongue with little coating, and thready and rapid pulse.

Explanation: This prescription is indicated for disorders due to kidney *yin* insufficiency and upward attack of deficiency fire. The lumbus houses the kidney, which controls the growth of bones, marrow and teeth, and so insufficient kidney *yin* may give rise to soreness and weakness of the lumbus and knees and loose teeth. The brain is the "sea of marrow," and kidney *yin* deficiency may impede the production of marrow and the function of the brain, causing dizziness. When kidney *yin* is deficient, the essence cannot be sent to the ears, resulting in tinnitus and deafness. Since the kidney stores the essence, the ministerial fire may disturb the spermatic room when kidney *yin* is deficient, leading to nocturnal emission. *Yin* deficiency may lead to internal heat generation, resulting in hectic fever, a hot sensation in the soles and palms, diabetes and night sweating. *Yin* deficiency in the lower body may induce an upward attack of deficiency fire, causing dry throat and red and dry tongue with little coating. The principle of treatment is to nourish *yin* and invigorate the kidney. In the prescription, Rehmanniae Preparata is the chief ingredient, used to nourish *yin*, invigorate the kidney, and replenish the essence and marrow; Corni and Dioscoreae serve as the adjuvant, the former used to nourish the liver and kidney in order to preserve essence, and the latter to invigorate spleen *yin* to strengthen essence. The above three drugs serve as the adjuvant and act together to nourish liver, spleen and kidney *yin*, particularly the latter. Moreover, Alismatis is added to purge turbid materials, promote diuresis and counteract the greasy character of Rehmanniae, Moutan Radicis purges liver fire and inhibits the warm character of Corni, and Poria purges the spleen dampness and enhances the ability of Dioscoreae to invigorate the spleen — the three, which form the so-called "three purgative drugs," serve as the assistant and guide. The six drugs together produce a tonic effect without causing any retention of pathogens and a purgative effect without damaging the antipathogenic *qi*. This is an ideal formula with both tonic and purgative effects, in which these two effects supplement each other. It was proposed by Qian Zhongyang and formed by omitting Ramulus Cinnamomi and Radix Aconiti Lateralis from Pill for Invigorating Kidney *Qi*, a prescription recorded in *Synopsis of the Golden Cabinet*. Formerly, it was used for delayed development in children, but is now widely applied in various syndromes due to deficient kidney *yin*.

Appendant Prescriptions

(1) Bolus of Anemarrhenae, Phellodendri and Rehmanniae Preparata

知柏地黄丸 *zhi bai di huang wan*

(from *Golden Mirror of Orthodox Medical Lineage*)

The prescription is composed of the same ingredients of Pill of Six Drugs Containing Rehmanniae Preparata with the addition of 6 g of Rhizoma Anemarrhenae and 6 g of Cortex Phellodendri. It is prepared into honeyed bolus, or else as an oral decoction. It acts to nourish *yin* and suppress fire, and is indicated for cases of deficient *yin* and hyperactive fire, exhibiting hectic fever, restlessness, night sweating, lumbago and nocturnal emission.

(2) Bolus of Lycii, Chrysanthemi and Rehmanniae Preparata

杞菊地黄丸 *qi ju di huang wan*

(from *Comprehensive Medical Collections*)

The prescription is composed of the same ingredients of Pill of Six Drugs Containing Rehmanniae Preparata with the addition of 9 g of Fructus Lycii and 9 g of Flos Chrysanthemi. To be prepared into honeyed bolus, or else as an oral decoction, it nourishes the liver and kidney, and is indicated for dizziness, poor vision or xerophthalmia and irritated epiphora.

(3) *Zuogui* Decoction

左归饮 *zuo gui yin*

(from *Complete Collection of Jingyue's Treatises*)

It is composed of 9 g of Radix Rehmanniae Preparata, 6 g of Rhizoma Dioscoreae, 6 g of Fructus Lycii, 3 g of Radix Glycyrrhizae Preparata, 4 g of Poria, and 5 g of Fructus Corni. To be prepared as an oral decoction, it invigorates and benefits kidney *yin*, and is indicated for cases of insufficient true *yin*, exhibiting lumbago, nocturnal emission, night sweating, dry mouth and throat, thirst, reddish tongue tip, and thready and rapid pulse.

The above three prescriptions are all modifications of Pill of Six Drugs Containing Rehmanniae Preparata, and act to nourish *yin* and invigorate the kidney. However, Bolus of Anemarrhenae, Phellodendri and Rehmanniae Preparata, tends to nourish *yin* and suppress fire, and is suitable for cases with hectic fever, nocturnal emission and night sweating due to deficient *yin* and hyperactive fire; Bolus of Lycii, Chrysanthemi and Rehmanniae Preparata tends to nourish the liver and kidney, and is appropriate for cases with dizziness and poor vision due to deficient liver and kidney *yin*; and *Zuogui* Decoction has a stronger action in invigorating the kidney than Pill of Six Drugs Containing Rehmanniae Preparata, and is indicated for cases of deficiency of true *yin*.

***Yiguan* Decoction**

一贯煎 *yi guan jian*

(from *Supplement to Classified Records of Cured Cases by Celebrated Physicians*)

Radix Glehniae	9 g

Radix Ophiopogonis	9 g
Radix Angelicae Sinensis (body part)	9 g
Radix Rehmanniae	18 g
Fructus Lycii	9 g
Fructus Toosendan	5 g

Administration: Decoct with water for oral administration.

Action: Nourishing *yin* and releasing liver *qi*.

Indications: Disorders with liver and kidney *yin* deficiency and liver *qi* stagnation, exhibiting pain in the chest, hypochondrium and epigastrium, acid regurgitation, dry mouth and throat, red and dry tongue, and thready and weak or feeble and taut pulse, or hernia.

Explanation: This prescription is indicated for disorders due to both liver and kidney *yin* deficiency, as well as liver *qi* stagnation. Since the liver is built as *yin* but functions as *yang*, liver *qi* is jeopardized when liver and kidney *yin* is deficient, producing pain in the chest, hypochondrium and epigastrium. Attack of the stomach by stagnant liver *qi* leads to acid regurgitation, and deficient *yin* and fluid results in dry mouth and throat as well as red and dry tongue. The treatment should be nourishing the liver and kidney, and releasing stagnant liver *qi*. In the prescription, Rehmanniae is used in large dosage and serves as the chief ingredient for nourishing *yin* and blood to invigorate the liver and kidney; Glehniae, Ophiopogonis, Angelicae Sinensis and Lycii, as the adjuvant ingredients, help the chief ingredient nourish *yin* and blood, promote fluid production and soften the liver; Toosendan serves as the assistant and guide to release stagnant liver *qi*; it is used in small dosage and its bitter and dry property is counteracted by the sweet and cold *yin*-nourishing drugs so that its impairment to *yin* is prevented. These drugs together nourish and soften the liver to release stagnant liver *qi*.

Pill for Replenishing *Yin* (formerly Invigoration Pill)

大补阴丸(大补丸) *da bu yin wan* (*da bu wan*)

(from *Danxi's Experience on Medicine*)

Cortex Phellodendri	120 g
Rhizoma Anemarrhenae (soaked in wine and then fried)	120 g
Radix Rehmanniae Preparata (steamed with wine)	180 g
Plastrum Testudinis (fried until crisp)	180 g

Administration: Grind the drugs into fine powder and prepare the powder with steamed pig's spinal cord and honey into pills, take 9 g each time, twice daily, or else as an oral decoction, with the dosages of the ingredients reduced proportionally.

Action: Nourishing *yin* and suppressing fire.

Indications: Disorders with deficient liver and kidney *yin* and an upward attack of deficiency fire, exhibiting hectic fever, night sweating, nocturnal emission, cough, hemoptysis, or irritability, liability to be hungry, pain and hotness of the feet and knees, red tongue with little coating, and rapid and forceful pulse in the *chi* region.

Explanation: This prescription is indicated for disorders with deficient liver and kidney *yin* and an upward attack by deficiency fire. Deficient liver and kidney *yin* leads to hyperactive ministerial fire, which gives rise to hectic fever, night sweating, irritability, hunger, and painful and hot feet and knees. The insufficient true *yin*, which leads to a flare-up of deficiency fire, damages the lung collaterals and induces cough and hemoptysis. Treatment aims at nourishing *yin* and suppressing fire. In the prescription, Rehmanniae Preparata and Plastrum Testudinis are used together to nourish true *yin* and suppress *yang* and fire; Phellodendri, bitter and cold, is included to purge kidney fire and strengthen kidney *yin*; Anemarrhenae nourishes *yin*, purges heat, promotes fluid production and protects true *yin*; honey and pig's spinal cord are tonics for essence and blood. All the above together nourish *yin*-essence and purge ministerial fire so as to strengthen body resistance.

This is a prescription frequently used to nourish *yin* and suppress deficiency fire, and clinical evidence calling for its application includes hectic fever, red tongue with little coating, and rapid forceful pulse in the *chi* region.

Decoction of Adenophorae and Ophiopogonis
沙参麦冬汤 *sha shen mai dong tang*
(from *Essentials of Seasonal Febrile Diseases*)

Radix Adenophorae	6 g
Rhizoma Polygonati Odorati	6 g
Radix Glycyrrhizae	3 g
Folium Mori	4.5 g
Radix Ophiopogonis	9 g
Semen Dolichoris Album	4.5 g
Radix Trichosanthis	4.5 g

Administration: Decoct with water for oral administration.

Action: Eliminating lung and stomach heat, promoting fluid production and moistening dryness.

Indications: Disorders due to deficient lung and stomach *yin*, manifested as dry throat, thirst and red tongue; or disorders due to affection by dryness-heat, marked by fever and dry cough.

Explanation: Long-standing cases of lung and stomach *yin* deficiency, or their consumption by dryness-heat, may give rise to the above manifestations. The treatment aims at purging lung and stomach heat, promoting fluid production and moistening dryness. In the prescription, Adenophorae and Ophiopogonis serve as the chief ingredients for purging lung and stomach heat; Polygonati Odorati and Trichosanthis are the adjuvant, promoting fluid production and moistening dryness; Dolichoris Album and Glycyrrhizae benefit *qi*, reinforce the middle *jiao* and regulate stomach *qi*; and Mori purges lung heat; they serve as the assistant and guide ingredients.

Decoction of Lilli for Strengthening the Lung
百合固金汤 *bai he gu jin tang*
(from *Variorum of Prescriptions*)

Radix Rehmanniae	6 g
Radix Rehmanniae Preparata	9 g
Radix Ophiopogonis	5 g
Bulbus Fritillariae Thunbergii	3 g
Radix Angelicae Sinensis	3 g
Bulbus Lilii	3 g
Radix Paeoniae Alba (fried)	3 g
Radix Glycyrrhizae	3 g
Radix Scrophulariae	2 g
Radix Platycodi	2 g

Administration: Decoct with water for oral administration.

Action: Nourishing *yin*, purging heat, moistening the lung and eliminating sputum.

Indications: Disorders due to lung and kidney *yin* deficiency and an upward attack by deficiency fire, manifested as dry throat, sore throat, cough with bloody sputum, dyspnea, a hot sensation in the palms and soles, red tongue with little coating, and thready and rapid pulse.

Explanation: This prescription is indicated for disorders due to lung and kidney *yin* deficiency. *Yin* deficiency leads to the formation of internal heat and the flare-up of deficiency fire, and causes dry throat and sore throat. Pathogenic fire damages the lung collaterals and leads to cough with bloody sputum and dyspnea. The hot sensation in the palms and soles, red uncoated tongue and thready and rapid pulse are indications of *yin* deficiency with internal heat. Treatment seeks to nourish *yin*, purge heat, moisten the lung and eliminate sputum. In the prescription, Lilli, Rehmanniae and Rehmanniae Preparata nourish the lung and kidney, and they act as the chief ingredients; Ophiopogonis and Fritillariae Thunbergii, serving as the adjuvant, moisten the lung, nourish *yin*, eliminate sputum and relieve cough. Scrophulariae, Angelicae Sinensis, Paeoniae Alba and Platycodi serve as the assistant ingredients: Scrophulariae nourishes *yin* and cools the blood to purge deficiency heat; Angelicae Sinensis and Paeoniae Alba nourish *yin* and benefit *qi*; Platycodi releases lung *qi* to relieve cough and eliminate sputum. Glycyrrhizae serves as the guide to coordinate the effects of other drugs, and also assists Platycodi in easing the throat. These drugs together enrich *yin*-fluid and nourish the lung and kidney, and eventually suppress deficiency fire.

Pill for Invigorating Kidney *Qi*
肾气丸 *shen qi wan*
(from *Synopsis of the Golden Cabinet*)

Radix Rehmanniae (dried)	240 g
Rhizoma Dioscoreae	120 g
Fructus Corni	120 g
Rhizoma Alismatis	90 g
Cortex Moutan Radicis	90 g
Poria	90 g
Ramulus Cinnamomi	30 g
Radix Aconiti Lateralis Preparata	30 g

Administration: Grind all the drugs into fine powder and prepare it into pills with honey, take 9 g each time and twice daily with warm water or salt water; or prepare them directly into an oral decoction, with their dosages reduced proportionally.

Action: Warming and invigorating kidney *yang*.

Indications: Disorders due to insufficient kidney *yang*, exhibiting lumbago, weak lower limbs, a cold sensation in the lower part of the body, lower abdominal spasm, difficulty in urination or polyuria, weak, deep and thready pulse in the *chi* region, and pale and corpulent tongue; also for beriberi, phlegm-fluid retention syndrome and diabetes due to insufficient kidney *yang*.

Explanation: Kidney is the prenatal basis that houses life-gate fire. Insufficient kidney *yang* causes failure to warm and nourish the lower *jiao*, exhibiting lumbago, weak lower limbs, a cold sensation in the lower part of the body and lower abdominal spasm. Kidney *yang* deficiency also disturbs *qi* activities and causes fluid stagnation, resulting in difficult urination, edema of the legs, or polyuria if the fluid is not well controlled; disturbance in fluid metabolism causes formation of phlegm, resulting in phlegm-fluid retention syndrome; diabetes occurs when fluid fails to go up. The therapeutic principle should be warming and invigorating kidney *yang*. In the prescription, Rehmanniae is applied to invigorate kidney *yin*; Corni and Dioscoreae invigorate the liver and kidney and help Rehmanniae invigorate kidney *yin*; a small amount of Aconiti Lateralis Preparata and Ramulus Cinnamomi warms kidney *yang* and activates kidney *qi*; and Alismatis, Moutan Radicis and Poria purge the turbid materials from the kidney. In summary, the prescription is used to strengthen both the water and fire and coordinate *yin* and *yang*, and eventually eliminate the pathogens, restore the antipathogenic *qi* and strengthen kidney *qi*. In the prescription, small dosages of drugs for warming kidney *yang* are added to drugs that nourish kidney *yin*, aiming to gradually generate the physiological fire to warm and nourish kidney *qi*.

Appendant Prescriptions

(1) *Jisheng* Pill for Invigorating Kidney *Qi*

(formerly Pill for Invigorating Kidney *Qi* with Modifications)
济生肾气丸 *ji sheng shen qi wan*
(from *Prescriptions for Life Saving*)

The prescription is composed of the same ingredients of Pill for Invigorating Kidney *Qi* with the addition of 15 g of Radix Achyranthis Bidentatae and 30 g of Semen Plantaginis. All the drugs are ground into fine powder and made into pills with honey. The patient is advised to take 9 g each time with warm water. It warms and invigorate kidney *yang*, promotes diuresis and reduces edema, and is indicated for insufficient kidney *yang*, exhibiting heaviness in the lumbus, edema of the lower limbs and difficulty in urination.

(2) Yougui Decoction
右归饮 *you gui yin*
(from *Complete Collection of Jingyue's Treatises*)

The prescription is composed of 6-30 g of Radix Rehmanniae Preparata, 6 g of Rhizoma Dioscoreae, 3 g of Fructus Corni, 6 g of Fructus Lycii, 6 g of Radix Glycyrrhizae Preparata, 6 g of Cortex Eucommiae, 6 g of Cortex Cinnamomi, and 3-9 g of Radix Aconiti Lateralis Preparata. To be decocted for oral administration, it warms the kidney to enrich the essence, and is indicated for cases of insufficient kidney *yang*, manifested as shortness of breath, fatigue, abdominal pain, lumbago, cold limbs, and thready pulse; or cases in which *yang* is kept outside by excessive *yin* (*yin sheng ge yang*) inside the body, or true-cold syndrome with false heat syndrome.

These two appendant prescriptions are modified versions of Pill for Invigorating Kidney *Qi*, and act to warm and invigorate kidney *yang*. In the *Jisheng* Pill for Invigorating Kidney *Qi*, Achyranthis Bidentatae and Semen Plantaginis are added to promote diuresis and reduce edema, and it is usually applied for edema due to insufficient kidney *yang*. The *Yougui* Decoction is formed by omitting the three "purgative" drugs—Alismatis, Moutan Radicis and Poria—and adding Cortex Eucommiae, Fructus Lycii and Radix Glycyrrhizae Preparata; it exerts a pure tonic action without purgative action. Its ability to benefit and support *yang* is more evident, and it is usually applied for cases of declination of the life-gate fire as a result of insufficient kidney *yang*.

Summary

Covered in this chapter are fifteen principal and thirteen appendant prescriptions. They are classified into five sub-categories according to their specific actions: invigorating *qi*, the blood, both *qi* and blood, *yin*, and *yang*.

(1) Prescriptions for invigorating *qi*:

They include Four Mild Drugs Decoction, Powder of Ginseng, Poria and Atractylodis Macrocephalae, Decoction for Strengthening the Middle *Jiao* and Benefiting *Qi*, and Powder for Restoring the Pulse, which are indicated for various disorders with *qi* deficiency. Four Mild Drugs Decoction is the basic formula for benefiting *qi* and invigorating the spleen, and is applicable to disorders with deficient spleen and stomach *qi*, as well as the organs' hypofunction. Aside from the above basic effects, Powder of Ginseng, Poria and Atractylodis Macrocephalae can also regulate the stomach and eliminate dampness, and is indicated for cases of spleen and stomach *qi* deficiency complicated by dampness. Decoction for Strengthening the Middle *Jiao* and Benefiting *Qi* is more effective at raising *yang qi*, and is appropriate for patients with impaired spleen and stomach, functional fever due to *qi* deficiency, or rectal prolapse and hysteroptosis due to insufficient middle *jiao qi* or the collapse of *qi*. Powder for Restoring the Pulse can also nourish *yin*, promote fluid production and arrest sweating, and is indicated for cases with consumption of *qi* and fluid by heat, as well as long-standing cough that impairs lung *qi* and *yin*.

(2) Prescriptions for invigorating blood:

Covered in this sub-category are Four Drugs Decoction, Decoction of Angelicae Sinensis for Enriching the Blood, and Decoction for Invigorating the Spleen and Nourishing the Heart; they are indicated for various disorders due to blood deficiency. Among them, Four Drugs Decoction is the basic recipe for enriching and regulating the blood, and is suitable for irregular menstruation, dysmenorrhea and metrorrhagia due to the deficiency and stagnation of *ying*-blood and weakness of the Chong and Ren meridians. Decoction of Angelicae Sinensis for Enriching the Blood possesses a blood-nourishing effect by invigorating *qi*, and is used for cases of impairment of the internal organs by overstrain, as well as fever due to blood deficiency. Decoction for Invigorating the Spleen and Nourishing the Heart acts as a *qi* and blood tonic to this effect, and is used for cases with palpitation, insomnia, hemafecia, metrorrhagia, and purpura due to heart and spleen deficiency.

(3) Prescriptions for invigorating both *qi* and blood:

They include Eight Precious Ingredients Decoction and Decoction of Glycyrrhizae Preparata, both of which are indicated for disorders due to deficiency of both *qi* and blood. The former is used for cases in which the disorder occurs after prolonged illness or excessive loss of blood. The latter additionally nourishes *yin* and restores the pulse, and is appropriate for cases of palpitation and bradyarrythmia due to deficient heart blood or declination of heart *qi* (*yang*).

(4) Prescriptions for invigorating *yin*:

They include Pill of Six Drugs Containing Rehmanniae Preparata, *Yiguan* Decoction, Pill for *Yin* Replenishing, Decoction of Adenophorae and Ophiopogonis, and Decoction of Lilli for Strengthening the Lung; they are indicated for various disorders due to *yin* deficiency. Here, Pill of Six Drugs Containing Rehmanniae Preparata is a representative one for invigorating the kidney and nourishing *yin*; it not only invigorates the liver and kidney but also spleen *yin*, and is indicated for cases of insufficient kidney *yin* and the flare-up of deficiency fire, which exhibit soreness and weakness of the lumbus and knees, tinnitus, night sweating and hectic fever. Pill for Invigorating *Yin* is mainly for nourishing kidney *yin* and suppressing fire, and applicable to cases of liver and kidney *yin* deficiency and hyperactive ministerial fire. *Yiguan* Decoction nourishes *yin* and releases liver *qi*, and is used for cases with pain in the chest, epigastrium and hypochondrium due to deficient liver and kidney *yin* and stagnant liver *qi*. Decoction of Adenophorae and Ophiopogonis is chiefly used for purging lung and stomach fire, promoting fluid production and moistening dryness, and is indicated for cases with dry mouth and tongue as well as dry cough due to deficient lung and stomach *yin*. Decoction of Lilli for Strengthening the Lung is a formula for nourishing *yin*, purging heat, moistening the lung and eliminating sputum, suitable for cases of deficient lung and kidney *yin* and the flare-up of deficiency fire exhibiting painful throat, cough with bloody sputum, a hot sensation in the palms and soles, red tongue with little coating, and thready and rapid pulse.

(5) Prescriptions for invigorating *yang*:

The example here is Pill for Invigorating Kidney *Qi*. It warms and invigorates kidney *yang*, and is indicated for various disorders with insufficient kidney *yang* and declination of the life-gate fire.

CHAPTER TWELVE
PRESCRIPTIONS WITH ASTRINGENT EFFECTS

Prescriptions with astringent effects (*gu se ji*) are mainly composed of astringent drugs. They are indicated for disorders of excessive loss of *qi*, blood, essence and fluid.

Due to differences in etiology and affected parts, disorders with excessive loss of *qi*, blood, essence and fluid may exhibit spontaneous sweating or night sweating, nocturnal emission or ejaculatio praecox, prolonged diarrhea or chronic dysentery, and metrorrhagia or leukorrhagia. Accordingly, the prescriptions may be classified as follows:

Prescriptions for strengthening the surface to stop perspiration (*gu biao zhi han ji*) are indicated for cases of spontaneous sweating and night sweating due to surface weakness, or insufficient *qi* and *yin* due to hyperactive heart *yang*. Common antihydrotics, working either by strengthening the surface or reinforcing *yin*, include Radix Astragali, Concha Ostreae, Radix Ephedrae and Fructus Tritici Levis (light). Jade Screen Powder and Powder of Concha Ostreae are two examples.

Prescriptions for preserving essence and controlling involuntary urination (*se jing zhi yi ji*) are indicated for cases of nocturnal emission and ejaculatio praecox due to kidney deficiency which causes failure in storing essence, or cases of frequent urination, incontinence of urine and enuresis due to kidney deficiency and bladder hypofunction which cause failure in controlling urination. The frequently used drugs for invigorating the kidney to preserve essence and control urination are Semen Astragali Complanati, Stamen Nelumbinis, Semen Euryales, Ootheca Mantidis, Fructus Alpiniae and Oxyphyllae. Golden Lock Bolus for Keeping Kidney Essence and Powder of Ootheca Mantidis are the examples.

Prescriptions for astringing the intestines to stop diarrhea (*se chang gu tuo ji*) are indicated for cases of lasting diarrhea and chronic dysentery due to deficiency cold in the spleen and kidney, resulting in failure to control defecation. The common drugs for warming and invigorating the spleen and kidney, astringing the intestines and arresting diarrhea are Semen Myristicae, Pericarpium Papaveris, Fructus Chebulae, and Fructus Psoraleae. *Zhenren* Decoction for Nourishing the Viscera and Pill of Four Miraculous Drugs are two typical examples.

Prescriptions for relieving metrorrhagia and leukorrhagia (*gu beng zhi dai ji*) are indicated for cases of abnormal uterine bleeding and profuse vaginal discharge. The common drugs are Os Draconis, Concha Ostreae, Galla Chinensis, and Os Sepielliae seu Sepiae. Decoction for Strengthening Chong Meridian and Decoction for Treating Leukorrhagia are two typical prescriptions of this type.

In traditional Chinese medicine, *qi*, blood, essence and fluid are regarded as the basic substances that nourish the human body; they are consumed and replenished continuously to maintain normal physiological activities. Insufficiency of the antipathogenic *qi* with weakened control may lead to loss of *qi*, blood, essence and fluid and, in turn, the continuous loss of these substances may aggravate the deficiency of the antipathogenic *qi*, or even threaten life. Hence, deficient antipathogenic *qi* is the primary cause of the disorders, and the various symptoms are secondary. Treatment aims at both the cause and the symptoms. Aside from the astringent drugs, various kinds of tonics may also be applied according to the severity of the loss of *qi*, blood, *yin*, *yang*, essence and fluid. In case of heavy loss, astringent drugs should be applied first and then followed by tonics. For cases with marked deficiency of primordial *qi* and exhaustion of *yang qi*, prescriptions for invigorating *qi* and restoring depleted *yang* (see Chpater "Prescriptions for Warming the Interior") should be immediately applied.

Prescriptions presented in this chapter are contraindicated for the following cases: sweating due to febrile diseases, cough due to affection by exogenous pathogens, nocturnal emission due to agitation of fire, diarrhea and dysentery due to improper diet, and metrorrhagia due to blood-heat. In addition, astringents may hold pathogens, if present, in the body, and so this kind of prescriptions should not be applied when exogenous pathogens are not completely eliminated.

Jade Screen Powder

玉屏风散 *yu ping feng san*

(from *Danxi's Experience on Medicine*)

Radix Ledebouriellae	30 g
Radix Astragali	30 g
Rhizoma Atractylodis Macrocephalae	60 g

Administration: Grind the drugs into fine powder for oral administration, take 6-9 g each time, twice daily; or prepare them into an oral decoction, with the dosages reduced proportionally.

Action: Benefiting *qi*, strengthening the surface and stopping sweating.

Indications: Cases with surface weakness, manifested as spontaneous sweating, aversion to wind, pale complexion, pale tongue with thin and white coating, and superficial, feeble and soft pulse; and for patients susceptible to the affection of wind.

Explanation: Weakness of *wei qi* (defensive *qi*) leads to weakening of the surface, causing failure in retaining *ying-yin*, resulting in spontaneous sweating; deficiency of *wei qi* makes the skin loose and susceptible to wind, exhibiting aversion to wind and superficial pulse, pale complexion, pale tongue with white coating, and feeble and soft pulse. Treatment should be benefiting *qi* and strengthening the surface to stop sweating. In the prescription, Astragali serves the chief ingredient for benefiting *qi* and strengthening the surface, while Atractylodis Macrocephalae acts as the adjuvant ingredient to enhance the effect of Astragali; the two together invigorate spleen *qi* and promote the generation of *qi* and blood, eventually strengthening the surface to arrest sweating. Ledebouriellae serves as the assistant drug, and its effect can go easily to the surface to dispel the pathogenic wind. Ledebouriellae helps Astragali strengthen the surface and prevents it from retaining pathogens, while Astragali prevents Ledebouriellae from damaging the antipathogenic *qi*. Hence, their combination produces both tonic and dispersive effects that promote each other. It is a common prescription for cases of spontaneous sweating due to surface weakness, and for patients susceptible to the affection by wind.

The prescription is called "Jade Screen" because it can function as a protective barrier to the attack by wind.

It has both tonic and dispersive effects, and the clinical evidence calling for its application is spontaneous sweating, aversion to wind, pale complexion, pale tongue with white coating, and feeble and soft pulse. For cases of unceasing spontaneous sweating, Fructus Tritici Levis and Concha Ostreae can be added to enhance the antihydrotic action. For cases due to affection by wind-cold that is not relieved after sweating, Ramulus Cinnamomi can be added to enhance the elimination of cold. For cases of nasal stuffiness due to weak *wei qi* and affection by wind, Flos Magnoliae and Fructus Xanthii can be added to eliminate wind and relieve the stuffiness.

This prescription and Decoction of Ramulus Cinnamomi are both indicated for exterior-weakness syndrome marked by spontaneous sweating and aversion to wind. But this is also good for benefiting *qi* and strengthening the surface to stop sweating, and is indicated for the syndrome marked by spontaneous sweating. Decoction of Ramulus Cinnamomi is good for dispersing cold from the surface and regulating *ying* and *wei*, and is indicated for exterior syndrome due to affection by wind-cold.

Powder of Concha Ostreae
牡蛎散 *mu li san*
(from *Benevolent Prescriptions from the Pharmaceutical Bureau of the Taiping Period*)

Radix Astragali	30 g
Radix Ephedrae	30 g
Concha Ostreae	30 g

Administration: Grind the drugs into granules, take 9 g of the granules and decoct it together 30 g of Fructus Tritici Levis (light) and take the decoction hot; or directly prepare them into an oral decoction, with the dosages reduced proportionally.

Action: Strengthening the surface and arresting sweating.

Indications: Disorders with insufficient heart *yin* and weakness of *wei qi*, manifested as spontaneous sweating that is more serious at night, palpitation, shortness of breath, fatigue, pink tongue, and thready and weak pulse.

Explanation: Disorders of sweating may be classified into spontaneous sweating and night sweating. The former is mostly caused by weak *wei qi* and insufficient *yang qi*, the latter mostly by deficient *yin*. This prescription is indicated for cases of both spontaneous sweating and night sweating. Sweat is considered the fluid derived from the heart and weak *wei qi* may lead to spontaneous sweating, while insufficient heart *yin* and hyperactive heart *yang* may lead to loss of *yin*-fluid and result in night sweating. Prolonged sweating may damage both *qi* and *yin* and cause failure in nourishing the heart, resulting in palpitation, shortness of breath and fatigue. The therapeutic principle should be strengthening the surface to arrest sweating and replenishing heart *yin* to suppress heart *yang*. In the prescription, Concha Ostreae, which is salty and cold, serves as the chief for replenishing heart *yin*, suppressing heart *yang* and arresting sweating; Astragali, sweet and warm, serves as the adjuvant for benefiting *qi* and strengthening the spleen and the surface to arrest sweating; Radix Ephedrae serves as the guide to distribute the effects of the other drugs to the surface and enhance the antihydrotic action; and Fructus Tritici Levis (light) serves as an assistant to nourish heart *yin* and purge heart fire to arrest sweating. These drugs together invigorate *wei qi*, strengthen the surface, suppress heart *yang* and retain *ying-yin*, so as to stop involuntary sweating.

This prescription is chiefly indicated for cases of spontaneous and night sweating due to insufficient heart *yin*, hyperactive heart *yang* and weak *wei qi*. For cases due to *yang* deficiency, Radix Aconiti Lateralis Preparata and Rhizoma Atractylodis Macrocephalae can be added to enhance the effects of supporting *yang* and strengthening the surface. For those cases with marked deficiency of *qi*, Radix Ginseng and Rhizoma Atractylodis Macrocephalae can be added to enhance the actions of invigorating the spleen, benefiting *qi* and strengthening the surface.

Golden Lock Bolus for Preserving Kidney Essence
金锁固精丸 *jin suo gu jing wan*
(from *Variorum of Prescriptions*)

Semen Astragali Complanati (fried)	60 g
Semen Euryales (steamed)	60 g
Stamen Nelumbinis	60 g
Os Draconis (fried)	30 g
Concha Ostreae (calcined)	30 g

Administration: Grind the drugs into fine powder and make the powder into bolus with the paste of Semen Nelumbinis, take 9 g each time, twice daily, with diluted salt water or warm water; or prepare them directly into an oral decoction by adding a certain amount of Semen Nelumbinis, with the dosages reduced proportionally.

Action: Invigorating the kidney and retaining essence.

Indications: Cases due to kidney deficiency, manifested as nocturnal emission, spiritlessness, fatigue, soreness and weakness of the limbs, lumbago, tinnitus, pale tongue with white coating, and thready and weak pulse.

Explanation: Nocturnal emission is a disorder which may be attributed to various causes. But, it is mainly related to the kidney. The kidney is responsible for storing essence, and so insufficient kidney *qi* may fail to retain essence and lead to nocturnal emission. Deficient kidney essence may produce spiritlessness, fatigue, and sore and weak limbs. The lumbus houses the kidney, and the ear is the orifice of the kidney, so that insufficient kidney essence may result in lumbago and tinnitus. Pale tongue with white coating, and thready and weak pulse are also indications of kidney deficiency. The therapeutic principle should be invigorating the kidney and retaining essence. In the prescription, Astragali Complanati serves as the chief drug for invigorating the kidney and retaining essence; Semen Nelumbinis and Stamen Nelumbinis invigorate the kidney to preserve essence; and Euryales invigorates the spleen and kidney to retain essence, and these serve as the adjuvant ingredients. Calcined Concha Ostreae and Os Draconis are used as assistant ingredients for their astringent effect, to relieve nocturnal emission. These ingredients form a prescription for both causative and symptomatic treatment of nocturnal emission due to kidney deficiency.

This prescription is particularly suitable for cases of nocturnal emission associated with lumbago, tinnitus, pale tongue with white coating, and thready and weak pulse. It is contraindicated for cases due to hyperactive ministerial fire, or disturbance of the lower *jiao* by dampness-heat.

Powder of Ootheca Mantidis
桑螵蛸散 *sang piao xiao san*
(from *Amplified Herbalism*)

Ootheca Mantidis	30 g
Radix Polygalae	30 g
Rhizoma Acori Graminei	30 g
Os Draconis	30 g
Radix Ginseng	30 g
Lignum Pini Poriaferum	30 g
Radix Angelicae Sinensis	30 g
Plastrum Testudinis (prepared with vinegar)	30 g

Administration: Grind the drugs into fine powder, and take 6 g of the powder with Ginseng decoction before sleep; or directly prepare them into an oral decoction, with the dosages reduced proportionally.

Action: Invigorating the heart and kidney, and relieving nocturnal emission.

Indications: Cases of heart and kidney deficiency, manifested as frequent micturition, enuresis or nocturnal emission, trance, amnesia, pale tongue with white coating, and thready and weak pulse.

Explanation: This prescription is suitable for cases of heart and kidney deficiency and imbalance between kidney fluid and heart fire. Insufficient heart *qi* may lead to a mental disorder, manifested as frequent micturition, enuresis, or nocturnal emission. The therapeutic principle is to invigorate both the heart and kidney to cure nocturnal emission. In the prescription, Ootheca Mantidis serves as the chief ingredient to invigorate the kidney, preserve essence, reduce the amount of urine and relieve spermatorrhea. Os Draconis and Plastrum Testudinis serve as the adjuvant ingredients: the former preserves essence and calms the mind, and the latter nourishes the kidney and heart. Ginseng and Angelicae Sinensis are applied to nourish *qi* and blood, Lignum Pini Poriaferum to calm the heart, Polygalae and Acori Graminei to appease heart fire and maintain balance between heart fire and kidney water—all act as assistant ingredients. The combined use of these drugs makes kidney fluid and heart fire support each other, so that nocturnal emission is relieved by restoring renal control, and trance and amnesia are relieved when the heart is nourished.

Zhenren Decoction for Nourishing the Viscera

真人养脏汤 *zhen ren yang zang tang*

(from *Benevolent Prescriptions from the Pharmaceutical Bureau of the Taiping Period*)

Radix Ginseng	18 g
Radix Angelicae Sinensis	18 g
Rhizoma Atractylodis Macrocephalae (fried)	18 g
Semen Myristicae (roasted)	15 g
Cortex Cinnamomi	24 g
Radix Glycyrrhizae Preparata	24 g
Radix Paeoniae Alba	48 g
Radix Aucklandiae	42 g
Fructus Chebulae	36 g
Pericarpium Papaveris (calyx and pedicel removed, and prepared with honey)	108 g

Administration: Grind these drugs into granules, decoct 6 g of the granules and take the decoction before meal.

Action: Astringing the intestines, warming and invigorating the spleen and kidney.

Indications: Chronic diarrhea and dysentery with deficiency cold in the spleen and kidney, manifested as frequent defecation, abdominal pain relieved by pressure and warmth, fatigue, poor appetite, pale tongue with white coating, and deep and slow pulse.

Explanation: Deficiency cold in the spleen and kidney leads to loss of intestinal control and *yang* dysfunction, thus giving rise to frequent defecation, abdominal pain relieved by pressure and warmth, fatigue, poor appetite, pale tongue with white coating, and deep and slow pulse. The therapeutic principle is to astringe the intestines, warm and invigorate the spleen and kidney. In the prescription, Papaveris is used in a large dosage as the chief drug to astringe the intestines. Chebulae, Myristicae and Cortex Cinnamomi are used as the adjuvant ingredients: Chebulae to relieve diarrhea, Myristicae to warm the kidney and spleen, and Cortex Cinnamomi to warm *yang qi* and eliminate cold. Ginseng and Atractylodis Macrocephalae are applied to benefit *qi* and strengthen the spleen, Angelicae Sinensis and Paeoniae Alba to nourish blood and regulate *ying*, Aucklandiae to activate *qi* and alleviate pain—they serve as the assistant ingredients to treat the consumption of *qi* and blood due to prolonged diarrhea and dysentery. Glycyrrhizae serves as the guide to promote the synergy of the other drugs, and alleviate pain when combined with Paeoniae Alba. These drugs together astringe the intestines, relieve diarrhea, warm the spleen and kidney, and nourish *qi* and blood to fortify the viscera. For cases with severe deficiency cold in the spleen and kidney, accompanied by cold limbs, and deep and feeble pulse, Rhizoma Zingiberis (dried) and Radix Aconiti Lateralis Preparata should be added to enhance the effect of warming the kidney and spleen. However, this prescription is contraindicated for cases of diarrhea and dysentery at the onset when the pathogens are still hyperactive and the intestinal stagnation has not yet been relieved. Furthermore, abstinence from raw food, fish and greasy food should be followed during the treatment.

Pill of Four Miraculous Drugs
四神丸 *si shen wan*
(from *Summary of Internal Medicine*)

Semen Myristicae	60 g
Fructus Psoraleae	120 g
Fructus Schisandrae	60 g
Fructus Evodiae	30 g

Administration: Grind these drugs into fine powder, mix the powder with 240 g of well boiled Rhizoma Zingiberis Recens and 100 pieces of Fructus Jujubae (with the stones removed and steamed) to form pills, take 6-9 g each time before meal, twice daily; or directly prepare them into an oral decoction, with the dosages reduced proportionally.

Action: Warming the kidney and spleen and astringing the intestines to stop diarrhea.

Indications: Cases due to deficiency cold in the spleen and kidney, manifested as morning diarrhea, poor appetite, or prolonged diarrhea, abdominal pain, lumbago, cold limbs, fatigue, pale tongue with white coating, and deep, slow and weak pulse.

Explanation: At dawn, *yin qi* in the human body is most active and *yang qi* is developing. Because of the declination of kidney *yang*, *yang qi* is deficient and *yin qi* is hyperactive and moves downward, resulting in morning diarrhea. Spleen *yang* deficiency gives rise to splenic and gastric dysfunction, resulting in poor appetite. The predominance of *yin*-cold in the interior due to spleen and kidney *yang* deficiency produces abdominal pain, lumbago, cold limbs and fatigue. Pale tongue with white coating, and deep and slow pulse are also indications of deficiency cold in the spleen and kidney. The therapeutic principle should be warming the spleen and kidney and arresting the intestines to stop diarrhea. In the prescription, Psoraleae serves as the chief drug to warm kidney *yang* and benefit the spleen. Myristicae warms the kidney and spleen, and astringes the intestines to stop diarrhea, and Evodiae warms the middle *jiao* and expel cold—they both serve as the adjuvant. Schisandrae produces an astringent effect, Zingiberis Recens warms the middle *jiao* and expels cold, and Jujubae invigorates the spleen and nourishes the stomach; together they serve as the assistant. These drugs together warm kidney *yang* and restore the spleen function, and gradually relieve morning diarrhea and anorexia.

This prescription is a combination of Pill of Two Miraculous Drugs, which contains Semen Myristicae and Fructus Psoraleae (from *Classified Effective Prescriptions*), and Powder of Schisandrae, which contains Fructus Schisandrae and Fructus Evodiae. Its warming, invigorating and astringing effects can be further strengthened by the combination. It is highly effective for cases of morning diarrhea and anorexia due to deficiency cold in the spleen and kidney.

Decoction for Strengthening the Chong Meridian

固冲汤 *gu chong tang*

(from *Discourse on Medical Problems Interpreted by Combining Chinese with Western Medicine*)

Rhizoma Atractylodis Macrocephalae (fried)	30 g
Radix Astragali (crude)	18 g
Os Draconis (roasted)	24 g
Concha Ostreae (roasted)	24 g
Fructus Corni	24 g
Radix Paeoniae Alba (crude)	12 g
Os Sepiae	12 g
Radix Rubiae	9 g
Vagina Trachycarpi Carbonisatus	6 g
Galla Chinensis (grind into fine powder and take with the decoction of the above drugs)	1.5 g

Administration: Decoct with water for oral administration.

Action: Benefiting *qi*, invigorating the spleen, consolidating the Chong Meridian, and controlling the blood.

Indications: Cases of weakened Chong Meridian, manifested as metrorrhagia or hypermenorrhea with pale and thin menstrual flow, palpitation, shortness of breath, pale tongue, and thready and weak or feeble and large pulse.

Explanation: The prescription is indicated for cases of metrorrhagia due to weakened spleen *qi* leading to weakened Chong Meridian. The Chong Meridian is the "sea of blood," and the spleen controls the blood. In cases of spleen deficiency, inadequate *qi* and blood are produced and the blood is uncontrollable, so that the Chong Meridian is weakened and metrorrhagia or hypermenorrhea ensues. Blood deficiency leads to pale and thin menses. Insufficient *qi* and blood causes poor nourishment to the heart, thus giving rise to palpitation, shortness of breath, thready and weak or feeble and large pulse, and pale tongue. Treatment aims at benefiting *qi*, invigorating the spleen, consolidating the Chong Meridian and controlling the blood. In the prescription, Atractylodis Macrocephalae and Astragali serve as the chief to benefit *qi*, invigorate the spleen, consolidate the Chong Meridian and control the blood, and are used in a larger dosage. The weakening of the Chong Meridian is usually related to liver and kidney functional disorder, and metrorrhagia or hypermenorrhea may induce *yin*-blood consumption, so Corni and Paeoniae Alba are used as the adjuvant drugs to benefit the liver and kidney, preserve *yin* and nourish the blood. Roasted Os Draconis and Concha Ostreae, Os Sepiae, Vagina Trachycarpi Carbonisatus and Galla Chinensis produce an astringent effect to stop bleeding, and enhance the hemostatic property of the chief and adjuvant ingredients; and Rubiae stops bleeding without inducing blood stasis. Drugs in the latter two groups serve as the assistant. All these drugs together benefit *qi*, nourish the blood and stop bleeding, and effect both a causative and a symptomatic treatment.

Decoction for Treating Leukorrhagia
完带汤 *wan dai tang*
(from *Fu Qingzhu's Obstetrics and Gynecology*)

Rhizoma Atractylodis Macrocephalae (fried with earth)	30 g
Rhizoma Dioscoreae (fried)	30 g
Radix Ginseng	6 g
Radix Paeoniae Alba (fried with wine)	15 g
Semen Plantaginis (fried with wine)	9 g
Rhizoma Atractylodis Preparata	9 g
Radix Glycyrrhizae	3 g
Pericarpium Citri Reticulatae	2 g
Spica Schizonepetae (charred)	2 g
Radix Bupleuri	2 g

Administration: Prepare as an oral decoction.

Action: Benefiting *qi*, invigorating the spleen, removing dampness and relieving leukorrhagia.

Indications: Cases of spleen deficiency, liver stagnation and a downward attack of dampness, manifested as leukorrhagia with whitish or yellowish thin discharge, pale complexion, fatigue, loose stools, pale tongue with white coating, and slow or soft, superficial and weak pulse.

Explanation: Leukorrhagia is mostly related to liver and spleen functional disorders. Dysfunction of the spleen itself or that resulting from liver *qi* stagnation leads to retention and downward attack of dampness, causing leukorrhagia. All other symptoms are also the result of spleen deficiency and retained dampness. For such cases, the treatment is to benefit *qi*, invigorate the spleen and remove dampness to relieve leukorrhagia. In the prescription, Atractylodis Macrocephalae and Dioscoreae, used in a larger dosage and together with Ginseng, serve as the chief ingredients for invigorating the middle *jiao*, benefiting *qi*, consolidating the spleen and removing dampness. Atractylodis and Pericarpium Citri Reticulatae remove dampness and regulate *qi* circulation, and Plantaginis promotes diuresis to eliminate dampness—they act as the adjuvant. The two groups of drugs together act to relieve leukorrhagia without retaining dampness and to eliminate dampness without damaging the antipathogenic *qi*. Paeoniae Alba eases the liver, consolidates the spleen and produces an astringent effect, whereas Bupleuri releases stagnant liver *qi* and raises lucid *yang*, and Schizonepetae relieves leukorrhagia—they together serve as the assistant ingredients. Glycyrrhizae acts as the guide to regulate the middle *jiao*, benefit *qi* and coordinate the effects of the other drugs.

This is a common prescription to treat leukorrhagia due to liver *qi* stagnation and spleen deficiency. Thin whitish and odorless vaginal discharge, pale complexion, pale tongue, and soft, superficial and weak pulse are clinical evidence calling for its application. For cases marked by obvious lumbago due to kidney deficiency, Semen Cuscutae and Cortex Eucommiae are added to invigorate the kidney.

Summary

Eight prescriptions are listed in this chapter, and according to their actions, they are classified into the following sub-categories.

(1) Prescriptions for strengthening the surface to stop sweating:

Jade Screen Powder and Powder of Concha Ostreae both produce this action and are indicated for cases of spontaneous and night sweating. The former strongly invigorates the spleen, benefits *qi* and strengthens the surface, and is appropriate for spontaneous sweating due to weak surface and *wei qi*. The latter has a strong antihydrotic effect and also benefits *yin* and suppresses *yang*; it is indicated for spontaneous and night sweating due to heart *yin* deficiency, hyperactive heart *yang* and weak *wei qi*.

(2) Prescriptions for preserving kidney essence to relieve enuresis and nocturnal emission:

Golden Lock Bolus for Keeping Essence and Powder of Ootheca Mantidis are indicated for cases of nocturnal emission and enuresis due to kidney hypofunction. The former is particularly effective for invigorating the kidney and essence, and is appropriate for cases of nocturnal emission due to kidney failure to preserve essence; while the latter produces the same effect by regulating the heart and kidney, and is indicated for cases of enuresis and frequent micturition due to insufficient heart *qi* and kidney hypofunction.

(3) Prescriptions with antidiarrheic effect:

Zhenren Decoction for Nourishing the Viscera and Pill of Four Miraculous Drugs both possess the antidiarrheic effect by warming *yang* and invigorating the kidney, and are indicated for cases of intractable diarrhea and chronic dysentery due to deficiency cold in the spleen and kidney. The former is good for benefiting *qi* and invigorating the spleen, and has a stronger astringent action; the latter exerts its astringent effect by warming the kidney and spleen.

(4) Prescriptions for relieving metrorrhagia and leukorrhagia:

Decoction for Strengthening the Chong Meridian acts to benefit *qi*, invigorate the spleen, consolidate the Chong Meridian and control the blood, and is designed for cases of metrorrhagia or hypermenorrhea due to weakened Chong Meridian and failure of *qi* to control the blood. Decoction for Treating Leukorrhagia invigorates the spleen and eliminates dampness, and is indicated for cases of leukorrhagia due to liver *qi* stagnation, spleen hypofunction and a downward attack of dampness.

CHAPTER THIRTEEN

PRESCRIPTIONS WITH SEDATIVE EFFECT

Prescriptions with sedative effect (*an shen ji*) are mainly composed of heavy sedatives or drugs that nourish the heart; they are indicated for mental disorders.

The causes for mental disorders vary and are clinically classified into two types—deficiency and excess. Those cases marked by irritability and vexation are mostly attributed to excess, and should be treated by calming with heavy sedatives and purging heart fire. Those cases marked by palpitation, amnesia, trance and insomnia are mostly attributed to deficiency, and should be treated by nourishing and invigorating the heart. These prescriptions are grouped accordingly.

Prescriptions composed of heavy sedatives (*zhong zhen an shen ji*), such as Cinnabaris, Magnetitum, Os Draconis, Dens Draconis and Concha Margaritifera Usta, are indicated for cases of fright, mania, epilepsy, etc. One example is Pill of Cinnabaris for Tranquilization.

Prescriptions composed of sedatives that nourish the heart (*zi yang an shen ji*), such as Semen Ziziphi Spinosae, Semen Biotae, Fructus Schisandrae, Fructus Tritici Levis and Lignum Pini Poriaferum, are indicated for cases of palpitation, amnesia, insomnia and dizziness. Examples: Heaven King Tonic Pill for Mental Discomfort and Decoction of Glycyrrhizae, Tritici Levis and Jujubae.

Heavy sedatives are metals, minerals or shells, which may affect digestion. Prolonged administration is therefore inadvisable, especially for patients with splenic and gastric dysfunction. It should also be emphasized that psyche factor is closely involved in mental disorders, and psychic therapy should be given along with medication.

Pill of Cinnabaris for Tranquilization
朱砂安神丸 *zhu sha an shen wan*
(from *Inventions of Medicine*)

Cinnabaris	15 g
Rhizoma Coptidis	18 g
Radix Glycyrrhizae Preparata	16 g
Radix Rehmanniae	8 g
Radix Angelicae Sinensis	8 g

Administration: Grind the drugs into fine powder, make the powder into pills, take 6-9 g before sleep; or prepare them directly into an oral decoction, with the dosages reduced proportionally (Cinnabaris is ground with water and mixed with the decoction).

Action: Tranquilizing the mind, calming the heart, purging heat and nourishing *yin*.

Indications: Cases due to dominant heart fire and insufficient *yin*-blood, exhibiting irritability, insomnia, dreaminess, fright, severe palpitation, nausea, chest upset, red tongue tip, and thready and rapid pulse.

Explanation: This is a common prescription containing a heavy sedative, and is indicated for cases of irritability, insomnia, severe palpitation, etc. due to dominant heart fire and insufficient *yin*-blood. Heart fire stirring inside may lead to feverishness in the chest, and insufficient *yin*-blood causes failure in nourishing the heart, manifesting severe palpitation and insomnia. The treatment is to tranquilize and calm the mind, purge heat and nourish *yin*. In the prescription, Cinnabaris, sweet and cold, serves as the chief ingredient for tranquilizing the mind; Coptidis, bitter and cold, serves as the adjuvant to purge heart fire. The two drugs constitute an ideal combination to purge fire and tranquilize the mind. Angelicae Sinensis nourishes the blood, and Rehmanniae nourishes *yin*—both serve as the assistant. Glycyrrhizae acts as the guide for coordinating the effects of the other drugs. These drugs together purge hyperactive fire on the one hand and enrich the insufficient *yin*-blood on the other, and eventually acquire a new balance between *yin* and *yang*.

Appendant Prescription

Decoction of Iron Scale

生铁落饮 *sheng tie luo yin*

(from *Insights into Medicine*)

The prescription is composed of 9 g of Radix Asparagi, 9 g of Radix Ophiopogonis, 9 g of Bulbus Fritillariae Thunbergii, 3 g of Arisaema cum Bile, 3 g of Exocarpium Citri Rubrum, 3 g of Radix Polygalae, 3 g of Rhizoma Acori Graminei, 3 g of Fructus Forsythiae, 3 g of Poria, 3 g of Lignum Pini Poriaferum, 5 g of Radix Scrophulariae, 5 g of Ramulus Uncariae cum Uncis, 5 g of Radix Salviae Miltiorrhizae, and 1 g of Cinnabaris. Decoct Iron Scale with water for one hour before adding other drugs. It possesses the ability to calm the heart, remove phlegm and tranquilize the mind, and is indicated for cases of mania due to upward attack of phlegm-fire.

Both this prescription and Pill of Cinnabaris for Tranquilization have a sedative effect. However, this contains phlegm-eliminating drugs and is suitable for manic syndrome resulting from phlegm-fire. Pill of Cinnabaris for Tranquilization, on the other hand, contains drugs that purge heat and nourish *yin*, and is appropriate for cases of palpitation, insomnia and dreaminess due to dominant heart fire and insufficient *yin*-blood.

Heavenly King Tonic Pill for Mental Discomfort
天王补心丹 *tian wang bu xin dan*
(from *Secret Recipes for Longevity*)

Radix Rehmanniae (crude)	120 g
Radix Ginseng	15 g
Radix Salviae Miltiorrhizae (slightly fried)	15 g
Radix Scrophulariae (slightly fried)	15 g
Poria	15 g
Fructus Schisandrae	15 g
Radix Polygalae	15 g
Radix Platycodi	15 g
Radix Angelicae Sinensis (body part)	60 g
Radix Asparagi	60 g
Radix Ophiopogonis	60 g
Semen Biotae (fried)	60 g
Semen Ziziphi Spinosae	60 g

Administration: Grind the drugs into fine powder, mix the powder with honey to produce pills coated with Cinnabaris, take 9 g each time with warm water; or directly prepare the drugs into an oral decoction, with the dosages reduced proportionally.

Action: Nourishing *yin* and blood, invigorating the heart and tranquilizing the mind.

Indications: Cases of insufficient *yin* and blood, manifested as irritability, insomnia, palpitation, spiritlessness, nocturnal emission, amnesia, dry stools, dry mouth and tongue or aphthae, red tongue with little coating, and thready and rapid pulse.

Explanation: This is a common prescription for nourishing *yin* and tranquilizing the mind, and is indicated for cases of irritability, insomnia, amnesia, nocturnal emission and spiritlessness due to heart and kidney hypofunction and deficient *yin* and blood. The therapeutic principle is to nourish *yin* and blood, invigorate the heart and tranquilize the mind. In the prescription, Rehmanniae is used as the chief ingredient to nourish *yin* and blood, and purge heat; Scrophulariae, Asparagi and Ophiopogonis are applied to enhance the effect of nourishing *yin*; and Angelicae Sinensis and Salviae Miltiorrhizae nourish and regulate the blood. Ginseng and Poria benefit *qi* and calm the heart; Ziziphi Spinosae, Schisandrae, Biotae and Polygalae nourish the heart; and Cinnabaris is a heavy sedative. These drugs together invigorate the heart and kidney, enrich *yin* and blood, and provide both a causative and symptomatic treatment. In addition, Platycodi is used to promote the circulation of *qi*, and it makes the other drugs produces a tonic effect without causing indigestion.

Appendant Prescription

Pill of Biotae for Nourishing the Heart
柏子养心丸 *bai zi yang xin wan*

(*from Tiren's Compilation*)

It is composed of 120 g of Semen Biotae, 90 g of Fructus Lycii, 30 g of Radix Ophiopogonis, 30 g of Radix Angelicae Sinensis, 30 g of Rhizoma Acori Graminei, 30 g of Lignum Pini Poriaferum, 60 g of Radix Scrophulariae, 60 g of Radix Rehmanniae Preparata, and 15 g of Radix Glycyrrhizae. The method of administration is: grind the drugs into fine powder and mix the powder with honey to produce pills as large as beans, take 40 pills each time with warm water. This prescription nourishes the heart, calms the mind, nourishes *yin* and invigorates the kidney, and is indicated for cases of palpitation, dreaminess, amnesia and night sweating due to insufficient *ying*-blood and imbalance between heart *yang* and kidney *yin*.

Decoction of Glycyrrhizae, Tritici Levis and Jujubae
甘麦大枣汤 *gan mai da zao tang*
(from *Synopsis of the Golden Cabinet*)

Radix Glycyrrhizae	9 g
Fructus Tritici Levis	15-30 g
Fructus Jujubae	10 pieces (big)

Administration: Decoct with water for oral use.

Action: Nourishing the heart, tranquilizing the mind, regulating the middle *jiao* and relieving irritability.

Indications: Cases of hysteria exhibiting lack of control over behavior and emotion, anxiety, frequent yawning, broken sleep, and red tongue with a little coating.

Explanation: Hysteria is a disorder resulting from poor nourishment of the heart and insufficient *yin* and blood. In the prescription, Glycyrrhizae acts as the chief to regulate the middle *jiao* and nourish the heart to relieve irritability; Tritici Levis, sweet and mild, serves as the adjuvant to nourish the heart and calm the mind; Jujubae, sweet and mild, is used to benefit spleen *qi*, nourish the heart and calm the mind. Their combination produces a tonic and tranquilizing effect. In clinical application, a proper amount of Semen Ziziphi Spinosae, Semen Biotae, Radix Angelicae Sinensis, Radix Salviae Miltiorrhizae, and Radix Polygoni Multiflori may be added to enhance the nourishing, calming and sedative effects.

Summary

Presented in this chapter are three principal and two appendant prescriptions, which are grouped into two sub-categories.

(1) Prescriptions composed of heavy sedatives:

Pill of Cinnabaris for Tranquilization is a typical example. It tranquilizes the mind, calms the heart, purges heat and nourishes *yin*, and is indicated for cases of mental disorder, insomnia, dreaminess, fright and severe palpitation due to hyperactive heart fire and insufficient *yin*-blood.

(2) Prescriptions composed of sedatives that nourish the heart:

Heaven King Tonic Pill for Mental Discomfort and Decoction of Glycyrrhizae, Tritici Levis and Jujubae are two examples. The former chiefly nourishes the heart to calm the mind, and is indicated for cases with palpitation, insomnia and amnesia due to heart and kidney *yin*-blood deficiency. The latter is particularly effective in nourishing the heart, regulating the middle *jiao* and relieving irritability, and is suitable for cases of hysteria due to insufficient visceral *yin*.

CHAPTER FOURTEEN

PRESCRIPTIONS WITH RESUSCITATIVE EFFECT

Prescriptions with resuscitative effect (*kai qiao ji*) are mainly composed of analeptics with aromatic flavor, which restore consciousness and are used in the treatment of coma.

In traditional Chinese medicine, coma is divided into two types—deficiency and excess. Excess-type coma usually results from blockage of the heart orifice by hyperactive pathogens; it can be further classified into the heat-type and the cold-type in line with the different pathogens. Those in which the pericardium is affected by heat and toxic pathogens are grouped under heat-type, and the treatment seeks to purge heat to induce resuscitation; while those caused by the blockage of the heart orifice by cold-dampness and phlegm-turbid pathogens are grouped under the cold-type, and the treatment aims at warming the meridians to induce resuscitation.

Prescriptions inducing resuscitation with cool drugs (*liang kai ji*) are indicated for heat-type coma, which is accompanied by high fever, delirium, or even convulsion. It is also applicable to other comatose cases associated with heat syndrome, such as apoplexy, phlegmatic collapse syndrome and affection by pestilent pathogens. Such prescriptions are usually composed of analeptics with aromatic flavor, such as Moschus, Borneolum Syntheticum, Radix Curcumae, in combination with drugs that purge heat and toxins, such as Cornu Rhinocerotis, Calculus Bovis, Rhizoma Coptidis and Gypsum Fibrosum. Bolus of Calculus Bovis for Resurrection, Purple-Snow Pellet and Bolus of Precious Drugs are few examples.

Prescriptions inducing resuscitation with warm drugs (*wen kai ji*) are indicated for cold-type coma, as seen in cases of apoplexy, cold-stroke, and phlegmatic cold-stroke collapse syndrome, all of which are marked by sudden loss of consciousness, lockjaw, white tongue coating, and slow pulse. Aside from analeptics with aromatic flavor, such as Storax, Borneolum Syntheticum, Moschus, such prescriptions also include drugs with warming and *qi*-activating actions. Pill of Storax is an example.

In writing out prescriptions with resuscitative effect, it is necessary first of all to make sure whether the syndrome is of the cold or heat type. Prescriptions covered in this chapter are only appropriate for excess-type coma. They are contraindicated for cases of collapse syndrome with sweating, cold limbs, feeble breathing, enuresis, open mouth and closed eyes, even when coma occurs. In addition, for cases of excess syndrome involving the Yangming *fu* organ, exhibiting coma and delirium, purgative prescriptions with cold drugs should be used rather than prescriptions with resuscitative effect. For cases complicated by affection of the pericardium, prescriptions covered in this chapter should be applied together with purgative prescriptions according to the severity of the cases.

Drugs that are used to form such prescriptions are mostly aromatic and can be readily distributed to the whole body. Hence, prolonged administration is inadvisable, for otherwise the primordial *qi* may be impaired. Other kinds of prescriptions should be given according to syndrome differentiation as soon as the patient recovers consciousness. Moreover, boiling may reduce the potency of aromatic drugs, so these prescriptions should be prepared into bolus (pill), powder or injection instead of decoction.

Bolus of Calculus Bovis for Resurrection
安宫牛黄丸 *an gong niu huang wan*
(from *Essentials of Seasonal Febrile Diseases*)

Calculus Bovis	30 g
Radix Curcumae	30 g
Cornu Rhinocerotis	30 g
Radix Scutellariae	30 g
Rhizoma Coptidis	30 g
Realgar	30 g
Fructus Gardeniae	30 g
Cinnabaris	30 g
Borneolum Syntheticum	7.5 g
Moschus	7.5 g
Margarita	15 g

Administration: Grind the drugs into fine powder and prepare the powder into boluses with honey, each weighing 3 g and wrapped with thin gold sheet and coated with wax; take one bolus (half for children) each time, thrice daily. For cases with feeble pulse, the bolus should be taken with decoction of Ginseng; and for cases with forceful pulse, take it with decoction of Lonicerae and Menthae.

Action: Eliminating heat and toxins, inducing resuscitation and removing phlegm.

Indications: Cases of seasonal febrile diseases with the pericardium attacked by heat and stagnant phlegm-heat in the heart orifice, manifested as high fever, irritability, coma, delirium, or apoplexy, or infantile convulsion due to internal heat stagnation.

Explanation: This is a common prescription for cases of coma or delirium due to affection of the pericardium by phlegm-heat. Treatment aims at purging heat and toxins from the pericardium and eliminating phlegm. In the prescription, Calculus Bovis purges toxins and heart fire and eliminates phlegm, and Moschus produces a resuscitative effect; both serve as the chief ingredients. Cornu Rhinocerotis purges heart fire, cools the blood and eliminates toxins, Coptidis, Scutellariae and Gardeniae purge heat and toxins and enhance the effect of Calculus Bovis, Curcumae and Borneolum Syntheticum are used to enhance the resuscitative effect—all serve as the adjuvant ingredients. Cinnabaris, Margarita and Aurum (gold) are used to calm the heart and tranquilize the mind, Realgar, to eliminate phlegm and purge toxins, and Mel (honey), to regulate the stomach and middle *jiao*—these serve as the assistant and guiding ingredients.

For cases with feeble pulse, the bolus may be taken with the decoction of Ginseng to benefit *qi* and strengthen the antipathogenic *qi*. For cases with forceful pulse, it may be taken with decoction of Lonicerae and Menthae to enhance the heat-eliminating effect.

Purple-Snow Pellet
紫雪丹 *zi xue dan*
(from *Clandestine Essentials from the Imperial Library*)

Gypsum Fibrosum	1,500 g
Talcum	1,500 g
Magnetitum	1,500 g
Calcitum	1,500 g
Cornu Rhinocerotis (scale)	150 g
Cornu Saigae Tataricae (scale)	150 g
Radix Aristolochiae	150 g
Lignum Aquilariae Resinatum	150 g
Radix Scrophulariae	500 g
Rhizoma Cimicifugae	500 g
Radix Glycyrrhizae Preparata	240 g
Flos Caryophylli	30 g
Natrii Sulfas (prepared)	5,000 g
Nitrum (refined)	96 g
Moschus	1.5 g
Cinnabaris	90 g
Aurum	3,100 g

Administration: Crush Gypsum Fibrosum, Calcitum, Talcum and Magnetitum into small pieces and decoct them with water three times; decoct Scrophulariae, Aristolochiae, Aquilariae Resinatum, Cimicifugae, Glycyrrhizae and Caryophylli with water three times; filter and mix the two decoctions and let the mixture condense into an extract; grind Natrii Sulfas and Nitrum into fine powder and mix the powder with the extract, let the mixture dry and then grind it into fine powder; file Cornu Rhinocerotis, Cornu Saigae Tataricae, Cinnabaris, Moschus and Aurum into powder and mix the two powders thoroughly. Take 1.5-3 g a time, twice daily. The dosage for children is reduced correspondingly.

Action: Eliminating heat, inducing resuscitation, relieving convulsion and tranquilizing the mind.

Indications: Seasonal febrile diseases with heat attacking the pericardium, exhibiting high fever, irritability, coma, delirium, convulsion, thirst, dry lips, deep-colored urine, and constipation.

Explanation: This is a common prescription that induces resuscitation with cool drugs, and is indicated for seasonal febrile diseases with high fever and convulsion due to affection of the pericardium by heat. Heat attacking the pericardium may lead to coma, delirium and irritability. Stagnant heat and toxins may lead to high fever, deep-colored urine, and constipation. Convulsion results from the irritation of endogenous wind by hyperactive heat, and thirst and dry lips from the consumption of fluid by heat. Treatment concentrates on purging heat, inducing resuscitation and relieving convulsion and tranquilizing the mind. In the prescription, Gypsum Fibrosum, Calcitum and Talcum, sweet and cold, are applied to purge heat; Scrophulariae, Cimicifugae and Glycyrrhizae are used to purge heat and toxins; Scrophulariae is used to nourish *yin* and promote fluid production; Glycyrrhizae is used to regulate the stomach; Cornu Rhinocerotis is used to purge heart fire and toxins; and Moschus, Aristolochiae, Caryophylli and Aquilariae Resinatum are included to promote *qi* circulation and induce resuscitation. All these drugs serve together as the chief ingredients to produce both the heat-eliminating and resuscitation-inducing effects. Drugs that purge heat selected for the prescription are sweet and cold instead of bitter and cold, so as to avoid the consumption of body fluid. Cornu Saigae Tataricae is used to purge liver fire and calm pathogenic wind to relieve convulsion, Cinnabaris and Magnetitum to tranquilize the mind, Natrii Sulfas and Nitrum to purge heat and remove stagnation—all serve as the adjuvant. Aurum is applied to tranquilize the mind and eliminate the toxins.

This prescription was first recorded in the *Supplement to Essentially Treasured Prescriptions*, in which Talcum was not included, and was used to treat serious heat syndrome due to traumatic injuries. Since the Song Dynasty, however, it has been used for febrile diseases with coma and convulsion.

Bolus of Precious Drugs

至宝丹 *zhi bao dan*

(from *Benevolent Prescriptions from the Pharmaceutical Bureau of the Taiping Period*)

Cornu Rhinocerotis (crude)	30 g
Carapax Eretmochelydis (crude)	30 g
Succinum	30 g
Cinnabaris	30 g
Realgar	30 g
Borneolum Syntheticum	7.5 g
Moschus	7.5 g
Calculus Bovis	15 g
Benzoinum	45 g
Gold sheet (half for coating, half for decoction)	50 pieces
Silver sheet	50 pieces

Administration: Grind the drugs into fine powder, pass the powder through a sieve and make it into boluses with honey, weighing 3 g each, take one bolus (half for children) daily with warm water, or dissolve the bolus in Ginseng decoction and take it.

Action: Eliminating heat and toxins, opening orifice and dissolving turbid substance.

Indications: Cases of sunstroke, apoplexy and seasonal febrile diseases with retention of phlegm-heat, exhibiting coma, delirium, fever, irritability, profuse expectoration, noisy breathing, red tongue with yellow, turbid and greasy coating, and smooth and rapid pulse, or infantile convulsion due to retained phlegm-heat.

Explanation: This prescription is indicated for cases with retained heat and affection of the pericardium by phlegm and turbid substance. Clinical evidence calling for its application includes coma, delirium, profuse expectoration and noisy breathing. Treatment primarily aims at opening the orifices and secondarily purging heat and toxins. In the prescription, Moschus, Borneolum Syntheticum and Benzoinum serve as the chief ingredients to induce resuscitation and eliminate phlegm and turbid substance. Rhinocerotis, Calculus Bovis and Carapax Eretmochelydis eliminate heat and toxins, and Calculus Bovis eliminates phlegm and relieves convulsion—they serve as the adjuvant ingredients. Realgar is used to eliminate phlegm and purge toxins, and Cinnabaris, Succinum, gold and silver sheets are used to calm the heart and the uneasiness of the body and mind; they together serve as the assistant and guiding ingredients.

The prescription can also be used for infantile convulsion due to retained phlegm-heat.

According to ancient medical literature, the bolus is dissolved in Ginseng decoction first as Ginseng benefits *qi* and reinforces the antipathogenic *qi*. This method of administration is especially appropriate for critical cases of exhausted antipathogenic *qi* and feeble pulse.

Bolus of Calculus Bovis for Resurrection and Purple-Snow Pellet and this one are known as "three precious prescriptions," but each has its own advantages. Bolus of Calculus Bovis for Resurrection is particularly effective in purging pathogenic heat and toxins, Purple-Snow Pellet in relieving convulsion, and the present prescription in inducing resuscitation. They may be applied alternately or in combination.

Pill of Storax

苏合香丸 *su he xiang wan*

(from *Clandestine Essentials from the Imperial Library*)

Rhizoma Atractylodis Macrocephalae	60 g
Radix Aristolochiae	60 g
Cornu Rhinocerotis	60 g
Rhizoma Cyperi	60 g
Cinnabaris (ground with water)	60 g
Pericarpium Chebulae	60 g
Lignum Santali Albi	60 g
Benzoinum	60 g
Lignum Aquilariae Resinatum	60 g

Moschus	60 g
Flos Caryophylli	60 g
Fructus Piperis Longi	60 g
Borneolum Syntheticum	15 g
Storax	15 g
Olibanum	15 g

Administration: Grind Cinnabaris with water, stew Storax and grind other drugs into fine powder, mix them and prepare the mixture into boluses with honey, weighing 3 g each, and take one bolus each time, twice daily.

Action: Warming and clearing the meridians, inducing resuscitation, promoting *qi* circulation and eliminating turbid substance.

Indications: Cases of apoplexy, cold-stroke, or phlegm retention and *qi* stagnation, exhibiting sudden loss of consciousness, lockjaw, or sudden cold pain in the chest and abdomen, cold limbs, deep and slow or taut and tense pulse, and white and smooth coating over the tongue.

Explanation: This is a representative prescription to induce resuscitation with warm drugs, and is indicated for cold-type excess coma due to stagnation of cold, phlegm and turbid substance. The therapeutic principle is to open the orifices, supplemented by dispersing cold, activating *qi* and eliminating turbid substance. In the prescription, Storax, Moschus, Benzoinum, Borneolum Syntheticum, Aristolochiae, Caryophylli, Aquilariae Resinatum, Santali, Olibanum and Cyperi are aromatics for inducing resuscitation, activating *qi*, relieving stagnation, expelling cold and eliminating turbid substance, and Piperis Longi enhances the effect of the aromatics. Cornu Rhinocerotis produces a resuscitative effect and purges toxins, Cinnabaris calms the uneasiness of the body and mind; Atractylodis Macrocephalae strengthens the spleen and regulates the middle *jiao* to dissolve turbid substance; and Chebulae eliminates phlegm and counteracts the effect of the aromatics which consume the antipathogenic *qi*. In sum, this prescription consists of aromatics with resuscitative effect along with acrid and fragrant drugs that activate *qi*. It is a common formula for cold-type coma of the excess syndrome and abdominal pain due to *qi* stagnation.

Since the acrid and fragrant drugs may damage the fetus, this prescription should be used cautiously with pregnant women.

Appendant Prescription

Bolus of Storax for Coronary Heart Diseases
冠心苏合丸 *guan xin su he wan*
(from *Proved Recipes*)

The prescription is composed of 50 g of Storax, 105 g of Borneolum Syntheticum, 210 g of Lignum Santali, 210 g of Radix Aristolochiae, and 105 g of Olibanum Preparata. The preparation is to grind all the drugs into fine powder and make it into boluses. One bolus each time (swallowing or chewing), thrice daily, or else before sleep or during the attack; it induces resuscitation, activates *qi* and kills pain, and is indicated for angina pectoris due to stagnant phlegm, turbid substance and *qi*.

Summary

Four principal and one appendant prescriptions are discussed in this chapter. Their resuscitative effect is accomplished by either cool drugs or warm drugs.

(1) Prescriptions for inducing resuscitation with cool drugs:

There are three such examples, i. e., Bolus of Calculus Bovis for Resurrection, Purple-Snow Pellet and Bolus of Precious Drugs. Yet, each of them has its own advantages. Bolus of Calculus Bovis for Resurrection is effective for seasonal febrile diseases with the pericardium attacked by heat and toxin; Purple-Snow Pellet is good for coma and convulsion; and the Bolus of Precious Drugs is indicated for coma due to retained phlegm-heat.

(2) Prescriptions for inducing resuscitation with warm drugs:

The one example cited here is Pill of Storax, which warms the meridians, promotes *qi* circulation and eliminates turbid substance. It is appropriate for cold-type coma of the excess syndrome and abdominal pain due to stagnant *qi*.

CHAPTER FIFTEEN

PRESCRIPTIONS FOR REGULATING *QI*

Prescriptions for regulating *qi* (*li qi ji*) are chiefly composed of drugs that regulate *qi* or suppress the abnormal rise of *qi*. They are indicated for diseases attributed to *qi* stagnation and the adverse flow of *qi*. The causes for the stagnation and adverse flow of *qi* are various. But the disturbance of *qi* activity and visceral dysfunction are generally responsible. Liver, spleen and stomach *qi* is usually involved in cases of *qi* stagnation, stomach and lung *qi* in cases of adverse flow of *qi*. The former should be treated by activating *qi*, and the latter by suppressing abnormally ascendant *qi*, and so the prescriptions are classified accordingly.

Prescriptions for activating *qi* (*xing qi ji*) are indicated for *qi* stagnation syndrome. Cases of spleen and stomach *qi* stagnation usually show abdominal fullness, eructation, acid regurgitation, vomiting, nausea, poor appetite and abnormal bowel movement, and the drugs commonly applied include Pericarpium Citri Reticulatae, Cortex Magnoliae Officinalis, Radix Aucklandiae and Fructus Amomi. Cases of liver *qi* stagnation usually exhibit distensive pain in the chest and hypochondrium, or hernial colic, or irregular menstruation, or dysmenorrhea, and drugs often prescribed are Rhizoma Cyperi Radix Linderae, Fructus Toosendan, Fructus Foeniculi, Pericarpium Citri Reticulatae Viride and Radix Curcumae. The representative prescriptions are *Yueju* Pill, Powder of Toosendan, Decoction of Pinelliae and Magnoliae Officinalis, and *Tiantai* Powder of Linderae.

Prescriptions for suppressing abnormally ascendant *qi* (*jiang qi ji*) are indicated for syndromes of abnormal *qi* flow. Cases of adversely ascendant lung *qi* are marked by cough and dyspnea, and the drugs commonly used include Fructus Perillae, Semen Armeniacae Amarum, Radix Asteris and Flos Farfarae. Cases of adversely ascendant stomach *qi* are characterized by hiccup and vomiting, and Flos Inulae, Haematitum, Rhizoma Pinelliae, Calyx Kaki and Caulis Bambusae in Taeniam are the drugs frequently applied. The representative prescriptions are Decoction of Perillae for Keeping *Qi* Downward, Decoction for Relieving Asthma, Decoction of Inulae and Haematitum, and Decoction of Caryophylli and Kaki.

With prescriptions for regulating *qi*, the syndromes of cold or heat, deficiency or excess should be differentiated, the presence or absence of complication should be determined, and the relevant drugs should be added. In addition, most of the drugs for regulating *qi* are aromatics, which are acrid and dry, and their long-term administration may induce fluid and *qi* consumption, and so overdosage should be avoided. For the aged, debilitated, pregnant women or patients with metrorrhagia, hematemesis and epistaxis, particular caution should be taken.

Yueju Pill

越鞠丸 *yue ju wan*

(from *Danxi's Experience on Medicine*)

Rhizoma Atractylodis
Rhizoma Cyperi
Rhizoma Chuanxiong
Massa Fermentata Medicinalis
Fructus Gardeniae
(in equivalent amount)

Administration: Grind the drugs into fine powder and prepare the powder into pills, take 6-9 g each time with warm water; or prepare them directly into an oral decoction.

Action: Promoting *qi* circulation and dispersing stagnation.

Indications: Cases of *qi* stagnation complicated by stagnant blood, phlegm, fire, dampness or food, exhibiting fullness of the chest, abdominal distensive pain, acid regurgitation, vomiting and indigestion.

Explanation: This is a common prescription for cases of various kinds of stagnation, particularly *qi* stagnation. Stagnant *qi* disturbs *qi* circulation as well as the transporting and digestive functions, and gives rise to the above symptoms. It is both the result and cause of stagnant blood, fire, dampness and food. This prescription aims to activate *qi* circulation, so that the other kinds of stagnation can be relieved. In this prescription, Cyperi serves as the chief ingredient to relieve *qi* stagnation. Chuanxiong is used to relieve blood stagnation, Gardeniae to remove fire stagnation, Atractylodis to remove dampness stagnation, and Massa Fermentata Medicinalis to remove food stagnation; and they together act as the adjuvant ingredients. There is no need to include drug(s) to remove phlegm stagnation, because it, if present, may be relieved after *qi* circulation is restored.

The prescription may be modified according to the predominant type of stagnation. For cases with predominant *qi* stagnation, Aucklandiae and Fructus Aurantii are added to enhance the action of promoting *qi* circulation. For cases with predominant blood stagnation, Chuanxiong is used as the chief ingredient, and Semen Persicae and Flos Carthami are added to promote blood circulation. For cases with predominant stagnation of dampness, Atractylodis is used as the chief ingredient, and Poria and Rhizoma Alismatis are added to eliminate dampness. For cases with predominant food stagnation, Massa Fermentata Medicinalis is used as the chief ingredient, and Fructus Hordei Germinatus and Fructus Crataegi are added to promote digestion. For cases with predominant fire stagnation, Gardeniae is used as the chief ingredient, and Radix Scutellariae and Rhizoma Coptidis are added to eliminate fire. And for cases with predominant phlegm stagnation, Pericarpium Citri Reticulatae and Rhizoma Pinelliae are added to eliminate phlegm.

Powder of Toosendan
金铃子散 *jin ling zi san*
(from *Basic Questions*: *Discourse on Mechanism for Preserving Life*)

Fructus Toosendan	30 g
Rhizoma Corydalis	30 g

Administration: Grind the drugs into fine powder, take 9 g each time with yellow wine or warm water; or directly prepare them into an oral decoction, with the dosages reduced correspondingly.

Action: Soothing the liver, purging heat, promoting *qi* circulation and alleviating pain.

Indications: Cases with liver *qi* stagnation and formation of fire, exhibiting intermittent pain in the precordial region, abdomen and hypochondrium, bitter taste, red tongue with yellow coating, and taut and rapid pulse.

Explanation: The liver controls the activity of *qi*, and its meridians traverse the hypochondria. Stagnant liver *qi* leads to sluggish blood circulation, giving rise to precordial, abdominal and hypochondriac pain. Liver *qi* is susceptible to emotional changes, so the pain comes and goes intermittently. The formation of fire produces a bitter taste, red tongue with yellow coating, and taut and rapid pulse. Treatment seeks to soothe the liver, purge heat, promote *qi* circulation and alleviate pain. In the prescription, Toosendan serves as the chief ingredient to disperse liver *qi* and purge liver fire; Corydalis, as the adjuvant, promotes *qi* and blood circulation. The two drugs form a common prescription for pains due to stagnant liver *qi* with the formation of fire, *qi*, and blood stagnation. Clinical evidence calling for its application includes pain in the precordial region, abdomen and hypochondrium that gets worse along with heat, red tongue with yellow coating, and taut and rapid pulse.

Decoction of Pinelliae and Magnoliae Officinalis
半夏厚朴汤 *ban xia hou pu tang*
(from *Synopsis of the Golden Cabinet*)

Rhizoma Pinelliae Preparata	9 g
Cortex Magnoliae Officinalis	9 g
Poria	12 g
Rhizoma Zingiberis Recens	15 g
Folium Perillae	6 g

Administration: Boil with water for oral administration.

Action: Promoting *qi* circulation, dispersing stagnation, suppressing adversely ascendant *qi* and eliminating phlegm.

Indications: Cases of globus hystericus, exhibiting a feeling of obstruction in the throat, a feeling of oppression in the chest and hypochondrium, cough, and vomiting.

Explanation: This prescription is designed for cases of globus hystericus resulting from emotional upset, stagnant liver *qi*, lung and stomach dysfunction, and accumulation of phlegm. The accumulation of phlegm and *qi* leads to lung dysfunction, giving rise to an oppressed feeling in the chest and hypochondrium, cough and dyspnea; or leads to adverse rising of stomach *qi*, causing nausea and vomiting. Treatment seeks to promote *qi* circulation, disperse stagnation, suppress the adverse rising of *qi* and eliminate phlegm. In the prescription, Magnoliae Officinalis is used to promote *qi* circulation and relieve fullness, while Pinelliae is used to eliminate phlegm, disperse stagnation, suppress the adversely ascendant *qi* and regulate the stomach—they both serve as the chief ingredients. Poria, sweet and bland, eliminates dampness through urination and assists Pinelliae in eliminating phlegm, and serves as the adjuvant. Zingiberis Recens is acrid and warm, regulates the stomach and stops vomiting, and Perillae is fragrant and soothes the chest and the middle *jiao*—they both serve as the assistant.

This is a common prescription for cases of globus hystericus due to affection by predominant phlegm-dampness. Clinical evidence calling for its application is a feeling of obstruction in the throat, white and greasy tongue coating, and taut and smooth pulse. For cases with marked *qi* stagnation, Radix Bupleuri, Radix Curcumae, Rhizoma Cyperi and Pericarpium Citri Reticulatae are added; or else modified *Xiaoyao* Powder is prescribed. The drugs in this prescription are mostly acrid, bitter, warm and dry, so it is only suitable for cases due to the accumulation of phlegm and *qi* but without internal heat. However, it is contraindicated for cases with flushed cheeks, bitter taste and red tongue with little coating resulting from *qi* stagnation and the formation of fire, which damages *yin* and consumes fluid, even though globus hystericus is present.

Decoction of Trichosanthis, Allii Macrostemi and Wine

瓜蒌薤白白酒汤 *gua lou xie bai bai jiu tang*

(from *Synopsis of the Golden Cabinet*)

Fructus Trichosanthis (crushed)	12 g
Bulbus Allii Macrostemi	9 g
Rice wine	30-60 ml

Administration: Decoct with water for oral administration.

Action: Activating *yang* and *qi*, relieving stagnation and eliminating phlegm.

Indications: Cases of chest *bi*-syndrome, exhibiting dull pain in the chest that refers to the back, dyspnea, cough, shortness of breath, white and greasy coating, and deep and taut or tense pulse.

Explanation: This prescription is indicated for cases of chest *bi*-syndrome due to the decline of *yang qi* in the chest as well as *qi* and phlegm stagnation, characterized by a dull pain in the chest which refers to the back. Stagnant *qi* and phlegm may lead to lung *qi* dysfunction and give rise to dyspnea, cough, shortness of breath, white and greasy tongue coating, and deep and taut or tense pulse. Treatment aims at activating *yang* and *qi*, dispersing stagnation and eliminating phlegm. In the prescription, Trichosanthis, which is cold and lubricant, serves as the chief ingredient for eliminating phlegm, removing stagnation and soothing the chest; Allii Macrostemi serves as the adjuvant for activating *yang* and *qi* and alleviating pain; and wine is conducive to *qi* and blood circulation and the distribution of the effects of the other drugs, and serves as the assistant and guide. They together activate *yang qi* in the chest and disperse phlegm, and eventually relieve the chest *bi*-syndrome.

Appendant Prescriptions

(1) Decoction of Trichosanthis, Allii Macrostemi and Pinelliae
瓜蒌薤白半夏汤 *gua lou xie bai ban xia tang*
(from *Synopsis of the Golden Cabinet*)

It is composed of 12 g of Fructus Trichosanthis, 9 g of Bulbus Allii Macrostemi, 12 g of Rhizoma Pinelliae, and 60 ml of rice wine. Prepared as an oral decoction, it activates *yang qi*, removes stagnation, eliminates phlegm and soothes the chest, and is indicated for chest *bi*-syndrome exhibiting pain in the chest that spreads to the back, and inability to lie flat.

(2) Decoction of Aurantii Immaturus, Allii Macrostemi and Cinnamomi
枳实薤白桂枝汤 *zhi shi xie bai gui zhi tang*
(from *Synopsis of the Golden Cabinet*)

It is composed of 12 g of Fructus Aurantii Immaturus, 12 g of Cortex Magnoliae Officinalis, 6 g of Bulbus Macrostemi, 3 g of Ramulus Cinnamomi, and 12 g of Fructus Trichosanthis. Prepared as an oral decoction, it activates *yang qi*, removes stagnation and relieves fullness, and is indicated for chest *bi*-syndrome marked by an oppressed and full feeling in the chest, the feeling of gas flowing from the hypochondrium to the heart, and white and greasy coating on the tongue.

The above three prescriptions are suitable for cases of chest *bi*-syndrome and possess similar actions, but Decoction of Trichosanthis, Allii Macrostemi and Wine is indicated for cases of chest *bi*-syndrome with a milder degree of phlegm accumulation, and Decoction of Trichosanthis, Allii Macrostemi and Pinelliae is appropriate for cases with marked phlegm accumulation, and Decoction of Aurantii Immaturus, Allii Macrostemi and Cinnamomi is better at activating *yang qi* and removing stagnation as well as suppressing the adversely ascendant *qi*, eliminating cold and relieving fullness, so it is indicated for cases of chest *bi*-syndrome with marked accumulation of phlegm and *qi*, characterized by fullness in the chest and a feeling of gas flowing from the hypochondrium to the heart.

Tiantai Powder of Linderae
天台乌药散 *tian tai wu yao san*
(from *Invention of Medicine*)

Tiantai's Radix Linderae	15 g
Radix Aucklandiae	15 g
Fructus Foeniculi (fried)	15 g
Pericarpium Citri Reticulatae Viride	15 g
Rhizoma Alpiniae Officinarum (fried)	15 g
Semen Arecae	15 g
Fructus Toosendan	12 g
Fructus Crotonis	15 g

Administration: Crush Crotonis and roast it and Toosendan with wheat bran until they turn brown, remove the Crotonis and wheat bran; grind the drugs into fine powder, take 3 g with warm wine (yellow wine for those with severe pain) each time; or directly prepare the drugs into an oral decoction, with the dosages reduced proportionally.

Action: Promoting *qi* circulation, releasing hepatic *qi*, dispersing cold and killing pain.

Indications: Cases of inguinal hernia, exhibiting pain in the lower abdomen that spreads to the testes, pale tongue with white coating, and deep and slow or taut pulse.

Explanation: This prescription is indicated for inguinal hernia resulting from stagnant cold in the liver meridian and disturbed *qi* activity. Since the liver meridian links the lower abdomen and the genitals, lower abdominal pain radiates to the testes when cold accumulates in the liver meridian and *qi* stagnates. The therapeutic principle is to promote *qi* circulation and disperse cold. In the prescription, Linderae serves as the chief ingredient to promote *qi* circulation, release hepatic *qi*, disperse cold and alleviate pain. Aucklandiae, Foeniculi, Citri Reticulatae Viride and Alpiniae Officinarum, fragrant, acrid and warm, serve as the adjuvant ingredients to enhance the action of Linderae. The effect of Arecae directly reaches the lower *jiao* to activate *qi* and eliminate stagnation, and Toosendan, bitter and cold, is used to promote *qi* circulation and disperse stagnation, and its cold nature is counteracted by roasting it with Crotonis, which is acrid and hot—these serve as assistant ingredients. The combination of these drugs relieves hernial pain through releasing stagnant *qi*, dispersing accumulated cold and regulating the liver collaterals.

Decoction of Perillae for Keeping _Qi_ Downwards
苏子降气汤 *su zi jiang qi tang*
(from *Benevolent Prescriptions from the Pharmaceutical Bureau of the Taiping Period*)

Fructus Perillae	9 g
Rhizoma Pinelliae Preparata	9 g
Radix Peucedani	6 g

Cortex Magnoliae Officinalis (fried with ginger juice)	6 g
Cortex Cinnamomi	3 g
Radix Angelicae Sinensis	6 g
Radix Glycyrrhizae Preparata	6 g

Administration: Decoct the drugs for oral administration by adding 2 pieces of Rhizoma Zingiberis Recens, 3 pieces of Fructus Jujubae and 2 g of Folium Perillae.

Action: Suppressing adversely ascendant *qi*, relieving dyspnea, eliminating sputum and relieving cough.

Indications: Cases with dyspneic cough, profuse expectoration, shortness of breath, fullness and oppression in the chest, lumbago, weak legs, fatigue, and white and greasy or smooth tongue coating.

Explanation: This prescription is indicated for dyspneic cough due to predominant excess in the upper part and deficiency in the lower part of the body. Excess in the upper part means an accumulation of sputum in the lung, which leads to inhibited lung *qi*, giving rise to a feeling of fullness and oppression in the chest, dyspneic cough and profuse expectoration. Deficiency in the lower part denotes renal *yang* deficiency with impeded inspiration, giving rise to lumbago, weak legs, fatigue, dyspnea and shortness of breath. Since the disorder mainly affects the lung and secondarily the kidney, major attention should be paid to treating the excess in the upper part of the body by suppressing the adversely ascendant *qi*, relieving dyspnea and cough and eliminating phlegm. At the same time, efforts should be made to warm the kidney and promote inspiration to treat deficiency in the lower part of the body. In the prescription, Fructus Perillae serves as the chief ingredient to suppress the adversely ascendant *qi*, eliminate sputum, relieve cough and dyspnea; Pinelliae, Magnoliae Officinalis and Peucedani serve as the adjuvant ingredients to enhance the action of Fructus Perillae. The combination of the chief and adjuvant drugs relieves the excess syndrome in the upper part of the body. Cortex Cinnamomi warms the kidney, expels cold and relieves dyspnea, Angelicae Sinensis nourishes the blood and liver, and helps Cinnamomi treat the deficiency syndrome in the lower part of the body, and Folium Perillae and Rhizoma Zingiberis Recens expel cold and release lung *qi*—these serve as the assistant drugs. The combination of all the drugs aims at both excess in the upper part and deficiency in the lower part of the body. When the adversely ascendant *qi* is suppressed and sputum eliminated, dyspneic cough is relieved.

In one ancient medical book, Pericarpium Citri Reticulatae is added to the prescription to enhance the effect of activating *qi* and eliminating sputum. In *Variorum of Prescriptions*, the prescription is modified by replacing Cortex Cinnamomi with Lignum Aquilariae Resinatum to enhance the promotion of inspiration and relief of dyspnea, and reduce the action of warming the kidney.

This prescription is warm and dry, and is contraindicated for cases of dyspneic cough due to lung and renal deficiency or lung heat.

Decoction for Relieving Asthma
定喘汤 *ding chuan tang*
(from *Wonderful Prescriptions for Keeping Health*)

Semen Ginkgo (nut discarded, crushed and fried)	9 g
Herba Ephedrae	9 g
Fructus Perillae	6 g
Radix Glycyrrhizae	3 g
Flos Farfarae	9 g
Semen Armeniacae Amarum	6 g
Cortex Mori Radicis	9 g
Radix Scutellariae	6 g
Rhizoma Pinelliae Preparata	9 g

Administration: Decoct with water for oral administration.

Action: Releasing inhibited lung *qi*, relieving asthma and eliminating sputum.

Indications: Cases of asthma, exhibiting wheezing cough, profuse expectoration of yellow and thick sputum, shortness of breath, or chills and fever, yellow and greasy tongue coating, and smooth and rapid pulse.

Explanation: This prescription is for cases of asthma due to attack of exogenous wind-cold and phlegm-heat retained in the interior. When wind-cold complicates retained phlegm and changes into heat, it may give rise to asthma, cough, profuse expectoration of thick yellow sputum, and chills and fever. The principle of treatment should be releasing the inhibited lung *qi*, relieving asthma, purging heat and eliminating sputum. In the prescription, Ephedrae is used to release the inhibited lung *qi*, relieve asthma and eventually treat exterior-cold syndrome; Ginkgo arrests the lung *qi*, relieves cough and asthma, eliminates sputum and prevents the consumption of lung *qi* by Ephedrae—both serve as the chief ingredients. Fructus Perillae, Armeniacae Amarum, Pinelliae and Farfarae, as the adjuvant drugs, suppress the adversely ascendant *qi*, relieve asthma and cough and eliminate sputum. Mori Radicis and Scutellariae, as the assistant ingredients, purge lung heat and relieve cough and asthma. Glycyrrhizae is the guide to coordinate the effects of the other drugs. Together, they release the inhibited lung *qi*, purge phlegm-heat and relieve wind-cold syndrome.

Clinical evidence calling for the application of this prescription is asthma with thick and yellow sputum, yellow and greasy tongue coating, and smooth and rapid pulse. For patients who have difficulty in expectoration, Fructus Trichosanthis and Rhizoma Arisaema cum Bile can be added; for those with a feeling of oppression in the chest, Fructus Aurantii and Cortex Magnoliae Officinalis can be added; and for those with marked lung heat syndrome, Gypsum Fibrosum and Herba Houttuyniae can be added.

Both this prescription and Small Blue Dragon Decoction can be applied for cases of asthma due to affection by wind-cold in the exterior and phlegm retained in the interior. But this one is better for cases with internal phlegm-heat, while Small Blue Dragon Decoction is more effective for cases with internal cold-phlegm marked by exterior cold syndrome.

Decoction of Inulae and Haematitum
旋复代赭汤 *xuan fu dai zhe tang*
(from *Treatise on Cold Diseases*)

Flos Inulae	9 g
Radix Ginseng	6 g
Rhizoma Zingiberis Recens	15 g
Haematitum	9 g
Radix Glycyrrhizae Preparata	9 g
Rhizoma Pinelliae Preparata	9 g
Fructus Jujubae	4 pieces

Administration: Decoct with water for oral administration.

Action: Suppressing the adversely ascendant *qi*, eliminating phlegm, benefiting *qi* and regulating the stomach.

Indications: Cases with retained phlegm and adversely rising stomach *qi*, exhibiting epigastric fullness, eructation, vomiting and nausea.

Explanation: The stomach receives food and its normal function is to send its content downward. When there is stomach deficiency and the stomach *qi* adversely goes up, eructation, vomiting and nausea occur. Retained phlegm may cause disturbance in the normal ascent and descent of *qi* and lead to epigastric fullness. The principle of treatment should be suppressing the adversely ascendant *qi*, eliminating phlegm, benefiting *qi* and regulating the stomach. In the prescription, Inulae is used to keep *qi* go down and eliminate phlegm, and Haematitum to suppress the adversely rising *qi*; both serve as the chief ingredients to relieve eructation and vomiting. Zingiberis Recens is used to warm the stomach, eliminate phlegm, expel cold and stop vomiting; and Pinelliae eliminates phlegm, disperses stasis, sends *qi* downward and regulates the stomach—they both serve as the adjuvant ingredients. Ginseng is a tonic to replenish *qi*, and Glycyrrhizae warms *qi* of the middle *jiao*; both serve as the assistant ingredients. Jujubae is used as the guiding ingredient to benefit *qi* and regulate *qi* of the middle *jiao*. All together act as a remedy for suppressing the adversely ascendant *qi*, eliminating phlegm, benefiting *qi* and regulating the stomach.

This prescription is usually used for cases of vomiting and regurgitation due to deficiency cold in the stomach *qi*, and cases of epigastric fullness and eructation. For cases of profuse expectoration, Poria and Pericarpium Citri Reticulatae are added to strengthen the effect to regulate the stomach and remove phlegm. For cases with marked gastric cold, dried Zingiberis is used to replace raw Zingiberis, and a proper amount of Flos Caryophylli and Calyx Kaki is added to enhance the effects of warming the stomach and suppressing *qi*.

Decoction of Citri Reticulatae and Bambusae in Taeniam

橘皮竹茹汤 *ju pi zhu ru tang*

(from *Synopsis of the Golden Cabinet*)

Pericarpium Citri Reticulatae	12 g
Caulis Bambusae in Taeniam	12 g
Fructus Jujubae	5 pieces
Rhizoma Zingiberis Recens	9 g
Radix Glycyrrhizae	6 g
Radix Ginseng	3 g

Administration: Decoct with water for oral administration.

Action: Suppressing the adversely rising *qi*, relieving hiccup, benefiting *qi* and purging heat.

Indications: Cases of stomach deficiency with heat and adversely ascending *qi*, manifested as hiccup or retching, tender and red tongue, and feeble and rapid pulse.

Explanation: Hiccup is considered a disorder of the stomach that may be grouped into cold, heat, deficiency and excess types. This prescription is designed for cases of stomach deficiency heat and the failure of *qi* to descend. Stomach deficiency should be relieved, heat eliminated, and the adversely ascending *qi* made to descend. In the prescription, Citri Reticulatae and Bambusae in Taeniam are used as the chief ingredients in larger dosages, the former to regulate stomach *qi* and suppress the adversely rising *qi* to stop vomiting, and the latter to purge heat and appease the stomach with the same effect. Ginseng, when used with Pericarpium Citri Reticulatae, activates and invigorates *qi*, and Zingiberis Recens used together with Bambusae in Taeniam produces both the clearing and warming actions in order to regulate the stomach and stop vomiting—they serve as the adjuvant ingredients. Glycyrrhizae and Jujubae, as assistant and guiding drugs, enhance the action of Ginseng and coordinate the effects of the other drugs. All the above together invigorate the stomach, purge stomach heat and suppress the adversely rising stomach *qi*, and at the same time produce a tonic effect without causing stagnation, and purge heat without causing cold.

This is a common prescription for relieving hiccup and retching; tender and red tongue and feeble rapid pulse are the clinical evidence calling for its application. For cases of vomiting due to insufficient stomach *yin* accompanied by thirst, red tongue with little and dry coating, and small and rapid pulse, Radix Ophiopogonis, Herba Dendrobii, Folium Eriobotryae and Rhizoma Phragmitis are added to nourish stomach *yin* and suppress the adversely ascendant stomach *qi* in order to stop vomiting. However, this prescription is contraindicated for cases of hiccup due to excess heat or deficiency cold.

Decoction of Caryophylli and Kaki

丁香柿蒂汤 *ding xiang shi di tang*

(from *Symptoms, Etiology, Pulse Condition and Treatment*)

Flos Caryophylli 6 g
Calyx Kaki 9 g
Radix Ginseng 3 g
Rhizoma Zingiberis Recens 6 g

Administration: Decoct with water for oral administration.

Action: Warming the middle *jiao*, benefiting *qi*, suppressing the adversely ascendant *qi* and relieving hiccup.

Indications: Cases of deficiency cold and failure of stomach *qi* to descend, exhibiting hiccup, vomiting, an oppressed feeling in the chest and epigastrium, pale tongue with white coating, and deep and slow pulse.

Explanation: Deficiency cold affecting the stomach *qi* may produce hiccup, vomiting, an oppressed feeling in the chest and epigastrium, pale tongue with white coating, and deep and slow pulse. Hence, the therapeutic principle is to warm the middle *jiao*, benefit *qi*, suppress the adversely ascendant *qi* and stop hiccup. In the prescription, Caryophylli is used to warm the stomach, expel cold, suppress the adversely ascendant *qi* and relieve hiccup, and Kaki suppresses the adverse flow of *qi*—both serve as the chief ingredients for treating hiccup due to stomach cold. Ginseng is used to benefit and invigorate *qi*, Zingiberis Recens warms the stomach and suppresses the adversely ascendant *qi*. The combination of these drugs expels stomach cold, suppresses the adversely rising *qi* and invigorates the stomach, so as to relieve hiccup.

This is a prescription frequently used for cases of hiccup and vomiting due to deficiency cold affecting stomach *qi*, and adversely rising *qi*. Hiccup, vomiting, pale tongue with white coating, and deep and slow pulse are key evidence calling for its application. For cases of severe cold accompanied by stagnation of *qi* and phlegm, Pericarpium Citri Reticulatae, Lignum Aquilariae Resinatum and Rhizoma Pinelliae are added to regulate *qi*, dissolve phlegm and enhance the action of warming the middle *jiao* and suppressing the adversely rising *qi*.

Summary

Ten principal and two appendant prescriptions are discussed in this chapter, which may be classified into two sub-categories.

(1) Prescriptions for promoting *qi* circulation:

Such prescriptions are indicated for cases of *qi* stagnation. *Yueju* Pill is a common prescription for mild cases in which *qi* stagnation is considered as the chief syndrome and is complicated by stagnation of blood, phlegm, fire, dampness and food. Powder of Toosendan is a basic prescription for promoting *qi* circulation to relieve pain, and is indicated for pain due to stagnant *qi* and blood. Decoction of Pinelliae and Magnoliae Officinalis and Decoction of Trichosanthis and Allii Macrostemi are both prescriptions to promote *qi* circulation and expel phlegm. However, the former can also disperse stagnation and suppress the adversely ascendant *qi*, and is chiefly indicated for globus hystericus due to *qi* and phlegm stagnation; the latter can also activate *yang qi* in order to relieve stagnation, and is mainly indicated for chest *bi*-syndrome due to the decline of chest *yang* and stagnation of *qi* and phlegm. *Tiantai* Powder of Linderae promotes *qi* circulation, soothes the liver and expels cold to reduce pain, and is indicated for inguinal hernia due to stagnant cold and *qi*.

(2) Prescriptions for suppressing adversely ascendant *qi*:

These prescriptions are indicated for cases of cough due to adversely rising lung *qi*, and cases of hiccup due to adversely ascendant stomach *qi*. Decoction of Perillae for Keeping *Qi* Downward and Decoction for Relieving Asthma both suppress adversely rising lung *qi*. The former, however, is good for warming and dissipating phlegm-dampness, and indicated for deficiency due to cold, dampness and phlegm stagnation, with excess in the upper and deficiency in the lower part of the body; the latter purges lung fire and expels exogenous pathogens, and is indicated for cases of asthma due to attack by wind-cold in the exterior and stagnant phlegm-heat in the interior. Decoction of Inulae and Haematitum, Decoction of Citri Reticulatae and Bambusae in Taeniam, and Decoction of Caryophylli and Kaki all suppress adversely ascendant stomach *qi* to relieve hiccup, and also invigorate *qi* and benefit the stomach. However, Decoction of Inulae and Haematitum is more effective in relieving vomiting, and is indicated for cases of vomiting, eructation and chest upset due to stomach deficiency and stagnant phlegm; Decoction of Citri Reticulatae and Bambusae in Taeniam and Decoction of Caryophylli and Kaki are good for relieving hiccup. Of the latter two, the former can also purge stomach heat and is indicated for heat-type hiccup due to stomach deficiency, while the latter warms and expels stomach cold and is indicated for hiccup of the cold type.

CHAPTER SIXTEEN

PRESCRIPTIONS FOR REGULATING THE BLOOD

Prescriptions for regulating the blood (*li xue ji*) are chiefly composed of drugs that activate blood circulation and remove blood stasis, or stop bleeding. They are indicated for blood-stasis syndromes and hemorrhagic diseases.

Blood diseases cover a wide range and their treatment is rather complicated. It includes the therapy of activating blood circulation to remove blood stasis, the therapy of stopping bleeding and the therapy of enriching the blood. The therapy of enriching the blood was dealt with in Chapter Eleven, and the other two therapies are discussed in the present chapter.

Prescriptions for activating blood circulation to remove blood stasis (*huo xue qu yu ji*) are indicated for blood-accumulation and blood-stasis syndromes, e.g., abdominal mass, hemiplegia due to stagnant blood in the meridians, amenorrhea and dysmenorrhea. The commonly used drugs include Rhizoma Chuanxiong, Semen Persicae, Flos Carthami, Radix Paeoniae Rubra and Radix Salviae Miltiorrhizae, and they can be used in combination with some drugs that regulate *qi*. Furthermore, some other drugs can also be added according to the nature of the disease (cold or heat, deficiency or excess). For example, for cases complicated by cold syndrome, drugs that warm the meridians and expel cold are added; for cases in which stagnant blood changes into heat, drugs that eliminate heat and remove blood stasis are added; and for chronic cases of blood stasis complicated by deficient antipathogenic *qi*, *qi* and blood tonics are added. Examples: Decoction of Persicae for Purgation, Decoction for Removing Blood Stasis in the Chest, Decoction for Invigorating *Yang*, and Decoction for Warming the Meridians.

Prescriptions for stopping bleeding (*zhi xue ji*) are indicated for hemorrhagic diseases, such as hematemesis, epistaxis, hemoptysis, hemafecia and hematuria. Drugs frequently used include Cacumen Biotae, Herba Cephalanoploris, Flos Sophorae and Terra Flava Usta. Since the cause, location and severity of bleeding vary, different prescriptions should be applied accordingly. For example, bleeding due to blood-heat should be treated by cooling the blood to stop bleeding, while treatment for bleeding due to deficient *yang* seeks to warm *yang* and benefit *qi* in order to control the blood. Examples: Powder of Ten Drugs' Ashes, Decoction of Cephalanoploris, and Decoction of Terra Flava Usta.

In applying prescriptions that regulate the blood, it is necessary to distinguish heat and cold syndromes as well as deficiency and excess syndromes, and determine the cause and severity of the disease. Generally speaking, a symptomatic treatment is given for acute cases and a causative treatment for chronic cases, or else both are applied simultaneously. However, long-term administration and large dosage of drugs that remove blood stasis are liable to impair the antipathogenic *qi*, so drugs that benefit *qi* and nourish the blood should also be used in such cases. Astringent hemostatics may lead to retained blood stasis, and so they should be combined with drugs that activate blood circulation and remove blood stasis. Moreover, the prescriptions for activating blood circulation to remove blood stasis may cause bleeding and induce abortion, and should be used cautiously in cases of menorrhagia and pregnancy.

Decoction of Persicae for Purgation
桃核承气汤 *tao he cheng qi tang*
(from *Treatise on Cold Diseases*)

Semen Persicae	12 g
Radix et Rhizoma Rhei	12 g
Ramulus Cinnamomi	6 g
Radix Glycyrrhizae Preparata	6 g
Natrii Sulfas	6 g

Administration: Decoct the first four drugs with water and mix their decoction with Natrii Sulfas for oral administration.

Action: Removing blood stasis.

Indications: Cases of blood accumulation in the lower *jiao*, exhibiting distensive pain in the lower abdomen, incontinent urine, delirium, extreme thirst, fever at night, or even mania.

Explanation: The prescription is formed by adding Semen Persicae and Ramulus Cinnamomi to Decoction for Purgation and Regulation of Stomach *Qi*. It is indicated for diseases due to the simultaneous accumulation of stagnant blood and heat. Stagnant blood and heat retained in the lower *jiao* may lead to distensive pain in the lower abdomen, accumulated stagnant blood may cause incontinent urine; stagnant heat in *xuefen* may result in delirium, thirst and fever at night; and serious blood stasis and high fever may elicit irritability or even mania. Hence, the key in the treatment of such diseases is to remove blood stasis with potent drugs. In the prescription, Persicae is a potent drug for eliminating blood stasis, and Rhei is a drug for purging stagnant blood and heat—both serve as the chief ingredients. Ramulus Cinnamomi dredges the blood vessels, and Natrii Sulfas purges heat and serves as the adjuvant ingredient to enhance the effects of Persicae and Rhei. Glycyrrhizae benefits *qi* and regulates the middle *jiao*, and serves as the assistant and guiding ingredient to counteract the potency of the other drugs and prevent their possible damage to the antipathogenic *qi*.

This prescription is also effective for cases of headache, heaviness in the head, congestion of conjunctiva and toothache due to hyperactive fire and stagnant blood in the head, epistaxis and hematemesis due to blood-heat; amenorrhea caused by blood stasis; or postpartum lochiostasis.

Decoction for Removing Blood Stasis in the Chest
血府逐瘀汤 *xue fu zhu yu tang*
(from *Correction of Medical Classics*)

Semen Persicae	12 g
Flos Carthami	9 g
Radix Angelicae Sinensis	9 g
Radix Rehmanniae (crude)	9 g
Rhizoma Chuanxiong	5 g
Radix Paeoniae Rubra	6 g
Rhizoma Achyranthis Bidentatae	9 g
Radix Platycodi	5 g
Radix Bupleuri	3 g
Fructus Aurantii	6 g
Radix Glycyrrhizae	3 g

Administration: Decoct with water for oral administration.

Action: Activating *qi* and blood circulation to remove blood stasis and alleviate pain.

Indications: Cases of blood stagnation in the chest, exhibiting prolonged and local pain in the chest or headache, stabbing pain, or continuous hiccup, irritability, palpitation, insomnia, hectic fever at night, dark-red tongue with petechiae on its fringe or surface, dark lips and eyes, and unsmooth or taut and tense pulse.

Explanation: The prescription was invented by the famous physician Wang Qingren (A.D. 1768-1831), and is indicated for cases of blood stagnation in the chest and stagnant hepatic *qi*. It is the combination of Four Drugs Decoction with Persicae and Carthami and Powder for Regulating the Liver and Spleen in addition to Radix Platycodi and Radix Achyranthis Bidentatae. The liver meridian passes through the chest and hypochondrium. Stagnant blood in the chest is likely to lead to stagnant hepatic *qi*, manifested as prolonged chest pain and irritability. Prolonged blood stagnation may produce heat and exhibit a feeling of oppression in the chest or hectic fever at night. When the heat goes to the head, there will be headache; when it affects the heart, there will be palpitation and insomnia; when it affects the stomach, hiccup will ensue. The dark-red tongue with petechiae on its fringe or surface, dark lips and eyes, and unsmooth or taut and tense pulse are also indications of blood stasis syndrome. For such cases, treatment aims at activating blood circulation to remove blood stasis in combination with activating *qi* circulation to disperse stagnation. In the prescription, the ingredients of Four Drugs Decoction are used along with Persicae and Carthami to activate blood circulation to remove blood stasis and nourish the blood; the ingredients of Powder for Regulating the Liver and Spleen are used to promote *qi* circulation and soothe the liver; Platycodi is used to release inhibited lung *qi*; and Aurantii soothes the chest, while Achyranthis Bidentatae opens the blood vessels and lets the blood flow downward. All the above drugs together promote the circulation of blood and *qi*, eliminate blood stasis and heat, and release inhibited lung *qi*.

This prescription activates blood circulation and removes blood stasis without consuming blood, and releases stagnant hepatic *qi* without consuming *qi*. It is only used for internal blood stasis.

Appendant Prescriptions

(1) Decoction for Opening the Orifices and Activating Blood Circulation
通窍活血汤 *tong qiao huo xue tang*
(from *Correction of Medical Classics*)

It is composed of 3 g of Radix Paeoniae Rubra, 3 g of Rhizoma Chuanxiong, 9 g of Semen Persicae (crushed), 9 g of Flos Carthami, 3 g of Herba Allii Fistulosi (crushed), 5 g of Fructus Jujubae, 0. 15 g of Moschus (wrapped with cloth), and 25 ml of yellow wine. The drugs are decocted with water for oral administration. It activates blood circulation and opens the orifices, and is indicated for headache, dizziness, deafness and alopecia due to stagnant blood in the head and infantile malnutrition.

(2) Decoction for Removing Blood Stasis Below the Diaphragm
膈下逐瘀汤 *ge xia zhu yu tang*
(from *Correction of Medical Classics*)

It is composed of 9 g of Faeces Trogopterori (fried), 9 g of Radix Angelicae Sinensis, 6 g of Rhizoma Chuanxiong, 9 g of Semen Persicae (crushed), 6 g of Cortex Moutan Radicis, 6 g of Radix Paeoniae Rubra, 6 g of Radix Linderae, 3 g of Rhizoma Corydalis, 9 g of Radix Glycyrrhizae, 5 g of Rhizoma Cyperi, 9 g of Flos Carthami, and 5 g of Fructus Aurantii. To be decocted with water for oral administration, it activates blood circulation to remove blood stasis and promotes *qi* circulation to relieve pain, and is indicated for cases with an accumulation of blood stasis below the diaphragm, infantile abdominal masses, local abdominal pain, or a weighted sensation in the abdomen upon lying down.

(3) Decoction for Removing Blood Stasis in the Lower Abdomen
少腹逐瘀汤 *shao fu zhu yu tang*
(from *Correction of Medical Classics*)

It is composed of 1. 5 g of Fructus Foeniculi (fried), 3 g of Rhizoma Zingiberis (fried), 3 g of Rhizoma Corydalis, 9 g of Radix Angelicae Sinensis, 3 g of Rhizoma Chuanxiong, 3 g of Cortex Cinnamomi, 6 g of Radix Paeoniae Rubra, 9 g of Pollen Typhae, and 6g of Faeces Trogopterori (fried). To be decocted with water for oral administration, it activates blood circulation to remove blood stasis and warms the meridians to relieve pain. It is indicated for cases of blood stasis in the lower abdomen, exhibiting lower abdominal pain and masses, lumbago and lower abdominal distention during the menstrual period, irregular menstruation with purple or dark clotted menses, or metrorrhagia accompanied by lower abdominal pain.

Angelicae Sinensis, Chuanxiong, Persicae and Carthami are the chief ingredients in all the above prescriptions, which activate blood circulation to remove blood stasis and relieve pain. All of them are applicable to treat blood stasis syndrome. However, Decoction for Removing Blood Stasis in the Chest contains Aurantii, Platycodi and Bupleuri to activate *qi* and soothe the chest, and Achyranthis Bidentatae to guide the blood downward, and so it is chiefly indicated for cases of blood stasis in the chest. Decoction for Opening the Orifice and Activating Blood Circulation contains Moschus and Allii Fistulosi for opening the orifices and activating *yang*, and is better at activating blood circulation and opening the orifices, and so it is chiefly indicated for cases of blood stasis in the head. Decoction for Removing Blood Stasis Below the Diaphragm contains Cyperi, Corydalis, Linderae and Aurantii to soothe the liver, activate *qi* circulation and relieve pain, and has a stronger effect in activating *qi* and killing pain, and so it is mainly indicated for cases of blood stasis below the diaphragm, exhibiting distensive pain and masses in the hypochondria and abdomen. Decoction for Removing Blood Stasis in the Lower Abdomen contains Foeniculi, Cinnamomi and Zingiberis to warm the meridians in order to relieve pain, and it is chiefly indicated for cases of blood stasis in the lower abdomen, manifested as masses in the lower abdomen, irregular menstruation and dysmenorrhea.

Decoction for Invigorating *Yang*

补阳还五汤 *bu yang huan wu tang*

(from *Correction of Medical Classics*)

Radix Astragali	30-120 g
Radix Angelicae Sinensis (tail part)	6 g
Radix Paeoniae Rubra	6 g
Lumbricus	3 g
Rhizoma Chuanxiong	3 g
Flos Carthami	3 g
Semen Persicae	3 g

Administration: Decoct with water for oral administration.

Action: Invigorating *qi*, activating blood circulation and dredging the collaterals.

Indications: Sequelae of stroke, exhibiting hemiplegia, facial deviation, aphasia, salivation, incontinent urine or frequent urination, white tongue coating, and slow pulse.

Explanation: This prescription is indicated for cases due to blood stagnation in the collaterals and deficient antipathogenic *qi*. Deficient antipathogenic *qi* and collateral obstruction lead to poor nourishment of the tendons and muscles, giving rise to hemiplegia and facial deviation. *Qi* deficiency and blood stagnation cause undernourishment of the tongue, exhibiting aphasia and salivation. Frequent or incontinent urination, white tongue coating and slow pulse are indications of *qi* deficiency. Hence, the principle of treatment should be invigorating *qi* primarily, and activating blood circulation and dredging the collaterals secondarily. In the prescription, Astragali serves as the chief ingredient and is used in a large dosage; it exerts a strong effect to invigorate *qi* so as to promote blood circulation and remove blood stasis, but without causing damage to the antipathogenic *qi*. Angelicae Sinensis is applied as an adjuvant ingredient to activate blood circulation in order to remove blood stasis, and so its tail part is used. Chuanxiong, Paeoniae Rubra, Persicae and Carthami enhance the action of Angelicae Sinensis, and Lumbricus dredges the collaterals—they serve as the assistant and guiding ingredients. All together activate *qi* and blood circulation, remove blood stasis and reopen the collaterals.

The dosage of Astragali should begin from 30-60 g and be increased gradually. When the disease is cured, the decoction should be taken continuously for a certain period of time.

Powder for Dissipating Blood Stasis

失笑散 *shi xiao san*

(from *Benevolent Prescriptions from the Pharmaceutical Bureau of the Taiping Period*)

Faeces Trogopterori (ground with wine)
Pollen Typhae (fried)
(in equivalent amount)

Administration: Grind both into fine powder and take 6 g each time with yellow wine or vinegar.

Action: Activating blood circulation to remove blood stasis, removing stagnation and relieving pain.

Indications: Cases of retained stagnant blood, exhibiting severe pain in the chest and abdomen, postpartum lochiostasis, or irregular menstruation with lower abdominal pain.

Explanation: This prescription is indicated for pains due to the retention of stagnant blood, obstruction of the vessels and impeded blood flow. The principle of treatment is to activate blood circulation and remove blood stasis to relieve pain. In the prescription, Faeces Trogopterori is a common drug for relieving pain due to blood stasis, Pollen Typhae removes blood stasis and stops bleeding; they act together to activate blood circulation and remove blood stasis, and produce an analgesic effect. Vinegar or yellow wine is applied to promote blood circulation and enhance the potency of the drugs.

This is a common prescription for killing pain, such as chest pain, stomachache and dysmenorrhea due to blood stasis. However, it is incapable of activating *qi*, so *qi*-activating drugs can be added when necessary.

Appendant Prescription

No. II Formula for Coronary Diseases

冠心Ⅱ号方 *guan xin er hao fang*

(A proved recipe)

The prescription is composed of 15 g of Rhizoma Chuanxiong, 15 g of Radix Paeoniae Rubra, 15 g of Flos Carthami, 15 g of Lignum Dalbergiae Odoriferae, and 30 g of Radix Salviae Miltiorrhizae. To be decocted with water for oral administration, it activates blood circulation, removes blood stasis, activates *qi* and kills pain, and is indicated for coronary diseases and angina pectoris due to blood stasis.

Decoction for Warming the Meridians
温经汤 *wen jing tang*
(from *Synopsis of the Golden Cabinet*)

Fructus Evodiae	5 g
Radix Angelicae Sinensis	9 g
Radix Lactiflorae	6 g
Rhizoma Chuanxiong	6 g
Radix Ginseng	6 g
Ramulus Cinnamomi	6 g
Colla Corii Asini	6 g
Cortex Moutan Radicis	6 g
Rhizoma Zingiberis Recens	6 g
Radix Glycyrrhizae	6 g
Rhizoma Pinelliae	6 g
Radix Ophiopogonis	9 g

Administration: Decoct with water for oral administration.

Action: Warming the meridians to expel cold, removing blood stasis and nourishing the blood.

Indications: Cases of deficiency cold in the Chong and Ren meridians, and blood stasis, exhibiting irregular or prolonged menstruation, evening fever, a hot sensation in the palms, dry lips and mouth, or else cold pain in the lower abdomen; also for sterility.

Explanation: The Chong Meridian is the "sea of blood," and the Ren Meridian controls the uterus. Both start from the lower abdomen and have a close relationship with menstruation. Deficiency cold in the Chong and Ren meridians and stagnant *qi* and blood may lead to irregular menstruation or cold pain in the lower abdomen, or else sterility. Blood stasis inhibits the generation of new blood, and leads to dry mouth and lips. Evening fever and the hot sensation in the palms are indications of *yin*-blood insufficiency. As deficiency and excess as well as heat and cold syndromes coexist, the therapeutic principle should be removing blood stasis along with warming the meridians, expelling cold and nourishing the blood. In the prescription, Evodiae and Ramulus Cinnamomi warm the meridians, expel cold and expand the blood vessels—they serve as the chief ingredients. Angelicae Sinensis, Chuanxiong and Lactiflorae are used to activate blood circulation, remove blood stasis, nourish the blood and regulate menstruation, while Moutan Radicis removes blood stasis, promotes menstruation and relieves deficiency fever—they serve as the adjuvant. Colla Corii Asini and Ophiopogonis nourish *yin*, moisten dryness and relieve deficiency heat, and the former also stops bleeding, Ginseng and Glycyrrhizae benefit *qi* and strengthen the spleen to promote the generation of blood, Pinelliae makes stomach *qi* go down, breaks stagnation and helps remove blood stasis and regulate menstruation, Zingiberis Recens warms the stomach and expels cold—all serve as the assistant ingredients. In addition, Glycyrrhizae serves as the guiding drug to coordinate the effects of the other drugs. Together, these drugs remove stagnant blood, expel cold, and invigorate *qi* and blood, and eventually reduce deficiency fever and restore normal menstruation.

Although the prescription can produce different effects simultaneously, it is mainly used to warm and nourish the Chong and Ren meridians. It is a common prescription for treating menstrual disorders, especially irregular menstruation and dysmenorrhea due to deficiency cold in the Chong and Ren meridians and stagnant blood.

Decoction for Ectopic Pregnancy

宫外孕方 *gong wai yun fang*

(A proved recipe developed by No. 1 Hospital Affiliated to the Shanxi Medical College)

Radix Salviae Miltiorrhizae	15 g
Radix Paeoniae Rubra	15 g
Semen Persicae	9 g
(No. 1 Prescription)	
Rhizoma Sparganii	1.5-6 g
Rhizoma Zedoariae	1.5-6 g
(added to form No. 2 Prescription)	

Administration: Decoct with water for oral administration.

Action: Activating blood circulation to remove blood stasis, removing abdominal masses and relieving pain.

Indications: Cases of ruptured ectopic pregnancy, exhibiting delayed menstruation with continuous and difficult discharge of dark red menses, acute and severe pain in the lower abdomen that occasionally extends to the whole abdomen.

Explanation: Masses in the lower abdomen with fixed local sharp pain that cannot be pressed belong to "*zheng*" (症) in traditional Chinese medicine. Discharge of dark and purplish blood clots from the uterus is an indication of blood-stasis syndrome. For such a case, the treatment is to activate blood circulation to remove blood stasis and abdominal masses, and relieve pain. In the prescription, Salviae Miltiorrhizae, Persicae, Sparganii and Zedoariae are used to activate blood circulation, remove stasis and relieve abdominal masses. Paeoniae Rubra activates blood circulation. These drugs together remove abdominal masses, kill pain and stop bleeding.

For cases of ectopic pregnancy complicated by shock, other emergency measures should be adopted. In cases of profuse bleeding and profound shock, timely surgery should be performed.

Powder of Ten Drugs' Ashes
十灰散 *shi hui san*
(from *Miraculous Books of Ten Effective Recipes*)

Herba seu Radix Cirsii Japonici
Herba Cephalanoploris
Folium Nelumbinis
Cacumen Biotae
Rhizoma Imperatae
Radix Rubiae
Fructus Gardeniae
Radix et Rhizoma Rhei
Cortex Moutan Radicis
Vagina Trachycarpi
(in equivalent amount)

Administration: Burn the drugs into charcoal and grind the ashes into fine powder, take 9 g each time with lotus-root juice, or juice of radish and Chinese ink; or prepare the ashes into pills, take 9 g each time, twice daily; or prepare them directly into an oral decoction, with dosages reduced proportionally.

Action: Cooling the blood and stopping bleeding.

Indications: Hematemesis, epistaxis and hemoptysis due to heat in the blood.

Explanation: This prescription is indicated for blood extravasation due to heat in the blood. Hyperactive fire damages the blood vessels, leading to hemorrhage, epistaxis and hemoptysis. The therapeutic principle should be cooling the blood and stopping bleeding. In the prescription, Cirsii Japonici, Cephalanoploris, Nelumbinis, Rubiae, Biotae and Imperatae cool the blood and stop bleeding; Trachycarpi produces an astringent effect; Gardeniae purges heat and fire; Rhei guides heat downward and suppresses fire to stop bleeding; Moutan Radicis is used with Rhei to cool the blood and remove blood stasis. The drugs are burnt into charcoal to enhance their astringent and hemostatic effects. The prescription's heat-eliminating, blood-cooling and hemostatic effects are enhanced by taking the charcoal ash with the juice of lotus root or else of radish and Chinese ink. In sum, cooling the blood and stopping bleeding are the chief actions of the prescription, along with those of purging heat and fire and removing blood stasis. Hence, this is a hemostatic prescription for emergency use.

In burning the drugs, attention must be paid to preserve their original properties. That is why they are only burned into charcoal. For bleeding due to severe heat, the drugs may be used in crude form and decocted for oral administration. Moreover, this prescription only provides a symptomatic treatment for bleeding in heat syndromes, causative treatment should be given after the bleeding is stopped. It may also be applied topically for epistaxis and trauma.

Decoction for Hemoptysis

咳血方 *ke xue fang*

(from *Danxi's Experience on Medicine*)

Indigo Naturalis (ground with water)	6 g
Semen Trichosanthis	9 g
Pumex	9 g
Fructus Gardeniae (fried until brown)	9 g
Fructus Chebulae	6 g

Administration: Decoct with water for oral administration.

Action: Purging fire, eliminating sputum, relieving cough and stopping bleeding.

Indications: Cases due to attack of the lung by liver fire, exhibiting cough with difficult expectoration of thick bloody sputum, or else irritability, sharp pain in the chest and hypochondrium, flushed cheeks, constipation, red tongue with yellow coating, and taut and rapid pulse.

Explanation: An attack of the lung by liver fire may lead to cough that damages the tissue of the lung and hemoptysis. When lung fluid is consumed by heat, sputum is produced and thick bloody expectoration ensues. Irritability, sharp pain in the chest and hypochondrium, constipation, flushed cheeks, red tongue with yellow coating, and taut and rapid pulse are indications of hyperactive liver fire. Although the diseases manifests itself as a lung disorder, its fundamental cause lies in the liver. Hence, the therapeutic principle should be suppressing liver fire. In the prescription, Indigo Naturalis and Gardeniae serve as the chief ingredients to purge liver fire and cool the blood. Trichosanthis and Pumex, as the adjuvant ingredients, eliminate heat, suppress fire, moisten dryness and remove sputum. Chebulae is used as an assistant drug to eliminate lung heat, relieve cough and remove sputum. The drugs are used together to purge liver fire, calm the lung and stop cough and bleeding.

In clinical practice, Semen Armeniacae Amarum, Bulbus Fritillariae Thunbergii, Concretio Silicea Bambusae may be added for cases with profuse expectoration, and Radix Adenophorae and Radix Ophiopogonis may be added for cases in which hyperactive fire leads to *yin* consumption.

Decoction of Cephalanoploris

小蓟饮子 *xiao ji yin zi*

(from *Prescriptions for Life Saving*)

Radix Rehmanniae (crude)	120 g
Herba Cephalanoploris	15 g
Talcum	15 g
Caulis Akebiae	15 g
Pollen Typhae (fried)	15 g

Nodus Nelumbinis Rhizomatis	15 g
Herba Lophatheri	15 g
Radix Angelicae Sinensis (soaked in wine)	15 g
Fructus Gardeniae (fried)	15 g
Radix Glycyrrhizae Preparata	15 g

Administration: Grind the drugs together into granules, decoct 15 g of the granules with water for oral administration before meals; or prepare them directly into an oral decoction, with dosages reduced proportionally.

Action: Cooling the blood, stopping bleeding, promoting diuresis and relieving stranguria.

Indications: Diseases due to stagnant blood and heat in the lower *jiao*, manifested as stranguria, hematuria, frequent discharge of reddish urine with a hot feeling, red tongue, and rapid pulse.

Explanation: This prescription is formed by adding certain drugs to Powder for Promoting Diuresis. Stagnant blood and heat in the lower *jiao* injure the blood vessels and lead to hematuria. Dysfunction of the urinary bladder results in dysuria and frequent discharge of reddish urine with a hot sensation. Red tongue and rapid pulse are also indications of stagnant heat in the lower *jiao*. Hence, treatment focuses on cooling the blood, stopping bleeding, promoting diuresis and relieving stranguria. In the prescription, Cephalanoploris is used as the chief ingredient to cool the blood and stop bleeding. Nodus Nelumbinis Rhizomatis and Typhae cool blood, stop bleeding and remove blood stasis, Talcum Lophatheri and Akebiae promote diuresis and expel heat, Gardeniae purges fire from the triple *jiao*, Rehmanniae nourishes *yin* and purges heat to prevent damage to *yin* caused by diuresis, and Angelicae Sinensis nourishes and regulates the blood to prevent the cold effect of other drugs—all serve as the adjuvant and assistant ingredients. Glycyrrhizae serves as the guiding ingredient to relieve pain and coordinate the effects of the other drugs. Together, they form a prescription whose chief action is to cool the blood and stop bleeding, and whose secondary effect is to promote diuresis and relieve stranguria.

This prescription produces a hemostatic effect while removing blood stasis, and a diuretic and heat-eliminating effect while nourishing *yin*. It is a common prescription for stranguria and hematuria due to excess heat. Dysuria, frequent discharge of reddish urine with a hot feeling, red tongue and rapid pulse are the clinical evidence calling for its application. For chronic hematuria along with obvious damage to both *qi* and *yin*, cold diuretics, such as Talcum and Akebiae, should be removed, and Radix Astragali and Colla Corii Asini should be added to benefit *qi* and nourish the blood and *yin*.

Decoction of Terra Flava Usta
黄土汤 *huang tu tang*
(from *Synopsis of the Golden Cabinet*)

Radix Glycyrrhizae	9 g

Radix Rehmanniae (dried)	9 g
Rhizoma Atractylodis Macrocephalae	9 g
Radix Aconiti Lateralis Preparata	9 g
Colla Corii Asini	9 g
Radix Scutellariae	9 g
Terra Flava Usta (ignited with yellow earth)	30 g

Administration: Decoct Terra Flava Usta with water first, then decoct the other drugs with its solution for oral administration.

Action: Warming *yang*, strengthening the spleen, nourishing the blood and stopping bleeding.

Indications: Cases due to spleen *yang* deficiency and deficiency cold in the middle *jiao*, exhibiting hemafecia, hematemesis, epistaxis or metrorrhagia with discharge of dull-colored blood, cold limbs, sallow complexion, pale tongue with white coating, and deep and thready weak pulse.

Explanation: Spleen *yang* deficiency affects the blood-controlling function of the spleen and leads to various kinds of bleeding. Discharge of dull-colored blood, cold limbs, sallow complexion, pale tongue with white coating, and deep and thready weak pulse are indications of deficiency cold affecting spleen *qi* and insufficient *yin*-blood. The principle of treatment should be warming *yang-qi* and stopping bleeding. In the prescription, Terra Flava Usta serves as the chief ingredient to warm the middle *jiao qi* and stop bleeding. Atractylodis Macrocephalae and Aconiti Lateralis Preparata, as the adjuvant, warm spleen *yang* and invigorate the middle *jiao qi*. Rehmanniae and Colla Corii Asini nourish *yin* and blood, and stop bleeding, and Scutellariae, bitter and cold, is used with the above two drugs to counteract the warm and dry nature of Atractylodis Macrocephalae and Aconiti Lateralis Preparata—they serve as the assistant ingredients. Glycyrrhizae is used as the guide to regulate the middle *jiao* and coordinate the effects of the other drugs. Together, these drugs form a prescription that warm the spleen and stop bleeding; it can warm *yang* without causing damage to *yin* and nourish *yin* without causing damage to *yang*.

Summary

Discussed in this chapter are ten principal and four appendant prescriptions, which can be divided into two sub-categories.

(1) Prescriptions for activating blood circulation to remove blood stasis:

These prescriptions are indicated for cases of impeded blood flow or retained blood stasis. Among them, Decoction of Persicae for Purgation is chiefly for eliminating blood stasis and heat, and is indicated for cases of blood accumulation in the lower *jiao* due to blood-heat. Decoction for Removing Blood Stasis in the Chest is effective in activating blood circulation to remove blood stasis and invigorating *qi* to relieve pain, and is indicated for cases of stagnant blood and *qi* in the chest. Decoction for Invigorating *Yang* invigorates *qi* and activates blood circulation, and is indicated for hemiplegia due to *qi* deficiency and blood stasis causing obstruction of the blood vessels. Powder for Dissipating Blood Stasis activates blood circulation to remove blood stasis and disperses stagnation to relieve pain, and is indicated for various kinds of chest and abdominal pain due to blood stasis. Decoction for Warming the Meridians warms the meridians, expels cold, nourishes blood and removes blood stasis, and is indicated for irregular menstruation due to deficiency cold in the Chong and Ren meridians and retained blood stasis. Decoction for Ectopic Pregnancy activates blood circulation, removes blood stasis, relieves abdominal pain and dissipates masses, and is indicated for ruptured ectopic pregnancy.

(2) Prescriptions for stopping bleeding:

Such prescriptions are indicated for various kinds of hemorrhagic diseases. Among them, Powder of Ten Drugs' Ashes cools the blood, stops bleeding, purges heat and removes blood stasis, and is indicated for bleeding of the heat syndrome. Decoction for Hemoptysis purges liver fire, and eliminates heat and sputum, and is indicated for hemoptysis due to attack of the lung by liver fire. Decoction of Cephalanoploris promotes diuresis and relieves stranguria, and is indicated for cases of stranguria complicated by hematuria, or hematuria. Decoction of Terra Flava Usta warms *yang*, and stops bleeding, and is indicated for bleeding due to deficient spleen *yang* and deficiency cold in the middle *jiao*, especially cases of hemafecia.

CHAPTER SEVENTEEN
PRESCRIPTIONS FOR DISPERSING STAGNATION

Prescriptions for dispersing stagnation (*xiao dao ji*) are composed of drugs that are effective to remove stagnation, and are applied to relieve dyspepsia and eliminate abdominal masses. They constitute the dispersive therapy, which is widely used for stagnation of *qi*, blood, phlegm, dampness and food, as well as abdominal masses. Discussed in this chapter are only prescriptions for relieving dyspepsia and eliminating masses, while those for regulating *qi* and blood and for eliminating phlegm and dampness are discussed in other related chapters.

Prescriptions for relieving dyspepsia (*xiao shi dao zhi ji*) are appropriate for food-stagnation syndrome, which exhibits fullness and oppression in the chest and epigastrium, acid regurgitation, poor appetite, and abdominal distention or diarrhea. Drugs commonly used are digestants, such as Fructus Crataegi, Mass Fermentata Medicinalis, Fructus Hordei Germinatus and Semen Raphani, in combination with drugs that invigorate the spleen, regulate *qi*, purge heat and eliminate dampness. Examples: Pill for Promoting Digestion, Pill of Aucklandiae and Arecae, and Pill for Invigorating the Spleen.

Prescriptions for eliminating masses (*xiao pi hua ji ji*) are indicated for syndromes that manifest epigastric and abdominal masses, anorexia and fatigue. They are mainly composed of drugs that activate *qi* and blood circulation, and eliminate dampness, phlegm and abdominal masses, such as Fructus Aurantii Immaturus, Cortex Magnoliae Officinalis and Rhizoma Pinelliae, Pericarpium Citri Reticulatae Viride and Rhizoma Zedoariae. An example cited here is Pill of Aurantii Immaturus for Removing Abdominal Mass.

Prescriptions discussed in this chapter and those purgative ones mentioned elsewhere in this book both eliminate tangible excess pathogens from the body. In clinical application, however, the former are recommended for mild and chronic diseases, the latter for acute and serious ones.

Pill for Promoting Digestion
保和丸 *bao he wan*
(from *Danxi's Experience on Medicine*)

Fructus Crataegi	180 g
Mass Fermentata Medicinalis	60 g
Rhizoma Pinelliae	90 g

Poria	90 g
Pericarpium Citri Reticulatae	30 g
Fructus Forsythiae	30 g
Semen Raphani	30 g

Administration: Grind the drugs into fine powder and mix the powder with water to make it into pills, take 6-9 g with boiled water or decoction of Fructus Hordei Germinatus; or prepare the drugs directly into an oral decoction, with dosages reduced proportionally.

Action: Promoting digestion and regulating stomach *qi*.

Indications: Various kinds of dyspepsia, manifested as epigastric and abdominal distention and pain, acid regurgitation, anorexia, nausea, vomiting or diarrhea, thick and greasy tongue coating, and smooth pulse.

Explanation: Dyspepsia is usually caused by immoderate eating and drinking. Overeating causes food retention which in turn disrupts the normal descent of stomach *qi*, resulting in oppression and distensive pain in the epigastrium and abdomen, acid regurgitation, anorexia and vomiting. Treatment aims at promoting digestion and regulating stomach *qi*. In the prescription, Crataegi is used as chief ingredient to promote digestion of all kinds of food, especially meat. Mass Fermentata Medicinalis strengthens the spleen and promotes digestion, and Raphani promotes digestion of cereals and removes phlegm or *qi* stagnation—both serve as the adjuvant ingredients. Pinelliae and Pericarpium Citri Reticulatae activate *qi* circulation, promote digestion, regulate stomach *qi* and suppress abnormally ascendant *qi*, Poria strengthens the spleen, eliminates dampness, regulates the middle *jiao* and relieves diarrhea, and Forsythiae purges heat and disperses stagnation—all serve as the assistant ingredients.

This is a mild prescription commonly used for various kinds of dyspepsia. Epigastric and abdominal distention, anorexia, acid regurgitation, thick tongue coating and smooth pulse are the clinical evidence calling for its application. For cases of severe abdominal distention, Fructus Aurantii Immaturus, Semen Arecae and Cortex Magnoliae Officinalis are added to strengthen the effects of promoting *qi* circulation and digestion. For cases with internal heat formed by retained food, yellow tongue coating and rapid pulse, Radix Scutellariae and Rhizoma Coptidis are added to eliminate heat and fire. For cases with constipation, Radix et Rhizoma Rhei and Semen Arecae are added to promote bowel movements. For cases associated with spleen deficiency, Rhizoma Atractylodis Macrocephalae is added to strengthen the spleen and replenish *qi*.

Pill of Aucklandiae and Arecae

木香槟榔丸 *mu xiang bing lang wan*

(from *Danxi's Experience on Medicine*)

Radix Aucklandiae	30 g
Semen Arecae	30 g

Pericarpium Citri Reticulatae Viride	30 g
Pericarpium Citri Reticulatae	30 g
Rhizoma Zedoariae	30 g
Fructus Aurantii	30 g
Radix Coptidis	30 g
Cortex Phellodendri	30 g
Radix et Rhizoma Rhei	15 g
Rhizoma Cyperi	60 g
Powder of Semen Pharbitidis	60 g

Administration: Grind the drugs together into fine powder, prepare the powder into pills, take 3-6 g with boiled water or ginger juice each time, twice daily; or prepare them into an oral decoction directly, with dosages reduced proportionally.

Action: Activating *qi* circulation, promoting digestion, eliminating stagnation and purging heat.

Indications: Stagnation syndrome with accumulated dampness that turns into heat, exhibiting epigastric and abdominal oppression, fullness and distensive pain, constipation, diarrhea with bloody or mucous stool, tenesmus, yellow and greasy tongue coating, and deep and forceful pulse.

Explanation: Stagnant food and dysfunctioning *qi* lead to epigastric and abdominal oppression, fullness and distensive pain. Dampness-heat and stagnant food in the interior block the intestinal *qi*, causing constipation, yellow and greasy tongue coating, and deep and forceful pulse. When dampness-heat affects the lower *jiao*, diarrhea with bloody and white mucous stools and tenesmus result. Hence, the treatment should seek to activate *qi* circulation, promote digestion, eliminate stagnation and purge heat. In the prescription, Aucklandiae and Arecae activate *qi* circulation, promote digestion, relieve abdominal distention and fullness; Aurantii relaxes the intestines and promotes the descent of *qi*; Cyperi, Zedoariae, Citri Reticulatae Viride and Citri Reticulatae help Aucklandiae and Arecae promote *qi* circulation and digestion; Zedoariae eliminates stagnation in the blood; Coptidis and Phellodendri dry dampness, purge heat and relieve diarrhea; Rhei and Pharbitidis remove stagnation, purge heat and promote bowel movements.

The clinical evidence calling for the application of this prescription is epigastric and abdominal distensive pain, constipation or diarrhea with bloody and white mucous stools, yellow and greasy tongue coating, and deep and forceful pulse.

This prescription has a potent action and is contraindicated for debilitated patients.

Pill for Invigorating the Spleen

健脾丸 *jian pi wan*

(from *Standards for Diagnosis and Treatment*)

Rhizoma Atractylodis Macrocephalae (fried)	75 g
Radix Aucklandiae	22 g

Rhizoma Coptidis (fried with wine)	22 g
Radix Glycyrrhizae	22 g
Poria	60 g
Radix Ginseng	45 g
Massa Fermentata Medicinalis (fried)	30 g
Pericarpium Citri Reticulatae	30 g
Fructus Amomi	30 g
Fructus Hordei Germinatus (fried)	30 g
Fructus Crataegi	30 g
Rhizoma Dioscoreae	30 g
Semen Myristicae	30 g

Administration: Grind the drugs into fine powder and prepare the powder as pills, take 6-9 g with boiled water each time, twice daily; or prepare them directly into an oral decoction, with dosages reduced proportionally.

Action: Invigorating the spleen, regulating stomach *qi*, promoting digestion and relieving diarrhea.

Indications: Hypofunction of the stomach and spleen due to stagnant food, manifested as anorexia, epigastric and abdominal fullness and distention, loose stools, yellowish and greasy tongue coating, and feeble and weak pulse.

Explanation: This prescription is indicated mainly for hypofunction of the spleen and stomach due to stagnant food which turns into heat. Gastric hypofunction affects the reception of food and splenic hypofunction disturbs the distribution of nutrients, resulting in anorexia and indigestion. Stagnant food in the middle *jiao* blocks the flow of *qi*, causing epigastric and abdominal distention and fullness. When the spleen fails in its transport function, dampness accumulates in the interior, affecting the ascent of lucid *yang* and resulting in the descent of turbid *yin*, thus loose stools appear. Yellow and greasy tongue coating indicates heat caused by food stagnation. Treatment aims at invigorating the spleen, regulating the stomach, promoting digestion, relieving diarrhea and purging heat. In the prescription, the ingredients of the Four Mild Drugs Decoction are used to invigorate *qi*, enforce the spleen and eliminate dampness; Crataegi, Massa Fermentata Medicinalis and Hordei Germinatus promote digestion and remove retained food; Aucklandiae Amomi and Pericarpium Citri Reticulatae regulate *qi* and the stomach and activate the spleen; Dioscoreae and Myristicae invigorate the spleen and relieve diarrhea; and Coptidis purges heat and dries dampness. All together strengthen the function of the spleen and promote digestion.

This is a common prescription for promoting digestion, invigorating the spleen and relieving diarrhea. Clinical evidence calling for its application includes epigastric and abdominal fullness and distention, anorexia, indigestion, yellowish and greasy tongue coating, and feeble and weak pulse. For cases without the symptoms of heat syndrome, Coptidis is removed, and Zingiberis Recens and Radix Aconiti Lateralis Preparata are added to warm the middle *jiao* and expel cold.

Pill of Aurantii Immaturus for Removing Abdominal Mass
枳实消痞丸 *zhi shi xiao pi wan*
(from *Secret Records of the Cabinet of Orchids*)

Rhizoma Zingiberis	3 g
Radix Glycyrrhizae Preparata	6 g
Massa Fermentata Fructus Hordei Germinatus	6 g
Poria	6 g
Rhizoma Atractylodis Macrocephalae	6 g
Massa Fermentata Rhizoma Pinelliae	9 g
Radix Ginseng	9 g
Cortex Magnoliae Officinalis (fried)	12 g
Fructus Aurantii Immaturus	15 g
Rhizoma Coptidis	15 g

Administration: Grind the drugs into fine powder and prepare the powder into pills, take 6-9 g with boiled water each time, twice daily; or prepare the drugs directly into an oral decoction, with dosages reduced proportionally.

Action: Relieving distention and fullness, invigorating the spleen and regulating the stomach.

Indications: *Qi* stagnation due to splenic hypofunction with retention of heat and cold, exhibiting epigastric fullness, anorexia, lassitude, or distention of the chest and abdomen, indigestion, and constipation.

Explanation: This prescription is indicated mainly for fullness and distention due to splenic and gastric hypofunction resulting from disturbance of the normal ascent and descent of *qi* and retention of cold and heat. The spleen controls the activity of the limbs, and its hypofunction may cause the stagnation of dampness and disorder of the middle *jiao*; this interferes with the distribution of *qi* to the limbs from the spleen and stomach, resulting in anorexia, indigestion and lassitude. Retained cold and heat, stagnant dampness and blocked *qi* lead to fullness and distention of the chest, epigastrium and abdomen, as well as constipation. Treatment seeks to relieve distention and fullness, invigorate the spleen, regulate the stomach and eliminate cold and heat. In the prescription, Aurantii Immaturus is used as the chief ingredient to activate *qi* and relieve distention and fullness, and Magnoliae Officinalis is used as the adjuvant to make *qi* descend, relieve fullness and strengthen the effects of the chief ingredient. Coptidis is used to purge heat and dry dampness, Massa Fermentata Rhizoma Pinelliae eliminates stagnation, regulates the stomach and suppresses the adversely ascendant *qi*; and Zingiberis warms the middle *jiao* and expels cold. These three enhance the ability of the chief and adjuvant ingredients to relieve stagnation. Ginseng invigorates *qi* and the spleen; Atractylodis Macrocephalae and Poria invigorate the spleen and eliminate dampness; Hordei Germinatus strengthens and regulates the stomach. Together, they serve as the assistant ingredients. Glycyrrhizae, which regulates the middle *jiao* and invigorates the spleen, serves as the guiding ingredient to coordinate the effects of the other drugs. The combination of these drugs produces both dispersive and tonic effects, and removes both cold and heat; it disperses stagnation without damaging the antipathogenic *qi*, and invigorates the antipathogenic *qi* without causing a retention of the pathogens.

This prescription is based on Decoction of Pinelliae for Purging Stomach-Fire and Four Mild Drugs Decoction. Although it is a prescription with both dispersive and tonic effects, it mainly activates *qi* circulation and relieves fullness and distention. It is therefore clinically appropriate for cases of splenic hypofunction and *qi* stagnation, in which the symptoms of heat and excess syndromes are predominant.

This prescription and Pill for Invigorating the Spleen both serve as therapy to disperse and invigorate. But the latter has a stronger tonic effect, and it is more effective in invigorating the spleen and promoting digestion, while the former has a stronger dispersive effect, and is more effective in activating *qi* circulation and dispersing stagnation.

Summary

Included in this chapter are four prescriptions, which are divided into two sub-categories.

(1) Prescriptions for promoting digestion:

They include Pill for Promoting Digestion, Pill of Aucklandiae and Arecae and Pill for Invigorating the Spleen. The first two are especially effective for dyspepsia when the antipathogenic *qi* is not injured. But Pill for Promoting Digestion is usually used to treat mild cases of dyspepsia, while Pill of Aucklandiae and Arecae is for dyspepsia with accumulated dampness resulting in the production of heat. Pill for Invigorating the Spleen is usually used for cases of dyspepsia due to splenic hypofunction.

(2) Prescription for dispersing stagnation:

Pill of Aurantii Immaturus for Removing Abdominal Mass is the only example cited. It activates *qi* circulation, disperses stagnation, invigorates the spleen and regulates the stomach, and is indicated for cases of epigastric fullness and anorexia due to *qi* stagnation, splenic hypofunction and retained cold and heat.

CHAPTER EIGHTEEN

PRESCRIPTIONS FOR EXPELLING DAMPNESS

Prescriptions for expelling dampness (*qu shi ji*) are mainly composed of drugs that remove dampness from the body, and have the effects of eliminating dampness, promoting diuresis, relieving stranguria and discharging turbidity.

As the pathogenic agent, dampness may be exogenous or endogenous in origin. An exogenous dampness syndrome means attack by exogenous dampness that usually results from prolonged living in a damp environment, drenching by rain or wading across water. The syndrome chiefly involves the body surface and the meridians. An endogenous dampness syndrome usually results from indulgence in raw or cold food and in alcohol, leading to splenic hypofunction, and often involving the *zang-fu* organs. But the surface and the *zang-fu* organs are interrelated, and so dampness in the surface may go inside to affect the *zang-fu* organs and dampness in the interior go to the surface. Therefore, exogenous and endogenous dampness syndromes may appear simultaneously. In addition, because of constitutional differences, the complication of pathogenic factors, the locations of the diseases, the vacillation between heat and cold, and the difference between deficiency and excess syndromes, therapy to expel dampness is rather complicated. In general, dampness affecting the surface and the upper part of the body should be expelled by mild diaphoretics; that affecting the interior and the lower part, by fragrant, bitter and dry drugs, or by sweet and bland drugs in order to promote diuresis; dampness that produces cold should be treated by warming *yang* to eliminate dampness, while that producing heat, by purging heat to eliminate dampness. For severe dampness in debilitated patients, therapies that expel dampness and invigorate healthy *qi* should be employed simultaneously. According to the therapeutic principle and their actions, these prescriptions are classified into the following sub-categories.

(1) Prescriptions for drying dampness and regulating the stomach:

Prescriptions for drying dampness and regulating the stomach (*zao shi he wei ji*) are indicated for cases with stagnant dampness and turbidity involving the spleen and stomach, manifested as epigastric and abdominal fullness and distention, eructation, acid regurgitation, vomiting, diarrhea, anorexia and lassitude. Bitter and warm drugs that dry dampness and fragrant drugs that disperse dampness are usually used, such as Rhizoma Atractylodis, Pericarpium Citri Reticulatae, Herba Agastaches and Fructus Amomi Rotundus; they are supplemented by drugs that regulate *qi* and relieve the exterior syndrome. Examples: Powder for Regulating the Function of the Stomach and Powder of Agastaches for Restoring Antipathogenic *Qi*.

(2) Prescriptions for purging heat and dampness:

Prescriptions for purging heat and dampness (*qing re qu shi ji*) are indicated for cases of retained dampness-heat in the interior or attack of the lower *jiao* by dampness-heat, manifested as dampness-warm disease, jaundice and heat-type stranguria. Such prescriptions are chiefly composed of drugs that purge heat and dampness, such as Semen Coicis, Fructus Gardeniae and Talcum, supplemented by fragrant drugs that disperse dampness, drugs that purge fire and promote bowel movements and drugs that promote diuresis and relieve stranguria. Examples: Decoction of Artemisiae Scopariae, Three Seeds Decoction and Powder for Dispersing Heat and Promoting Urination.

(3) Prescriptions for promoting diuresis and eliminating dampness:

Prescriptions for promoting diuresis and eliminating dampness (*li shui shen shi ji*) are indicated for cases of accumulated fluid and dampness in the body, exhibiting dysuria, stranguria with turbid urine, edema and diarrhea. Such prescriptions are mainly composed of drugs that promote diuresis and eliminate dampness, such as Poria, Rhizoma Alismatis and Polyporus Umbellatus, in combination with drugs that invigorate *qi* and the spleen, warm *yang* and regulate *qi*. Examples: Powder of Five Drugs Containing Poria and Powder Containing Five Kinds of Peel.

(4) Prescriptions for warming and dispersing dampness:

Prescriptions for warming and dispersing dampness (*wen hua shui shi ji*) are indicated for dampness syndrome along with production of cold and failure of *yang* to eliminate water, manifested as edema, discharge of whitish and turbid urine and stranguria with chyluria. They are chiefly composed of drugs that warm *yang* and diuretics, such as Radix Aconiti Lateralis Preparata, Rhizoma Zingiberis, Poria and Rhizoma Atractylodis Macrocephalae. Examples: *Zhenwu* Decoction, Powder for Invigorating the Spleen and Decoction of Dioscoreae Septemlobae for Clearing Turbid Urine.

(5) Prescriptions for expelling wind and eliminating dampness:

Prescriptions for expelling wind and eliminating dampness (*qu feng sheng shi ji*) are indicated for cases in which wind-cold-dampness affect the body surface, manifested as headache and general achiness; or cases in which wind-cold-dampness affects the tendons and knees, manifested as numbness and pain of the lumbus and knees. Such prescriptions are chiefly composed of drugs that expel wind and cold, such as Rhizoma seu Radix Notopterygii, Radix Angelicae Pubescentis, Radix Ledebouriellae and Radix Gentianae Macrophyllae, in combination with drugs that invigorate the blood, activate blood circulation, invigorate *qi* and the spleen, kidney and liver. Examples: Decoction of Notopterygii for Eliminating Dampness and Decoction of Angelicae Pubescentis and Taxilli.

Water and dampness fall into the same category of pathogenic factors. In the human body, the kidney controls water metabolism, the spleen inhibits the accumulation of water, and the lung regulates water distribution. Hence, diseases due to affection of water and dampness are closely related to the functions of these organs. Splenic dysfunction may lead to the generation of dampness, renal dysfunction may cause edema, and pulmonary dysfunction may affect water distribution. Therefore, the treatment should be based on both the disorders of the relevant *zang-fu* organs and the differentiation of syndromes. In addition, the triple *jiao* and the urinary bladder are also related to affection by water and dampness; hence their normal functioning is also important for the elimination of accumulated water and dampness. Furthermore, dampness is heavy, turbid and viscous, and is likely to affect the functional activity of *qi*; in prescriptions that eliminate dampness, drugs for regulating *qi* should therefore be added.

Prescriptions for eliminating dampness are usually composed of drugs that are acrid and fragrant, and warm and dry, or else drugs that are sweet and bland with diuretic effect. Since these drugs are liable to consume *yin* fluid, they should be used with caution for patients with constitutional *yin*-fluid deficiency, patients debilitated after a long illness, and pregnant women.

Powder for Regulating Stomach Function

平胃散 *ping wei san*

(from *Benevolent Prescriptions from the Pharmaceutical Bureau of the Taiping Period*)

Rhizoma Atractylodis	2,500 g
Cortex Magnoliae Officinalis (fried with ginger juice)	1,560 g
Pericarpium Citri Reticulatae	1,560 g
Radix Glycyrrhizae Preparata	900 g

Administration: Grind the drugs into fine powder and take 6-9 g each time with ginger and date decoction; or prepare them directly into an oral decoction, with dosages reduced proportionally.

Action: Drying dampness, strengthening the spleen, invigorating *qi* flow and regulating the stomach.

Indications: Cases of stagnant dampness in the spleen and stomach, exhibiting epigastric and abdominal distention and fullness, anorexia, tastelessness, vomiting, nausea, eructation, acid regurgitation, heaviness in the body, fatigue, loose stools, white and thick greasy tongue coating, and slow pulse.

Explanation: The spleen is responsible for the transportation and transformation of nutrients and fluid; it prefers dryness and is averse to dampness. Retained dampness in the spleen and stomach may lead to visceral dysfunction, causing anorexia and loose stools. Stagnant dampness and *qi* give rise to epigastric and abdominal distention and fullness. Gastric dysfunction results in vomiting, nausea, eructation and acid regurgitation. An affection of dampness on the limbs may cause heaviness and lassitude. White and greasy tongue coating and slow pulse are indications of retained dampness. The therapeutic principle should be to dry dampness, strengthen splenic function, promote *qi* circulation and regulate the stomach. In the prescription, Atractylodis, bitter, warm and dryness, is used as the chief ingredient to eliminate dampness and strengthen splenic function. Magnoliae Officinalis serves as the adjuvant ingredient to promote *qi* circulation and eliminate dampness to relieve distention and fullness. Pericarpium Citri Reticulatae, as the assistant, regulates *qi* and relieves stagnation. Glycyrrhizae, which is sweet, regulates the middle *jiao* and coordinates the effects of the other drugs. Zingiberis Recens and Jujubae are applied to regulate splenic and gastric function. All together eliminate dampness, normalize *qi* activity and restore splenic and gastric function, so that all the symptoms subside.

This is a prescription frequently used to dry dampness, strengthen splenic function, invigorate *qi* circulation and regulate the stomach. Clinical evidence calling for its application includes epigastric and abdominal distention and fullness, and white, thick and greasy tongue coating. For cases of anorexia and indigestion, Massa Fermentata Medicinalis and Fructus Hordei Germinatus are added to promote digestion; for cases of dampness-heat, Rhizoma Coptidis and Radix Scutellariae are added to purge heat and dry dampness; and for cases of cold-dampness, Rhizoma Zingiberis and Cortex Cinnamomi are added to warm and relieve cold-dampness.

Powder of Agastaches for Restoring Antipathogenic *Qi*
藿香正气散 *huo xiang zheng qi san*
(from *Benevolent Prescriptions from the Pharmaceutical Bureau of the Taiping Period*)

Herba Agastaches	90 g
Pericarpium Arecae	30 g
Radix Angelicae Dahuricae	30 g
Folium Perillae	30 g
Poria	30 g
Massa Fermentata Rhizoma Pinelliae	60 g
Rhizoma Atractylodis Macrocephalae	60 g
Pericarpium Citri Reticulatae	60 g
Radix Platycodi	60 g
Cortex Magnoliae Officinalis (prepared with ginger juice)	60 g
Radix Glycyrrhizae Preparata	75 g

Administration: Grind the drugs into fine powder, take 3-9 g with ginger and date decoction; or prepare the powder into pills and take 3-9 g with warm water; or directly prepare them into an oral decoction, with dosages reduced proportionally.

Action: Relieving exterior syndrome, eliminating dampness, and regulating *qi* and the middle *jiao*.

Indications: Cases of affection by exogenous wind and cold, and stagnant dampness in the interior, exhibiting fever, chills, headache, chest upset, epigastric and abdominal pain, vomiting, nausea, increased borborygmus, diarrhea, and white and greasy tongue coating.

Explanation: Affection by wind-cold depresses the activity of *wei-yang* and leads to chills, fever and headache. Stagnant dampness in the interior disrupts the function of *qi* and causes chest upset and pain in the epigastrium and abdomen. Stagnant dampness in the gastrointestinal tract leads to nausea, vomiting, increased borborygmus and diarrhea. White and greasy tongue coating is an indication of retained dampness. The principle of treatment should be to expel wind-cold from the surface, eliminate internal dampness and regulate the middle *jiao* and *qi*. In the prescription, Agastaches is used in a larger dosage and acts as the chief ingredient to expel wind-cold, eliminate dampness, regulate the stomach and relieve vomiting. Perillae and Angelicae Dahuricae, acrid and fragrant, help the chief ingredient eliminate wind-cold and dampness, Massa Fermentata Pinelliae and Pericarpium Citri Reticulatae dry dampness, regulate the stomach, suppress the adversely ascendant *qi* and relieve vomiting, Atractylodis Macrocephalae and Poria strengthen the spleen to eliminate dampness, regulate the middle *jiao* and relieve diarrhea, Magnoliae Officinalis and Pericarpium Arecae activate *qi* circulation to disperse dampness and ease the middle *jiao* so as to relieve fullness, and Platycodi releases stagnant lung *qi*—all serve as the adjuvant ingredients. Zingiberis Recens, Jujubae and Glycyrrhizae regulate splenic and gastric function, and serve as the assistant and guide ingredients. All together eliminate wind-cold, disperse dampness, normalize *qi* activity and restore splenic and gastric function.

This prescription is appropriate for common cold in all seasons, especially cases due to affection by cold and dampness, and splenic and gastric disorders in summer.

Decoction of Artemisiae Scopariae
茵陈蒿汤 *yin chen hao tang*
(from *Treatise on Cold Diseases*)

Herba Artemisiae Scopariae	18 g
Fructus Gardeniae	12 g
Radix et Rhizoma Rhei	6 g

Administration: Decoct with water for oral administration.

Action: Eliminating heat, promoting diuresis to eliminate dampness and relieving jaundice.

Indications: Jaundice of dampness-heat type, manifested as bright yellowish color of the eyes and skin, slight fullness sensation in the abdomen, thirst, dysuria, yellow and greasy tongue coating, and deep and forceful or smooth and rapid pulse.

Explanation: This prescription is indicated for cases of jaundice due to the accumulation of dampness-heat in the interior. Stagnant dampness-heat leads to general jaundice. Internal accumulated dampness-heat disrupts *qi* activity, causing dysuria, abdominal fullness, thirst, yellow and greasy tongue coating, and smooth and rapid pulse. The treatment should be to eliminate heat and dampness and relieve jaundice. In the prescription, Artemisiae Scopariae is a special agent for relieving jaundice, and is used in a larger dosage as the chief ingredient to eliminate heat and dampness. Gardeniae serves as the adjuvant ingredient to purge dampness-heat from the triple *jiao* through urination. Rhei is applied as the assistant ingredient to purge accumulated heat and promote bowel movements. The three drugs together eliminate dampness-heat through urination and defecation, thus relieving jaundice.

In traditional Chinese medicine, jaundice is further classified into *yin* jaundice and *yang* jaundice. This prescription is indicated for jaundice of dampness-heat type, which is attributed to the latter. Clinical evidence calling for its application includes bright yellowish color of the eyes and skin, dysuria, and yellow and greasy tongue coating.

Appendant Prescription

Decoction of Ephedrae, Forsythiae and Phaseoli
麻黄连翘赤小豆汤 *ma huang lian qiao chi xiao dou tang*
(from *Treatise on Cold Diseases*)

It is composed of 6 g of Herba Ephedrae, 6 g of Radix Forsythiae, 9 g of Semen Armeniacae Amarum, 24 g of Semen Phaseoli, 3 pieces of Fructus Jujubae, 6 g of Cortex Catalpae Ovatae Radicis, 6 g of Rhizoma Zingiberis Recens, and 6 g of Radix Glycyrrhizae Preparata. It relieves exterior syndrome, induces sweating, purges heat and dampness, and is indicated for cases of jaundice due to stagnant dampness-heat in the interior when the exterior syndrome has not yet relieved.

This prescription and Decoction of Artemisiae Scopariae are both used for jaundice of dampness-heat type. But, the former is applied to cases due to stagnant dampness-heat in the interior complicated by exterior syndrome, while the latter is better for cases with predominance of both dampness and heat.

Three Seeds Decoction
三仁汤 *san ren tang*
(from *Essentials of Seasonal Febrile Diseases*)

Semen Armeniacae Amarum	15 g
Talcum	18 g
Medulla Tetrapanacis	6 g
Fructus Amomi Rotundus	6 g
Herba Lophatheri	6 g
Cortex Magnoliae Officinalis	6 g
Semen Coicis	18 g
Rhizoma Pinelliae	15 g

Administration: Decoct with water for oral administration.

Action: Activating *qi* circulation, purging heat and eliminating dampness.

Indications: The initial stage of dampness-warm syndrome with affection of *qifen* by summer-heat and dampness, manifested as headache, chills, general achiness, yellowish complexion, chest upset, afternoon fever, absence of thirst, white tongue, and taut, thready, soft and superficial pulse.

Explanation: This is a prescription frequently used for the initial stage of dampness-warm syndrome, with the pathogens attacking *qifen* and dampness predominant over heat. Although headache, chills and general achiness appear as an exterior syndrome of exogenous febrile diseases, the presence of taut, thready, soft and superficial pulse indicates that the *wei qi* and *yang qi* are retrained by dampness. Stagnant dampness in the muscles causes general achiness. Dampness is considered a *yin* pathogen and when it is restrained by accumulated heat, afternoon fever occurs. When *qi* activity is disturbed by dampness, chest upset and poor appetite result. Finally, white tongue, absence of thirst and yellowish complexion are indications of stagnant dampness. Therefore, if only bitter and acrid, and dry and warm drugs are used to eliminate dampness, heat will become predominant, and if only bitter and cold drugs are used to purge heat, dampness will persist. Fragrant, bitter and acrid drugs that activate *qi* and possess the diuretic effect are therefore recommended. In the prescription, Semen Armeniacae Amarum, which is bitter and acrid, releases lung *qi* to disperse dampness; Amomi Rotundus, which is fragrant, disperses dampness, activates *qi* and soothes the chest; Coicis, acrid and bland, eliminates dampness-heat by promoting diuresis; Pinelliae and Magnoliae Officinalis promote *qi* flow, eliminate dampness and relieve distention and fullness and also help Armeniacae Amarum and Amomi Rotundus remove obstructions in the upper and middle *jiao*; and Talcum, Medulla Tetrapanacis and Herba Lophatheri enhance the effects of Coicis. These drugs, when used together, eliminate dampness-heat by releasing the upper *jiao*, soothe the middle *jiao* and promote diuresis from the lower *jiao*.

Appendant Prescription

Decoction of Agastaches, Magnoliae Officinalis, Pinelliae and Poria

藿朴夏苓汤 *huo pu xia ling tang*

(from *Causative Treatment of Diseases*)

It is composed of 6 g of Herba Agastaches, 4.5 g of Rhizoma Pinelliae, 9 g of Poria Rubra, 9 g of Semen Armeniacae Amarum, 12 g of Semen Coicis, 2 g of Fructus Amomi Rotundus, 4.5 g of Polyporus Umbellatus, 9 g of Semen Sojae Preparatum, 4.5 g of Rhizoma Alismatis, and 3 g of Cortex Magnoliae Officinalis. To be prepared as an oral decoction, it relieves the exterior syndrome and eliminates dampness, and is indicated for the initial stage of dampness-heat syndrome, exhibiting fever, chills, lassitude, chest upset, greasy feeling in the mouth, white and thin tongue coating, and soft, superficial and slow pulse.

This prescription and Three Seeds Decoction are both applicable to dampness-warm syndrome. But the former not only eliminates dampness but also relieves exterior syndrome, and is indicated for the initial stage of dampness-warm syndrome with predominant exterior syndrome; the latter purges dampness and heat, and is good for the initial stage of dampness-warm syndrome with more dampness than heat.

Sweet Dew Pill for Detoxification
甘露消毒丹 *gan lu xiao du dan*
(from *Compendium of Seasonal Febrile Diseases*)

Talcum	450 g
Herba Artemisiae Scopariae	330 g
Radix Scutellariae	300 g
Rhizome Acori Graminei	180 g
Bulbus Fritillariae Cirrhosae	150 g
Caulis Akebiae	150 g
Herba Agastaches	120 g
Rhizoma Belamcandae	120 g
Fructus Forsythiae	120 g
Herba Menthae	120 g
Fructus Amomi Rotundus	120 g

Administration: Grind the drugs into fine powder, take 9 g of the powder each time, or prepare it with Massa Fermentata Medicinalis as pills, take 9 g for one dose; or prepare the drugs directly as an oral decoction, with dosages reduced proportionally.

Action: Eliminating heat and dampness, dispersing turbidity and eliminating toxins.

Indications: Dampness-warm syndrome involving *qifen*, exhibiting fever, lassitude, chest upset, abdominal distention, sore limbs, swelling of the throat and lower cheek, yellow skin, thirst, scanty urine, vomiting, diarrhea, stranguria with turbid urine, whitish, or thick and greasy, or dry and yellowish tongue coating.

Explanation: This prescription is indicated for dampness-warm syndrome with predominant dampness and heat and the involvement of *qifen*. The simultaneous attack by dampness and heat leads to fever, fatigue and sore limbs. A disturbance of lucid *yang* and *qi* by dampness causes chest upset, abdominal fullness and even vomiting and diarrhea. When noxious heat attacks upward, swelling and pain of the throat and cheek occur. When heat is retained in the interior by dampness, a yellowish color of the skin results. Finally, scanty dark urine and yellowish greasy tongue coating are indications of stagnant dampness-heat in the interior. The principle of treatment is to purge heat and dampness, disperse turbidity and eliminate toxins. In the prescription, Talcum purges heat and dampness to relieve summer-heat syndrome; Artemisiae Scopariae and Caulis Akebiae produce the same result through promoting urination; Scutellariae purges heat and dries dampness; Forsythiae purges heat and toxins; Fritillariae Cirrhosae and Belamcandae ease the throat and relieve stagnation; and Acori Graminei, Amomi Rotundus, Agastaches and Menthae are all fragrant and applied to disperse turbidity, activate the spleen and *qi* circulation.

This is a prescription often used in summer for dampness-warm syndrome and summer-heat syndrome, whenever both dampness and heat are predominant and the *qifen* is involved. Clinical evidence calling for its application includes fever, fatigue, thirst, reddish urine, whitish thick and greasy or dry and yellowish tongue coating.

Powder for Dispersing Heat and Promoting Urination

八正散 *ba zheng san*

(from *Benevolent Prescriptions from the Pharmaceutical Bureau of the Taiping Period*)

Semen Plantaginis	500 g
Herba Dianthi	500 g
Herba Polygoni Avicularis	500 g
Talcum	500 g
Fructus Gardeniae	500 g
Radix Glycyrrhizae Preparata	500 g
Caulis Akebiae	500 g
Radix et Rhizoma Rhei Preparata	500 g

Administration: Grind the drugs into fine powder, decoct 9 g of the powder together with 2 g of Medulla Junci in water and take the decoction at bedtime; or directly prepare the drugs as an oral decoction, with dosages reduced proportionally.

Action: Eliminating heat and fire, promoting diuresis and relieving stranguria.

Indications: Stranguria of the heat type due to a downward attack by dampness-heat, exhibiting frequent and painful micturition, dripping discharge of urine, or even retention of urine, lower abdominal fullness, dry mouth and throat, red tongue with yellow coating, and rapid pulse.

Explanation: This prescription is mainly indicated for cases due to the downward attack by dampness and heat on the urinary bladder. Dampness-heat retained in the bladder blocks the water passage, causing frequent, difficult and painful micturition, dripping discharge or even urine retention, along with fullness in the lower abdomen. An internal accumulation of heat causes dry mouth and throat, yellow tongue coating and rapid pulse. These cases should be treated by purging heat and relieving stranguria. In the prescription, Akebiae, Talcum, Plantaginis, Dianthi and Polygoni Avicularis are effective in promoting diuresis to relieve stranguria, and they are used for purging dampness-heat. Gardeniae eliminates dampness-heat from the triple *jiao*; Rhei eliminates heat and purges fire; and Medulla Junci guides heat downward. Glycyrrhizae coordinates the effects of the other drugs and relieves the urgency in micturition.

This is a prescription often used to treat heat-type stranguria manifested along with excess-heat syndrome. For cases of stranguria complicated by hematuria, Herba Cephalanoploris and Rhizoma Imperatae are added to cool the blood and arrest bleeding; for stranguria caused by urinary stones, Herba Lysimachiae and Spora Lygodii are added to remove the stones and relieve stranguria.

This prescription is composed of bitter and cold drugs and possesses the diuretic effect. It is appropriate for cases due to excess fire. For chronic cases, debilitated patients and pregnant women, it should be used with caution.

Powder of Five Drugs Containing Poria
五苓散 *wu ling san*
(from *Treatise on Cold Diseases*)

Polyporus Umbellatus	9 g
Rhizoma Alismatis	15 g
Rhizoma Atractylodis Macrocephalae	9 g
Poria	9 g
Ramulus Cinnamomi	10 g

Administration: Decoct with water for oral administration.

Action: Promoting diuresis, eliminating dampness, warming *yang* and activating *qi* flow.

Indications: (1) Exterior syndrome with water and dampness retained in the interior, exhibiting headache, fever, thirst with a desire to drink, or vomiting upon drinking, dysuria, white tongue coating, and superficial pulse. (2) Internal retention of water and dampness, manifested as edema, diarrhea, dysuria and vomiting. (3) Phlegm-fluid retention syndrome, exhibiting throbbing in the lower abdomen, salivation, dizziness, shortness of breath and cough.

Explanation: This prescription is designed for the simultaneous occurrence of a Taiyang Meridian disease and a Taiyang *fu* organ disease. When the Taiyang exterior syndrome is not yet relieved and the urinary bladder (Taiyang *fu* organ) is affected, it causes bladder dysfunction and fluid retention in the lower *jiao*. The attack by the exogenous pathogens on the body surface leads to fever, headache and superficial pulse. Bladder dysfunction causes difficulty in urination and fluid retention. Fluid retained in the lower *jiao* disrupts fluid distribution, resulting in thirst with a desire to drink; when retained in the interior, it causes vomiting upon drinking. These cases should be treated by promoting diuresis, activating *qi* circulation and relieving exterior syndrome. In the prescription, Alismatis, sweet, bland and cold, directly acts upon the bladder, and so is used as the chief ingredient to promote diuresis and eliminate dampness. Poria and Polyporus Umbellatus, both bland, are used as the adjuvant ingredients to strengthen the effect of promoting diuresis. Atractylodis Macrocephalae, which invigorates the spleen and eliminates dampness, and Ramulus Cinnamomi, which relieves Taiyang exterior syndrome and restores bladder function, are used as assistant ingredients. In addition, this prescription can also be used to treat cases of edema, diarrhea, vomiting and phlegm-fluid retention due to splenic dysfunction and an overflow of fluid and dampness.

Powder Containing Five Kinds of Peel
五皮散 *wu pi san*
(from *Hua's Treasured Classics*)

Cortex Zingiberis Recens	9 g

Cortex Mori Radicis	9 g
Pericarpium Citri Reticulatae	9 g
Pericarpium Arecae	9 g
Poria	9 g

Administration: Decoct with water for oral administration.

Action: Promoting diuresis to reduce edema, regulating *qi* and strengthening the spleen.

Indications: Edema due to spleen deficiency and accumulated dampness, exhibiting anasarca, heaviness of the limbs, fullness in the chest and abdomen, shortness of breath, dysuria, and edema during pregnancy.

Explanation: Accumulated dampness caused by splenic hypofunction gives rise to anasarca and heaviness of the limbs. Disturbance of *qi* activity by dampness leads to fullness in the chest and abdomen, and the abnormal flow of *qi* to the lung causes shortness of breath. Accumulated dampness obstructing the passage of water results in dysuria. Treatment aims at invigorating the spleen, regulating *qi*, eliminating dampness and relieving edema. In the prescription, Poria promotes diuresis, eliminates dampness and invigorates the spleen; Pericarpium Arecae relieves fluid retention with its acrid flavor; Cortex Mori Radicis suppresses the adverse flow of lung *qi* and clears the water passage; Pericarpium Arecae makes adversely ascendant *qi* downward and promotes diuresis to relieve distention and fullness; and Pericarpium Citri Reticulatae regulates *qi* and the middle *jiao*, activates the spleen *qi* and eliminates dampness. The combination of the five drugs invigorates the spleen, regulates *qi*, eliminates dampness and relieves edema.

A prescription of the same name is recorded in *A Complete Book of Measles*, in which Mori Radicis and Citri Reticulatae are removed and Cortex Acanthopanacis Radicis is added. Since Acanthopanacis Radicis is warm, the prescription can, in addition to invigorating the spleen, regulating *qi*, eliminating dampness and relieving edema, dredge the meridians to eliminate wind-dampness.

Another prescription of the same name is recorded in *Benevolent Prescriptions from the Pharmaceutical Bureau of the Taiping Period*; in it Mori Radicis and Citri Reticulatae are removed and Cortex Acanthopanacis Radicis and Cortex Lycii Radicis are added. It has the same effects as the prescription recorded in *Hua's Treasured Classics*, but has a weaker effect to activate *qi*.

Decoction of Stephaniae Tetrandrae and Astragali

防己黄芪汤 *fang ji huang qi tang*

(from *Synopsis of the Golden Cabinet*)

Radix Stephaniae Tetrandrae	12 g
Radix Astragali	15 g
Rhizoma Atractylodis Macrocephalae	9 g
Radix Glycyrrhizae	6 g

Administration: Decoct the drugs together with an appropriate amount of Rhizoma Zingiberis Recens and Fructus Jujubae for oral administration.

Action: Supplementing *qi*, expelling wind, invigorating the spleen and promoting diuresis.

Indications: Edema caused by wind or wind-dampness marked by sweating, chills, a feeling of heaviness, dysuria, pale tongue with white coating, and superficial pulse.

Explanation: This prescription is indicated for cases due to deficient antipathogenic *qi*, weak *wei qi*, and an attack by wind with fluid retention in the body. Exterior deficiency leads to sweating and chills, fluid retention on the surface heaviness in the body, and fluid retention in the interior gives rise to dysuria. A superficial pulse indicates exterior syndrome. The principle of treatment is to invigorate *qi*, strengthen the surface, expel wind and promote diuresis. In the prescription, Stephaniae Tetrandrae expels wind and promotes diuresis; Astragali invigorates *qi*, strengthens the surface and also promotes diuresis to relieve edema; both serve as the chief ingredients. Atractylodis Macrocephalae supplements *qi* and invigorates the spleen, and serves as the adjuvant ingredient to enhance *wei qi* and strengthen the effect of Astragali. Glycyrrhizae reinforces the spleen, regulates the middle *jiao* and coordinates the effects of the other drugs; Zingiberis Recens and Jujubae regulate *ying qi* and *wei qi*—these serve as the guiding ingredients. These six drugs together strengthen the surface, expel wind, normalize splenic function and distribute body fluid freely.

Zhenwu Decoction

真武汤 *zhen wu tang*

(from *Treatise on Cold Diseases*)

Poria	9 g
Radix Paeoniae Lactiflorae	9 g
Rhizoma Atractylodis Macrocephalae	6 g
Rhizoma Zingiberis Recens	9 g
Radix Aconiti Lateralis Preparata	9 g

Administration: Decoct with water for oral administration.

Action: Warming *yang* and promoting diuresis.

Indications: (1) Retention of fluid in the interior due to deficient spleen and kidney *yang*, exhibiting dysuria, heaviness and pain in the limbs, abdominal pain, diarrhea, or edema in the limbs, absence of thirst, white tongue coating and deep pulse. (2) Taiyang disease characterized by sweating, fever, palpitation, dizziness and muscular twitching.

Explanation: This prescription is indicated for cases of dysuria and fluid accumulation due to deficient kidney *yang* with a disorder in *qi* and fluid circulation as well as deficient spleen *yang* with a failure in fluid transportation. If the fluid accumulates in the skin and muscles, heaviness and pain in the limbs and even edema occur; if it flows downward, diarrhea and loose stools result; if it attacks upward, cough and vomiting occur. When lucid *yang* fails to go up, there will be dizziness, and palpitation follows if the heart is affected. In case of Taiyang disease, excessive sweating may consume *yang qi* and lead to failure in warming the meridians, causing severe muscular twitching. The principle of treatment should be warming kidney *yang* to improve the functional activity of *qi*, and opening the water passage to eliminate accumulated fluid. In the prescription, Aconiti Lateralis Preparata, strongly acrid and hot, serves as the chief ingredient to warm and strengthen kidney *yang*, activate *qi* circulation and promote diuresis. Atractylodis Macrocephalae invigorates the spleen and eliminates dampness, and Poria promotes diuresis and regulates water passage to eliminate water dampness through urination—both serve as the adjuvant ingredients. Zingiberis Recens, which is acrid and warm, helps Aconiti Lateralis Preparata warm *yang* and expel cold, and helps Poria and Atractylodis Macrocephalae eliminate fluid, Paeoniae Lactiflorae not only induces diuresis, relieves abdominal spasm and pain, astringes *yin* and regulates *ying*, but also counteracts the *yin*-consuming effect of Zingiberis Recens and Aconiti Lateralis Preparata—both serve as the assistant ingredients.

Powder for Invigorating the Spleen
实脾散 *shi pi san*
(from *Revised Edition of Yan's Prescriptions for Life Saving*)

Cortex Magnoliae Officinalis (fried with ginger juice)	6 g
Rhizoma Atractylodis Macrocephalae	6 g
Fructus Chaenomelis	6 g
Radix Aucklandiae	6 g
Fructus Tsaoko	6 g
Fructus Arecae	6 g
Radix Aconiti Lateralis Preparata	6 g
Poria	6 g
Rhizoma Zingiberis	6 g
Radix Glycyrrhizae Preparata	3 g

Administration: Decoct the drugs together with five pieces of ginger and one date for oral administration.

Action: Warming *yang*, invigorating the spleen, activating *qi* circulation and promoting diuresis.

Indications: Edema due to *yang* deficiency, exhibiting predominant edema in the lower part of the body, cold limbs, absence of thirst, fullness in the chest and abdomen, loose stools, thick greasy tongue coating, and deep and slow pulse.

Explanation: This prescription is indicated for *yin*-type edema caused by the failure of deficient spleen and kidney *yang* to eliminate water. Water is considered as a *yin* pathogen, and tends to go downward; edema is thus more serious in the lower part of the body. The spleen controls the limbs; if *yang qi* fails to warm them, cold hands and feet result. Retained water and dampness disrupt *qi* activity, causing distention and fullness in the chest and abdomen. Absence of thirst, loose stools, thick greasy tongue coating and deep and slow pulse all indicate predominant dampness. These cases should be treated by warming *yang*, invigorating the spleen, activating *qi* circulation and promoting diuresis. In the prescription, Aconiti Lateralis Preparata and Zingiberis act as the chief ingredients to warm and nourish the spleen and stomach, enforce *yang* and suppress *yin*. Poria and Atractylodis Macrocephalae invigorate the spleen, dry dampness and promote diuresis, Chaenomelis promotes diuresis and eliminates dampness by means of inducing urination, and Magnoliae Officinalis, Aucklandiae, Arecae and Tsaoko guide *qi* downward, relieve stagnation, eliminate dampness and promote diuresis—they all act as the adjuvant ingredients. Glycyrrhizae, Zingiberis and Jujubae, as the guiding ingredients, regulate the effects of the other drugs and benefit the spleen and regulate the middle *jiao*.

This is an important prescription for *yin*-type edema, especially for patients with fluid accumulation and *qi* stagnation. Clinical evidence calling for its application includes severe edema in the lower part of the body, abdominal distention, anorexia, oliguria, loose stools, pale tongue with greasy coating, and deep and slow pulse.

Decoction of Dioscoreae Septemlobae for Clearing Turbid Urine
萆薢分清饮 *bi xie fen qing yin*
(from *Danxi's Experience on Medicine*)

Fructus Alpiniae Oxyphyllae	10 g
Rhizoma Dioscoreae Septemlobae	10 g
Rhizoma Acori Graminei	10 g
Radix Linderae	10 g

Administration: Decoct the drugs with water and take the decoction warm by adding a small amount of salt.

Action: Warming the kidney, eliminating dampness and separating the clear from the turbid.

Indications: Stranguria with discharge of white turbid urine, manifested as frequent micturition, discharge of white, thick and viscous urine resembling rice water.

Explanation: This prescription is indicated for cases due to deficient kidney *yang* and the downward attack by dampness-turbidity. Kidney deficiency may lead to failure to control body fluid, thus giving rise to frequent micturition. Insufficient kidney *yang* may lead to the disorder of *qi* activity and failure to separate the clear from the turbid, thus causing the discharge of turbid urine. Such disorders should be treated by warming kidney *yang*, eliminating dampness and separating the clear from turbid fluid. In the prescription, Dioscoreae Septemlobae acts as the chief ingredient to eliminate dampness and disperse turbidity. Alpiniae Oxyphyllae, as the adjuvant ingredient, warms kidney *yang* and reduces the frequency of micturition. Linderae, which warms the kidney and activates *qi* circulation, and Acori Graminei, which disperses turbidity and benefits the orifices, are used as the assistant drugs. Salt is used to guide the effects of the other drugs towards the kidney, the key organ in charge of water metabolism. According to another medical work, the prescription also includes Poria and Radix Glycyrrhizae to enhance its effect of separating the clear from the turbid.

Another prescription of the same name is recorded in *Insight into Medicine*, in which Alpiniae Oxyphyllae and Linderae are removed and Cortex Phellodendri, Rhizoma Atractylodis Macrocephalae, Poria, Plumula Nelumbinis, Radix Salviae Miltiorrhizae and Semen Plantaginis are added. It purges heat and eliminates dampness, and is indicated for stranguria with discharge of white and turbid urine due to a downward attack of dampness and heat.

Decoction of Notopterygii for Expelling Dampness

羌活胜湿汤 *qiang huo sheng shi tang*

(from *Differentiation of Endogenous and Exogenous Diseases*)

Rhizoma seu Radix Notopterygii	6 g
Radix Angelicae Pubescentis	6 g
Rhizoma Ligustici	3 g
Radix Ledebouriellae	3 g
Radix Glycyrrhizae Preparata	3 g
Rhizoma Chuanxiong	3 g
Fructus Viticis	2 g

Administration: Decoct with water for oral administration.

Action: Eliminating wind and dampness.

Indications: Cases of affection of the body surface by wind-dampness, exhibiting headache, heaviness in the head, severe pain in the waist and back, general achiness, chills, low fever, whitish tongue coating, and superficial pulse.

Explanation: The affection of the body surface by wind-dampness usually occurs as a result of exposure to wind when sweating, or prolonged residence in a damp place. Stagnant wind and dampness in the skin and muscles lead to headache, heaviness in the head, pain in the back and waist, and general achiness. Since dampness attacks the body surface, treatment should expel wind and dampness by relieving exterior syndrome. In the prescription, Notopterygii and Angelicae Pubescentis serve as the chief ingredients to eliminate wind-dampness in the upper and lower part of the body respectively. The two together eliminate wind-dampness from anywhere in the body and ease movements of the joints to relieve pain. Ligustici and Ledebouriellae serve as adjuvant ingredients to expel wind-dampness and relieve headache. Chuanxiong activates *qi* and blood circulation, expels wind and relieves pain, while Viticis expels wind-dampness in the upper part of the body and relieves headache; both serve as the assistant ingredients. Glycyrrhizae acts as the guiding drug to coordinate the effects of the other drugs. It is advisable to let the patient perspire slightly after taking the decoction, so that the wind-dampness can be expelled and pain relieved.

Decoction of Angelicae Pubescentis and Taxilli
独活寄生汤 *du huo ji sheng tang*
(from *Essentially Treasured Prescriptions for Emergencies*)

Radix Angelicae Pubescentis	9 g
Ramulus Taxilli	6 g
Cortex Eucommiae	6 g
Radix Achyranthis Bidentatae	6 g
Herba Asari	6 g
Radix Gentianae Macrophyllae	6 g
Poria	6 g
Lignum Cinnamomi	6 g
Radix Ledebouriellae	6 g
Rhizoma Chuanxiong	6 g
Radix Ginseng	6 g
Radix Glycyrrhizae	6 g
Radix Angelicae Sinensis	6 g
Radix Paeoniae Lactiflorae	6 g
Radix Rehmanniae	6 g

Administration: Decoct with water for oral administration.

Action: Expelling wind-dampness, relieving arthralgia, benefiting the liver and kidney and invigorating *qi* and blood.

Indications: Chronic *bi*-syndrome due to hepatic and splenic hypofunction and insufficient *qi* and blood, exhibiting lumbago, pain in the knees, hampered mobility in the joints or numbness, aversion to cold and desire for warmth, pale tongue with whitish coating, and small and thready pulse.

Explanation: This prescription is indicated for prolonged exposure to wind, cold and dampness, which affect the liver and kidney as well as *qi* and blood. The kidney controls the bones and lies in the lumbar region, the liver controls the activity of the tendon, and the knees are considered the "house of the tendon." Hepatic and splenic hypofunction leads to malnutrition of the tendons and bones and insufficient *qi* and blood, and so lumbago, pain in the knees, hampered mobility and numbness occur. Treatment should eliminate the pathogens and reinforce the antipathogenic *qi*, that is, expel wind-dampness, relieve arthralgia, reinforce the liver and kidney and invigorate *qi* and blood. In the prescription, Angelicae Pubescentis, Gentianae Macrophyllae, Ledebouriellae and Asari expel wind-cold and wind-dampness and relieve arthralgia; Eucommiae, Achyranthis Bidentatae and Ramulus Taxilli invigorate the liver and kidney and eliminate wind-dampness; Angelicae Sinensis, Paeoniae Lactiflorae, Rehmanniae and Chuanxiong nourish the blood and activate blood circulation; Ginseng, Poria and Glycyrrhizae invigorate *qi* and strengthen the spleen; and Cinnamomi warms the blood and promotes blood circulation. By combining these drugs, this prescription provides both a causative and symptomatic treatment for the syndrome.

Summary

This chapter examines fourteen principal and two appendant prescriptions, which, according to their specific actions, are further classified into the following sub-categories.

(1) Prescriptions for drying dampness and regulating the stomach:

Powder for Regulating the Function of the Stomach is a prescription for dampness retained in the spleen and stomach. Epigastric and abdominal distention and fullness, and thick and greasy tongue coating are the clinical evidence calling for its application. Powder of Agastaches for Restoring Antipathogenic *Qi* relieves exterior syndrome, eliminates dampness, regulates *qi* and the middle *jiao*, and is used for cases characterized by headache, chills, fever, distention in the chest and stomach, abdominal pain and vomiting caused by attack of exogenous wind and retention of cold and dampness in the interior.

(2) Prescriptions for purging heat and dampness:

Decoction of Artemisiae Scopariae is effective in relieving jaundice, and is indicated for jaundice of the dampness-heat type. Three Seeds Decoction and Sweet Dew Pill for Detoxification can both treat dampness-warm syndrome. But the former is more effective in eliminating dampness than purging heat, and it is better for the initial stage of dampness-warm syndrome with pathogen in *qifen* and more predominant dampness than heat, the latter is effective at both purging heat and eliminating dampness, and is indicated for dampness-warm syndrome with the epidemic pathogen in *qifen* and a predominance of both dampness and heat. Powder for Dispersing Heat and Promoting Urination is more effective at relieving stranguria by diuresis, and is indicated for heat-type stranguria caused by the downward attack on the bladder by dampness-heat.

(3) Prescriptions for promoting diuresis and eliminating dampness:

Powder of Five Drugs Containing Poria promotes diuresis and relieves exterior syndrome, warms *yang* and activates *qi* circulation, and is applicable to cases of water retention, edema, diarrhea and dysuria caused by bladder dysfunction and accumulated dampness. Powder Containing Five Kinds of Peel invigorates the spleen, regulates *qi* and promotes diuresis to reduce edema, and is indicated for cases of general anasarca. Decoction of Stephaniae Tetrandrae and Astragali supplements *qi*, strengthens the surface, expels wind and activates fluid circulation, and is indicated for wind-dampness syndrome and edema caused by wind attributed to weak surface and predominant dampness.

(4) Prescriptions for warming and eliminating dampness:

Zhenwu Decoction and Powder for Invigorating the Spleen warm the spleen and kidney, restore *yang* and promote diuresis, and are indicated for edema due to *yang* deficiency. The former is more effective in warming the kidney, astringing *yin* and relieving spasm, and is indicated for edema due to deficient kidney *yang*. The latter is more effective in warming the spleen, and indicated for edema due to *yang* deficiency accompanied by distention and fullness in the chest and abdomen. Decoction of Dioscoreae Hypoglaucae for Clearing Turbid Urine warms the kidney, activates *qi* circulation and separates the clear from the turbid, and is especially effective in treating stranguria with discharge of whitish and turbid urine due to *yang* deficiency.

(5) Prescriptions for expelling wind and dampness:

Decoction of Notopterygii for Expelling Dampness expels and disperses wind-dampness, and is indicated for wind-dampness syndrome involving the surface. Decoction of Angelicae Pubescentis and Taxilli expels wind-dampness and has a tonic effect, and is suitable for chronic *bi*-syndrome with hepatic and renal hypofunction and insufficient *qi* and blood.

CHAPTER NINETEEN

PRESCRIPTIONS FOR EXPELLING PHLEGM

Prescriptions for expelling phlegm (*qu tan ji*) are composed of drugs that eliminate retained phlegm, and are indicated for various types of phlegm syndrome.

Cases of phlegm syndrome are caused by many factors, and the method of treatment should be decided accordingly. For instance, cases due to splenic dysfunction should be treated by drying dampness; those due to fire-heat retained in the interior, by purging heat; those due to dryness in the lung, deficient *yin* and a flare-up of deficiency fire, by moistening dryness; those due to deficient spleen *yang* or coldness in the lung with retained cold phlegm, by warming and dispersing phlegm; those due to the upward attack of wind-phlegm, by calming the wind; and those due to an affection of exogenous pathogens which leads to cough and pulmonary dysfunction, by dispersing wind.

Tan (phlegm) and *yin* (accumulated fluid) fall into the same category of pathogenic factors. Generally speaking, phlegm is turbid and thick, while fluid is clear and diluted. The pathogenesis of phlegm syndrome is related to the internal organs, especially the spleen, lung and kidney. The spleen is the origin of phlegm production, the lung a container of phlegm, and the kidney a controller of phlegm distribution. Hence, the treatment for phlegm syndrome should not be limited to eliminating phlegm. Attention should also be given to the organ which is responsible for its pathogenesis.

Prescriptions for drying dampness and eliminating phlegm (*zao shi hua tan ji*) are indicated for dampness-phlegm syndrome, exhibiting profuse expectoration, chest upset, epigastric fullness, vomiting, nausea, dizziness, white and smooth tongue coating, and slow or taut and smooth pulse. They are chiefly composed of drugs that dry dampness and eliminate phlegm, such as Rhizoma Pinelliae and Rhizoma Arisaematis, in combination with drugs that activate *qi* circulation, promote diuresis and invigorate the spleen. One example is *Erchen* Decoction.

Prescriptions for purging heat and eliminating phlegm (*qing re hua tan ji*) are indicated for heat-phlegm syndrome, exhibiting cough with yellow sticky sputum, difficulty in expectoration, red tongue with yellow greasy coating, and smooth and rapid pulse. They are chiefly composed of drugs that purge heat and eliminate phlegm, such as Fructus Trichosanthis and Arisaemacum Bile, in combination with drugs that purge heat, activate *qi* circulation, promote diuresis and relieve cough. Examples: Pill for Purging Heat in *Qifen* and Dispersing Phlegm and Pill for Chronic Phlegm Syndrome.

Prescriptions for moistening dryness and eliminating phlegm (*run zao hua tan ji*) are for dryness-phlegm syndrome marked by difficulty in expectoration of thick and sticky sputum, dry throat, and even choking cough and hoarseness. They are mainly composed of drugs that moisten the lung and eliminate phlegm, such as Bulbus Fritillariae Thunbergii and Fructus Trichosanthis, in combination with drugs that promote fluid production, moisten dryness and activate *qi* circulation. Example: Powder of Fritillariae Thunbergii and Trichosanthis.

Prescriptions for warming and eliminating cold-phlegm (*wen hua han tan ji*) are indicated for cold-phlegm syndrome, exhibiting cough with profuse whitish watery sputum, chills, cold limbs, and white and smooth tongue coating. They are chiefly composed of drugs that warm and disperse cold phlegm, such as Rhizoma Pinelliae, Rhizoma Zingiberis and Semen Sinapis Albae, in combination with drugs that invigorate the spleen, promote digestion and suppress adversely ascendant *qi*. Examples: Decoction of Poria, Glycyrrhizae, Schisandrae, Zingiberis and Asari, and Decoction Containing Three Kinds of Seed for the Aged.

Prescriptions for dispelling wind and eliminating phlegm (*zhi feng hua tan ji*) are indicated for wind-phlegm syndrome that is either exogenous or endogenous. Exogenous wind-phlegm syndrome is characterized by productive cough, chills and fever. Prescriptions indicated for it are usually composed of antitussives and expectorants in combination with drugs that dispel wind and relieve the surface. One example is Powder for Relieving Cough. Endogenous wind-phlegm syndrome is marked by dizziness, headache, chest upset, vomiting and nausea. Prescriptions for such cases are composed of drugs that eliminate phlegm, in combination with drugs that calm the liver and suppress endogenous wind. One example is Decoction of Pinelliae, Atractylodis Macrocephalae and Gastrodiae.

Erchen Decoction

二陈汤 *er chen tang*

(from *Benevolent Prescriptions from the Pharmaceutical Bureau of the Taiping Period*)

Rhizoma Pinelliae Preparata	12 g
Pericarpium Citri Rubrum	10 g
Poria	9 g
Radix Glycyrrhizae Preparata	5 g

Administration: Decoct in water together with three pieces of Rhizoma Zingiberis Recens and one piece of Fructus Mume for oral administration.

Action: Drying dampness, eliminating phlegm, activating circulation and regulating the middle *jiao*.

Indications: Cases of accumulated dampness-phlegm, manifested as productive cough with whitish sputum, chest upset, nausea, vomiting, lassitude or dizziness, palpitation, whitish and moist tongue coating, and smooth pulse.

Explanation: Dampness-phlegm syndrome is caused by splenic dysfunction, which leads to the accumulation of dampness and turbidity and disturbs *qi* activity. An attack of phlegm-dampness on the lung results in productive cough. Stagnant phlegm and *qi* disrupts normal gastric functioning, resulting in fullness in the chest, nausea and vomiting.

Accumulated phlegm-turbidity blocks lucid *yang* and affects the heart, causing dizziness and palpitation. It should be treated chiefly by drying dampness and eliminating phlegm, supplemented by activating *qi* circulation and regulating the middle *jiao*. In the prescription, Pinelliae Preparata, acrid, warm and dry, serves as the chief ingredient to dry dampness, eliminate phlegm, regulate the stomach and suppress adversely ascendant *qi*. Citri Rubrum is used as the adjuvant ingredient to activate *qi* circulation so as to disperse phlegm. Poria eliminates dampness and invigorates the spleen, and serves as the assistant ingredient. Glycyrrhizae serves as the guiding drug to coordinate the effects of the other drugs, and help Poria invigorate the spleen and regulate the middle *jiao*. A few pieces of Zingiberis Recens are added to suppress the adversely ascendant *qi* and disperse phlegm, and also reduce the toxicity of Pinelliae. Synergic with Pinelliae Preparata and Citri Rubrum, Mume is used to enhance the elimination of phlegm and to astringe lung *qi*, so as to protect the antipathogenic *qi*. The drugs composing the prescription are few, but the principle of its composition is strict, so that it is considered a basic prescription for eliminating phlegm.

Clinical evidence calling for its application includes productive cough with whitish sputum, chest upset, whitish and moist tongue coating, and smooth pulse. Aside from the dampness-phlegm syndrome, this prescription may also be modified for other types of phlegm syndrome. For instance, for wind-phlegm syndrome, Rhizoma Arisaematis Preparata and Rhizoma Typhonii are added to expel wind and eliminate phlegm; for cold-phlegm syndrome, Rhizoma Zingiberis and Herba Asari are added to warm the lung and eliminate phlegm; for heat-phlegm syndrome, Radix Scutellariae and Fructus Trichosanthis are added to purge heat and eliminate phlegm; for phlegm syndrome complicated by indigestion, Fructus Crataegi and Semen Raphani are added to promote digestion and eliminate phlegm.

Appendant Prescriptions

(1) Decoction for Purging Gallbladder Heat

温胆汤 *wen dan tang*

(from *Treatise on the Tripartite Pathogenesis of Diseases*)

It is composed of 6 g of Rhizoma Pinelliae Preparata, 6 g of Caulis Bambusae in Taeniam, 6 g of Fructus Aurantii Immaturus, 9 g of Pericarpium Citri Reticulatae, 3 g of Radix Glycyrrhizae Preparata, 5 g of Poria, 5 pieces of Rhizoma Zingiberis Recens, and one piece of Fructus Jujubae. To be decocted with water for oral administration, this prescription purges gallbladder heat, regulates stomach *qi* and activates *qi* circulation to eliminate phlegm. It is indicated for disorders of *qi* in the gallbladder and stomach as well as disturbance of phlegm-heat in the interior, marked by restlessness, insomnia, palpitation, vomiting, salivation or epilepsy, bitter taste, and yellow greasy tongue coating.

This prescription was originally recorded in *Essentially Treasured Prescriptions for Emergencies*, but Poria was not used. Compared with the *Erchen* Decoction, Caulis Bambusae in Taeniam and Aurantii Immaturus are added in this prescription. The former is acrid and cool, and purges heat, eliminates phlegm and relieves vomiting and restlessness. The latter is bitter and cold, and activates *qi* circulation, eliminates phlegm, relieves distention and disperses stagnation. These two drugs, when used together with Citri Reticulatae and Pinelliae, enhance the effects of eliminating phlegm and activating *qi* circulation.

(2) Decoction for Eliminating Phlegm
导痰汤 *dao tan tang*
(from *Revised Edition of Yan's Prescriptions for Saving Life*)

It is composed of 10 g of Rhizoma Pinelliae Preparata, 6 g of Rhizoma Arisaematis Preparata, 6 g of Exocarpium Citri Rubrum, 6 g of Fructus Aurantii Immaturus (fried with wheat bran), 6 g of Poria Rubra, 3 g of Radix Glycyrrhizae Preparata, and 5 pieces of Rhizoma Zingiberis Recens. To be boiled with water for oral administration, it dries dampness, eliminates phlegm, activates *qi* circulation and relieves stagnation, and is indicated for cases with marked accumulation of phlegm, exhibiting fullness in the chest and distention in the hypochondrium, or cough with thick and sticky sputum and nausea, or headache and dizziness, or even syncope. Compared with the *Erchen* Decoction, this prescription includes Arisaematis Preparata and Aurantii Immaturus, so that its effects in drying dampness, eliminating phlegm, activating *qi* circulation and relieving stagnation are improved. It is especially effective in treating cases with marked phlegm accumulation.

Pill for Purging Heat in *Qifen* and Dispersing Phlegm
清气化痰丸 *qing qi hua tan wan*
(from *Study on Prescriptions*)

Semen Trichosanthis	30 g
Pericarpium Citri Reticulatae	30 g
Radix Scutellariae (fried with wine)	30 g
Semen Armeniacae Amarum	30 g
Fructus Aurantii Immaturus (fried with wheat bran)	30 g
Poria	30 g
Arisaema cum Bile	45 g
Rhizoma Pinelliae Preparata	45 g

Administration: Grind the drugs into fine powder and mix the powder with ginger juice to produce pills, take 6 g each time with warm water; or prepare them directly as an oral decoction, with dosages reduced proportionally.

Action: Eliminating heat, dispersing phlegm, activating *qi* circulation and relieving cough.

Indications: Cases of accumulated heat-phlegm in the interior, exhibiting cough with yellow, thick and sticky sputum, fullness in the chest or shortness of breath, vomiting, nausea, red tongue with yellowish greasy coating, and smooth and rapid pulse.

Explanation: Heat-phlegm syndrome usually is caused by fluid consumption by fire and accumulated phlegm and heat in the interior, which leads to cough with difficult expectoration of yellow sticky sputum. When lung *qi* is blocked by phlegm and fails to descend, chest upset or shortness of breath, vomiting and nausea result. Treatment should be chiefly purging heat and dispersing phlegm, aided by activating *qi* circulation and relieving cough. In the prescription, Arisaema cum Bile and Trichosanthis, bitter and cold, serve as the chief ingredients to purge heat and disperse phlegm. Scutellariae and Pinelliae Preparata are used as the adjuvant ingredients to suppress lung fire and eliminate phlegm-dampness, so as to enhance the effects of purging heat and dispersing phlegm. Armeniacae Amarum and Pericarpium Citri Reticulatae, as assistant ingredients, disperse phlegm and stagnation by activating *qi* circulation; Poria and Armeniacae Amarum also serve as assistant drugs to eliminate dampness by invigorating the spleen, and to relieve cough by releasing lung *qi* respectively.

This prescription is frequently used for heat-phlegm syndrome. Clinical evidence calling for its application includes cough with difficult expectoration of yellow sticky sputum, red tongue with yellowish greasy coating, and smooth and rapid pulse. For cases of predominant lung heat, Flos Lonicerae, Fructus Forsythiae and Herba Houttuyniae are added to purge heat and remove toxins; and for cases of constipation due to accumulated heat, Radix et Rhizoma Rhei is added to purge heat and relax the bowels.

Pill for Chronic Phlegm Syndrome
滚痰丸 *gun tan wan*
(from *Danxi's Experience on Medicine*)

Radix et Rhizoma Rhei (steamed with wine)	24 g
Radix Scutellariae	24 g
Lapis Chloriti (crashed)	30 g
Nitrum (calcined with Lapis Chloriti)	30 g
Lignum Aquilariae Resinatum	15 g

Administration: Grind the drugs into fine powder and prepare the powder as pills, take 5-9 g each time, twice daily.

Action: Purging fire and eliminating phlegm.

Indications: Chronic phlegm syndrome due to excess-heat, exhibiting manic-depressive psychosis, palpitation, or dyspneic cough with thick sputum, chest and epigastric fullness, dizziness or insomnia, unbearable arthralgia, constipation, yellow and thick greasy tongue coating, and smooth, rapid and strong pulse.

Explanation: The manifestations of chronic phlegm syndrome vary when the different parts of the body are affected. When phlegm affects the head, manic-depressive psychosis occurs; when it disturbs the heart, palpitation or insomnia takes place; when it accumulates in the lung, cough with sticky sputum, dyspnea and chest upset result; and when it stays in the joints, arthralgia occurs. Yet, all these manifestations are associated with yellow and thick greasy tongue coating, constipation, and smooth, rapid and strong pulse. In the prescription, Lapis Chloriti and Nitrum, which are calcined together, serve as the chief ingredients to eliminate phlegm that has accumulated for a long time, Rhei, bitter and cold, serves as the adjuvant ingredient to purge excess-heat and relax the bowels; they are used together to purge phlegm-fire from the intestines. Scutellariae acts as the assistant ingredient to purge heat and eliminate phlegm in order to suppress the fire. Lignum Aquilariae Resinatum keeps adversely ascendant *qi* going downward. These four drugs together eliminate phlegm and stagnation, and compose a potent prescription for chronic cases of phlegm syndrome due to excess-heat. Since the prescription is likely to damage the antipathogenic *qi*, it should be used with caution for the aged and the debilitated. It is contraindicated for pregnant women.

Powder of Fritillariae Thunbergii and Trichosanthis
贝母瓜蒌散 *bei mu gua lou san*
(from *Insight into Medicine*)

Bulbus Fritillariae Thunbergii	5 g
Fructus Trichosanthis	12 g
Radix Trichosanthis	2. 5 g
Poria	2. 5 g
Exocarpium Citri Rubrum	2. 5 g
Radix Platycodi	2. 5 g

Administration: Decoct with water for oral administration.

Action: Nourishing the lung, dispersing phlegm, purging heat and promoting fluid production.

Indications: Lung dryness syndrome with expectoration, exhibiting cough, difficult expectoration, dry throat, sore throat, red tongue, and rapid pulse.

Explanation: All the above symptoms are the result of lung dryness due to fluid consumption. The therapeutic principle should be to moisten dryness, purge heat, promote fluid production and disperse phlegm. In the prescription, Bulbus Fritillariae Thunbergii, bitter, sweet and cool, is used as the chief ingredient to nourish the lung, purge heat, eliminate phlegm and relieve cough. Fructus Trichosanthis and Platycodi, as the adjuvant ingredients, purge heat, moisten dryness, activate lung *qi* and eliminate phlegm. Radix Trichosanthis purges heat, eliminates phlegm, promotes fluid production and nourishes the lung, Poria invigorates the spleen and eliminates dampness to prevent phlegm production, and Citri Rubrum activates *qi* circulation and eliminates phlegm—these serve together as the assistant ingredients.

In clinical application, expectorant agents that moisten the lung, such as Radix Adenophorae and Radix Ophiopogonis, may be added to the prescription. For cases with cough and sore throat, Semen Armeniacae Amarum and Fructus Arctii are added to release lung *qi* and ease the throat.

Another prescription of the same name was recorded in the same book. Its composition differs with this one in that it does not include Fructus Trichosanthis, Poria and Platycodi, but includes Arisaema cum Bile, Radix Scutellariae, Rhizoma Coptidis, Fructus Gardeniae and Radix Glycyrrhizae. Among these additional drugs, the first three, bitter and cold, are used to purge heat and fire, while Arisaema cum Bile eliminates phlegm and calms the wind. It is therefore applicable to cases of apoplexy resulting from an upward attack of phlegm-fire.

Decoction of Poria, Glycyrrhizae, Schisandrae, Zingiberis and Asari
苓甘五味姜辛汤 *ling gan wu wei jiang xin tang*
(from *Synopsis of the Golden Cabinet*)

Poria	12 g
Radix Glycyrrhizae	9 g
Rhizoma Zingiberis	9 g
Herba Asari	6 g
Fructus Schisandrae	6 g

Administration: Decoct with water for oral administration.

Action: Warming the lung and eliminating retained phlegm.

Indications: Cases due to cold-phlegm retained in the interior, exhibiting productive cough with thin clear sputum, chest upset, and white and smooth tongue coating.

Explanation: Insufficient spleen *yang* with production of endogenous cold disrupts the function of the spleen and leads to dampness retention. In addition, when the lung is affected by cold and fails to distribute fluid, a phlegm-fluid retention syndrome occurs. Hence, productive cough with thin clear sputum, chest upset, and white and smooth tongue coating are the result of cold-phlegm retained in the interior. For such cases, treatment seeks to warm *yang* and relieve retained phlegm-fluid by taking into consideration of both the spleen and lung. In the prescription, Zingiberis, sweet, acrid and hot, is used as the chief ingredient to warm the lung and disperse cold to eliminate the accumulated phlegm, and also to warm spleen *yang* to eliminate dampness. Asari, as the adjuvant ingredient, warms the lung to disperse cold and helps Zingiberis to disperse accumulated cold-phlegm. Poria, sweet and bland, invigorates the spleen, eliminates dampness, removes accumulated phlegm and prevents the phlegm production, Schisandrae has an astringent effect on the lung and relieves cough—both are used as the assistant ingredients. When the two are used together with Zingiberis and Asari, they produce a dispersive effect without causing damage to the antipathogenic *qi*, and an astringent effect without retaining pathogens. Glycyrrhizae invigorates the spleen and regulates the middle *jiao*, and serves as the guide to coordinate the effects of the other drugs. As a whole, the prescription produces both dispersive and astringent effects. For cases of profuse sputum and nausea, Rhizoma Pinelliae Preparata is added to suppress adversely ascendant *qi*, relieve nausea, dry dampness and eliminate phlegm; for upward rushing of *qi*, Ramulus Cinnamomi is added to warm the middle *jiao* and suppress the *qi*; and for frequent cough and puffy face, Semen Armeniacae Amarum is added to activate lung *qi* and relieve cough.

Decoction Containing Three Kinds of Seed for the Aged
三子养亲汤 *san zi yang qin tang*
(from *Han's Treatise on Medicine*)

Semen Sinapis Albae	6 g
Fructus Perillae	9 g
Semen Raphani	9 g

Administration: Crush the drugs into granules, wrap 9 g with a piece of gauze and prepare them into a decoction and drink as tea. For cases with dry stools, add honey. And add a few pieces of ginger when it is cold.

Action: Dissolving phlegm, promoting digestion, suppressing adversely rising *qi* and relieving dyspnea.

Indications: Cases of stagnant phlegm and *qi*, exhibiting productive cough, dyspnea, chest upset, anorexia, indigestion, white and greasy tongue coating, and smooth pulse.

Explanation: This prescription is indicated for old patients with poor appetite, much phlegm, and cough and dyspnea, which result from pulmonary dysfunction with stagnant phlegm and *qi*. The principle of treatment is to eliminate phlegm, promote digestion and regulate *qi*. In the prescription, Sinapis Albae, acrid and warm, eliminates cold-phlegm, regulates *qi* in the chest; Perillae suppresses the adversely rising *qi*, eliminates phlegm, relieves cough and dyspnea; and Raphani relieves dyspepsia, activates *qi* circulation and eliminates phlegm. When these three are used together, they are effective in relieving all the symptoms mentioned above. In clinical application, the chief ingredient is decided according to whether expectoration, indigestion or dyspnea is more predominant, so as to achieve a better result. Yet, this prescription only serves as a symptomatic treatment regardless of age, and causative treatment should be given after the symptoms relieved.

Powder for Relieving Cough
止嗽散 *zhi sou san*
(from *Insight into Medicine*)

Radix Platycodi	1,000 g
Herba Schizonepetae	1,000 g
Radix Asteris	1,000 g
Radix Stemonae	1,000 g
Rhizoma Cynanchi Stauntonii	1,000 g
Radix Glycyrrhizae Preparata	375 g
Pericarpium Citri Reticulatae	500 g

Administration: Grind the drugs into fine powder, take 6 g with warm water or ginger decoction each time; or prepare as concentrated pills, take 3 g each time, two or three times daily; or prepare them directly as an oral decoction, with dosages reduced proportionally.

Action: Eliminating phlegm, relieving cough, dispelling pathogenic wind from the exterior.

Indications: Lung disorders due to affection by wind, exhibiting cough with white sputum, itching of the throat, chills and fever, and white and thin tongue coating.

Explanation: The prescription is indicated for cough due to exogenous pathogens, which cannot be relieved by remedies that relieve exterior syndrome and regulate lung *qi*. In this case, although the exogenous pathogen is mostly eliminated, it still remains and lung *qi* is not released, and so cough is predominant and there is a large amount of sputum. Hence, antitussives and expectorants should be applied as the chief remedy, and supplemented by drugs that expel exogenous wind. In the prescription, Asteris, Platycodi, Cynanchi Stauntonii and Stemonae are antitussives and expectorants which can be applied to relieve both new and chronic cases of productive cough. Schizonepetae disperses wind from the surface and eliminates the remnant pathogen. Citri Reticulatae activates *qi* circulation, eliminates sputum and relieves cough. Glycyrrhizae coordinates the effects of the other drugs and also regulates the middle *jiao* and relieves cough. These drugs are warm, moist and mild, and are neither hot nor cold—they are ideal to disperse wind and release lung *qi*. For cases with severe wind-cold in the surface, Radix Ledebouriellae, Folium Perillae and Rhizoma Zingiberis Recens are added to induce perspiration and eliminate the superficial pathogens; and for cough with thick sputum, Rhizoma Pinelliae, Fructus Trichosanthis and Bulbus Fritillariae Thunbergii are added to disperse sputum.

Decoction of Pinelliae, Atractylodis Macrocephalae and Gastrodiae

半夏白术天麻汤 *ban xia bai zhu tian ma tang*

(from *Insight into Medicine*)

Rhizoma Pinelliae	9 g
Rhizoma Gastrodiae	6 g
Poria	6 g
Exocarpium Citri Rubrum	6 g
Rhizoma Atractylodis Macrocephalae	15 g
Radix Glycyrrhizae	3 g
Rhizoma Zingiberis Recens	1 piece
Fructus Jujubae	2 pieces

Administration: Decoct with water for oral administration.

Action: Drying dampness, eliminating phlegm, calming the liver and inhibiting wind.

Indications: Cases of upward attack by wind-phlegm, exhibiting headache, dizziness, chest upset, vomiting, nausea, copious expectoration, white and greasy tongue coating, and taut and smooth pulse.

Explanation: This prescription is composed of all the ingredients of *Erchen* Decoction in addition to Rhizoma Atractylodis Macrocephalae and Gastrodiae. It is indicated for cases of spleen deficiency with accumulated dampness forming phlegm, and accompanied by internal stirring of liver wind. The attack of wind-phlegm on the head causes dizziness and headache. Stagnant phlegm affects the normal circulation of *qi* and leads to the adverse rise of stomach *qi*, thus chest upset, vomiting and nausea occur. For such cases, the treatment should be to eliminate phlegm and suppress wind. In the prescription, Pinelliae dries dampness, eliminates phlegm, suppresses the adversely rising *qi* and relieves vomiting, and Gastrodiae calms the liver and inhibits wind—both serve as the chief ingredients, and are frequently used to relieve dizziness and headache due to attacks by wind-phlegm. Atractylodis Macrocephalae serves as the adjuvant ingredient to invigorate the spleen and eliminate dampness, and it is used together with Pinelliae and Gastrodiae to strengthen the effects of eliminating phlegm and suppressing wind. Poria and Citri Rubrum serve as assistant ingredients: the former eliminates dampness and invigorates the spleen, and forms together with Atractylodis Macrocephalae a remedy for phlegm syndrome; the latter activates *qi* circulation and eliminates phlegm. Glycyrrhizae is used as the guiding ingredient to regulate the middle *jiao* and coordinates the effects of the other drugs. Clinical evidence calling for the application of this prescription is dizziness or heaviness of the head and headache, profuse expectoration, nausea, vomiting, and greasy tongue coating. For cases with severe dizziness, Ramulus Uncariae cum Uncis, Bombyx Batryticatus and Succus Bambusae are added to strengthen the effects of eliminating phlegm and suppressing wind; for cases with deficient *qi*, Radix Codonopsis Pilosulae and Radix Astragali are added to invigorate *qi*. In another prescription of the same name recorded in the chapter on headache, Fructus Viticis is added to the above formula. It is used for headache due to an adverse rise of phlegm and rotatory vertigo.

Summary

This chapter examines eight principal and two appendant prescriptions, which can be grouped into five sub-categories according to their actions.

(1) Prescriptions for drying dampness and eliminating phlegm:

Erchen Decoction dries dampness, eliminates phlegm, activates *qi* circulation and regulates the middle *jiao*, and is indicated for cases of productive cough due to accumulated dampness-phlegm.

(2) Prescriptions for purging heat and eliminating phlegm:

Pill for Purging Heat in *Qifen* and Dispersing Phlegm and Pill for Chronic Phlegm Syndrome are the representative prescriptions. The former activates *qi* circulation and relieves cough, and is often used for cases of difficult expectoration of thick yellow sputum due to accumulated phlegm-heat; the latter purges fire, and is indicated for chronic phlegm syndrome, exhibiting manic-depressive psychosis, palpitation, dyspneic cough and dizziness.

(3) Prescriptions for moistening dryness and eliminating phlegm:

Powder of Fritillariae Thunbergii and Trichosanthis is one example. It is used for lung dryness syndrome with cough, difficulty in expectoration and dry throat.

(4) Prescriptions for warming and eliminating cold-phlegm:

Decoction of Poria, Glycyrrhizae, Schisandrae, Zingiberis and Asari warms the lung and eliminates phlegm, and is indicated for cases of retained cold-phlegm exhibiting productive cough with profuse thin and white sputum. Decoction Containing Three Kinds of Seed for the Aged promotes digestion, eliminates phlegm, suppresses adversely ascendant *qi* and relieves dyspnea, and is indicated for cases with the symptoms of cough, dyspnea, poor appetite and indigestion due to accumulated phlegm and stagnant *qi*.

(5) Prescriptions for dispelling wind and eliminating phlegm:

Powder for Relieving Cough eliminates phlegm, relieves cough and expels wind from the surface, and is a prescription frequently used for cough due to attack by exogenous wind when the pathogen is still present. Decoction of Pinelliae, Atractylodis Macrocephalae and Gastrodiae dries dampness, eliminates phlegm, calms the liver and suppresses wind, and is a major prescription for dizziness and headache due to an upward attack of wind-phlegm.

CHAPTER TWENTY

PRESCRIPTIONS FOR RELIEVING WIND DISORDER

Prescriptions for relieving wind disorder (*zhi feng ji*) are composed of drugs that expel exogenous wind and suppress endogenous wind to relieve convulsion.

Wind disorders cover a wide range of diseases and their development is quite complicated. In brief, wind disorders can be divided into exogenous- and endogenous-wind syndromes. The former results from an attack by exogenous wind on the surface, meridians, muscles and joints, and it should be treated by expelling exogenous wind. The latter is due to disorders of the internal organs, including the stirring of wind by excessive heat, the upward attack of liver wind, and the irritation of wind by *yin* deficiency, and it should be treated by suppressing endogenous wind. Accordingly, two types of prescriptions are used to relieve wind disorders.

Prescriptions for dispersing exogenous wind (*shu san wai feng ji*) are applied to various kinds of diseases caused by exogenous wind. A person with insufficient antipathogenic *qi* and weak surface is susceptible to affection by exogenous wind, and the diseases thus caused usually show the symptoms of headache, aversion to wind, itching, numb limbs, arthralgia, hampered mobility of the joints or distortion of the face. Drugs usually used to form such prescriptions include Rhizoma seu Radix Notopterygii, Radix Angelicae Pubescentis, Radix Ledebouriellae, Rhizoma Chuanxiong, Radix Angelicae Dahuricae and Radix Typhonii, in combination with drugs that nourish the blood, purge heat, warm the interior, eliminate phlegm and activate blood circulation. Examples: Powder for Dispelling Wind, Powder of Chuanxiong with Folium Camelliae Sinensis, Powder for Treating Face Distortion and Bolus for Mildly Activating the Meridians.

Prescriptions for suppressing endogenous wind (*ping xi nei feng ji*) are for the endogenous-wind syndrome, which is a disorder with different pathogens and clinical manifestations. Disorders due to the stirring of wind by excessive heat may show unconsciousness and spasms; while those due to hyperactive liver *yang* and the stirring of liver wind inside the body may exhibit dizziness, fever, headache, flushed complexion and even coma, deviation of the mouth and hemiplegia. They should be treated by calming the liver and suppressing wind. Drugs frequently used in such prescriptions include Cornu Saigae Tataricae, Ramulus Uncariae cum Uncis, Concha Haliotidis, Rhizoma Gastrodiae and Concha Ostreae, in combination with drugs that purge heat, eliminate phlegm, nourish *yin* and blood. Examples: Decoction of Cornu Saigae Tataricae and Ramulus Uncariae cum Uncis, and Decoction for Calming Liver-Wind. In the late stage of seasonal febrile diseases when *yin* is consumed by heat and deficiency wind is produced, spasms in the tendons and involuntary movements of the hands and feet ensue. Drugs commonly used include Radix Paeoniae Alba, Colla Corii Asini and yolk, in combination with drugs that calm the liver, suppress wind, purge heat and eliminate phlegm. Example: Bolus for Serious Endogenous-Wind Syndrome.

Clinically, it is necessary first of all to determine whether a wind-syndrome is endogenous or exogenous, cold or hot, and deficiency or excess. For exogenous-wind syndrome, the wind should be dispersed rather than suppressed, while for endogenous-wind syndrome, the converse applies. If a wind syndrome is complicated by cold, heat, dampness, phlegm or blood-stasis syndrome, corresponding treatment should be given simultaneously. In addition, exogenous and endogenous wind may affect and evoke each other, it is therefore necessary to differentiate the primary from the secondary syndrome in cases of a complicated wind disorder.

Powder for Dispelling Wind

消风散 *xiao feng san*

(from *Orthodox Treatise on External and Surgical Disorders*)

Radix Angelicae Sinensis	6 g
Radix Rehmanniae	6 g
Radix Ledebouriellae	6 g
Periostracum Cicadae	6 g
Radix Anemarrhenae	6 g
Radix Sophorae Flavescentis	6 g
Semen Sesami	6 g
Herba Schizonepetae	6 g
Rhizoma Atractylodis	6 g
Fructus Arctii	6 g
Gypsum Fibrosum	6 g
Radix Glycyrrhizae	3 g
Caulis Akebiae	3 g

Administration: Decoct with water and take the decoction on an empty stomach.

Action: Dispelling wind, nourishing the blood, purging heat and eliminating dampness.

Indications: Rubella or eczema, characterized by reddish itching rashes or patches which exude after broken, white or yellow tongue coating, and superficial and rapid strong pulse.

Explanation: It is a prescription frequently used to treat rubella and eczema due to wind-heat or wind-dampness attacking *qi* and blood and stagnating in the skin and muscles. Since itching is caused by wind, it should be mainly treated by dispelling wind, purging heat and eliminating dampness. In the prescription, Schizonepetae, Ledebouriellae, Arctii and Periostracum Cicadae are used as the chief ingredients to dispel wind from the surface. Atractylodis disperses wind and dampness, and Sophorae Flavescentis purges heat and dries dampness; Akebiae eliminates dampness-heat, and Gypsum Fibrosum and Anemarrhenae purge heat and fire—they all serve as the adjuvant ingredients. Since wind attacks the blood vessels and impairs *yin*-blood, Angelicae Sinensis, Rehmanniae and Sesami are used as assistant drugs to nourish the blood, promote blood circulation, nourish *yin* and moisten dryness. Glycyrrhizae serves as the guide to purge heat, remove toxins and coordinate the effects of the other drugs. When used in combination, these drugs prove to be effective in dispelling wind, eliminating dampness and heat, and nourishing *yin*-blood.

Clinically, for cases with predominant wind-heat, Flos Lonicerae and Fructus Forsythiae are added to eliminate heat and remove toxins; for cases with predominant dampness-heat, Fructus Kochiae and Semen Plantaginis are added to eliminate heat and dampness; for cases with predominant heat in *xuefen*, Radix Paeoniae Rubra and Radix Arnebiae seu Lithospermi are added to purge heat and cool the blood. Moreover, spicy and hot food, fish, cigarette, wine and tea should be avoided during the administration of the prescription. Otherwise, the therapeutic effect may be weakened.

Powder of Chuanxiong with Folium Camelliae Sinensis

川芎茶调散 *chuan xiong cha tiao san*

(from *Benevolent Prescriptions from the Pharmaceutical Bureau of the Taiping Period*)

Rhizoma Chuanxiong	120 g
Herba Schizonepetae	120 g
Radix Angelicae Dahuricae	60 g
Rhizoma seu Radix Notopterygii	60 g
Radix Glycyrrhizae (broiled)	60 g
Radix Ledebouriellae	45 g
Herba Asari	30 g
Herba Menthae	240 g

Administration: Grind the drugs into fine powder, take 9 g with tea each time, twice daily; or prepare them directly into an oral decoction, with dosages reduced proportionally.

Action: Dispelling wind and relieving pain.

Indications: Headache due to attack of exogenous wind, exhibiting general or regional headache, chills, fever, dizziness, stuffy nose, thin and white tongue coating, and superficial pulse.

Explanation: Headache may be due to various causes. This prescription is indicated only for headache due to the attack by exogenous wind, which goes along the meridians up to the head, resulting in headache. Pathogenic wind that stagnates on the surface and fights with the antipathogenic *qi* leads to chills, fever, dizziness, stuffy nose, and superficial pulse. General or regional headache which occurs intermittently for a long period is known as head-wind syndrome. The exogenous wind-syndrome should be treated by dispelling wind in order to relieve headache. In the prescription, Chuanxiong, Angelicae Dahuricae and Notopterygii are used as the chief ingredients to dispel wind and relieve pain. Chuanxiong is better for headache involving the Shaoyang and Jue*yin* meridians (parietal or temporal headache), Notopterygii for headache involving the Taiyang Meridian (occipital headache), and Angelicae Dahuricae for headache involving the Yangming Meridian (frontal headache). Asari dispels cold and relieves pain, and is good for Shaoyang headache, Menthae, used in a heavy dosage, relieves headache and dizziness and dispels wind, Schizonepetae and Ledebouriellae dispel wind in the upper part of the body—they are used as the adjuvant ingredients to enhance the dispersive and analgesic effects of the chief ingredients, and also to expel pathogens from the surface. Glycyrrhizae coordinates the effects of the other drugs. The powder should be taken with tea, which is bitter and cold, relieves headache and dizziness and counteracts the warming, drying, ascending and dispelling actions of the acrid wind-dispelling drugs. The latter two serve as the assistant and guiding ingredients.

Drugs used to form the prescription are mostly acrid and dry, so the prescription is not suitable for headache due to blood and *qi* deficiency, or hyperactive liver *yang*.

Appendant Prescription

Powder of Chrysanthemi with Folium Camelliae Sinensis
菊花茶调散 *ju hua cha tiao san*
(from *Variorum of Prescriptions*)

It is composed of all the ingredients of the Powder of Chuanxiong with Folium Camelliae Sinensis in addition to Flos Chrysanthemi and Bombyx Batryticatus. It dispels wind, stops pain and relieves headache and dizziness, and is indicated for headache and dizziness due to an upward attack of wind-heat.

Powder for Treating Facial Distortion
前正散 *qian zheng san*
(from *Yang's Family Prescriptions*)

Rhizoma Typhonii
Bombyx Batryticatus
Scorpio
(in equivalent amount)

Administration: Grind the drugs into fine powder, take 3 g each time with warm wine or water.

Action: Dispelling wind, eliminating phlegm and relieving convulsion.

Indications: Apoplexy and distortion of the face.

Explanation: Apoplexy may involve either the meridians or the *zang-fu* organs. This prescription is indicated only for cases due to the blockage of the meridians of the head and face by wind-phlegm. The Foot-Yangming Meridian passes through the mouth, curving around the lips, and the Foot-Taiyang Meridian starts from the inner canthus. Accumulated phlegm in Yangming and an attack of wind on Taiyang block the meridians, disrupt *qi* and blood circulation, and disable the corresponding muscles and tendons, resulting in deviation of the mouth and eyes. The treatment aims at eliminating wind-phlegm, removing the obstruction and relieving convulsions. In the prescription, Typhonii dispels wind and eliminates phlegm, especially that involving the head and face. Bombyx Batryticatus and Scorpio dispel wind and relieve convulsion; the former also eliminates phlegm, and the latter also removes obstruction from the meridians. Warm wine can promote *qi* and blood circulation and guide the effects of the other drugs to the affected parts.

In the prescription, Typhonii is warm and dry and only applicable to the cold-type wind-phlegm syndrome. It is not suitable for facial distortion or hemiplegia caused by *qi* deficiency, blood stasis or an upward stirring of liver wind. Since Typhonii and Scorpio are poisonous, overdose should be avoided.

Bolus for Mildly Activating the Meridians
小活络丹 *xiao huo luo dan*
(from *Benevolent Prescriptions from the Pharmaceutical Bureau of the Taiping Period*)

Radix Aconiti (roasted)	180 g
Radix Aconiti Kusnezoffii (roasted)	180 g
Lumbricus	180 g
Rhizoma Arisaematis Preparata	180 g
Olibanum	66 g
Myrrha	66 g

Administration: Grind the drugs into fine powder and prepare into boluses with honey, each weighing 5 g, take one bolus with wine or warm water, twice daily.

Action: Dispelling wind, eliminating dampness and phlegm, removing obstruction from the meridians and collaterals, activating blood circulation and relieving pain.

Indications: Cases of stagnant wind, cold and dampness in the meridians, manifested as cramps in the limbs, wandering arthralgia with hampered movement; or apoplexy due to stagnant phlegm, dampness and blood in the meridians, manifested as protracted numbness of the hands and feet, heavy sensation in the loins and lower limbs, or pain in the limbs.

Explanation: Stagnant wind, cold and dampness, or phlegm, dampness and blood in the meridians interfere with *qi* and blood circulation and affect the nourishment of tendons and muscles, thus producing cramps in the limbs and hampered movement of the joints. The treatment concentrates on eliminating dampness, and is supplemented by eliminating phlegm and activating blood circulation. In the prescription, Aconiti and Aconiti Kusnezoffii, which are acrid and hot, serve as the chief ingredients to expel wind, eliminate dampness, warm and dredge the meridians and relieve pain. Arisaematis dries dampness, eliminates phlegm from the meridians and relieves pain; it serves as the adjuvant ingredient. Olibanum and Myrrha, as assistant ingredients, activate *qi* and blood circulation and remove blood stasis from the meridians. Lumbricus reopens and activates the meridians, and old wine strengthens the effects of the drugs and guides them directly to the affected parts.

This prescription has a potent action, and is recommended for patients with strong constitution. For patients with heat due to *yin* deficiency, and pregnant women, it should be applied with caution.

Decoction of Cornu Saigae Tataricae and Ramulus Uncariae cum Uncis
羚角钩藤汤 *ling jiao gou teng tang*
(from *Popular Treatise on Cold Diseases*)

Cornu Saigae Tataricae (sliced and decocted first)	4.5 g
Folium Mori	6 g
Bulbus Fritillariae Cirrhosae	12 g
Radix Rehmanniae (fresh)	15 g
Ramulus Uncariae cum Uncis (decocted later)	9 g
Flos Chrysanthemi	9 g
Lignum Pini Poriaferum	9 g
Radix Paeoniae Alba	9 g
Radix Glycyrrhizae	2.5 g
Caulis Bambusae in Taeniam (decocted first)	15 g

Administration: Decoct with water for oral administration.

Action: Cooling the liver, suppressing wind, increasing fluid production and relaxing the muscles and tendons.

Indications: Cases of excessive heat in the liver meridian complicated by wind disturbance, exhibiting persistent high fever, fidgetiness, spasm or convulsion of the limbs, or even coma, dry and crimson tongue with rough and prickly coating, and taut and rapid pulse.

Explanation: This prescription is indicated for cases of accumulated heat in the liver meridian which produces wind. When internal heat is excessive, high fever persists; when the heat disturbs the heart, fidgetiness and even coma occur; when heat produces wind, and fire and wind interact, convulsion ensues. Dry crimson tongue and taut, rapid pulse are indications of excessive heat in the liver meridian. In the prescription, Cornu Saigae Tataricae and Ramulus Uncariae cum Uncis are used as the chief ingredients to cool the liver, expel wind, purge heat and relieve convulsion. Mori and Chrysanthemi, as the adjuvant ingredients, strengthen the effects of calming the liver and expelling wind. Paeoniae Alba and Rehmanniae are used to nourish *yin* and promote fluid production, so as to soften the liver and relax the muscles and tendons, since the interaction of wind and fire is liable to consume *yin* and body fluid, Bulbus Fritillariae Cirrhosae and Caulis Bambusae in Taeniam are used to purge heat and eliminate phlegm, and Lignum Pini Poriaferum is included to calm the liver and heart and tranquilize the mind—they all act as the assistant drugs. Crude Radix Glycyrrhizae serves as the guide to coordinate the effects of the other drugs and relax the muscles and relieve spasm when used together with Paeoniae Alba.

This is a typical prescription for cases in which wind is produced by excessive heat. It is used for seasonal febrile diseases when high fever, irritability and convulsion occur. It is also for cases of headache, dizziness and tremor caused by hyperactive liver *yang*. For coma due to the blockage of the heart by heat, remedies that purge heat and induce resuscitation, such as Bolus of Calculus Bovis for Resurrection, and Purple-Snow Pellet, may be used simultaneously.

Decoction for Calming Liver Wind

镇肝熄风汤 *zhen gan xi feng tang*

(from *Discourse on Medical Problems Interpreted by Combining Chinese and Western Medicine*)

Radix Achyranthis Bidentatae	30 g
Haematitum	30 g
Os Draconis (crushed)	15 g
Concha Ostreae (crushed)	15 g
Plastrum Testudinis (crushed)	15 g
Radix Paeoniae Alba	15 g
Radix Scrophulariae	15 g
Radix Asparagi	15 g
Fructus Toosendan (crushed)	6 g
Fructus Hordei Germinatus	6 g
Herba Artemisiae Scopariae	6 g
Radix Glycyrrhizae	4.5 g

Administration: Decoct with water for oral administration.

Action: Calming the liver, suppressing wind, nourishing *yin* and suppressing excess *yang*.

Indications: Cases of deficient liver and kidney *yin*, hyperactive liver *yang* and disordered *qi* and blood, exhibiting dizziness, tinnitus, a hot sensation and pain in the head, fidgetiness, flushed cheeks, frequent eructation, hampered mobility, deviation of the mouth, or even fainting or coma, listlessness, and long and strong pulse.

Explanation: This is a typical prescription for calming the liver and suppressing wind. Deficient liver and kidney *yin*, hyperactive liver *yang*, and an upward attack of wind-*yang* lead to dizziness, blurred vision, tinnitus, flushed face and a hot sensation and pain in the head. Disharmony between the liver and spleen, along with the adverse ascent of stomach *qi*, leads to eructation. Hyperactive liver *yang* causes the adverse ascent of *qi* and blood, giving rise to fainting or coma, hampered mobility and hemiplegia. A taut, long and strong pulse is also an indication of hyperactive liver *yang*. Treatment should be concentrated on calming the liver and suppressing wind, and supplemented by nourishing liver and kidney *yin* fluid. In the prescription, Achyranthis Bidentatae, which exerts its effects through the liver and kidney meridians, is used in a large dosage as the chief ingredient to nourish the liver and kidney and guide the blood downward. Haematitum, Os Draconis and Concha Ostreae are used as the adjuvant ingredients to suppress the adverse ascent of *qi*, inhibit the excess *yang*, calm the liver and suppress wind. Plastrum Testudinis, Scrophulariae, Asparagi and Paeoniae Alba nourish *yin* fluid to inhibit hyperactive *yang*, and Artemisiae Scopariae, Toosendan and Hordei Germinatus disperse stagnant liver *qi* and purge heat—they serve as the assistant ingredients to help the chief and adjuvant ingredients calm and suppress liver *yang*. Glycyrrhizae serves as the guide to coordinate the effects of the other drugs, regulates the stomach and the middle *jiao* and prevents the stomach from being injured by the mineral drugs when used with Hordei Germinatus. In clinical application, for cases with predominant heat in the heart, Gypsum Fibrosum is added; for cases with much phlegm, Arisaema cum Bile is added; for cases with weak pulse in the *chi* region, Rhizoma Rehmanniae Preparata and Fructus Corni are added; and for cases with loose stools, Plastrum Testudinis and Haematitum are removed and Halloysitum Rubrum is added.

Appendant Prescription

Decoction of Gastrodiae and Ramulus Uncariae cum Uncis

天麻钩藤饮 *tian ma gou teng yin*

(from *New Concepts About Diagnosis and Treatment of Miscellaneous Diseases*)

It is composed of 9 g of Rhizoma Gastrodiae, 12 g of Ramulus Uncariae cum Uncis (decocted later), 18 g of Concha Haliotidis (decocted first), 9 g of Fructus Gardeniae, 9 g of Radix Scutellariae, 9 g of Radix Cyathulae, 9 g of Cortex Eucommiae, 9 g of Herba Leonuri, 9 g of Ramulus Taxilli, 9 g of Caulis Polygoni Multiflori, and 9 g of Lignum Pini Poriaferum. To be prepared as an oral decoction, the prescription calms the liver, suppresses wind, purges heat, activates blood circulation and nourishes the liver and kidney. It is indicated for cases due to hyperactive liver *yang* and an upward disturbance of liver wind, exhibiting such symptoms as headache, fainting and insomnia.

In this prescription, Gastrodiae, Uncariae cum Uncis and Concha Haliotidis are applied as the chief ingredients to calm the liver and suppress wind. Gardeniae and Scutellariae, as the adjuvant ingredients, purge heat and fire from the liver meridian. Leonuri activates blood circulation and promotes diuresis, Cyathulae guides the blood downward and nourishes the liver and kidney when used together with Eucommiae and Taxilli, and Polygoni Multiflori and Lignum Pini Poriaferum tranquilize the mind—they act as the assistant and guiding ingredients. For serious cases, Cornu Saigae Tataricae is added.

Bolus for Serious Endogenous Wind Syndrome
大定风珠 *da ding feng zhu*
(from *Essentials of Seasonal Febrile Diseases*)

Radix Paeoniae Alba	18 g
Colla Corii Asini	9 g
Plastrum Testudinis	12 g
Radix Rehmanniae	18 g
Semen Cannabis	6 g
Fructus Schisandrae	6 g
Concha Ostreae	12 g
Radix Ophiopogonis	18 g
Radix Glycyrrhizae Preparata	12 g
Yolk	2 pieces
Carapax Trionycis	12 g

Administration: Boil the drugs to produce a decoction, mix the decoction with yolks and take it warm.

Action: Nourishing *yin* and suppressing wind.

Indications: Long-standing seasonal febrile diseases with impairment of true *yin* by heat or consumption of *yin*-fluid due to misuse of diaphoretic and purgative drugs, exhibiting listlessness, clonic convulsion, feeble pulse, crimson tongue with scanty coating, and tendency to collapse.

Explanation: In the late stage of seasonal febrile diseases, when true *yin* is severely impaired by heat, listlessness, feeble pulse, crimson tongue with scanty coating and the tendency to collapse occur. When *yin*-blood is consumed, accompanied by failure to nourish the tendons and vessels and an internal stirring of deficiency wind, clonic convulsion results. In such cases, the pathogen is mostly eliminated but true *yin* is also damaged, and thus tonics with strong flavor should be used to invigorate the exhausted true *yin* and suppress internal deficiency wind. In the prescription, yolk and Colla Corii Asini are used as chief ingredients to nourish fluid as well as the tendons and vessels to suppress the endogenous wind. Rehmanniae, Ophiopogonis and Paeoniae Alba nourish *yin* and blood and soften the liver, Plastrum Testudinis and Carapax Trionycis nourish *yin* and inhibit *yang*—they all serve as the adjuvant ingredients. Cannabis nourishes *yin* and moistens dryness, Concha Ostreae calms the liver and inhibits excess *yang*, Schisandrae and Glycyrrhizae produce *yin* with their sour and sweet flavor—they serve as assistant and guiding ingredients.

This prescription is developed on the basis of Decoction for Restoring the Pulse Beating and Nourishing *Yin* recorded in *Essentials of Seasonal Febrile Diseases*, which is composed of Radix Glycyrrhizae, Radix Rehmanniae, Radix Paeoniae Alba, Radix Ophiopogonis, Colla Corii Asini and Semen Cannabis. If heat persists and *yin* is injured, yolk, Fructus Schisandrae, Plastrum Testudinis and Carapax Trionycis are added to form a remedy that nourishes *yin* and suppresses wind.

Clinical evidence calling for the application of this prescription includes clonic convulsion, feeble pulse and crimson tongue with scanty coating, all of which result from serious consumption of true *yin* by heat and the internal stirring of deficiency wind. For cases along with dyspnea, Radix Ginseng is added to invigorate *qi* and promote fluid production; for cases with spontaneous perspiration, Os Draconis and Fructus Tritici Levis (light) are added to astringe and arrest it; and for cases with palpitation, Radix Ginseng and Lignum Pini Poriaferum are added to replenish *qi* and tranquilize the mind. This prescription is not indicated for cases in which pathogens are still predominant, even though *yin*-fluid is deficient.

Summary

This chapter has selected seven principal and two appendant prescriptions, which are classified into two sub-categories.

(1) Prescriptions for driving out exogenous wind:

Powder for Dispelling Wind dispels wind, nourishes the blood, and eliminates heat and dampness, and is usually used to treat urticaria and eczema. Powder of Chuanxiong with Folium Camelliae Sinensis effectively disperses wind in the upper part of the body, and is used for general or regional headache due to the affection by exogenous wind. Powder for Treating Facial Distortion expels wind, eliminates phlegm and relieves convulsion, and is indicated for distortion of the face due to accumulated wind and phlegm in the meridians. Bolus for Mildly Activating the Meridians expels wind and dampness, eliminates phlegm, dredges the meridians, activates blood circulation and relieves pain, and is applicable to cases with arthralgia and hampered movement of the joints due to accumulated wind, cold and dampness, or else phlegm, dampness and blood stasis in the meridians.

(2) Prescriptions for suppressing endogenous wind:

Both Decoction of Cornu Saigae Tataricae and Ramulus Uncariae cum Unicis and Decoction for Calming Liver Wind calm the liver and suppress wind. But the former vigorously purges heat and cools the liver, and is indicated for cases of wind irritation by excessive heat in the liver meridian; while the latter is better at inhibiting liver *yang*, and is used for cases of hyperactive liver *yang* and disturbance of liver wind. Bolus for Serious Endogenous Wind Syndrome nourishes *yin* and suppresses wind, and is indicated for the late stage of seasonal febrile diseases when *yin* is consumed by heat and liver wind is irritated.

CHAPTER TWENTY-ONE

PRESCRIPTIONS FOR EXPELLING INTESTINAL PARASITES

Prescriptions for expelling intestinal parasites (*qu chong ji*) are composed of drugs that expel or kill parasites. They are used for parasitic diseases.

There are many kinds of parasitic diseases, and the methods of treatment also vary accordingly. Prescriptions selected in this chapter are mainly those for expelling and killing intestinal parasites, such as roundworm, pinworm, cestode and hookworm. The common manifestations of parasitic diseases are intermittent abdominal pain with voracious appetite, sallow or pale complexion, whitish patches or reddish lines over the face, grinding of the teeth during sleep, eructation, vomiting, exfoliated tongue coating and alternately large and small pulse; or emaciation, loss of appetite, listlessness, blurred vision, withered hair, and abdominal distention with engorged veins over the body surface in chronic cases. In addition, different kinds of parasitosis may show different characteristics, such as itching of ears and nose and whitish and reddish spots on the mucosa of the lips in case of ascariasis; itching around the anus in cases of enterobiasis; discharge of white parasite segments in cases of cestodiasis; and heterorexia, sallow complexion and edema in cases of ancylostomiasis.

The major drugs used in antiparasitic prescriptions include Fructus Mume, Pericarpium Zanthoxyli, Omphalia, Semen Arecae, Fructus Carpesii and Fructus Quisqualis. However, the treatment of parasitosis should vary with the different syndromes. For instance, Rhizoma Zingiberis and Pericarpium Zanthoxyli should be used to warm the middle *jiao* and expel cold for cases attributed to cold syndrome; Rhizoma Coptidis and Cortex Phellodendri should be included to eliminate heat for cases of heat syndrome; and these drugs should be used together for cases attributed to the coexistence of cold and heat syndromes. Moreover, for cases of malnutrition and spleen dysfunction, Massa Fermentata Medicinalis, Fructus Hordei Germinatus, Semen Myristicae and Radix Aucklandiae, or Radix Ginseng, Radix Scutellariae, Rhizoma Atractylodis Macrocephalae and Radix Glycyrrhizae should be added.

In the administration of antiparasitic prescriptions, it is necessary to (1) avoid fatty food and take the medicine on an empty stomach; (2) avoid overdoses of some antiparasitic drugs since they are poisonous; (3) take care not to prescribe or prescribe with caution the potent drugs to the aged, the debilitated and the pregnant; (4) to prescribe remedies that invigorate the spleen and stomach for cases in which spleen and stomach hypofunction appears because of the administration of antiparasitic prescriptions; and (5) to examine the feces before writing out the antiparasitic prescriptions to confirm there are parasites.

Bolus of Fructus Mume
乌梅丸 *wu mei wan*
(from *Treatise on Cold Diseases*)

Fructus Mume	480 g
Herba Asari	180 g
Rhizoma Zingiberis	300 g
Rhizoma Coptidis	480 g
Radix Angelicae Sinensis	120 g
Radix Aconiti Lateralis Preparata	180 g
Pericarpium Zanthoxyli	120 g
Ramulus Cinnamomi	180 g
Radix Ginseng	180 g
Cortex Phellodendri	180 g

Administration: Soak Mume in vinegar for one night, crush it with the kernel removed and mix it with other drugs, dry and grind them together into fine powder, prepare the powder as boluses with honey, take 9 g with warm water empty-stomached each time, three times daily; or prepare the drugs directly as oral decoction, with dosages reduced proportionally.

Action: Warming the viscera and expelling ascarides.

Indications: Colic due to ascariasis, characterized by fidgetiness, vomiting of ascarides, cold limbs and abdominal pain; or chronic cases of dysentery and diarrhea.

Explanation: This is a prescription often used for colic due to ascariasis. When heat and cold in the stomach and intestines are not properly regulated and irritate ascarides in the intestines, fidgetiness, vomiting of ascarides and abdominal pain occur intermittently. When abdominal pain becomes serious, *yin qi* and *yang qi* counteract each other and cold limbs occur. In the treatment, drugs of both hot and cold nature are used simultaneously to warm the viscera and calm ascarides. Since sour flavor can restrain ascarides, a large dose of Mume, soaked in vinegar, is used to inhibit their activity. Zanthoxyli and Asari expel ascarides with their acrid flavor and warm the viscera and eliminate cold with their warm property. Coptidis and Phellodendri are bitter and cold, and promote the discharge of ascarides and purge heat. In addition, Ramulus Cinnamomi, Zingiberis and Aconiti Lateralis Preparata warm the viscera and dispel cold, and Ginseng and Angelicae Sinensis nourish *qi* and blood. As a whole, the prescription relieves both cold and heat syndromes, eliminates pathogens and invigorates antipathogenic *qi* in order to warm the viscera and calm the ascarides. This prescription is also indicated for long-standing cases of dysentery and diarrhea due to simultaneous presence of cold and heat syndromes and deficient antipathogenic *qi*. But it is not suitable for acute cases of diarrhea and dysentery due to dampness-heat.

Appendant Prescription

Decoction of Picrorhizae and Mume for Calming Ascarides
连梅安蛔汤 *lian mei an hui tang*
(from *Popular Treatise on Cold Diseases*)

It is composed of 3 g of Rhizoma Picrorhizae, 1.5 g of Pericarpium Zanthoxyli (fried), 9 g of Omphalia, 5 g of Fructus Mume (with the kernel removed), 2.5 g of Cortex Phellodendri, and 10 g of Semen Arecae. To be boiled with water three times and divided into three doses, take the decoction twice in the morning on an empty stomach and once in the afternoon. It purges heat and calms ascarides, and is indicated for abdominal pain due to parasitic infection, exhibiting anorexia, even vomiting of ascarides, or irritability, cold limbs, flushed face, dry mouth, red tongue, and rapid pulse and fever.

Decoction for Expelling Cestode
驱绦汤 *qu tao tang*
(from *Proved Recipes*)

Semen Cucurbitae	60-120 g
Semen Arecae	30-60 g

Administration: Take Semen Cucurbitae first, then take the concentrated decoction of Arecae two hours later. After 4-5 hours, diarrhea may occur with the parasite discharged. When diarrhea is absent, 9 g of Natrii Sulfas Exsiccatus can be administered. For children the dosage should be reduced according to age. If the head of the cestode is not discharged, repeat the treatment after half a month. If only part of the cestode comes out of the anus, do not pull it by hand; sitting in warm water would make the cestode come out eventually.

Action: Expelling cestode.

Explanation: Semen Cucurbitae, especially its middle and posterior segments, paralyzes the parasite. Arecae contains several kinds of alkaloid and its antiparasitic ingredient is arecoline, which can paralyze the head and immature segments. It is more effective for Taeniasolium and Taenia murina, Diphyllobothrium latum and Fasciolopsis. It can also serve as a purgative. These two drugs, when used together, mutually enhance each other.

Baby Fattening Bolus
肥儿丸 *fei er wan*
(from *Benevolent Prescriptions from the Pharmaceutical Bureau of the Taiping Period*)

Massa Fermentata Medicinalis (fried)	300 g
Rhizoma Coptidis	300 g

Semen Myristicae	150 g
Fructus Quisqualis	150 g
Fructus Hordei Germinatus (fried)	150 g
Semen Arecae	120 g
Radix Aucklandiae	60 g

Administration: Grind the drugs into fine powder and prepare the powder into boluses with pig bile, each weighing 3 g; take one bolus after dissolving it in water on an empty stomach. The dosage for infants under one year old may be reduced accordingly.

Action: Killing parasites, promoting digestion, invigorating the spleen and purging heat.

Indications: Parasitic infection with abdominal pain and indigestion, along with sallow complexion, emaciation, abdominal distention, fever, halitosis and loose stools.

Explanation: The therapeutic principle for such cases is to expel parasites, promote digestion, invigorate the spleen and purge heat. In the prescription, Massa Fermentata Medicinalis and Hordei Germinatus regulate the middle *jiao*, invigorate the spleen and promote digestion. Coptidis purges stagnant heat. Myristicae, which is fragrant, invigorates the stomach and relieve diarrhea. Aucklandiae regulates *qi* in the middle *jiao* and relieves abdominal pain. Arecae and Quisqualis expel parasites. Bile is used together with Coptidis to eliminate stagnant heat in the liver and stomach. This prescription is designed for infant malnutrition due to parasitosis.

Summary

This chapter examines three principal and one appendant prescriptions. Although they all produce an antiparasitic effect, they have different indications because of their different compositions. Pill of Mume warms the viscera and calms ascarides, and is indicated for colic due to taeniasis with the simultaneous occurrence of cold and heat syndromes. It is a major prescription for Jueyin diseases with symptoms of both cold and heat syndromes, and so is used for vomiting and chronic dysentery thus resulted. Baby Fattening Bolus invigorates the spleen, promotes indigestion, purges heat and kills parasites, and is indicated for infant malnutrition caused by parasitic infection arising from spleen deficiency accompanied by stagnant heat. Decoction for Expelling Cestode is especially effective for taeniasis.

Appendix I

A List of Common Patent Medicines

A. Remedies to Relieve Exterior Syndrome

1. Bolus of Cornu Saigae Tataricae and Forsythiae for Detoxification

羚翘解毒丸 (*ling qiao jie du wan*)

Composition: Cornu Saigae Tataricae, Fructus Forsythiae, Radix Puerariae, Flos Lonicerae, Radix Trichosanthis, Cortex Phellodendri, Folium Isatidis, Gypsum Fibrosum, Fructus Gardeniae, Ramulus Uncariae cum Uncis, Radix Paeoniae Rubra, Lasiosphaera seu Calvatis, Bulbus Fritillariae Thunbergii, Folium Mori, Fructus Aurantii, Radix Scutellariae, Rhizoma Anemarrhenae, Herba Menthae, Radix Scrophulariae, and Borneolum Syntheticum.

Action: Dispersing wind from the surface, eliminating heat and toxins.

Indications: Common cold, exhibiting high fever, sore throat, headache, cough, sore limbs, thirst and dry throat.

Administration and Dosage: Oral use; one bolus with warm water, twice daily.

Specification: 9 g per bolus.

2. Bolus for Releasing and Regulating Lung *Qi*

通宣理肺丸 (*tong xuan li fei wan*)

Composition: Folium Perillae, Radix Scutellariae, Fructus Aurantii, Radix Glycyrrhizae, Pericarpium Citri Reticulatae, Radix Platycodi, Poria, Semen Armeniacae Amarum, Radix Peucedani, Herba Ephedrae, and Rhizoma Pinelliae Preparata.

Action: Dispelling cold, relieving exterior syndrome, releasing lung *qi* and relieving cough.

Indications: Cough due to exogenous pathogens, exhibiting fever, chills, headache, anhidrosis, sore limbs and runny nose.

Administration and Dosage: Oral use; two boluses with warm water, twice or three times daily.

Specification: 6 g per bolus.

3. Liquor Agastaches for Restoring Antipathogenic *Qi*

藿香正气水 (*huo xiang zheng qi shui*)

Composition: Rhizoma Atractylodis, Pericarpium Citri Reticulatae, Cortex Magnoliae Officinalis, Radix Angelicae Dahuricae, Poria, Pericarpium Arecae Rhizoma Pinelliae, Extract of Glycyrrhizae, Oleum Agastaches, and Oleum Perillae Folium.

Action: Eliminating summer-heat, relieving exterior syndrome, removing dampness and regulating the middle *jiao*.

Indications: Sunstroke, exhibiting dizziness, distensive pain in the epigastrium and abdomen, vomiting and diarrhea.

Administration and Dosage: Oral use; 2-10 ml, twice or three times daily.

Specification: 10 ml per ampoule.

4. Medicated Tea for Common Cold
午时茶 (*wu shi cha*)

Composition: Folium Camelliae Sinensis, Fructus Forsythiae, Rhizoma Atractylodis, Radix Bupleuri, Radix Ledebouriellae, Fructus Aurantii Immaturus, Radix Peucedani, Radix Platycodi, Fructus Crataegi, Rhizoma Chuanxiong, Rhizoma seu Radix Notopterygii, Pericarpium Citri Reticulatae, Herba Agastaches, Folium Perillae, Massa Fermentata Medicinalis, Cortex Magnoliae Officinalis, Radix Glycyrrhizae, Fructus Hordei Germinatus, and Radix Angelicae Dahuricae.

Action: Relieving exterior syndrome, regulating the middle *jiao*, promoting digestion and invigorating the stomach.

Indications: Common cold of wind-cold type with indigestion, exhibiting chills, fever, headache, nasal stuffiness, cough, abdominal pain, vomiting, and diarrhea.

Administration and Dosage: Oral use; mix two pieces in water, twice daily; or drink it as tea every day.

Specification: 9 g per piece.

5. Instant Granules for Common Cold and Eliminating Heat
感冒清热冲剂 (*gan mao qing re chong ji*)

Composition: Spica Schizonepetae, Radix Ledebouriellae, Herba Menthae, Folium Perillae, Radix Angelicae Dahuricae, Radix Bupleuri, Rhizoma Phragmitis, Radix Puerariae, Radix Platycodi, Semen Armeniacae Amarum, and Herba Corydalis Bungeanae.

Action: Relieving exterior syndrome and purging heat.

Indications: Common cold, exhibiting headache, fever, chills, general achiness and heaviness, runny nose, cough and dry throat.

Administration and Dosage: Mix it in boiled water for oral use; 12 g per dose, twice daily.

Specification: 12 g per package.

6. Pill of Ledebouriellae for Dispersing Wind from the Surface

防风通圣丸 (*fang feng tong sheng wan*)

Composition: Radix Ledebouriellae, Herba Schizonepetae, Fructus Forsythiae, Herba Ephedrae, Herba Menthae, Rhizoma Chuanxiong, Radix Angelicae Sinensis, Radix Paeoniae Alba (fried), Fructus Gardeniae, Radix et Rhizoma Rhei (prepared with wine), Natrii Sulfas, Gypsum Fibrosum, Radix Scutellariae, Radix Platycodi, Radix Glycyrrhizae, Talcum, and Rhizoma Atractylodis Macrocephalae.

Action: Expelling wind, relieving exterior syndrome, purging heat and relieving constipation.

Indications: Affection by exogenous wind and accumulated heat with excess syndrome in both the exterior and interior, exhibiting chills, high fever, headache, dry throat, constipation, deep-colored urine, skin infection and eczema.

Administration and Dosage: Oral use; take 6 g with warm water each time, one or two times daily.

Specification: 18 g per package.

B. Remedies to Purge Heat

1. Tablet of Calculus Bovis for Detoxification

牛黄解毒片 (*niu huang jie du pian*)

Composition: Calculus Bovis, Borneolum Syntheticum, Realgar, Radix Platycodi, Radix Scutellariae, Radix Glycyrrhizae, Radix et Rhizoma Rhei, and Gypsum Fibrosum.

Action: Purging heat and toxins.

Indications: Heat-toxic syndrome with stagnant fire, exhibiting sore throat, toothache, gingival swelling, aphthae, conjunctivitis and constipation.

Administration and Dosage: Oral use; two tablets each time, twice or three times daily.

Specification: 0.4 g per tablet.

2. Bolus of Calculus Bovis for Purging Heat

牛黄上清丸 (*niu huang shang qing wan*)

Composition: Calculus Bovis, Radix et Rhizoma Rhei, Rhizoma Coptidis, Radix Scutellariae, Cortex Phellodendri, Gypsum Fibrosum, Fructus Gardeniae, Fructus Forsythiae, Borneolum Syntheticum, Radix Paeoniae Rubra, Radix Rehmanniae, Radix Angelicae Sinensis, Herba Menthae, Flos Chrysanthemi, Rhizoma Chuanxiong, Spica Schizonepetae, Radix Angelicae Dahuricae, Radix Platycodi, and Radix Glycyrrhizae.

Action: Purging heat and fire, reducing swelling and relieving pain.

Indications: Headache, dizziness, acute conjunctivitis, aphthae, gingival swelling and pain, constipation.

Administration and Dosage: Oral use; one bolus each time, twice daily.

Specification: 6 g per bolus.

3. Pill of Coptidis and Aucklandiae

香连丸 (*xiang lian wan*)

Composition: Rhizoma Coptidis (prepared with Fructus Evodiae), and Radix Aucklandiae.

Action: Purging heat, drying dampness, activating *qi* circulation and dispersing stagnation.

Indications: Dysentery due to dampness-heat, exhibiting discharge of bloody and mucous stools, abdominal pain and tenesmus.

Administration and Dosage: Oral use; 3-6 g each time, twice or three times daily; reduced dosage for children.

Specification: 18 g per package.

4. *Zijin* Troche

紫金锭 (*zi jin ding*)

Composition: Pseudobulbus Cremastrae Appendiculatae, Radix Knoxiae, Semen Euphorbiae Lathyridis, Galla Chinensis, Moschus, Realgar, and Cinnabaris.

Action: Removing toxins, eliminating phlegm, inducing resuscitation, reducing swelling and relieving pain.

Indications: Affection by phlegm-turbidity, exhibiting distention and pain in the epigastrium and abdomen, vomiting, diarrhea; phlegm-syncope syndrome in children; and furuncles (external application).

Administration and Dosage: Oral use; 0.6-1.5 g each time, twice daily; or grind with vinegar for external application. Contraindicated for pregnant women.

Specification: 0.3 or 3 g per troche.

5. Pill of Two Wonder Drugs

二妙丸 (*er miao wan*)

Composition: Cortex Phellodendri, and Rhizoma Atractylodis.

Action: Purging heat and drying dampness.

Indications: Cases of downward attack by dampness-heat, exhibiting redness, swelling, heat and pain in the knees and feet, leucorrhagia and eczema of scrotum.

Administration and Dosage: Oral use; 9 g each time, one or two times daily.

Specification: 3 g per 50 pills; 9 g per package.

6. Pill of Six Precious Drugs

六神丸 (*liu shen wan*)

Composition: Calculus Bovis, Moschus, Borneolum Syntheticum, Venenum Bufonis,

Margarita, and Realgar.

Action: Purging heat, removing toxins, reducing swelling and relieving pain.

Indications: Tonsillitis, acute pharyngeal diseases, sore throat and pharyngitis in scarlet fever.

Administration and Dosage: Oral use (slowly dissolved in the mouth); 10 pills each time, one or two times daily; one pill for each year of age in children. External use: dissolve 10 pills in water or vinegar and apply topically, several times daily. Contraindicated for pregnant women.

Specification: 3 g per 100 pills; 30 pills per bottle.

7. *Zuojin* Pill

左金丸 (*zuo jin wan*)

Composition: Rhizoma Coptidis, and Fructus Evodiae.

Action: Purging heat and fire, regulating the stomach and relieving pain.

Indications: Cases of hyperactive liver and stomach fire, exhibiting epigastric and hypochondriac pain, acid regurgitation, bitter taste and epigastric upset.

Administration and Dosage: Oral use; 3-6 g each time, twice daily.

8. Powder of Borneolum Syntheticum and Borax

冰硼散 (*bing peng san*)

Composition: Borneolum Syntheticum, Borax, Natrii Sulfas Exsiccatus, and Cinnabaris.

Action: Purging heat, removing toxins, reducing swelling and relieving pain.

Indications: Sore throat, gingival swelling and pain, and aphthae.

Administration and Dosage: External use; several times daily.

9. *Xilei* Powder

锡类散 (*xi lei san*)

Composition: Indigo Naturalis, Calculus Bovis, Borneolum Syntheticum, Urocteae (charred), Margarita, ivory slices, and finger nails.

Action: Purging heat, removing toxins and necrotic tissue and promoting granulation.

Indications: Erosion, swelling and pain of the throat, mouth, tongue and gums.

Administration and Dosage: External use; several times daily.

Specification: 0.3 g per bottle.

10. Powder of Margarita, Calculus Bovis for Throat Disorders

珠黄吹喉散 (*zhu huang chui hou san*)

Composition: Margarita, Calculus Bovis, Pulvis Citrulli, Borax, Realgar, Catechu, Rhizoma Coptidis, Cortex Phellodendri, and Borneolum Syntheticum.

Action: Removing toxins, reducing swelling, removing necrotic tissue and promoting granulation.

Indications: Swelling, pain and blister in the throat, mouth and tongue.

Administration and Dosage: External use; 3-5 times daily.

C. Tonics

1. Capsule of Two Precious Drugs
双宝素 (*shuang bao su*)

Composition: Fresh Queen Bee Jelly, Radix Ginseng, and Glucose.

Action: Strengthening the resistance, and invigorating the liver and spleen.

Indications: General debility with palpitation, lassitude and anorexia.

Administration and Dosage: Oral use; one or two capsules each time, three times daily.

Specification: 30 capsules per package.

2. *Erzhi* Pill
二至丸 (*er zhi wan*)

Composition: Fructus Ligustri Lucidi, and Herba Ecliptae.

Action: Invigorating the liver and kidney, nourishing *yin* and blood.

Indications: Cases of deficient liver and kidney *yin*, exhibiting dizziness, insomnia, dreaminess, flaccidity of lower limbs, and precocious gray discoloration of hairs.

Administration and Dosage: Oral use; 6-9 g each time, twice daily.

3. Pill of Mori and Sesami Nigrum
桑麻丸 (*sang ma wan*)

Composition: Folium Mori, and Semen Sesami Nigrum.

Action: Nourishing the liver and kidney, expelling wind and improving vision.

Indications: Cases of liver and kidney deficiency, exhibiting dizziness, poor vision, and irritative epiphora.

Administration and Dosage: Oral use; 6 g each time, two or three times daily.

4. Extract of Asparagi and Ophiopogonis
二冬膏 (*er dong gao*)

Composition: Radix Asparagi, and Radix Ophiopogonis.

Action: Nourishing *yin* and eliminating lung heat.

Indications: Cases of dryness-heat in the lung and stomach, exhibiting sore throat and dry cough.

Administration and Dosage: Oral use; 9-15 g each time, twice daily.

5. Tonic Bolus (Pill) of Placenta Hominis
河车大造丸 (*he che da zao wan*)

Composition: Placenta Hominis, Rhizoma Rehmanniae Preparata, Radix Asparagi, Radix Ophiopogonis, Cortex Eucommiae, Radix Achyranthis Bidentatae, Cortex Phellodendri, and Plastrum Testudinis.

Action: Invigorating the lung and kidney, nourishing *yin* and purging heat.

Indications: Cases of deficient lung and kidney *yin*, exhibiting hectic fever, cough, night sweating, nocturnal emission and weakness of the loins and knees.

Administration and Dosage: Oral use; water-honeyed pills, 6 g each time; small honeyed pills, 9 g each time; and large honeyed bolus, one piece each time, twice daily.

Specification: 9 g per bolus.

6. Bolus of Ginseng and Cornu Cervi Pantotrichum
参茸丸 (*shen rong wan*)

Composition: Radix Ginseng, Cornu Cervi Pantotrichum, Rhizoma Rehmanniae Preparata, Radix Morindae Officinalis, Radix Salviae Miltiorrhizae, Radix Codonopsis Pilosulae, Fructus Lycii, Herba Cistanches, Semen Nelumbinis, Semen Euryales, Arillus Longan, Radix Polygalae, and Rhizoma Dioscoreae.

Action: Invigorating *qi*, strengthening *yang*, enriching the blood and promoting the generation of vital essence.

Indications: Cases of deficiency of both *yin* and *yang*, exhibiting listlessness, shortness of breath, tinnitus, palpitation, nocturnal emission, praecox ejaculation, sore loins and knees, metrorrhagia and leukorrhagia.

Administration and Dosage: Oral use; one bolus each time, twice daily.

Specification: 9 g per bolus.

7. Pill of Deer
全鹿丸 (*quan lu wan*)

Composition: Fresh deer meat, Colla Cornu Cervi, Cornu Cervi pantotrichum, kidney and tail of deer, Radix Ginseng, Radix Astragali, Rhizoma Atractylodis Macrocephalae (fried), Poria, Radix Glycyrrhizae, Rhizoma Dioscoreae, Rhizoma Rehmanniae Preparata, Radix Rehmanniae (dried), Radix Angelicae Sinensis, Rhizoma Chuanxiong, Fructus Lycii, Semen Cuscutae, Fructus Broussonetiae, Fructus Rubi, Semen Trigonellae, Cortex Eucommiae, Radix Dipsaci, Radix Achyranthis Bidentatae, Fructus Psoraleae, Radix Morindae Officinalis, Herba Cistanches, Herba Cynomorii, Halitum, Depositum Urinae Preparatum, Radix Asparagi, Radix Ophiopogonis, Fructus Foeniculi, Pericarpium Zanthoxyli, Lignum Aquilariae Resinatum, Pericarpium Citri Reticulatae, Semen Euryales, and Fructus Schisandrae.

Action: Strengthening *yang*, invigorating *yin*, and enriching *qi* and blood.

Indications: Cases of deficiency of both *yin* and *yang*, exhibiting general debility, dizziness, tinnitus, nocturnal emission, sore loins and knees, anorexia, lassitude, spontaneous perspiration, night sweating, metrorrhagia and leukorrhagia.

Administration and Dosage: Oral use; one bolus each time, twice daily.

Specification: 9 g per bolus.

8. *Guiling* Powder

龟龄集 (*gui ling ji*)

Composition: Cornu Cervi Pantotrichum, Radix Ginseng, Radix Rehmanniae, Radix Rehmanniae Preparata, Hippocampus, Cortex Eucommiae (charred), Herba Cistanches, Herba Cynomorii, Fructus Psoraleae, Semen Cuscutae, Fructus Lycii, Radix Asparagi, Radix Aconiti Lateralis (soaked in salt solution), brain of sparrow, silk moth (legs and wings removed), dragonfly, Flos Caryophylli, Radix Glycyrrhizae, Herba Epimedii, Halitum, Herba Asari, Fossilia Spiriferis, Fructus Amomi, Semen Impatientis, Squama Manitis, Cortex Lycii Radicis, Cinnabaris, and Radix Achyranthis Bidentatae.

Action: Invigorating the kidney and strengthening *yang*.

Indications: Cases of kidney *yang* deficiency, exhibiting impotence, nocturnal emission, dyspneic cough, dizziness, tinnitus, cold and pain in the loins and knees, spasm of the lower abdomen, hypomensis, metrorrhagia, leukorrhea and morning diarrhea.

Administration and Dosage: Oral use; 0.3 g daily.

Specification: 3 g per bottle.

9. Bolus (Pill) of Black-Bone Chicken

乌鸡白凤丸(*wu ji bai feng wan*)

Composition: Black-bone chicken (with feather, paws and intestines removed), Radix Ginseng, Colla Cornu Cervi, Concha Ostreae, Radix Paeoniae Alba, Radix Angelicae Sinensis, Radix Astragali, Carapax Trionycis, Ootheca Mantidis, Radix Rehmanniae, Radix Rehmanniae Preparata, Rhizoma Chuanxiong, Radix Glycyrrhizae, Radix Salviae Miltiorrhizae, Semen Euryales, Rhizoma Dioscoreae, Radix Stellariae, Cornu Cervi Degelatinatum, Radix Asparagi and Rhizoma Cyperi Preparata.

Action: Invigorating *qi*, enriching the blood, regulating menstruation and relieving leukorrhagia.

Indications: Cases of deficiency of both *qi* and blood, exhibiting general debility, sore loins and knees, irregular menstruation, metrorrhagia and leukorrhagia.

Administration and Dosage: Oral use; one bolus each time, twice daily.

Specification: 9 g per bottle.

10. Pill of Five Kinds of Seed for Invigorating the Kidney

五子补肾丸(*wu zi bu shen wan*)

Composition: Fructus Lycii, Semen Cuscutae, Fructus Rubi, Fructus Schisandrae, and Semen Plantaginis.

Action: Invigorating the kidney and replenishing vital essence.

Indications: Lumbago due to kidney deficiency, and dribbling urination.

Administration and Dosage: Oral use; water-honeyed pills, 6 g each dose; small honeyed pills, 9 g each dose; or one large honeyed bolus each dose, twice daily.

Specification: 9 g per large bolus.

11. *Zuoci* Bolus for Deafness
耳聋左慈丸 (*er long zuo ci wan*)

Composition: Magnetitum Usta, Rhizoma Rehmanniae Preparata, Fructus Corni, Rhizoma Dioscoreae, Poria, Rhizoma Alismatis, Cortex Moutan Radicis, and Radix Bupleuri.

Action: Nourishing the kidney and calming the liver.

Indications: Cases of liver and kidney *yin* deficiency, exhibiting tinnitus, deafness and dizziness.

Administration and Dosage: Oral use; water-honeyed pills, 6 g each dose; small honeyed pills, 9 g each dose; or one large honeyed bolus; twice daily.

Specification: 9 g per large honeyed bolus.

12. Bolus for Invigorating the Spleen
启脾丸 (*qi pi wan*)

Composition: Radix Ginseng, Rhizoma Atractylodis Macrocephalae (fried), Poria, Radix Glycyrrhizae, Pericarpium Citri Reticulatae, Rhizoma Dioscoreae, Semen Nelumbinis, Fructus Crataegi (fried), Massa Fermentata Medicinalis (fried), Fructus Hordei Germinatus (fried), and Rhizoma Alismatis.

Action: Invigorating the spleen and regulating the stomach.

Indications: Cases of spleen and stomach deficiency, exhibiting anorexia, indigestion, abdominal distention and loose stools.

Administration and Dosage: Oral use; one bolus each time, two or three times daily. For children under three years old, the dosage is to be reduced accordingly.

Specification: 3 g per bolus.

13. Eight-Ingredient Bolus Containing Leonuri
八珍益母丸(*ba zhen yi mu wan*)

Composition: Herba Leonuri, Radix Codonopsis Pilosulae, Rhizoma Atractylodis Macrocephalae (fried), Poria, Radix Glycyrrhizae, Radix Angelicae Sinensis, Radix Paeoniae Alba (fried), Rhizoma Chuanxiong, and Radix Rehmanniae Preparata.

Action: Invigorating *qi* and blood and regulating menstruation.

Indications: Disorders in women due to deficiency of both *qi* and blood, exhibiting general debility, lassitude and irregular menstruation.

Administration and Dosage: Oral use; water-honeyed pills, 6 g each dose, and large honeyed bolus, one piece each dose, twice daily.

Specification: 9 g per large bolus.

D. Remedies to Expel Wind-Dampness

1. Bolus of Gastrodiae

天麻丸 (*tian ma wan*)

Composition: Rhizoma Gastrodiae, Rhizoma seu Radix Notopterygii, Radix Angelicae Pubescentis, Rhizoma Dioscoreae Hypoglaucae, Cortex Eucommiae Preparata, Radix Achyranthis Bidentatae, Radix Aconiti Lateralis Preparata, Radix Rehmanniae, Radix Scrophulariae, and Radix Angelicae Sinensis.

Action: Expelling wind and dampness, relaxing muscles and tendons, dredging the meridians, activating blood circulation and relieving pain.

Indications: Arthralgia due to wind-dampness, exhibiting spasms of the limbs, numb hands and feet, and sore loins and knees.

Administration and Dosage: Oral use; water-honeyed pills, 6 g each dose, and large honeyed bolus, one piece each dose, two or three times daily; contraindicated for pregnant women.

Specification: 9 g per bolus.

2. Pill of Chaenomelis

木瓜丸 (*mu gua wan*)

Composition: Fructus Chaenomelis, Radix Angelicae Sinensis, Rhizoma Chuanxiong, Radix Angelicae Dahuricae, Radix Clematidis, Rhizoma Cibotii Preparata, Radix Achyranthis Bidentatae, Caulis Spatholobi, Caulis Piperis Futokadsurae, Radix Ginseng, Radix Aconiti Preparata and Radix Aconiti Kusnezoffii Preparata.

Action: Expelling wind and cold, dredging the meridians and relieving pain.

Indications: Arthralgia due to wind-cold-dampness, exhibiting numb limbs, general achiness, pain and weakness in the loins and difficulty in walking.

Administration and Dosage: Oral use; 30 pills each dose, twice daily; contraindicated for pregnant women.

Specification: 18 g per 10 pills.

3. Bolus of Siegesbeckiae

豨莶丸 (*xi xian wan*)

Composition: Herba Siegesbeckiae.

Action: Expelling wind and dampness, and easing the joints.

Indications: Arthralgia due to wind-dampness, exhibiting sore and weak loins and knees, and numb limbs.

Administration and Dosage: Oral use; one bolus each time, two or three times daily.

Specification: 9 g per bolus.

4. ***Shiguogong*** **Medicated Wine**

史国公药酒 (*shi guo gong yao jiu*)

Composition: Radix Glycyrrhizae, Rhizoma seu Radix Notopterygii, Rhizoma Chuanxiong, Radix Angelicae Sinensis, Radix Angelicae Pubescentis, Radix Dipsaci, Excrementum Bombycis, Fructus Chaenomelis, Radix Achyranthis Bidentatae, Radix Ledebouriellae, Rhizoma Polygonati Odorati, Ramulus Taxilli, Rhizoma Atractylodis Macrocephalae, Flos Carthami, Colla Cornu Corvi, Colla Carapax Trionycis, and Massa Fermentata Medicinalis.

Action: Expelling wind and dampness, enriching the blood and activating the meridians.

Indications: Arthralgia due to wind-cold-dampness, exhibiting numb limbs.

Administration and Dosage: Oral use; 9-10 ml each dose, twice or three times daily.

5. Medicated Wine of Centropus Sinensis

毛鸡药酒 (*mao ji yao jiu*)

Composition: Centropus Sinensis, Radix Angelicae Sinensis, Rhizoma Chuanxiong, Radix Angelicae Dahuricae, Flos Carthami, Radix Paeoniae Rubra, Semen Persicae, Rhizoma Homalomenae, and Poria.

Action: Warming the meridians, expelling wind, activating blood circulation and removing blood stasis.

Indications: Puerperant with dizziness, sore and weak limbs, dysmenorrhea due to blood stasis.

Administration and Dosage: Oral use; 15-30 ml each dose, twice or three times daily.

6. Medicated Wine of Os Tigris and Chaenomelis

虎骨木瓜酒 (*hu gu mu gua jiu*)

Composition: Os Tigris Preparata, Fructus Chaenomelis, Rhizoma Chuanxiong, Radix Cyathulae, Radix Angelicae Sinensis, Rhizoma Gastrodiae, Cortex Acanthopanacis Radicis, Flos Carthami, Radix Dipsaci, Radix Solani Melongenae, Rhizoma Polygonati Odorati, Radix Gentianae Macrophyllae, Radix Ledebouriellae, and Ramulus Mori.

Action: Expelling wind, relieving pain, eliminating dampness and cold.

Indications: Arthralgia due to wind-cold-dampness, exhibiting muscular spasm, numb limbs, arthralgia, deviation of the eyes and mouth, or acute arthritis.

Administration and Dosage: Oral use; 15-30 ml each dose, twice daily.

7. Dog-Skin Plaster
狗皮膏 (*gou pi gao*)

Composition: Fructus Aurantii, Pericarpium Citri Reticulatae Viride, Semen Hydnocarpi, Halloysitum Rubrum, Radix Paeoniae Rubra, Rhizoma Gastrodiae, Radix Glycyrrhizae, Radix Linderae, Radix Achyranthis Bidentatae, Rhizoma seu Radix Notopterygii, Cortex Phellodendri, Fructus Psoraleae, Radix Clematidis, Radix Aconiti, Radix Dipsaci, Radix Cynanchi Atrati, Semen Persicae, Radix Aconiti Lateralis, Rhizoma Chuanxiong, Radix Aconiti Kusnezoffii, Cortex Eucommiae, Radix Polygalae, Squama Manitis, Rhizoma Cyperi, Rhizoma Atractylodis Macrocephalae, Fructus Toosendan, Bombyx Batryticatus, Fructus Foeniculi, Fructus Cnidii, Radix Angelicae Sinensis, Herba Asari, Semen Cuscutae, Pericarpium Citri Reticulatae, Caulis Sinomenii, Radix Aucklandiae, Cortex Cinnamomi, Calomelae, Catechu, Flos Caryophylli, Olibanum, Myrrha, Resina Draconis, and Camphora.

Action: Expelling wind and cold, relaxing the tendons, activating the meridians, improving blood circulation and relieving pain.

Indications: Arthralgia due to wind-cold-dampness, exhibiting lumbago, pain of legs, and numbness; trauma.

Administration and Dosage: External use after being softened by heat; change the plaster every 5-7 days.

Specification: 15 g for small pieces, 30 g for large pieces.

8. Plaster for Rheumatism
伤湿止痛膏 (*shang shi zhi tong gao*)

Composition: Radix Aconiti Kusnezoffii, Radix Aconiti, Olibanum, Myrrha, Semen Strychni, Flos Caryophylli, and Cortex Cinnamomi.

Action: Expelling wind and dampness, activating blood circulation and alleviating pain.

Indications: Rheumatism with arthralgia and muscular pain.

Administration and Dosage: External use.

E. Remedies to Regulate *Qi*

1. Bolus for Soothing the Liver
舒肝丸 (*shu gan wan*)

Composition: Fructus Toosendan, Radix Corydalis, Radix Paeoniae Alba (fried), Rhizoma Curcumae Longae, Radix Aucklandiae, Lignum Aquilariae Resinatum, Semen Myristicae, Fructus Amomi, Cortex Magnoliae Officinalis Preparata, Pericarpium Citri Reticulatae, Fructus Aurantii (fried), Poria, and Cinnabaris.

Action: Soothing the liver, regulating *qi* and alleviating pain.

Indications: Cases of liver *qi* stagnation, exhibiting distention and fullness in the chest and hypochondrium, epigastric pain, vomiting, stomach upset and acid regurgitation.

Administration and Dosage: Oral use; one bolus each dose, two or three times daily.

Specification: 6 g per bolus.

2. Pill Containing Nine Drugs for Relieving Pain
九气拈痛丸 (*jiu qi nian tong wan*)

Composition: Rhizoma Cyperi Preparata, Radix Aucklandiae, Rhizoma Alpiniae Officinarum, Pericarpium Citri Reticulatae, Radix Curcumae, Rhizoma Zedoariae Preparata, Radix Corydalis Preparata, Semen Arecae, Radix Glycyrrhizae, and Faeces Trogopterori.

Action: Regulating *qi*, activating blood circulation, dispersing masses and relieving pain.

Indications: Epigastric pain, distention in the hypochondriac region and abdominal masses.

Administration and Dosage: Oral use; 6-9 g each dose, twice daily.

Specification: 20 pills per g.

3. Pill of Foeniculi and Citri Reticulatae
茴香橘核丸 (*hui xiang ju he wan*)

Composition: Fructus Foeniculi, Fructus Anisi Stellati, Semen Citri Reticulatae (fried), Semen Litchi, Fructus Psoraleae, Cortex Cinnamomi, Fructus Toosendan, Radix Corydalis Preparata, Rhizoma Zedoariae Preparata, Radix Aucklandiae, Rhizoma Cyperi Preparata, Pericarpium Citri Reticulatae Viride (fried), Thallus Eckloniae, Semen Arecae, Olibanum Preparata, Semen Persicae, and Squama Manitis.

Action: Activating *qi* circulation, expelling cold, reducing swelling and alleviating pain.

Indications: Hernia and testalgia.

Administration and Dosage: Oral use; 6-9 g per dose, twice daily.

Specification: 20 pills per g.

4. Pill for Regulating *Qi* in the Chest
开胸顺气丸 (*kai xiong shun qi wan*)

Composition: Semen Arecae, Semen Pharbitidis, Pericarpium Citri Reticulatae, Radix Aucklandis, Cortex Magnoliae Officinalis Preparata, Rhizoma Sparganii Preparata, Rhizoma Zedoariae Preparata, and Fructus Gleditsiae Abnormalis.

Action: Promoting digestion, activating *qi* circulation and alleviating pain.

Indications: Dyspepsia due to stagnant *qi*, exhibiting distention and fullness of the chest and abdomen, and epigastric pain.

Administration and Dosage: Oral use; 3-9 g each time, one or two times daily.

5. Bolus of Ten Fragrant Drugs
十香丸 (*shi xiang wan*)

Composition: Lignum Aquilariae Resinatum, Radix Aucklandiae, Semen Litchi, Fructus Gleditsiae Abnormalis, Flos Caryophylli, Fructus Foeniculi, Rhizoma Cyoeri, Pericarpium Citri Reticulatae, Radix Linderae, and Rhizoma Alismatis.

Action: Activating *qi* circulation, dispersing stagnant *qi*, expelling cold and alleviating pain.

Indications: Abdominal pain due to stagnant *qi*, hernial pain and dysmenorrhea.

Administration and Dosage: Oral use; one bolus per dose, twice daily.

F. Remedies to Activate the Blood and Remove Blood Stasis

1. Bolus for Regulating Menstruation
调经丸 (*tiao jing wan*)

Composition: Radix Angelicae Sinensis, Radix Paeoniae Alba Preparata, Rhizoma Chuanxiong, Radix Rehmanniae Preparata, Folium Artemisiae Argyi (fried), Rhizoma Cyperi Preparata, Pericarpium Citri Reticulatae, Rhizoma Pinelliae Preparata, Poria, Radix Glycyrrhizae, Rhizoma Atractylodis Macrocephalae (fried), Fructus Evodiae, Fructus Foeniculi, Radix Corydalis Preparata, Myrrha Preparata, Herba Leonuri, Cortex Moutan Radicis, Radix Dipsaci, Radix Scutellariae (fried), Radix Ophiopogonis, and Colla Corii Asini.

Action: Regulating *qi*, blood and menstruation, and alleviating pain.

Indications: Cases of *qi* and blood stagnation, exhibiting irregular menstruation, dysmenorrhea, metrorrhagia and leukorrhagia.

Administration and Dosage: Oral use; one bolus per dose, two or three times daily.

Specification: 9 g per bolus.

2. Tablet for Removing Abdominal Masses
化症四生片 (*hua zheng si sheng pian*)

Composition: Radix Ginseng, Radix Rehmanniae Preparata, Cortex Cinnamomi, Moschus, Rhizoma Curcumae Longae, Flos Caryophylli, Pericarpium Zanthoxyli, Fructus Evodiae, Rhizoma Alpiniae Officinarum, Fructus Foeniculi, Nudus Bambusae, Rhizoma Cyperi, Flos Carthami, Semen Persicae, Rhizoma Sparganii, Tabanus, Pollen Typhae, Lignum Dalbergiae Odoriferae, Faeces Trogopterori, Radix Angelicae Sinensis, Radix Paeoniae Alba, Lacca Toxicodendri Verniciflne, Olibanum, Myrrha, Hirudo, Rhizoma Chuanxiong, Herba Leonuri, Colla Carapax Trionycis, Radix et Rhizoma Rhei, Rhizoma Corydalis, Folium Artemisiae Argyi, Lignum Sappan, Resina Ferulae, Fructus Perillae and Semen Armeniacae Amarum, and Rhizoma Cyperi.

Action: Dispersing abdominal masses, removing blood stasis and promoting tissue regeneration.

Indications: Abdominal masses due to blood disorder, puerperal abdominal pain due to blood stasis, consumptive disease in women and dysmenorrhea due to blood stasis.

Administration and Dosage: Oral use; 5-6 tablets each time, twice daily. Contraindicated for pregnant women.

3. Bolus of Leonuri

益母丸 (*yi mu wan*)

Composition: Herba Leonuri, Radix Angelicae Sinensis, Radix Chuanxiong, and Radix Aucklandiae.

Action: Activating blood circulation, regulating menstruation, promoting *qi* circulation and alleviating pain.

Indications: Cases of *qi* and blood stagnation, exhibiting irregular menstruation, dysmenorrhea, and postpartum abdominal pain due to blood stasis.

Administration and Dosage: Oral use; one bolus each time, twice daily. Contraindicated for pregnant women and cases with menorrhagia.

Specification: 9 g per bolus.

4. Bolus For Trauma

跌打丸 (*die da wan*)

Composition: Radix Notoginseng, Radix Angelicae Sinensis, Radix Paeoniae Alba, Radix Paeoniae Rubra, Semen Persicae, Flos Carthami, Resina Draconis, Herba Artemisiae Anomalae, Rhizoma Drynariae, Radix Dipsaci, Lignum Sappan, Cortex Moutan Radicis, Olibanum Preparata, Myrrha Preparata, Rhizoma Curcumae Longae, Rhizoma Sparganii Preparata, Semen Melo, Radix Ledebouriellae, Fructus Aurantii Immaturus (fried), Radix Platycodi, Radix Glycyrrhizae, Caulis Akebiae, Pyritum Usta, and Eupolyphaga seu Steleophaga.

Action: Activating blood circulation, removing blood stasis, reducing swelling and alleviating pain.

Indications: Trauma, fracture, traumatic ecchymosis and sprain.

Administration and Dosage: Oral use; one bolus each time, twice daily. Contraindicated for pregnant women.

Specification: 3 g per bolus.

5. Plaster for Regulating *Yang* to Remove Stagnation

阳和解凝膏 (*yang he jie ning gao*)

Composition: Herba Arctii (fresh), Folium Impatientis (fresh), Radix Aconiti (fresh), Ramulus Cinnamomi, Radix et Rhizoma Rhei, Radix Angelicae Sinensis, Radix Aconiti Kusnezoffii (fresh), Radix Aconiti Lateralis (fresh), Lumbricus Bombyx Batryticatus, Radix Paeoniae Rubra, Radix Angelicae Dahuricae, Radix Ampelopsis, Rhizoma Bletillae, Radix Chuanxiong, Radix Dipsaci, Radix Ledebouriellae, Herba Schizonepetae, Faeces Trogopterorum, Radix Aucklandiae, Fructus Citri, Pericarpium Citri Reticulatae, Cortex Cinnamomi, Olibanum, Myrrha, Storax, and Moschus.

Action: Dispersing cold and dampness, and activating *qi* and blood circulation.

Indications: The early stage of deep-rooted *yin*-type carbuncle, and scrofula and arthralgia due to wind-dampness.

Administration and Dosage: External use after being softened by heat.,

Specification: 1.5 g, 3 g, 6 g or 9 g per plaster.

6. White Medicated Powder

白药 (*bai yao*)

(The composition is considered a secret and thus omitted.)

Action: Alleviating pain, stopping bleeding, removing blood stasis and promoting tissue regeneration.

Indications: Trauma, incised wound, internal impairment caused by strain, hemoptysis, hematemesis, swelling and pain of the muscles and bones, numbness due to attack by wind and dampness, stomachache and puerperal abdominal pain.

Administration and Dosage: Oral use; two or three times daily, or administer under doctor's guidance; half a bottle for people 5-10 years old and one bottle for people over 10; avoid sour and cold food and turnip when the medicine is taken. Mixed it with wine for external use.

G. Remedies to Tranquilize and Resuscitate

1. Bolus of Calculus Bovis for Relieving Convulsion

牛黄镇惊丸 (*niu huang zhen jing wan*)

Composition: Calculus Bovis, Scorpio, Bombyx Batryticatus (fried), Margarita, Moschus, Cinnabaris, Realgar, Rhizoma Gastrodiae, Ramulus Uncariae cum Uncis, Radix Ledebouriellae, Succinum, Arisaema cum Bile, Rhizoma Typhonii Preparata, Rhizoma Pinelliae Preparata, Concretio Silicea Bambusae, Borneolum Syntheticum, Herba Menthae, and Radix Glycyrrhizae.

Action: Relieving convulsion, tranquilizing the mind, expelling wind and eliminating phlegm.

Indications: Infantile convulsion with high fever, lockjaw and irritability.

Administration and Dosage: Oral use; water-honeyed pills, 1 g per dose, and large honeyed bolus, one piece per dose, one to three times daily. For children under three years old, the dosage should be reduced accordingly.

Specification: 1.5 g per bolus.

2. Pill for Tranquilizing the Mind and Invigorating the Heart
安神补心丹 (*an shen bu xin dan*)

Composition: Radix Salviae Miltiorrhizae, Fructus Schisandrae, Rhizoma Acori Graminei, Cortex Albiziae, Fructus Ligustri Lucidi, Radix Rehmanniae, Semen Cuscutae, Caulis Polygoni Multiflori, Herba Ecliptae, and Concha Margaritifera Usta.

Action: Invigorating the heart and tranquilizing the mind.

Indications: Cases of palpitation, insomnia, dizziness and tinnitus.

Administration and Dosage: 15 pills each time, three times daily.

Specification: 2 g per 15 pills.

3. *Baolong* Bolus of Calculus Bovis
牛黄抱龙丸 (*niu huang bao long wan*)

Composition: Calculus Bovis, Arisaema cum Bile, Concretio Silicea Bambusae, Poria, Succinum, Moschus, Scorpio, Bombyx Batryticatus (fried), Realgar, and Cinnabaris.

Action: Eliminating heat, relieving convulsion, expelling wind and eliminating phlegm.

Indications: Infantile convulsion with high fever, coma and abundant expectoration.

Administration and Dosage: Oral use; one bolus each time, one or two times daily. The dosage for children under one year old should be reduced accordingly.

Specification: 1. 5 g per bolus.

4. Powder of Calculus Macacae Mulattae
猴枣散 (*hou zao san*)

Composition: Calculus Macacae Mulattae, Concretio Silicea Bambusae, Borax, Lapis Chloriti, Bulbus Fritillariae Cirrhosae, Cornu Saigae Tataricae, and Lignum Aquilariae Resinatum.

Action: Eliminating heat and phlegm, promoting resuscitation and relieving convulsion.

Indications: Infantile convulsion with abundant expectoration, shortness of breath and irritability.

Administration and Dosage: Oral use; 0. 3-0. 6 g each time, twice daily.

Specification: 0. 3 g per bottle.

H. Antitussive and Expectorant Remedies

1. Bolus of Exocarpium Citri Rubrum
橘红丸 (*ju hong wan*)

Composition: Exocarpium Citri Rubrum, Pericarpium Citri Reticulatae, Rhizoma Pinelliae Preparata, Poria, Radix Glycyrrhizae, Radix Platycodi, Semen Armeniacae Amarum, Fructus Perillae, Radix Asteris, Flos Farfarae, Pericarpium Trichosanthis, Bulbus Fritillariae Thunbergii, Radix Rehmanniae, Radix Ophiopogonis, and Gypsum Fibrosum.

Action: Eliminating heat, moistening the lung, removing sputum and relieving cough.

Indications: Cough due to lung heat, exhibiting profuse expectoration, dyspnea, chest upset, dry mouth and tongue.

Administration and Dosage: Oral use; small honeyed bolus, 12 g each dose; or large honeyed bolus, two pieces each time, twice daily.

Specification: 6 g per large honeyed bolus.

2. Antitussive Syrup of Armeniacae Amarum and Perillae
杏苏止咳糖浆（*xing su zhi ke tang jiang*）

Composition: Folium Perillae, Semen Armeniacae Amarum, Radix Platycodi, Radix Peucedani, Pericarpium Citri Reticulatae, and Radix Glycyrrhizae.

Action: Releasing lung *qi*, expelling cold, eliminating sputum and relieving cough.

Indications: Common cold of wind-cold type with productive cough.

Administration and Dosage: Oral use; 10-15 ml each time, two or three times daily.

3. Powder of Snake's Bile and Fritillariae Cirrhosae
蛇胆川贝散（*she dan chuan bei san*）

Composition: Snake's bile, and Bulbus Fritillariae Cirrhosae.

Action: Eliminating lung heat and eliminating phlegm.

Indications: Cough due to lung heat with profuse expectoration.

Administration and Dosage: Oral use; 0. 3-0. 6 g each time, one to three times daily.

Specification: 0. 3 g per bottle.

4. Powder of Snake's Bile and Citri Reticulatae
蛇胆陈皮散（*she dan chen pi san*）

Composition: Snake's bile and Pericarpium Citri Reticulatae.

Action: Regulating *qi*, eliminating phlegm, expelling wind and strengthening the stomach.

Indications: Cough due to wind-cold with profuse expectoration and vomiting.

Administration and Dosage: Oral use; 0. 3-0. 6 g each time, two or three times daily.

Specification: 0. 3 g per bottle.

I. Remedies to Improve Digestion

1. Bolus of Crataegi

大山楂丸 (*da shan zha wan*)

Composition: Fructus Crataegi, Massa Fermentata Medicinalis and Fructus Hordei Germinatus (fried).

Action: Improving appetite and relieving dyspepsia.

Indications: Cases of anorexia, dyspepsia, and epigastric and abdominal distention.

Administration and Dosage: Oral use; one or two boluses each time, one to three times daily. The dosage for children is cut by half.

Specification: 9 g per bolus.

2. Pill of Aurantii Immaturus for Promoting Digestion

枳实导滞丸 (*zhi shi dao zhi wan*)

Composition: Fructus Aurantii Immaturus (fried), Radix et Rhizoma Rhei, Rhizoma Coptidis, Radix Scutellariae, Massa Fermentata Medicinalis (fried), Rhizoma Atractylodis Macrocephalae (fried), Poria, and Rhizoma Alismatis.

Action: Promoting digestion, purging dampness and heat.

Indications: Distensive pain in the epigastrium and abdomen, loss of appetite, constipation, and dysentery with tenesmus.

Administration and Dosage: Oral use; 6-9 g each time, twice daily.

3. *Baochi* Powder

保赤散 (*bao chi san*)

Composition: Massa Fermentata Medicinalis (fried), Semen Crotonis Pulveratum, Rhizoma Arisaematis Preparata, and Cinnabaris.

Action: Promoting digestion, eliminating phlegm and relieving convulsion.

Indications: Infantile indigestion with abdominal distention and fullness, constipation, profuse expectoration, palpitation and restlessness.

Administration and Dosage: Oral use; 0. 09 g for children six months to one year old, and 0. 18 g for children two to four years old.

Specification: 0. 09 g per bottle.

J. Remedies to Improve Vision

1. Bolus of Coptidis and Sheep's Liver

黄连羊肝丸 (*huang lian yang gan wan*)

Composition: Rhizoma Coptidis, Radix Picrorhizae, Radix Scutellariae, Cortex Phellodendri, Radix Gentianae, Radix Bupleuri, Pericarpium Citri Reticulatae Viride (fried), Herba Equiseti Hiemalis, Flos Buddlejae, Fructus Leonuri, Semen Cassiae, Concha Haliotidis, Faeces Vespertilionis, and fresh sheep's liver.

Action: Purging liver fire, improving acuity of vision and removing nebula.

Indications: Cases due to preponderant liver fire, exhibiting poor vision, photophobia, conjunctivitis and pterygium.

Administration and Dosage: Oral use; one bolus each time, one or two times daily.

Specification: 9 g per bolus.

2. Bolus of Dendrobii for Improving Acuity of Vision

石斛夜光丸 (*shi hu ye guang wan*)

Composition: Herba Dendrobii, Radix Ginseng, Rhizoma dioscoreae, Poria, Radix Glycyrrhizae, Herba Cistanches, Fructus Lycii, Semen Cuscutae, Radix Rehmanniae, Radix Rehmanniae Preparata, Fructus Schisandrae, Radix Asparagi, Radix Ophiopogonis, Semen Armeniacae Amarum, Radix Ledebouriellae, Rhizoma Chuanxiong, Fructus Aurantii (fried), Radix Coptidis, Radix Achyranthis Bidentatae, Flos Chrysanthemi, Fructus Tribuli (fried), Semen Celosiae, Semen Cassiae, Cornu Rhinocerotis, and Cornu Saigae Tataricae.

Action: Nourishing *yin*, suppressing fire, nourishing the liver and improving the acuity of vision.

Indications: Cases due to liver and kidney deficiency, *yin* deficiency and fire hyperactivity, exhibiting poor and blurred vision, photophobia, lacrimation and mydriasis.

Administration and Dosage: Oral use; water-honeyed pills, 3-6 g per dose, and small honeyed pills, 4.5-9 g per dose, or large honeyed bolus, one piece per dose, twice daily.

Specification: 9 g per large bolus.

3. *Babao* Eyedrop

八宝眼药 (*ba bao yan yao*)

Composition: Margarita, Moschus, Fel Ursi, Os Spiellae seu Sepiae, Borax, Cinnabaris, Borneolum Syntheticum, Calamina, and Pulvis Cornu Heleocharis Dulcis.

Action: Eliminating heat, reducing swelling and improving vision.

Indications: Conjunctivitis, tarsitis, photophobia and sensation of a foreign body in the canthus.

Administration and Dosage: Two or three times daily.

Appendix II

A List of Chinese Drugs Appeared in Volume II

Agkistrodon seu Bungarus 白花蛇
Aloe 芦荟
Alumen 白矾
Arillus Longan 龙眼肉
Arisaema cum Bile 胆南星
Arsenicum 砒霜
Aurum 金

Benzoinum 安息香
Bombyx Batryticatus 僵蚕
Borax 硼砂
Borneolum Syntheticum 冰片
Bulbus Allii Fistulosi 葱白
Bulbus Allii Macrostemi 薤白
Bulbus Fritillariae Cirrhosae 川贝母
Bulbus Fritillariae Thunbergii 浙贝母
Bulbus Lilii 百合

Cacumen Biotae 侧柏
Calamina 炉干石
Calcitum 寒水石
Calculus Bovis 牛黄
Calculus Macacae Mulattae 猴枣
Calomelae 轻粉
Calyx Kaki 柿蒂
Camphora 樟脑
Carapax Eretmochelydis 玳瑁
Carapax Trionycis 鳖甲
Catechu 儿茶
Caulis Akebiae 木通
Caulis Bambusae in Taeniam 竹茹
Caulis Lonicerae 忍冬藤
Caulis Perillae 紫苏梗
Caulis Piperis Futokadsurae 海风藤
Caulis Polygoni Multiflori 夜交藤
Caulis Sargentodoxae 红藤
Caulis Sinomenii 清风藤
Caulis Spatholobi 鸡血藤
Centropus Sinensis 毛鸡
Cinnabaris 朱砂
Colla Carapax Trionycis 鳖甲胶
Colla Corii Asini 阿胶
Colla Cornus Cervi 鹿角胶
Concha Haliotidis 石决明
Concha Margaritifera Usta 珍珠母
Concha Meretricis 海蛤
Concha Ostreae 牡蛎
Concretio Silicae Bambusae 天竹黄
Cordyceps 冬虫夏草
Cormus Heleocharis Dulcis 地栗(荸荠)
Cornu Bubali 水牛角
Cornu Cervi 鹿角
Cornu Cervi Degelatinatum 鹿角霜
Cornu Cervi Pantotrichum 鹿茸
Cornu Naemorhedi 山羊角
Cornu Rhinocerotis 犀角
Cornu Saigae Tataricae 羚羊角
Cortex Acanthopanacis 五加皮
Cortex Ailanthi 椿根皮
Cortex Albiziae 合欢皮
Cortex Catalpae Ovatae 梓白皮
Cortex Cinnamomi 肉桂
Cortex Eucommiae 杜仲
Cortex Fraxini 秦皮
Cortex Lycii Radicis 地骨皮
Cortex Magnoliae Officinalis 厚朴
Cortex Meliae 苦楝皮
Cortex Mori Radicis 桑白皮

Cortex Mori Radicis Preparata 炙桑皮
Cortex Moutan Radicis 牡丹皮
Cortex Phellodendri 黄柏
Crinis Carbonisatus 血余炭

Den Draconis 龙齿
Depositum Urinae Preparatum 秋石

Endothelium Corneum Gigeriae Galli 鸡内金
Eupolyphaga seu Steleophaga 土鳖虫
Exocarpium Benicasae 冬瓜皮
Exocarpium Citri Rubrum 橘红
Exocarpium Citrulli 西瓜翠衣
Excrementum Bombycis 蚕沙

Faeces Trogopterori 五灵脂
Faeces Vespertilionis 夜明沙
Fel Ursi 熊胆
Flos Buddlejae 密蒙花
Flos Carthami 红花
Flos Caryophylli 丁香
Flos Chrysanthemi 菊花
Flos Chrysanthemi Indici 野菊花
Flos Dolichoris 扁豆花
Flos Eriocauli 谷精草
Flos Farfarae 款冬花
Flos Genkwa 芫花
Flos Inulae 旋复花
Flos Lonicerae 银花
Flos Magnoliae 辛夷花
Flos Sophorae 槐花
Folium Artemisiae Argyi 艾叶
Folium Callicarpae Pedunculatae 紫珠
Folium Camelliae Sinensis 茶叶
Folium Eriobotryae 枇杷叶
Folium Impatientis 凤仙叶
Folium Isatidis 大青叶
Folium Mori 桑叶
Folium Nelumbinis 荷叶
Folium Perillae 苏叶
Folium Pyrrosiae 石苇
Folium Sennae 番泻叶

Fossilia Spiriferis 石燕
Fructus Alpiniae Oxyphyllae 益智仁
Fructus Amomi 砂仁
Fructus Amomi Rotundus 豆蔻
Fructus Anisi Stellati 八角茴香
Fructus Arctii 牛蒡子
Fructus Aristolochiae 青木香
Fructus Aurantii 枳壳
Fructus Aurantii Immaturus 枳实
Fructus Broussonetiae 实子
Fructus Cannabis 火麻仁
Fructus Carotae 南鹤虱
Fructus Carpesii 鹤虱
Fructus Chaenomelis 木瓜
Fructus Chebulae 诃子
Fructus Citri 香橼
Fructus Citri Sarcodactylis 佛手
Fructus Cnidii 蛇床子
Fructus Crataegi 山楂
Fructus Crotonis 巴豆
Fructus Evodiae 吴茱萸
Fructus Foeniculi 茴香
Fructus Forsythiae 连翘
Fructus Gardeniae 栀子
Fructus Gleditsiae Abnormalis 猪牙皂
Fructus Hordei Germinatus 麦芽
Fructus Jujubae 大枣
Fructus Kochiae 地肤子
Fructus Leonuri 茺蔚子
Fructus Ligustri Lucidi 女真子
Fructus Lycii 枸杞子
Fructus Meliae 苦楝子
Fructus Mume 乌梅
Fructus Oryzae Germinatus 谷芽
Fructus Oryzae Sativae 粳米
Fructus Perillae 紫苏子
Fructus Piperis Longi 荜拨
Fructus Psoraleae 补骨脂
Fructus Pyri 梨
Fructus Quisqualis 使君子
Fructus Rosae Laevigatae 金樱子
Fructus Rubi 复盆子
Fructus Schisandrae 五味子

Fructus Sophorae 槐角
Fructus Toosendan 川楝子
Fructus Tribuli 蒺藜
Fructus Trichosanthis 瓜蒌
Fructus Tritici Levis 小麦
Fructus Tritici Levis (light) 浮小麦
Fructus Tsaoko 草果
Fructus Viticis 蔓荆子
Fructus Xanthii 苍耳子

Galla Chinensis 五倍子
Gecko 蛤蚧
Gemma Agrimoniae 鹤草芽
Gemma Bambusae 竹叶心
Gypsum Fibrosum 石膏

Haematitum 代赭石
Halitum 大青盐
Halloysitum Rubrum 赤石脂
Herba Agastaches 藿香
Herba Agrimoniae 仙鹤草
Herba Allii Fistulosi 葱
Herba Andrographitis 穿心莲
Herba Artemisiae Annuae 青蒿
Herba Artemisiae Anomalae 刘寄奴
Herba Artemisiae Scopariae 茵陈蒿
Herba Asari 细辛
Herba Cephalanoploris 小蓟
Herba Cistanches 肉苁蓉
Herba Corydalis Bungeanae 苦地丁
Herba Cynomorii 锁阳
Herba Dendrobii 石斛
Herba Dianthi 瞿麦
Herba Ecliptae 旱莲草
Herba Elsholtziae 香薷
Herba Ephedrae 麻黄
Herba Epimedii 仙灵脾(淫羊草)
Herba Equiseti Hiemalis 木贼
Herba Eupatorii 佩兰
Herba Hedyotis Diffusae 白花蛇舌草
Herba Houttuyniae 鱼腥草
Herba Leonuri 益母草
Herba Lobeliae Chinensis 半边莲

Herba Lophatheri 淡竹叶
Herba Lysimachiae 金钱草
Herba Menthae 薄荷
Herba Patriniae 败酱草
Herba Polygoni Avicularis 萹蓄
Herba Polygoni Hydropiperis 辣蓼
Herba Portulacae 马齿苋
Herba Schizonepetae 荆芥
Herba seu Hadix Cirsii Japonici 大蓟
Herba Siegesbeckiae 豨莶草
Herba Taraxaci 蒲公英
Herba Violae 紫花地丁
Hippocampus 海马
Hirudo 水蛭
Hydrargyrum 水银

Indigo Naturalis 青黛

Lacca Toxicodendri Verniciflne 干漆
Lapis Chloriti 礞石
Lasiosphaera seu Calvatia 马勃
Lignum Aquilariae Resinatum 沉香
Lignum Cinnamomi 桂心
Lignum Dalbergiae Odoriferae 降香
Lignum Pini Poriaferum 茯神
Lignum Santali Albi 檀香
Lignum Sappan 苏木
Lithargyrum 密陀僧
Lumbricus 地龙

Magnetitum 磁石
Margarita 珍珠
Massa Fermentata Fructus Hordei Germinatus 麦芽曲
Massa Fermentata Medicinalis 神曲
Massa Fermentata Rhizoma Pinelliae 半夏曲
Medulla Junci 灯心草
Medulla Tetrapanacis 通草
Mel 蜂蜜
Moschus 麝香
Mylabris 斑蝥
Myrrha 没药

Natrii Sulfas 芒硝
Natrii Sulfas Exsiccatus 玄明粉
Nitrum 硝石
Nitrum Depuratum 牙硝
Nodus Nelumbinis Rhizomatis 藕节
Nudus Bambusae 竹节

Olibanum 乳香
Omphalia 雷丸
Otheca Mantidis 桑螵蛸
Ophicalcitum 花蕊石
Os Draconis 龙骨
Os Sepiae 海螵蛸
Os Tigris 虎骨

Pericarpium Arecae 大腹皮
Pericarpium Chebulae 诃子皮
Pericarpium Citri Reticulatae 陈皮
Pericarpium Citri Reticulatae Viride 青皮
Pericarpium Granati 石榴皮
Pericarpium Papaveris 罂粟壳
Pericarpium Trichosanthis 瓜蒌皮
Pericarpium Zanthoxyli 川椒(花椒)
Periostracum Cicadae 蝉蜕
Petiolus Nelumbinis 荷梗
Placenta Hominis 紫河车
Plastrum Testudinis 龟板
Plumula Nelumbinis 莲子心
Pollen Typhae 蒲黄
Polyporus Umbellatus 猪苓
Poria 茯苓
Poria Rubra 赤茯苓
Pseudobulbus Cremastrae Appendiculatae 山慈姑
Pumex 海浮石
Pyritum 自然铜

Radix Achyranthis Bidentatae 牛膝
Radix Aconiti 乌头
Radix Aconiti Lateralis 生附子
Radix Aconiti Lateralis Preparata 附子
Radix Aconiti Kusnezoffii 草乌
Radix Adenophorae 沙参
Radix Ampelopsis 白蔹子
Radix Angelicae Dahuricae 白芷
Radix Angelicae Pubescentis 独活
Radix Angelicae Sinensis 当归
Radix Arnebiae seu Lithospermi 紫草
Radix Asparagi 天冬
Radix Asteris 紫菀
Radix Astragali 黄芪
Radix Aucklandiae 木香
Radix Boehmeriae 苎麻根
Radix Bupleuri 柴胡
Radix Clematidis 威灵仙
Radix Codonopsis Pilosulae 党参
Radix Curcumae 郁金
Radix Cyathulae 川牛膝
Radix Cynanchi Atrati 白薇
Radix Dichroae 常山
Radix Dipsaci 续断
Radix Ephedrae 麻黄根
Radix et Rhizoma Rhei 大黄
Radix Euphorbiae Fischerianae 狼毒
Radix Euphorbiae Pekinensis 大戟
Radix Forsythiae 连翘根
Radix Gentianae 龙胆草
Radix Gentianae Macrophyllae 秦艽
Radix Ginseng 人参
Radix Glehniae 北沙参
Radix Glycyrrhizae 甘草
Radix Glycyrrhizae Preparata 炙甘草
Radix Isatidis 板蓝根
Radix Kansui 甘遂
Radix Knoxiae 红大戟
Radix Ledebouriellae 防风
Radix Linderae 乌药
Radix Morindae Officinalis 巴戟天
Radix Notoginseng 三七
Radix Ophiopogonis 麦冬
Radix Oryzae Glutinosae 糯稻根
Radix Paeoniae Alba 白芍
Radix Paeoniae Lactiflorae 芍药
Radix Paeoniae Rubra 赤芍
Radix Panacis Quinquefolii 西洋参

Radix Peucedani 前胡
Radix Platycodi 桔梗
Radix Polygalae 远志
Radix Polygoni Multiflori 首乌
Radix Pseudostellariae 太子参
Radix Puerariae 葛根
Radix Pulsatillae 白头翁
Radix Rehmanniae 生地
Radix Rehmanniae Preparata 熟地
Radix Rubiae 茜草
Radix Salviae Miltiorrhizae 丹参
Radix Sanguisorbae 地榆
Radix Scrophulariae 玄参
Radix Scutellariae 黄芩
Radix Solani Melongenae 茄根
Radix Sophorae Flavescentis 苦参
Radix Sophorae Tonkinensis 山豆根
Radix Stellariae 银柴胡
Radix Stemonae 百步
Radix Stephaniae Tetrandrae 防己
Radix Trichosanthis 天花粉
Ramulus Cinnamomi 桂枝
Ramulus Mori 桑枝
Ramulus Taxilli 桑寄生
Ramulus Uncariae cum Uncis 钩藤
Realgar 雄黄
Resina Draconis 血竭
Resina Ferulae 阿魏
Retinervus Luffae Fructus 丝瓜络
Rhizoma Acori Graminei 石菖蒲
Rhizoma Alismatis 泽泻
Rhizoma Alpiniae Officinarum 高良姜
Rhizoma Anemarrhenae 知母
Rhizoma Arisaematis 天南星
Rhizoma Atractylodis 苍术
Rhizoma Atractylodis Macrocephalae 白术
Rhizoma Belamcandae 射干
Rhizoma Bletillae 白及
Rhizoma Chuanxiong 川芎
Rhizoma Cibotii 狗脊
Rhizoma Cimicifugae 升麻
Rhizoma Coptidis 黄连
Rhizoma Corydalis 延胡索
Rhizoma Curculiginis 仙茅
Rhizoma Curcumae Longae 姜黄
Rhizoma Cynanchi Stauntonii 白前
Rhizoma Cyperi 香附
Rhizoma Dioscoreae 山药
Rhizoma Dioscoreae Septemlobae 萆薢
Rhizoma Drynariae 骨碎补
Rhizoma Dryopteris Crassirhizomae 贯众
Rhizoma et Radix Veratri 藜芦
Rhizoma Fagopyri Cymosi 金荞麦
Rhizoma Gastrodiae 天麻
Rhizoma Homalomenae 千年健
Rhizoma Imperatae 茅根
Rhizoma Ligustici 藁本
Rhizoma Nelumbinis 藕
Rhizoma Phragmitis 芦根
Rhizoma Picrorhizae 胡黄连
Rhizoma Pinelliae 半夏
Rhizoma Pinelliae Preparata 法半夏
Rhizoma Polygonati 黄精
Rhizoma Polygonati Odorati 虎杖
Rhizoma Polygoni Cuspidati 玉竹
Rhizoma seu Radix Notopterygii 羌活
Rhizoma Sparganii 三棱
Rhizoma Typhonii 白附子
Rhizoma Zedoariae 莪术
Rhizoma Zingiberis 干姜
Rhizoma Zingiberis Recens 生姜

Saccharum Granorum 饴糖
Sargassum 海藻
Scolopendra 蜈蚣
Scorpio 全蝎
Semen Alpiniae Katsumadai 草豆蔻
Semen Amomi Rotundus 白蔻仁
Semen Arecae 槟榔
Semen Armeniacae Amarum 杏仁
Semen Astragali Complanati 沙苑蒺藜
Semen Begoniae Laciniatae 石莲子
Semen Benincasae 冬瓜子
Semen Biotae 柏子仁
Semen Cassiae 决明子
Semen Celosiae 青葙子

Semen Citri Reticulatae 橘核
Semen Coicis 薏苡仁
Semen Crotonis Pulveratum 巴豆霜
Semen Cucurbitae 南瓜子
Semen Cuscutae 菟丝子
Semen Dolichoris Album 白扁豆
Semen Euphorbiae Lathyridis 千金子
Semen Euryales 芡实
Semen Ginkgo 白果
Semen Hydnocarpi 大风子
Semen Impatientis 急性子
Semen Juglandis 胡桃
Semen Lepidii seu Descurainiae 葶苈子
Semen Litchi 荔枝核
Semen Melo 甜瓜子
Semen Myristicae 肉豆蔻
Semen Nelumbinis 莲子肉
Semen Persicae 桃仁
Semen Pharbitidis 牵牛子
Semen Phaseoli 赤小豆
Semen Phaseoli Radiati 绿豆
Semen Plantaginis 车前子
Semen Pruni 郁李仁
Semen Raphani 莱服子
Semen Sesami 胡麻仁
Semen Sesami Nigrum 黑芝麻
Semen Sinapis Albae 白芥子
Semen Sojae Preparatum 淡豆豉
Semen Strychni 马钱子
Semen Torreyae 榧子
Semen Trichosanthis 瓜蒌仁
Semen Trigonellae 葫芦巴
Semen Vaccariae 王不留行
Semen Ziziphi Spinosae 酸枣仁
Spica Prunellae 夏枯草
Spica Schizonepetae 荆芥穗
Spina Gleditsiae 皂角刺
Spora Lygodii 海金沙
Squama Manitis 穿山甲
Stamen Nelumbinis 莲须
Storax 苏合香
Succinum 琥珀
Succus Bambusae 竹沥
Sulfur 硫磺

Tabanus 虻虫
Talcum 滑石
Terra Flava Usta 灶心土
Thallus Eckloniae 昆布
Thallus Laminariae 海带

Urocteae 壁钱

Vagina Trichycarpi Carbonisatus 棕榈炭
Venenum Bufonis 蟾酥

Zaocys 乌梢蛇

Appendix III

A List of Traditional Chinese Prescriptions Appeared in Volume II

Antiphlogistic Powder 败毒散

Antiphlogistic Powder with Schizonepetae and Ledebouriellae 荆防败毒散

Antitussive Syrup of Armeniacae Amarum and Perillae 杏苏止咳糖浆

Babao Eyedrop 八宝眼药

Baby Fattening Bolus 肥儿丸

Baijiang Dan (White Reducing Powder) 白降丹

Baochi Powder 保赤散

Baolong Bolus of Calculus Bovis 牛黄抱龙丸

Bolus for Invigorating the Spleen 启脾丸

Bolus for Mildly Activating the Meridians 小活络丹

Bolus for Regulating Menstruation 调经丸

Bolus for Regulating the Middle Jiao 理中丸

Bolus for Releasing and Regulating Lung *Qi* 通宣理肺丸

Bolus for Serious Endogenous Wind Syndrome 大定风珠

Bolus for Soothing the Liver 舒肝丸

Bolus for Trauma 跌打丸

Bolus of Anemarrhenae, Phellodendri and Rehmanniae Preparata 知柏地黄丸

Bolus of Calculus Bovis for Eliminating Heart Fire 牛黄清心丸

Bolus of Calculus Bovis for Purging Heat 牛黄上清丸

Bolus of Calculus Bovis for Relieving Convulsion 牛黄镇惊丸

Bolus of Calculus Bovis for Resurrection 安宫牛黄丸

Bolus of Cannabis 麻子仁丸

Bolus of Coptidis and Sheep's Liver 黄连羊肝丸

Bolus of Cornu Saigae Tataricae and Forsythiae for Detoxification 羚翘解毒丸

Bolus of Crataegi 大山楂丸

Bolus of Dendrobii for Improving Acuity of Vision 石斛夜光丸

Bolus of Exocarpium Citri Rubrum 橘红丸

Bolus of Four Fresh Drugs 四生丸

Bolus of Gastrodiae 天麻丸

Bolus of Ginseng and Cornu Cervi Pantotrichum 参茸丸

Bolus of Leonuri 益母丸

Bolus of Lycii, Chrysanthemi and Rehmanniae Preparata 杞菊地黄丸

Bolus of Mume 乌梅丸

Bolus of Precious Drugs 至宝丹

Bolus of Storax for Coronary Heart Diseases 冠心苏合丸

Bolus of Ten Fragrant Drugs 十香丸

Bolus (Pill) of Black-Bone Chicken 乌鸡白凤丸

Capsule of Two Precious Drugs 双宝素

Cock-Waking Powder 鸡苏散

Decoction Containing Three Kinds of Seeds

for the Aged 三子养亲汤
Decoction for Calming Liver Wind 镇肝息风汤
Decoction for Discharging Blood Stasis 下瘀血方
Decoction for Ectopic Pregnancy 宫外孕方
Decoction for Eliminating Gallbladder Heat 温胆汤
Decoction for Eliminating Heat in the *Yingfen* 清营汤
Decoction for Eliminating Phlegm 导痰汤
Decoction for Eliminating Summer-Heat and Benefiting *Qi* 清暑益气汤
Decoction for Expelling Cestode 驱绦汤
Decoction for Fluid Increase and Purgation 增液承气汤
Decoction for General Antiphlogistic 普济消毒饮
Decoction for Hemoptysis 咳血方
Decoction for Invigorating the Middle *Jiao* and Benefiting *Qi*
Decoction for Invigorating the Spleen and Nourishing the Heart 归脾汤
Decoction for Invigorating *Yang* 补阳还五汤
Decoction for Mild Purgation 小承气汤
Decoction for Mildly Warming the Middle *Jiao* 小建中汤
Decoction for Opening the Orifices and Activating Blood Circulation 通窍活血汤
Decoction for Potent Purgation 大承气汤
Decoction for Purgation and Regulation of Stomach 调胃承气汤
Decoction for Purging Stomach Fire 泻心汤
Decoction for Regulating the Middle *Jiao* 理中汤
Decoction for Relieving Asthma 定喘汤
Decoction for Removing Blood Stasis Below the Diaphragm 膈下逐瘀汤
Decoction for Removing Blood Stasis in the Chest 血府逐瘀汤
Decoction for Removing Blood Stasis in the Lower Abdomen 少腹逐瘀汤
Decoction for Rescuing Collapse 升陷汤
Decoction for Restoring the Pulse and Nourishing *Yin* 复脉汤
Decoction for Strengthening the Middle *Jiao* and Benefiting *Qi* 补中益气汤
Decoction for Strengthening the Chong Meridian 固冲汤
Decoction for Treating Leukorrhagia 完带汤
Decoction for Treating *Yang* Exhaustion 四逆汤
Decoction for Warming the Meridians 温经汤
Decoction for Warming the Spleen 温脾汤
Decoction for Warming *Yang* 阳和汤
Decoction of Adenophorae and Ophiopogonis 沙参麦冬汤
Decoction of Agastaches, Magnoliae Officinalis, Pinelliae and Poria 藿朴夏苓汤
Decoction of Alismatis 泽泻汤
Decoction of Allii Fistulosi and Sojae Preparatum 葱豉汤
Decoction of Angelicae Pubescentis and Taxilli 独活寄生汤
Decoction of Angelicae Sinensis for Enriching the Blood 当归补血汤
Decoction of Angelicae Sinensis for Warming Cold Limbs 当归四逆汤
Decoction of Artemisiae Annuae and Carapax Trionycis 青蒿鳖甲汤
Decoction of Artemisiae Annuae and Scutellariae for Eliminating Dampness-Heat from the Gallbladder 蒿芩清胆汤
Decoction of Artemisiae Scopariae 茵陈蒿汤
Decoction of Artemisiae Scopariae for Treating *Yang* Exhaustion 茵陈四逆汤
Decoction of Astragali for Strengthening the Middle *Jiao* 黄芪建中汤
Decoction of Aurantii Immaturus, Allii Macrostemi and Cinnamomi 枳实薤白桂枝汤

Decoction of Biotae 侧柏汤
Decoction of Bupleuri for Regulating Shaoyang 小柴胡汤
Decoction of Bupleuri for Regulating Shaoyang and Yangming 大柴胡汤
Decoction of Caryophylli and Kaki 丁香柿蒂汤
Decoction of Cephalanoploris 小蓟子饮
Decoction of Citri Reticulatae and Bambusae in Taeniam 橘皮竹茹汤
Decoction of Colla Corii Asini and Artemisiae Argyi 胶艾汤
Decoction of Coptidis for Detoxification 黄连解毒汤
Decoction of Coptidis for Regulating the Middle *Jiao* 连理汤
Decoction of Cornu Rhinocerotis and Rehmanniae 犀角地黄汤
Decoction of Cornu Saigae Tataricae and Ramulus Uncariae cum Unis 羚羊钩藤汤
Decoction of Dioscoreae Septemlobae for Clearing Turbid Urine 萆薢分清饮
Decoction of Dredging the Maridians for Cold Extremities 通脉四逆汤
Decoction of Elsholtziae 香薷饮
Decoction of Ephedrae 麻黄汤
Decoction of Ephedrae, Aconiti Lateralis and Asari 麻黄附子细辛汤
Decoction of Ephedrae, Armeniacae Amarum, Glycyrrhizae and Gypsum Fibrosum 麻杏甘石汤
Decoction of Ephedrae, Forsythiae and Phaseoli 麻黄连翘赤小豆汤
Decoction of Evodiae 吴茱萸汤
Decoction of Four Drugs with Persicae and Carthami 桃红四物汤
Decoction of Gardeniae and Sojae Preparatum 栀子豉汤
Decoction of Gastrodiae and Ramulus Uncariae cum Uncis 天麻钩藤汤
Decoction of Gentianae for Purging Liver Fire 龙胆泻肝汤
Decoction of Ginseng and Aconiti Lateralis 参附汤
Decoction of Ginseng and Juglandis 人参胡桃汤
Decoction of Ginseng for Nourishing *Qi* and *Ying* 人参养荣汤
Decoction of Ginseng for Treating *Yang* Exhaustion 四逆加人参汤
Decoction of Glycyrrhizae, Tritici Levis and Jujubae 甘麦大枣汤
Decoction of Glycyrrhizae Preparata 炙甘草汤
Decoction of Inulae and Haematitum 旋复代赭汤
Decoction of Iron Scale 生铁落饮
Decoction of Jujubae 十枣汤
Decoction Lepidii seu Descurainiae and Jujubae for Purging Lung Heat 葶苈大枣泻肺汤
Decoction of Lilli for Strengthening the Lung 百合固金汤
Decoction of Lophatheri and Gypsum Fibrosum 竹叶石膏汤
Decoction of Mori and Chrysanthemi 桑菊饮
Decoction of Nine Ingredients Containing Notopterygii 九味羌活汤
Decoction of Notopterygii for Expelling Dampness 羌活胜湿汤
Decoction of Paeoniae Alba and Glycyrrhizae 芍药甘草汤
Decoction of Perillae for Keeping *Qi* Downwards 苏子降气汤
Decoction of Persicae for Purgation 桃核承气汤
Decoction of Phragmitis 苇茎汤
Decoction of Picrorrhizae and Mume for Calming Ascarides 连梅安蛔汤
Decoction of Pinelliae, Atractylodis Macrocephalae and Gastrodiae 半夏白术天麻汤
Decoction of Pinelliae and Magnoliae Officinalis 半夏厚朴汤
Decoction of Pinelliae for Purging Stomach

Fire 半夏泻心汤
Decoction of Platycodi 桔梗汤
Decoction of Poria, Glycyrrhizae, Schisandrae, Zingiberis and Asari 苓甘五味姜辛汤
Decoction of Poria, Ramulus Cinnamomi, Atractylodis Macrocephalae and Glycyrrhizae 苓桂术甘汤
Decoction of Puerariae, Scutellariae and Coptidis 葛根黄芩黄连汤
Decoction of Pulsatillae 白头翁汤
Decoction of Ramulus Cinnamomi 桂枝汤
Decoction of Rhei and Aconiti Lateralis Preparata 大黄附子汤
Decoction of Rhei and Moutan Radicis 大黄牡丹汤
Decoction of Sargentodoxae 红藤煎
Decoction of Six Mild Drugs 六君子汤
Decoction of Six Mild Drugs with Cyperi and Amomi 香砂六君子汤
Decoction of Stephaniae Tetrandrae and Astragali 防己黄芪汤
Decoction of Ten Powerful Tonic Drugs 十全大补汤
Decoction of Terra Flava Usta 黄土汤
Decoction of Three Drugs Containing Magnoliae Officinalis 厚朴三物汤
Decoction of Trichosanthis, Allii Macrostemi and Pinelliae 瓜蒌薤白半夏汤
Decoction of Trichosanthis, Allii Macrostemi and Wine 瓜蒌薤白白酒汤
Detoxification Pill 甘露消毒丹
Distillate of Artemesiae Annuae 青蒿露
Distillate of Flos Lonicerae 银花露
Dog-Skin Plaster 狗皮膏

Eight Precious Ingredients Decoction 八珍汤
Eight-Ingredient Bolus Containing Leonuri 八珍益母丸
Erchen Decoction 二陈汤
Erzhi Pill 二至丸
Extract of Asparagi and Ophiopogonis 二冬膏
Eyedrop with Eight Ingredients 八宝眼药

Fine Jade Extract 琼玉膏
Four Drugs Decoction 四物汤
Four Mild Drugs Decoction 四君子汤

Golden Lock Bolus for Preserving Kidney Essence 金锁固精丸
Green Jade Powder 碧玉散
Guiling Powder 龟龄集
Gushen Pill 谷神丸

Heavenly King Tonic Pill for Mental Discomfort 天王补心丹
Huagai Powder 华盖散
Huqian Pill 虎潜丸

Instant Granules for Common Cold and Eliminating Heat 感冒清热冲剂

Jade Maid Decoction 玉女煎
Jade Screen Powder 玉屏风散
Jade Spring Pill 玉泉丸
Jisheng Pill for Invigorating Kidney *Qi* 济生肾气丸

Liquor Agastaches for Restoring Antipathogenic *Qi* 藿香正气水

Medicated Tea for Common Cold 午时茶
Medicated Wine of Centropus Sinensis 毛鸡药酒
Medicated Wine of Os Tigris and Chaenomelis 虎骨木瓜酒
Modified Decoction for Restoring the Pulse and Nourishing *Yin* 加减复脉汤
Modified Decoction of Polygonati Odorati 加减葳蕤汤
Modified *Xiaoyao* Powder 加减逍遥散

No. II Formula for Coronary Diseases 冠心II号方

Pill Containing Nine Drugs for Relieving Pain 九气拈痛丸
Pill Containing Two Drugs 水陆二仙丹
Pill for Chronic Phlegm Syndrome 滚痰丸
Pill for Decreasing Urination 缩泉丸
Pill for Eliminating Heat in *Qifen* and Dispersing Phlegm 清气化痰丸
Pill for Invigorating Kidney *Qi* 金匮肾气丸
Pill for Invigorating Kidney *Qi* with Modifications 加减肾气丸
Pill for Invigorating the Spleen 健脾丸
Pill for Promoting Digestion 保和丸
Pill for Regulating *Qi* in the Chest 开胸顺气丸
Pill for Replenishing *Yin* 大补阴丸
Pill for Resolving Scrofula 消瘰丸
Pill for Tranquilizing the Mind and Invigorating the Heart 安神补心丹
Pill for Treating Phlegm Syndrome 控涎丹
Pill of Aconiti Lateralis and Cinnamomi for Regulating the Middle *Jiao* 附桂理中丸
Pill of Aconiti Lateralis for Regulating the Middle *Jiao* 附子理中丸
Pill of Alpiniae Officinarum and Cyperi 良附丸
Pill of Alumen and Lysimachiae 白金丸
Pill of Artemisiae Argyi and Cyperi for Warming the Uterus 艾附暖宫丸
Pill of Aucklandiae and Arecae 木香槟榔丸
Pill of Aucklandiae and Coptidis 香连丸
Pill of Aucklandiae and Sophorae Flavescentis 香参丸
Pill of Aurantii Immaturus and Atractylodis Macrocephalae 枳术丸
Pill of Aurantii Immaturus for Promoting Digestion 枳实导滞丸
Pill of Aurantii Immaturus for Removing Abdominal Mass 枳实消痞丸
Pill of Biotae for Nourishing the Heart 柏子养心丸
Pill of Calculus Bovis for Detoxification 牛黄解毒丸
Pill of Chaenomelis 木瓜丸
Pill of Cinnabaris for Tranquilization 朱砂安神丸
Pill of Coptidis and Aucklandiae 香连丸
Pill of Cornu Rhinocerotis and Calculus Bovis 犀角牛黄片
Pill of Deer 全鹿丸
Pill of Eight Ingredients Containing Cinnamomi and Aconiti Lateralis 桂附八味丸
Pill of Five Kinds of Seed for Invigorating the Kidney 五子补肾丸
Pill of Five Seeds 五仁丸
Pill of Foeniculi and Citri Reticulatae 茴香橘核丸
Pill of Four Miraculous Drugs 四神丸
Pill of Four Wonderful Ingredients 四妙丸
Pill of Lapis Chloriti Usta for Expelling Phlegm 礞石滚痰丸
Pill of Ledebouriellae for Dispersing Wind from the Surface 防风通圣丸
Pill of Magnetitum and Cinnabaris 磁朱丸
Pill of Mori and Sesami Nigrum 桑麻丸
Pill of Pharbitidis and Arecae 牛槨丸
Pill of Rehmanniae 地黄丸
Pill of Six Drugs Containing Rehmanniae Preparata 六味地黄丸
Pill of Six Precious Drugs 六神丸
Pill of Stephaniae Tetrandrae, Zanthoxyli, Lepidii seu Descurainiae and Rhei 己椒苈黄丸
Pill of Storax 苏合香丸
Pill of Storax and Borneolum Syntheticum 苏冰滴丸
Pill of Two Miraculous Drugs 二神丸
Pill of Two Wonder Drugs 二妙丸
Plaster for Regulating *Yang* to Remove Stagnation 阳和解凝膏
Plaster for Rheumatism 伤湿止痛膏
Powder Containing Five Kinds of Peel 五皮散
Powder for Dispelling Wind 消风散
Powder for Dispersing Heat and Promoting

Urination 八正散
Powder for Dissipating Blood Stasis 失笑散
Powder for Eliminating Stomach-Heat 清胃散
Powder for Eliminating Summer-Heat and Dampness 益元散
Powder for Expelling Lung Heat 泻白散
Powder for Invigorating the Spleen 实脾散
Powder for Promoting Diuresis 导赤散
Powder for Promoting Tissue Regeneration 生肌散
Powder for Regulating Stomach Function 平胃散
Powder for Regulating the Liver and Spleen 四逆散
Powder for Relieving Cough 止嗽散
Powder for Relieving Deficiency-Heat Syndrome 清骨散
Powder for Restoring the Pulse 生脉散
Powder for Treating Diarrhea with Abdominal Pain 痛泻要方
Powder for Treating Dysentery Associated with Loss of Appetite 开噤散
Powder for Treating Facial Distortion 前正散
Powder of Agastaches for Restoring Antipathogenic *Qi* 藿香正气散
Powder of Borneolum Syntheticum 冰硼散
Powder of Borneolum Syntheticum and Borax 冰硼散
Powder of Calculus Macacae Mulattae 猴枣散
Powder of Caryophylli and Kaki 丁香柿蒂散
Powder of Chrysanthemi with Folium Camelliae Sinensis 菊花茶调散
Powder of Chuanxiong with Folium Camelliae Sinensis 川芎茶调散
Powder of Coicis, Aconiti Lateralis and Patriniae 薏苡附子败酱散
Powder of Concha Ostreae 牡蛎散
Powder of Elsholtziae 香薷散
Powder of Five Drugs Containing Poria 五苓散
Powder of Flos Sophorae 槐花散
Powder of Fritillariae and Anemarrhenae 二母散
Powder of Fritillariae Thunbergii and Trichosanthis 贝母瓜蒌散
Powder of Fructus Xanthii 苍耳散
Powder of Ginseng, Poria and Atractylodis Macrocephalae 参苓白术散
Powder of Indigo Naturalis and Concha Meretricis 黛蛤散
Powder of Lonicerae and Forsythiae 银翘散
Powder of Margarita and Calculus Bovis for Throat Disorders 珠黄吹喉散
Powder of Olibanum and Myrrha 海浮散
Powder of Otheca Mantidis 桑螵蛸散
Powder of Os Sepiae and Bletillae 乌及散
Powder of Os Sepiae and Fritillariae 乌贝散
Powder of Phellodendri and Atractylodis 二妙散
Powder of Schisandrae 五味子散
Powder of Snake's Bile and Citri Reticulatae 蛇胆陈皮散
Powder of Snake's Bile and Fritillariae Cirrhosae 蛇胆川贝散
Powder of Ten Drugs' Ashes 十灰散
Powder of Toosendan 金铃子散
Powder (Decoction) for Restoring the Pulse 复脉散(饮)
Purple-Snow Pellet 紫雪丹

Seven *Li* Powder 七厘散
Shiguogong Medicated Wine 史国公药酒
Six-to-One Powder 六一散
Small Blue Dragon Decoction 小青龙汤
Spasmolitic Power 止痉散

Tablet for Removing Abdominal Masses 化症四生片
Tablet of Calculus Bovis for Detoxification

牛黄解毒片
Taohua Decoction 桃花汤
Three Crude Drugs Decoction 三拗汤
Three Seeds Decoction 三仁汤
Tiantai Powder of Linderae 天台乌药散
Tonic Bolus (Pill) of Placenta Hominis 河车大造丸
Tonic Wine of Ten Drugs 十全大补酒

White Medicated Powder 白药
White Tiger Decoction 白虎汤
White Tiger Decoction with Atractylodis 白虎加苍术汤
White Tiger Decoction with Ginseng 白虎加人参汤
White Tiger Decoction with Ramulus Cinnamomi 白虎加桂枝汤
Wine of Os Tigris and Chaenomelis 虎骨木瓜酒

Xiaoyao Powder 逍遥散
Xiaoyao Powder with Moutan Radicis and Gardeniae 丹栀逍遥散
Xilei Powder 锡类散

Yellow Dragon Decoction 黄龙汤
Yiguan Decoction 一贯煎
Yougui Decoction 右归饮
Yueju Pill 越鞠丸
Yuzhen Powder 玉真散

Zhenren Decoction for Nourishing the Viscera 真人养脏汤
Zhenwu Decoction 真武汤
Zuoci Bolus for Deafness 耳聋左慈丸
Zijin Troche 紫金锭
Zuogui Decoction 左归饮
Zuojin Pill 左金丸

Appendix IV

A List of Traditional Chinese Medicine Terms Appeared in Volume II

adjuvant ingredient 臣药
anthelmintics 驱虫药
aromatic drugs for dispelling dampness 芳香化湿药
ascending 升
assistant ingredient 佐药
astringents 收涩药
attributive meridian 归经

boiling 煮

calcining 煅
chest *bi*-syndrome 胸痹
chief ingredient 君药
compatibility of drugs 药物配伍

dan 丹剂
decocted first 先煎
decocted later 后下
decocted with wrappings 包煎
decoction 汤剂
descending 降
diaphoretic therapy 汗法
digestives 消食药
diuretics 利水渗湿药
drastic purgatives 峻下逐水药
drugs for activating blood circulation and removing blood stasis 活血祛瘀药
drugs for breaking up blood stasis 破血药
drugs for calming the liver and suppress wind 平肝息风药
drugs for dispelling wind-cold 发散风寒药
drugs for dispelling wind-heat 发散风热药
drugs for eliminating heat and toxins 清热解毒药
drugs for nourishing the blood 养血药
drugs for nourishing *yin* 养阴药
drugs for promoting analepsia 开窍药
drugs for purgation (cathartics) 泻下药
drugs for purging deficiency heat 清虚热药
drugs for purging heat 清热药
drugs for purging heat and fire 清热泻火药
drugs for regulating *qi* 理气药
drugs for relieving cough and dyspnea 止咳平喘药
drugs for relieving exterior syndrome 解表药
drugs for resolving phlegm 化痰药
drugs for replenishing *qi* 补气药
drugs for replenishing the blood 补血药
drugs for replenishing *yin* 补阴药
drugs for strengthening *yang* 补阳药
drugs for warming the interior 温里药

eight therapeutic methods 八法
eighteen incompatible drugs 十八反
emetic therapy 吐法
epidemic diseases with swollen head 大头瘟
expectorants, autitussives and dyspnea-relieving drugs 化痰止咳平喘药
extract 膏剂

five tastes 五味

floating 浮
fluid-retention syndrome in the thorax 悬饮
four *qi* 四气

grinding in water 水飞
guiding ingredient 使药

heat-purging therapy 清法
hemostatics 止血药
high temperature stir-baking 炮

incompatibility 相反
injection 针剂
instant granule 冲剂

lubricant purgatives 润下药
lung abscess 肺痈

medicinal tea 茶剂
mutual antagonism 相恶
mutual detoxification 相杀
mutual enhancement 相使

nineteen antagonistic drugs 十九反

ointment 软剂

paper strip 条剂
pill 丸剂
plaster 硬膏
potent purgatives 攻下药
powder 散剂
prescriptions composed of heart-nourishing sedatives 滋养安神剂
prescriptions composed of heavy sedatives 重镇安神剂
prescriptions exerting resuscitative effect by cooling 凉开剂
prescriptions exerting resuscitative effect by warming 温开剂
prescriptions for activating blood circulation to remove blood stasis 活血祛瘀剂
prescriptions for activating *qi* 行气剂
prescriptions for astringing the intestine to stop diarrhea 涩肠固脱剂
prescriptions for dispelling wind and eliminating phlegm 治风化痰剂
prescriptions for dispersing exogenous wind 疏散外风剂
prescriptions for dispersing stagnation 消导剂
prescriptions for drying dampness and eliminating phlegm 燥湿化痰剂
prescriptions for drying dampness and regulating the stomach 燥湿和胃剂
prescriptions for expelling dampness 祛湿剂
prescriptions for expelling intestinal parasites 驱虫剂
prescriptions for expelling phlegm 祛痰剂
prescriptions for invigorating both *qi* and blood 气血双补剂
prescriptions for invigorating *qi* 补气剂
prescriptions for invigorating the blood 补血剂
prescriptions for invigorating *yang* 补阳剂
prescriptions for invigorating *yin* 补阴剂
prescriptions for moistening dryness and eliminating phlegm 润燥化痰剂
prescriptions for promoting diuresis and eliminating dampness 利水渗湿剂
prescriptions for purgation 泻下剂
prescriptions for purgation associated with invigoration 攻补兼施剂
prescriptions for purgation by cold drugs 寒下剂
prescriptions for purgation by warm drugs 温下剂
prescriptions for purgation composed by lubricant drugs 润下剂
prescriptions for purging deficiency heat 清虚热剂
prescriptions for purging heat 清热剂
prescriptions for purging heat and dampness 清热祛湿剂

prescriptions for purging heat and eliminating phlegm 清热化痰剂
prescriptions for purging heat and toxins 清热解毒剂
prescriptions for purging heat from *qifen* 清气分热剂
prescriptions for purging heat from the viscera 清脏腑热剂
prescriptions for purging heat from *yingfen* and cooling the blood 清热凉血剂
prescriptions for purging summer-heat 清热祛暑剂
prescriptions for recuperating the depleted *yang* and rescuing the patient from danger 回阳救逆剂
prescriptions for regulating *qi* 理气剂
prescriptions for regulating *Shaoyang* 和解少阳剂
prescriptions for regulating the blood 理血剂
prescriptions for regulating the liver and spleen 调和肝脾剂
prescriptions for regulating the stomach and intestines 调和肠胃剂
prescriptions for relieving dyspepsia 消食导滞剂
prescriptions for relieving exterior syndrome 解表剂
prescriptions for relieving exterior syndrome and supporting antipathogenic *qi* 扶正解表剂
prescriptions for relieving exterior syndrome with acrid and cool drugs 辛凉解表剂
prescriptions for relieving exterior syndrome with acrid and warm drugs 辛温解表剂
prescriptions for relieving metrorrhagia and leukorrhagia 固崩止带剂
prescriptions for relieving wind disorder 治风剂
prescriptions for stopping bleeding 止血剂
prescriptions for strengthening the surface to stop perspiration 固表止汗剂
prescriptions for suppressing endogenous wind 平息内风剂
prescriptions for warming and dispersing dampness 温化水湿剂
prescriptions for warming and eliminating cold-phlegm 温化寒痰剂
prescriptions for warming the interior 温里剂
prescriptions for warming the meridians to expel cold 温经散寒剂
prescriptions for warming the middle *jiao* and eliminating cold 温中祛寒剂
prescriptions with astringent effect 固涩剂
prescriptions with reconciliatory action 和解剂
prescriptions with resuscitative effect 开窍剂
prescriptions with sedative effect 安神剂
prescriptions with tonic effect 补益剂
purgative therapy 下法

regulative therapy 和法
resolving therapy 清法

sedatives 安神药
seven prescriptions 七方
single application 单行
sinking 沉
spirit 酒剂
steaming 蒸
stir-baking 炒
stir-baking with adjuvant 炙
synergism 相须
syrup 糖浆剂

tablet 片剂
ten prescriptions 十剂
thread 线剂
tonics 补虚药
toxicity 毒性
troche 锭剂

中医中药教材第二卷：英文/国家中医药管理局编.
北京：新世界出版社，1995.5
ISBN 7-80005-262-1

Ⅲ. 中国医药学-教材-英文
Ⅳ. R2

国家中医药管理局 编

新世界出版社出版
(北京百万庄路24号)
北京大学印刷厂印刷
[illegible]
(中国北京车公庄西路35号)
北京邮政信箱第399号 邮政编码100044

ISBN 7-80005-262-1
05800
14-E-2838SB